Preface

The development of pediatric cardiac surgical programs has had a profound effect on the specialty of pediatric critical care medicine, and as a result, the field of pediatric cardiac intensive care is rapidly emerging as a separate subspecialty of pediatric critical care medicine. The ability to provide care for the critically ill child with congenital heart disease clearly separates pediatric intensivists from our adult colleagues. A thorough understanding and knowledge of the unique physiology of the child with congenital heart disease are therefore absolutely crucial for anyone working in the pediatric intensive care unit. Once again, we would like to dedicate this textbook to our families and to the physicians and nurses who provide steadfast care every day in pediatric intensive care units across the globe.

Derek S. Wheeler
Hector R. Wong
Thomas P. Shanley

Preface to *Pediatric Critical Care Medicine: Basic Science and Clinical Evidence*

The field of critical care medicine is growing at a tremendous pace, and tremendous advances in the understanding of critical illness have been realized in the last decade. My family has directly benefited from some of the technological and scientific advances made in the care of critically ill children. My son Ryan was born during my third year of medical school. By some peculiar happenstance, I was nearing completion of a 4-week rotation in the newborn intensive care unit (NICU). The head of the pediatrics clerkship was kind enough to let me have a few days off around the time of the delivery—my wife, Cathy, was 2 weeks past her due date and had been scheduled for elective induction. Ryan was delivered through thick meconium-stained amniotic fluid and developed breathing difficulty shortly after delivery. His breathing worsened over the next few hours, so he was placed on the ventilator. I will never forget the feelings of utter helplessness my wife and I felt as the NICU transport team wheeled Ryan away in the transport isolette. The transport physician, one of my supervising third-year pediatrics residents during my rotation the past month, told me that Ryan was more than likely going to require extracorporeal membrane oxygenation (ECMO). I knew enough about ECMO at that time to know that I should be scared! The next 4 days were some of the most difficult moments I have ever experienced as a parent, watching the blood being pumped out of my tiny son's body through the membrane oxygenator and roller pump, slowly back into his body (Figures 1 and 2). I remember the fear of each day when we would be told of the results of his daily head ultrasound, looking for evidence of intracranial hemorrhage, and then the relief when we were told that there was no bleeding. I remember the hope and excitement on the day Ryan came off ECMO, as well as the concern when he had to be sent home on supplemental oxygen. Today,

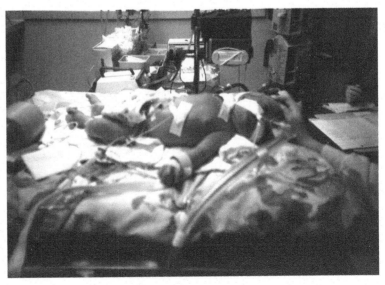

FIGURE 1

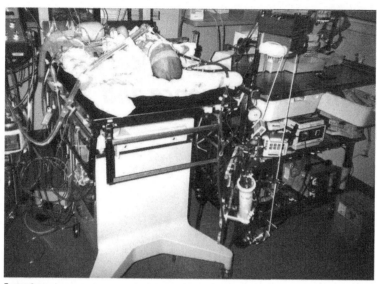

Figure 2

Ryan is happy, healthy, and strong. We are thankful to all the doctors, nurses, respiratory therapists, and ECMO specialists who cared for Ryan and made him well. We still keep in touch with many of them. Without the technological advances and medical breakthroughs made in the fields of neonatal intensive care and pediatric critical care medicine, things very well could have been much different. I made a promise to myself long ago that I would dedicate the rest of my professional career to advancing the field of pediatric critical care medicine as payment for the gifts with which we, my wife and I, have been truly blessed. It is my sincere hope that this textbook, which has truly been a labor of joy, will educate a whole new generation of critical care professionals and in so doing help make that first step toward keeping my promise.

Derek S. Wheeler

Contents

Contributors

Shamel Abd-Allah, MD
Associate Professor of Pediatrics
Loma Linda University School of Medicine
Director, Division of Critical Care Medicine
Loma Linda University Children's Hospital
Loma Linda, CA, USA

Andrew M. Atz, MD
Associate Professor of Pediatrics
Medical University of South Carolina
Director, Pediatric Cardiac Intensive Care
MUSC Children's Hospital
Charleston, SC, USA

Carl L. Backer, MD
Professor of Surgery
Northwestern University Feinberg School of
   Medicine
A.C. Buehler Professor of Surgery
Children's Memorial Hospital
Chicago, IL, USA

Robert H. Beekman III, MD
Professor of Pediatrics
University of Cincinnati College of Medicine
Samuel Kaplan Chair of Pediatric Cardiology
Cincinnati Children's Hospital Medical
   Center
Cincinnati, OH, USA

Desmond J. Bohn, MB, BCh, MRCP, FRCPC
Professor of Anaesthesia and Paediatrics
University of Toronto School of Medicine
Chief, Department of Critical Care Medicine
The Hospital for Sick Children
Toronto, Ontario, Canada

William L. Border, MBChB
Assistant Professor of Clinical Pediatrics
University of Cincinnati College of Medicine
Division of Cardiology
Cincinnati Children's Hospital Medical Center
Cincinnati, OH, USA

John R. Charpie, MD, PhD
Clinical Associate Professor of Pediatrics and
   Communicable Diseases
University of Michigan

Associate Director, Pediatric Cardiothoracic
   Intensive Care Unit
University of Michigan Congenital Heart
   Center
C.S. Mott Children's Hospital
Ann Arbor, MI, USA

Paul A. Checchia, MD
Assistant Professor of Critical Care and
   Cardiology
Washington University School of Medicine
Director, Pediatric Cardiac Intensive Care
   Program
Co-Director, Pediatric Intensive Care Unit
St. Louis Children's Hospital
St. Louis, MO, USA

John M. Costello, MD
Clinical Instructor in Pediatrics
Harvard Medical School
Department of Cardiology
Children's Hospital Boston
Boston, MA, USA

Dennis C. Crowley, MD
Clinical Professor of Pediatrics and
   Communicable Diseases
University of Michigan Medical Center
Co-Director, Pediatric Heart Transplant
   Program
Michigan Congenital Heart Disease Center
Division of Cardiology
C.S. Mott Children's Hospital
Ann Arbor, MI, USA

Heidi J. Dalton, MD, FCCM
Professor of Pediatrics
George Washington University
Department of Critical Care Medicine and
   Anesthesiology
Director, PICU and Pediatric ECMO
Children's National Medical Center
Washington, DC, USA

Catherine L. Dent, MD
Assistant Professor of Pediatrics
University of Cincinnati College of Medicine
Director, Cardiac Intensive Care Unit

Division of Cardiology
Cincinnati Children's Hospital Medical
  Center
Cincinnati, OH, USA

Jodie Y. Duffy, PhD
Assistant Professor of Pediatrics and Surgery
University of Cincinnati College of Medicine
Co-Director, Cardiothoracic Surgery
  Research Laboratory
Children's Hospital Research Foundation
Cincinnati Children's Hospital Medical
  Center
Cincinnati, OH, USA

Brian W. Duncan, MD
Surgical Director
Pediatric Cardiac Failure and
  Heart Transplant
Pediatric and Congenital Heart Surgery
The Children's Hospital
The Cleveland Clinic
Cleveland, OH, USA

Michael H. Gewitz, MD
Professor and Vice Chair of Pediatrics
New York Medical College
Physician-in-Chief and Director,
  Pediatric Cardiology
Maria Fareri Children's Hospital at
  Westchester Medical Center
Valhalla, NY, USA

Ana Lia Graciano, MD
Assistant Professor of Pediatrics
University of California, San Francisco
Division of Critical Care Medicine
Children's Hospital of Central California
Fresno, CA, USA

Joseph N. Graziano, MD
Clinical Instructor of Pediatrics and
  Communicable Diseases
University of Michigan Medical Center
Michigan Congenital Heart Disease Center
Division of Cardiology
C.S. Mott Children's Hospital
Ann Arbor, MI, USA

John A. Hawkins, MD
Associate Professor of Surgery
University of Utah Medical Center
Division of Cardiothoracic Surgery
Primary Children's Medical Center
Salt Lake City, UT, USA

Russell Hirsch, MD
Assistant Professor of Pediatrics
University of Cincinnati College of Medicine
Director, Cardiac Catheterization Laboratory
Division of Cardiology
Cincinnati Children's Hospital Medical
  Center
Cincinnati, OH, USA

Lauren D. Holinger, MD
Paul H. Holinger Professor of
  Otolaryngology-Head and Neck Surgery

Northwestern University Feinberg School of
  Medicine
Head, Pediatric Otolaryngology
Children's Memorial Hospital
Chicago, IL, USA

Kan Hor, MD
Division of Cardiology
Cincinnati Children's Hospital Medical
  Center
Cincinnati, OH, USA

Timothy K. Knilans, MD
Associate Professor of Clinical Pediatrics
University of Cincinnati College of Medicine
Director, Clinical Cardiac Electrophysiology
  and Pacing
Cincinnati Children's Hospital Medical
  Center
Cincinnati, OH, USA

Keith C. Kocis, MD, MS
Professor of Pediatrics
The University of North Carolina at
  Chapel Hill
Chief, Pediatric Critical Care Medicine
North Carolina Children's Hospital
Chapel Hill, NC, USA

Neil W. Kooy, MD
Associate Professor of Pediatrics
University of Cincinnati College of Medicine
Director, Fellowship Training Program
Division of Critical Care Medicine
Cincinnati Children's Hospital Medical
  Center
Cincinnati, OH, USA

Peter C. Laussen, MBBS
Associate Professor of Anesthesia
Harvard Medical School
D.D. Hansen Professor of
  Pediatric Anesthesia
Director, Cardiac Intensive Care Unit
Department of Cardiology
Children's Hospital Boston
Boston, MA, USA

John P. Lombardi, CCP
Perfusionist, Division of Cardiothoracic
  Surgery
Cincinnati Children's Hospital Medical
  Center
Cincinnati, OH, USA

Marianne N. Majdalani, MD
Assistant Professor of Pediatrics
Division of Critical Care Medicine
American University of Beirut
Beirut, Lebanon

Peter B. Manning, MD
Professor of Surgery and Pediatrics
University of Cincinnati College of Medicine
Co-Director, The Heart Center
Director, Division of Cardiothoracic Surgery
Cincinnati Children's Hospital Medical Center
Cincinnati, OH, USA

Constantine Mavroudis, MD
Professor of Surgery
Northwestern University Feinberg School of
  Medicine
Willis J. Potts Professor of Surgery
Surgeon-in-Chief
Children's Memorial Hospital
Chicago, IL, USA

Kelly M. McLean, MD
Research Fellow
Division of Cardiothoracic Surgery
Department of Surgery
University of Cincinnati College of
  Medicine
Cincinnati, OH, USA

Jon N. Meliones, MD, MS
Professor of Pediatrics
Duke University
Durham, NC, USA

Dianna S. Meredith, RDCS
The Heart Center
Cincinnati Children's Hospital
  Medical Center
Cincinnati, OH, USA

Erik C. Michelfelder, MD
Associate Professor of Pediatrics
University of Cincinnati College of
  Medicine
Director, Fetal Cardiac Center
Division of Cardiology
Cincinnati Children's Hospital
  Medical Center
Cincinnati, OH, USA

L. LuAnn Minich, MD
Professor of Pediatrics
University of Utah Medical Center
Division of Pediatric Cardiology
Primary Children's Medical Center
Salt Lake City, UT, USA

Ndidi L. Musa, MD
Assistant Professor of Pediatrics
Medical College of Wisconsin
Division of Critical Care Medicine
Children's Hospital of Wisconsin
Milwaukee, WI, USA

David P. Nelson, MD, PhD
Associate Professor of Pediatrics
Baylor College of Medicine
Director, Cardiovascular
  Intensive Care
Division of Pediatric Cardiology
Texas Children's Hospital
Houston, TX, USA

Jeffrey M. Pearl, MD
Associate Professor of Surgery
University of Cincinnati College of Medicine
Surgical Director, Pediatric Heart Transplant
  Program
Division of Cardiothoracic Surgery
Cincinnati Children's Hospital Medical
  Center
Cincinnati, OH, USA

Gary M. Satou, MD
Assistant Professor of Pediatrics
New York Medical College
Section of Pediatric Cardiology
Children's Hospital of Westchester Medical
  Center
Valhalla, NY, USA

Mark A. Scheurer, MD
Division of Pediatric Cardiology
Medical University of South Carolina
MUSC Children's Hospital
Charleston, SC, USA

Steven M. Schwartz, MD
Associate Professor of Anaesthesia and
  Paediatrics
University of Toronto School of Medicine
Director, Cardiac Intensive Care Unit
Department of Critical Care Medicine
The Hospital for Sick Children
Toronto, Ontario, Canada

James D. St. Louis, MD, PhD
Assistant Professor of Surgery
Medical College of Georgia
Director, Pediatric Cardiothoracic Surgery
MCG Children's Medical Center
Augusta, GA, USA

Shane M. Tibby, MRCP
Pediatric Intensive Care Unit
Evelina Children's Hospital
Guy's and St. Thomas' NHS Hospital Trust
London, UK

Derek S. Wheeler, MD
Assistant Professor of Clinical Pediatrics
University of Cincinnati College of Medicine
Division of Critical Care Medicine
Cincinnati Children's Hospital Medical
  Center
Cincinnati, OH, USA

Henry B. Wiles, MD
Professor of Pediatrics
Medical College of Georgia
Chief, Section of Cardiology
MCG Children's Medical Center
Augusta, GA, USA

1
Developmental Cardiac Physiology

Keith C. Kocis, Ana Lia Graciano, and Jon N. Meliones

A Primer on Cardiac Embryology

During the third week of gestation, the forming embryo divides into the three primary germ layers, of which the mesodermal cells will form the heart and blood vessels [1,2]. The angiogenic clusters form anterior to the neural plate in a horseshoe shape, while the primitive streak is forming and migrating posteriorly. As the brain quickly enlarges, it ventrally and caudally moves these cells that have now formed a tube. These structures finally merge in the midline, forming the primitive heart tube. The heart tube from caudal to cranial has five parts, which will later form all aspects of the normal cardiac anatomy (Figure 1.1). These structures are the (1) sinus venosus; (2) atrium; (3) ventricle; (4) bulbus cordis divided into (a) proximal conus cordis and (b) distal truncus arteriosus and; and (5) aortic sac. The sinus venosus forms the superior and inferior vena cavae. The primitive atrium and ventricle divide into right and left portions, with distinct structural features attributable to each unique chamber. The two atrioventricular valves (tricuspid and mitral valves) form from the endocardial cushions, which also form the primum atrial septum and the inlet portion of the ventricles. The bulbus cordis gives rise to the right ventricular outflow track defined at its origin by the septal and parietal muscle bundles. The truncus arteriosus forms both semilunar valves and the proximal ascending aorta and pulmonary trunk. The aortic sac will form the bulk of the ascending aorta, while the third and fourth aortic arches form the carotid arteries and transverse aorta. Finally, the sixth arch forms the ductus arteriosus and junction of the pulmonary arteries.

The primitive heart tube is fixed at either end, the aortic sac (cranial) and the sinus venosus (caudal) within the pericardial sac. As the other cardiac structures grow, the heart must rotate and bend in an important set of events, called *cardiac looping*. Normally the tube rotates to the right (dexter or D-loop), placing the structural right ventricle anterior and to the right, while the structural left ventricle is rotated leftward and posterior. Abnormalities in these complex sequence of events results in the vast majority of congenital cardiac defects.

Cardiomyocytes

Cardiomyocytes differ significantly from striated muscle types in several specific ways [3,4]. Cardiomyocytes are elongated specialized striated muscle cells, 100–150 µm in length × 20–35 µm in width. These cells branch because of differing lengths of the individual myofibrils (see later), which are made up of the contractile proteins actin and myosin and the regulatory proteins (troponin and tropomyosin). Individual myofibrils are structurally bound within the cell by a network of desmin filaments, which are linked to the inner wall of the cell membrane at the costamere. The ends of individual cells communicate with each other through the intercalated disc, which is made up of three specialized areas: (1) fascia adherens, (2) desmosome, and (3) gap junction [5,6]. These structures allow for electromechanical synchrony and complex cell signaling between the individual cells.

Cardiomyocytes are able to spontaneously depolarize and conduct electrical impulses from cell to cell over a long duration in order to coordinate contraction within and between the different chambers (i.e., left ventricle) of the heart in an efficient manner. These cells begin to acquire spontaneous and coordinated contraction at a very early stage in cardiac development. No neural innervation is required for the heart to contract (i.e., denervated organs after cardiac transplantation). Apart from the working myocardial cells, specialized cardiac conduction cells containing few contractile elements that stain for glycogen compose the cells of the sinoatrial node (pacemaker), atrioventricular node, and Purkinje cells [3,7,8].

Spontaneous depolarization (Figure 1.2) occurs during phase 4 (diastolic depolarization) as L-type (long-lasting) calcium channels allow influx of this essential cation until reaching a threshold voltage, which results in phase 0 depolarization (or systole). Phase 1 occurs as the voltage within the cell becomes positive (overshoot) and is followed by phase 2 or the plateau phase, where voltage remains slightly less than 0. There is then progressive return to resting maximal negative potential during phase 3. During specific time periods within phase 3 are the absolute refractory (AF) and the relative refractory (RR) periods, whereby depolarization cannot (AF) and can occur only with supramaximal stimulation (RR).

D.S. Wheeler et al. (eds.), *Cardiovascular Pediatric Critical Illness and Injury*,
DOI 10.1007/978-1-84800-923-3_1, © Springer-Verlag London Limited 2009

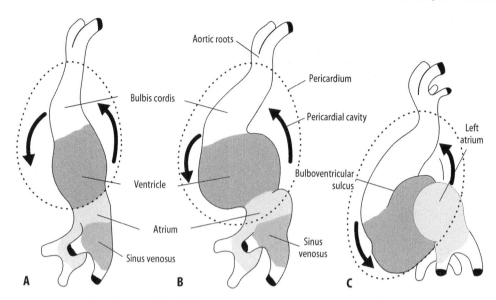

FIGURE 1.1. Primitive heart tube is shown with the five embryologic structures that will form all future cardiac anatomy. From caudal to cranial these structures are the (1) sinus venosus; (2) atrium; (3) ventricle; (4) bulbus cordis divided into a proximal (a) conus cordis and distal (b) truncus arteriosus; and (5) aortic sac. The progression from panels **A-C** illustrate the normal looping in which the heart tube rotates to the right to form the normal heart structures.

Finally, onset of phase 4 begins when there is a fairly stable maximally negative potential within the cardiomyocyte. Pacemaker cells have more phase 4 depolarization occurring and thus are ready to reenter phase 1 again for the next cardiac contraction.

The basic unit of contraction is the sarcomere (Figure 1.3) [9–19]. It contains the contractile proteins actin and myosin with the regulatory proteins α-tropomyosin binding troponins T, I, and C [19–23]. The thin filaments (F [filamentous] form) contain two strands of α-actin-cardiac composed of multiple monomers spiraled in a helix with α-tropomyosin entwined between the two strands. The double-stranded α-tropomyosin binds the troponin complex, made up three individual proteins, I, T, and C [22,24,25]. Tropomyosin also blocks actin myosin cross-bridging, which is necessary for ATPase activity to take place. Troponin I inhibits the interaction between the myosin head in the thick filament and actin. Troponin T is responsible for binding the tropomyosin chain to actin, adding to the structural integrity of the thin filament. Finally, troponin C contains four binding sites for calcium (although at basal state only one site is usually bound) [24,25], which results in movement of the troponin I protein so that it is no longer able to inhibit actin and myosin cross-bridges from forming. The thick filament is composed of the contractile protein myosin, which is made up of six protein chains, two heavy and four light [8–12,14–18,26,27]. Each myosin heavy chain is associated with two distinct myosin light chains, one essential (LC1) and one regulatory (LC2). The heavy chains form the rod and head of the myosin filament, while the four light chains are found in the head alone. The head of the myosin chain is the portion that after binding with the thin filament can enzymatically cleave adenosine triphosphate (ATP) into adenosine diphosphate (ADP) and phosphoinositide (Pi).

Spatially, each thick filament interacts with six thin filaments, allowing for the cross bridges to occur and the power stroke to shorten the sarcomere [18]. The sarcomere extends from one z line to the next, with the thin filaments attached at the z line [3]. The A (anisotropic) band spans the length of the thick filament, while the I (isotropic) band is composed of thin filaments alone. Actin and myosin are overlapping in most of the region of the A band, although the central portion, referred to as the H zone, contains only thick filaments. The M line is the middle of the thick filament. When contraction begins, there is movement of actin and myosin and more cross-bridges occur so that the I zone becomes smaller. The sarcomere cannot shorten to less than the length of the A band.

Developmentally, there are significant changes in the contractile proteins in the heart that occur during the transition from fetal to neonatal to adult life stages [5,10,12,26–31]. α-*Actin-cardiac* exists throughout fetal and adult life in one filamentous form made of

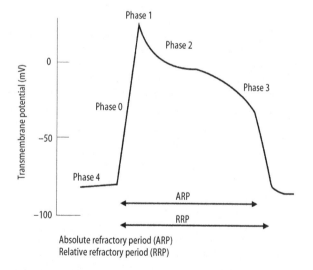

FIGURE 1.2. Phases of cardiomyocyte action potential. Diastolic depolarization occurs during phase 4 until threshold is met, initiating phase 0 depolarization (systole). Phase 1 follows as an overshoot of the voltage within, followed by phase 2 or the plateau phase when voltage remains slightly less than 0. Phase 3 begins the return to resting maximal negative potential (−90 mV). During specific time periods within phase 3 are the absolute refractory period (AFP) and relative refractory period (RRP). Finally, onset of phase 4 begins, when there is maximally negative potential within the cardiomyocyte.

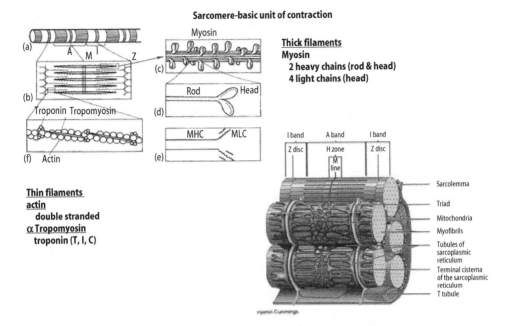

FIGURE 1.3. Anatomy of the sarcomere, the basic unit of contraction (see text for full explanation).

globular protein monomers. *Tropomyosin* exists in the human heart during fetal, neonatal, and adult life as the homodimer (α,α). *Troponin* has three different proteins expressed in a developmentally regulated manner [31–37]. In the human heart there are four isoforms of troponin T (TnT1 through TnT4). TnT1 and TnT2 are the two isoforms present in the fetal heart, whereas TnT3 is found in the adult heart. Troponin I has 2 isoforms, a slow skeletal troponin I (ssTnI) found in the fetus, neonate, and infants (<1 year of life) and the adult cardiac form (cTnI) expressed after birth through adulthood. These isoforms have significantly different functional responses to calcium and pH. Troponin C exists as a single protein throughout gestation and postnatal life. Mutations in thin filament proteins (tropomyosin, actin, troponins I and T) have been identified and are associated with familial hypertrophic and restrictive cardiomyopathies [19,23,31,38–40]. There exist three isoforms of the *myosin* heavy chain protein, V1 to V3 [8–10,12,26,28,41,42]. V1 (the adult form), with the highest ATPase activity, is composed of two homodimer α strands of myosin heavy chain, whereas V3 (the fetal form) (~50% less ATPase activity) is composed of two β-chains. V2, a heterodimer, is intermediate in function. The transition from V3 to V1 occurs largely at birth with the large increase in thyroid hormone (T_3) that occurs at that time [42–46]. Thyroid hormone plays a prominent role in transitioning several important cardiac proteins into their adult isoforms, which is discussed later. In the fetal ventricle, the myosin light chains undergo developmental changes from a fetal form (ALC1 and ALC2) to the adult form (VLC1, VLC2) [15]. The presence of the atrial isoform (ALC) in the fetal ventricle is quite intriguing. As a side note, there can be a reversion back to the fetal isoforms in the diseased adult ventricle (e.g., aortic stenosis) [15].

Actin–Myosin Interactions During the Power Stroke

Having described the contractile proteins, it is next necessary to discuss their interaction through one contractile cycle (Figure 1.4) [19,24,25,47]. Cardiomyocyte membrane depolarization causes an influx of calcium through the sarcolemma and t tubules, which are intimately related to the ryanodine (RyR) receptor in the junctional sarcoplasmic reticulum (SR) [48–55]. This calcium-initiated calcium release (CICR) results in a rapid release of calcium into the cytosol. This cytosolic calcium binds to troponin C, which results in conformational changes in troponin I, releasing it from actin binding sites while also moving tropomyosin, thereby promoting cross-bridge formation to occur between actin and myosin. Energy previously stored in myosin from ATP hydrolysis now powers the movement of the myosin head at the hinge point, allowing for shortening of the sarcomere (movement of the z lines toward one another). Adenosine diphosphate and Pi are now released, and a new molecule of ATP is bound to myosin head before the actin–myosin cross-bridges are broken and then hydrolyzed. The energy from this reaction is stored in conformational changes in the myosin head for later use in the power stroke. Calcium is removed from troponin C back into the longitudinal SR. This moves tropomyosin and troponin I back into blocking positions, and actin and myosin now become disengaged. The cycle then repeats itself.

Developmental Changes in the Structure of the Heart

Developmentally, in the fetal heart there is a decrease in ratio of contractile elements to collagen, extracellular matrix, and vascular elements. In the fetal cardiomyocyte only 30% of the volume is composed of myofibrils, whereas this increases to 60% in the adult [56,57]. In addition, the structural organization of the mitochondria to the myofibrils is quite different [58]. In the adult, these structures are compacted and intimately related to the sarcomere. These anatomic variations place the fetal and neonatal heart at a distinct disadvantage to generating force per cell. This also relates to the noncompliance of the immature heart, which is not alterable with current therapies [59–61]. This is different from the abnormalities in diastolic relaxation present in the fetus, neonate, and a variety of diseased cardiac states, which is related to the SR and ATP-dependent calcium reuptake (see later) [59–62].

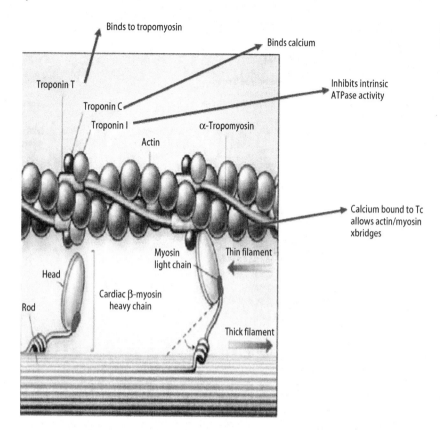

Binds to tropomyosin

Binds calcium

Inhibits intrinsic ATPase activity

Troponin T

Troponin C

Troponin I

α-Tropomyosin

Actin

Calcium bound to Tc allows actin/myosin xbridges

Myosin light chain

Thin filament

Head

Cardiac β-myosin heavy chain

Rod

Thick filament

Figure 1.4. Magnified view of the actin myosin cross-bridges and proteins necessary for the power stroke (cardiac cycle).

Calcium Regulation in the Cardiomyocyte

Critical to excitation and contraction is the entry of calcium into the cardiomyocyte from across the sarcolemma, and its deep invaginations called the transverse (t) tubules and then cytosolic release from the SR (see Figure 1.3) [48–55]. The sarcolemma has several types of calcium channels connecting extracellular calcium to the intracellular environment, although this predominantly occurs through the L (long-lasting) channels [48–55]. These voltage-gated L channels are also referred to as the *dihydropyridine* (DHP) channels because of their binding of these calcium blocking agents. These receptors are the same in both neonates and adults. The t tubule system is an extension of the cell membrane deep into the cell and, along with the terminal cisternae of the junctional SR, forms the triad. The t tubules are nearly absent in the fetus but develop invaginations into the cell at the level of the z lines in the first week of postnatal life [48].

The SR is an intracellular organelle that appears as a network of channels that surround the myofibrils and is responsible for the release and reuptake of calcium necessary for contraction and relaxation [3]. There are two regions of the SR, the junctional SR and the longitudinal SR, which have distinctly different roles in calcium handling. The junctional SR located near the z lines contains the protein calsequestrin in terminal cisternae for calcium storage and rapid release during systole. Release is triggered by influx of calcium through the L-type calcium channels located on the sarcolemma and t tubules after membrane depolarization. This then triggers a calcium-induced calcium release (CICR) through the ryanodine receptor (RyR) located in the junctional SR. Anatomically, theses channels and the junctional SR are closely linked, and rapid calcium flow between these two receptors has been referred to as *calcium sparks* [49]. Another mechanism for this

rapid release of calcium after depolarization involves reverse transport through the sarcolemma sodium/calcium exchanger [51,52]. The longitudinal SR located around the M line is critical for calcium reuptake during diastole. This diastolic relaxation is an active process requiring ATP [60,61]. Abnormalities in this SR Ca^{2+}/ATPase pump enzyme occurs in many diseased states (e.g., ventricular hypertrophy), resulting in abnormal relaxation during diastole that typically precedes abnormal diastolic function caused by decreased compliance (e.g., fibrosis) [60,61]. Phospholamban is another important regulatory protein that inhibits the Ca^{2+}/ATPase pump and thus delays reuptake of calcium into longitudinal SR. Phosphorylation of phospholamban inhibits its function and thus increases calcium reuptake and diastolic relaxation [63].

Neonatal cardiomyocytes are much more dependent on extracellular calcium influx for contraction because of the immaturity of the SR [48]. In the fetus, there are fewer cisternae in the junctional SR, and the t tubules are absent, resulting in decreased contraction during systole. There is decreased Ca^{2+}/ATPase in the longitudinal SR resulting in decreased relaxation during diastole.

Energy Metabolism in the Cardiomyocyte

Energy in the form of ATP derived from aerobic metabolism is necessary for the contraction and relaxation of the heart. This energy is derived from several sources (Figure 1.5), which are significantly different in the fetus, neonate, and adult [64–66]. The fetus uses carbohydrates in the form of lactate (60%), glucose (35%), and pyruvate (5%), whereas the adult heart consumes free fatty acids (90%) with little from carbohydrate and amino acids. At birth, a glucagon surge occurs that switches the utilization of energy substrates from carbohydrates to fatty acids. This occurs by

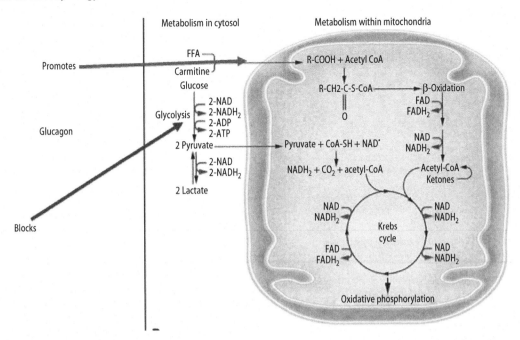

FIGURE 1.5. Energy substrates for the generation of adenosine triphosphate in the cardiomyocyte come predominantly from glycolysis (fetus) and B oxidation of free fatty acids (adult). These energy sources create acetyl CoA, which then generates the nicotinamide adenine dinucleotide (NADH) and flavin adenine dinucleotide ($FADH_2$) necessary for oxidative phosphorylation in the mitochondria. The glucagon surge at birth shifts the cardiomyocytes into utilizing free fatty acids rather than glucose.

blocking both (1) fructose-2,6-bisphosphate 2-phosphatase, a promotor of the glycolytic pathway, and (2) malonyl CoA, an inhibitor of free fatty acid transport into the mitochondria. By either metabolic pathway, NADH and $FADH_2$ are produced in the Krebs cycle and pass through the electron chain transport system, ultimately transferring electrons to oxygen. Oxidative phosphorylation takes place in the cristae of the mitochondria after a hydrogen ion gradient is established, thus producing ATP, which is then transported out of the mitochondria.

The adult heart consumes 8–15 mL O_2/min/100 g tissue, which can increase to 70 mL O_2/min/100 g tissue with exercise [64]. These needs can only be met by aerobic metabolism. Myocardial oxygen consumption is directly proportional to wall tension generated by the ventricle, defined best by the pressure volume area (PVA) [67], and to heart rate. According to Laplace's law, wall tension is directly proportional to the pressure generated within the ventricle and the radius of the ventricle and inversely proportional to the thickness of the ventricular wall. Many disease states result in increased oxygen consumption by dilating the ventricle (e.g., ventricular septal defect) or generating increased pressure within the ventricle (e.g., aortic stenosis). Cardiac hypertrophy is an adaptive process to decrease wall tension in certain disease states.

Autonomic Innervation of the Heart

The parasympathetic (vagus nerve) nervous system innervates the heart prior to the sympathetic (T1–T4) nervous system, although both are present by the age of fetal viability (20 weeks). There is a relative dominance to the parasympathetic system over the sympathetic in the neonatal ages. The right vagus innervates the sinoatrial node (SA node), while the left vagus innervates the atrioventricular node (AV node). The preganglionic fibers are short for the sympathetic nerves, which synapse with longer postganglionic fibers in the superior cervical, middle cervical, and inferior (stellate) ganglions before passing to the posterior part of the heart into the cardiac plexus innervating the SA node, AV node, and myocardium. The vagus nerve has a very long preganglionic fiber with a short postganglionic fiber. Visceral afferents run in both the sympathetic and parasympathetic nerves.

Adrenergic Receptor Physiology

There are numerous age-dependent changes in the autonomic responsiveness of ventricular myocardial or conducting tissue. Although some of these involve a simple quantitative difference in the magnitude or sensitivity of the response, in other cases a more complex qualitative alteration is observed. Receptors include a group of proteins responsible for the transduction of a signal from a circulating hormone, or neurotransmitter. Myocardial receptors include adrenergic and muscarinic cholinergic receptors.

All of the adrenergic receptors mediate their actions through interaction with a group of intracellular proteins called *G proteins* (Figure 1.6). G proteins are a large family of regulatory proteins whose activities are determined by their interaction with guanine nucleotides. G proteins cycle between an inactive guanosine diphosphate (GDP) bound form and an active guanosine triphosphate (GTP) bound form. G proteins can be divided into two groups: (1) a *heterotrimeric* form consisting of three subunits, α, β, and γ, which are membrane bound and linked to *G-protein–coupled receptors* (GPCR); and (2) *monomeric* cytoplasmic G proteins, which are involved in the regulation of various intracellular processes. G-protein–coupled receptor structure consists of seven transmembrane domains linked by extracellular and intracellular loops, with an extracellular amino (N) terminus and an intracellular carboxy (C) terminus. The extracellular domains contribute

A

B

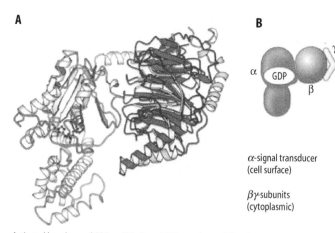

α-signal transducer
(cell surface)

βγ-subunits
(cytoplasmic)

Activated by release of GDP and binding of GTP → release of βγ-subunits
Deactivated by hydrolysis of GTP → reassociation of α to βγ subunits

FIGURE 1.6. Structure of G proteins. GDP, guanosine diphosphate; GTP, guanosine triphosphate. **(A)** 3-D structure. **(B)** Senematic depicting the various subunits.

to ligand recognition and binding, and secondary messenger coupling is determined mainly by interactions with intracellular domains [68].

G proteins can be divided into three main classes: Gs (stimulatory), Gi (inhibitory), and Gq. Gs and Gi are coupled to the adenyl cyclase pathway, and Gq is coupled to phospholipase C. Gs stimulates adenyl cyclase to hydrolyze ATP to cyclic adenosine monophosphate (cAMP), the secondary messenger. The specific cellular response that follows the change in the concentration of cAMP depends on the specialized function of the target cell. Typically, an increase in concentration of *cAMP* leads to *cAM- dependent protein kinase* activation, which phosphorylates and activates other key regulatory proteins in cardiac myocytes. Gi proteins inhibit adenyl cyclase and secondary phosphorylation [68].

β_1- and β_2-receptors are associated with stimulatory (Gs) proteins, and α_2 and cholinergic receptors are coupled with inhibitory (Gi) proteins. α_1-Receptors are coupled to Gq proteins. Binding of the ligand to the α_1-receptor activates phospholipase C, which converts phosphoinositol diphosphate into diacylglycerol (DAG) and inositol triphosphate (IP3). Diacylglycerol activates the enzyme protein kinase C, which phosphorylates cellular enzymes, leading to an increase in intracellular calcium by opening ion channels. The increase in calcium activates excitation contraction coupling and stimulates muscle contraction. α_1-Agonists and β-agonists increase contractility via different pathways [69–71].

Persistent exposure of receptors to an agonist results in the loss of receptor-activated function or *desensitization*. Desensitization is cell specific and dependent on both the expression and the subcellular localization of specific components that function in desensitization processes. *Homologous desensitization* refers to the loss of stimulatory activity in the pathway that is involved with the specific receptor that is being stimulated. *Heterologous desensitization* refers to the decreased activity in all the pathways involved in the receptor stimulation. Three general mechanisms are associated with desensitization of GPCRs: (1) phosphorylation, (2) internalization or sequestration, and (3) downregulation. Receptor phosphorylation occurs in an agonist-dependent manner that is correlated (with respect to both time and dose) with a decreased

affinity of receptors for the agonist, as well as attenuated receptor function. Agonist-induced receptor phosphorylation by GPCR kinases increases the affinity of receptor binding to an *arrestin* molecule, resulting in uncoupling of the G protein from the receptor. Arrestin receptor binding prevents further signal transduction between receptor and G proteins [72,73]. Another process associated with agonist-induced receptor desensitization is *sequestration* of cell-surface receptors into an intracellular membrane compartment. Receptor sequestration may involve different membrane trafficking pathways. Sequestered receptors can either recycle to the cell surface or enter the endolysosomal pathway and eventually be degraded. Both receptor phosphorylation and sequestration are associated primarily with more rapid receptor desensitization, which occurs over a period of only a few minutes [74].

With more persistent exposure to agonist, a slower phase (typically hours) of receptor *downregulation* occurs in which the steady-state level of receptor protein is decreased. Mechanisms responsible for the agonist-induced reduction in the cellular density of receptors (homologous receptor downregulation) remain largely unclear but involve appropriate changes in either receptor synthesis (i.e., reduction in the steady-state level of receptor mRNA) and/or receptor degradation. Receptor downregulation is also cell specific and involves the complex interaction between multiple cellular events to influence receptor expression. The decreased response to inotropic agents in the failing heart has been related to β-receptor downregulation [75,76].

β-Adrenergic receptors on the neonatal myocardium are pharmacologically identical to their adult form and are approximately 80% β_1 and 20% β_2. β-Adrenergic receptors and the adenyl cyclase system are well developed by late fetal life; receptor density peaks at birth and decreases with advancing post conceptional age. β-Adrenergic receptor responsiveness is markedly decreased with aging; this occurs by multiple mechanisms, including downregulation and decreased agonist binding of β_1-receptors, uncoupling of β_2-receptors, and abnormal G-protein–mediated signal transduction [77]. These changes in the β-adrenergic receptors are primarily modulated by increases in both thyroid hormone and adrenocorticosteroids that occur with birth. At birth, these differences in β-receptor function along with higher circulating catecholamine levels result in a lower responsiveness to exogenously administered catecholamines. α_1-Adrenergic receptors appear early in gestation and in many species reach their highest density in the newborn period.

Vagal tone influences contractility via cholinergic receptors, operating through Gi proteins. In humans, acetylcholine inhibits sinoatrial pacemaker activity in hearts as young as 3–7 weeks gestation, and parasympathetic cholinergic nerves are found in the atria very early in gestation. Sensitivity to acetylcholine increases up to week 9 and then remains stable until the eighteenth week. Vagal myelination progresses throughout fetal development in humans and reaches adult levels by about 50 weeks postconceptual age. Expression of cholinergic receptors, which appear to be similar to adult receptors, is maximal at birth, remains high for several weeks, and then declines to adult levels, at least in the rat.

Although the innervation of the mammalian heart has been study extensively in animals, much less is known about the innervation of these tissues in humans. The initial sympathetic dominance in the neural supply to the human heart in infancy and its gradual transition into a sympathetic and parasympathetic codominance in adulthood correlate with the changes in heart rate observed during postnatal development.

Transition from Fetus to Neonate

Separation of the fetus from the mother is a complex physiologic process that has multiple effects on cardiac function, cardiopulmonary interactions, and the processes that bring about the ontogenic changes in cardiac structure described earlier [46,48,56,78–82].

Fetal Oxygen Saturation

After blood circulates through the placenta, the highest oxygen saturation ($SaO_2 = 80\%$; $PaO_2 = 35\,mm\,Hg$) in the fetal circulation is found in the single umbilical vein, which continues into the fetus as the ductus venosus (Figure 1.7). This highly oxygenated blood enters the right atrium where it is preferentially shunted across the foramen ovale into the left atrium. There is subsequent admixture of desaturated blood from the inferior vena cava and ($SaO_2 = 70\%$), superior vena cava SVC ($SaO_2 = 40\%$), hepatic veins, coronary sinus, leading to a left ventricle (LV) $SaO_2 = 65\%$. This LV blood is preferentially flows via the ascending aorta into the developing brain and coronary system. The desaturated blood preferentially enters the right ventricle (RV) with a saturation of 55%, which ejects into the uninflated lungs, and ductus arteriosus, which leads to the descending aorta. There is a step up in oxygen saturations in the descending aorta (60%) because of a small amount of blood crossing the isthmus of the aorta from the ascending aorta. This blood then flows to the right and left internal iliac arteries, which then give

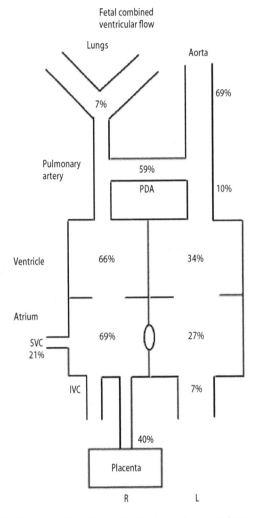

FIGURE 1.8. Flow through the various cardiac chambers and great vessels as a percentage of combined ventricular output (both right and left ventricles). IVC, inferior vena cava; PDA, patent ductus arteriosus; SVC, superior vena cava.

rise to the two umbilical arteries that will bring this desaturated blood to the placenta for oxygenation [56,79–81].

Fetal Blood Flow

Blood flow in the fetus (Figure 1.8) is best described as combined ventricular output (CVO) (both RV and LV) in contrast to postnatal blood flow, which is described as LV cardiac output (because the two circulations are normally in series). Following the same blood pathway as described earlier, the combined ventricular output (both RV and LV) is approximately 500 mL/kg with 40% of this blood flowing to (and from) the placenta. Roughly two thirds of the CVO enters the RV, with 59% passing through the ductus arteriosus on its way to the descending aorta while only 7% perfuses the collapsed lungs. The LV, in contrast, receives only one third of the CVO and ejects 31% out the aortic valve into the ascending aorta, where 3% enters the coronary circulation and 21% perfuses the brain. The remainder (10%) crosses the isthmus of the aorta into the descending aorta. Obviously, dramatic changes occur in blood flow when congenital heart defects are present in utero. Two defects with drastically (and opposite) blood flows occur in fetuses with hypoplastic left heart syndrome and tricuspid atresia [56,79–81].

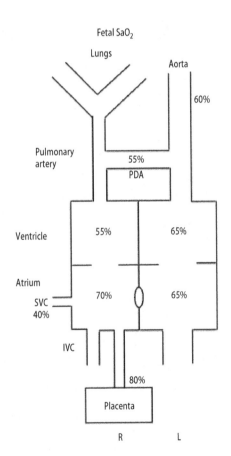

FIGURE 1.7. Oxygen saturations found in the various cardiac chambers and great vessels of the fetus. IVC, inferior vena cava; PDA, patent ductus arteriosus; SVC, superior vena cava.

Fetal Hemoglobin

It is important to understand the characteristics of the fetal hemoglobin (HbF) oxygen disassociation curve (Figure 1.9). First, the P50 (or partial pressure of oxygen where hemoglobin is 50% saturated) is lower (21 mm Hg) than adult hemoglobin (HbA) (27 mm Hg). Thus, the HbF disassociation curve is shifted *leftward* of the HbA curve. Acidic pH, PCO_2, and 2,3-DPG all shift the curves to the right. Importantly, HbA production begins at 34 weeks' gestation, with a half life of 6 weeks, such that at birth 60% of the neonate's blood is HbF. These characteristics of HbF allow for transfer of oxygen from the placenta to the fetal circulation and unloading of relatively desaturated blood in the tissue beds of the fetus. In addition, HbF has a lower viscosity than HbA at the same level of hematocrit.

Pulmonary Vascular Resistance

Because in utero the fetal lungs are not inflated with gas, but distended by pulmonary fluid [83], and only 7% of CVO perfuses them, the pulmonary vascular resistance (PVR) is very high (Figure 1.10) [56,79–81,84–86]. Even in this state, the pulmonary bed has been shown to be reactive to relative hypoxemia ($PaO_2 < 18$ mm Hg) and acidosis, which increases PVR, and relative hyperoxia and alkalosis, which decreases PVR [84–86]. With normal vaginal delivery and baby's first breath there is a tremendous decrease in PVR predominantly because of lung inflation with air. Again, hypoxemia, acidosis, hypothermia, and polycythemia serve to increase PVR, whereas hyperoxia, alkalosis, hyperthermia, prostaglandin (E_2 and I_2), and nitric oxide (among many other things) decrease PVR [85,86].

The central nervous system influences PVR in several ways, mostly, although not entirely, mediated through the sympathetic nervous system. First, stimulation of baroreceptors located in the carotid bodies and in the pulmonary arteries themselves result in pulmonary vasoconstriction. Chemoreceptors located in the carotid and aortic bodies sense both oxygen and carbon dioxide tensions (while the sensors in the respiratory center of the brain stem only detect carbon dioxide). These sensors affect PVR in the fashions described earlier [86].

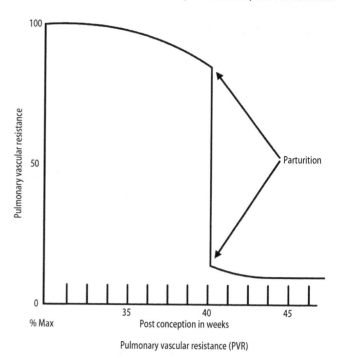

FIGURE 1.10. The changes in pulmonary artery pressure, pulmonary blood flow, and pulmonary vascular resistance (PVR) that occur during fetal development, parturition, and neonatal life. Note that the most dramatic decrease in PVR occurs with the infant's first breath.

The Ductus Arteriosus

The ductus arteriosus (DA) [87–93] connects the main pulmonary artery to the descending aorta at the level just beyond the isthmus and takeoff of the subclavian artery. Embryologic origin is from the sixth aortic arch. During fetal life, the DA allows blood to bypass the fluid-filled lungs and perfuse the lower body via the right ventricle. This ultimately returns deoxygenated blood back to the placenta for renewal of oxygen and metabolic substrates from the mother. The main anatomic differences between the DA and pulmonary artery (PA) reside in spiraling layers of smooth muscle in the media (DA) rather than circumferentially oriented ones (PA), which then migrate into the subintimal areas during late gestation. The media is also filled with hyaluronic acid (DA). The intima is also noticeably thicker (DA) than in the PA.

Postnatal closure of the ductus involves two phases. The *first phase* occurs within the first 12 hr after birth. The mechanism responsible for this is contraction of the smooth muscle fibers in the media, resulting in a narrowing of the ductal lumen and shortening of the ductus. This leads to increased ductal wall thickness with protrusion of intimal *cushions* into the lumen. The *second phase* is normally completed in the first few weeks of life. The mechanisms involved in this phase include endothelial infolding with disruption and fragmentation of the subintimal layers with fibrous proliferation resulting in formation of the ligamentum arteriosum.

Ductal vasoreactivity is affected predominantly by oxygen, prostaglandins, and other substances. During fetal life, the ductus is exposed to relatively hypoxemic blood coming from the RV. As gestation advances, increases in PaO_2 cause vasoconstriction. The more advanced the gestational age, the lower the level of oxygen necessary to cause vasoconstriction. Bradykinin, acetylcholine catecholamines and endothelin are all potent DA vasoconstrictors. The best-studied mediators of ductal patency are the prostaglandins (PGs) derived

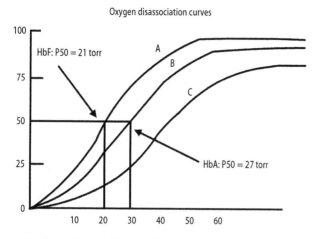

FIGURE 1.9. Oxygen disassociation curve of fetal hemoglobin (HbF) (curve A) compared with adult hemoglobin (HbA) (curve B) as well as a rightward shift of the HbA curve (curve C) associated with several physiologic processes, including 2,3-diphosphoglycerate.

from the cyclooxygenase-mediated products of arachidonic acid metabolism. These are produced by the DA itself and also by the placenta. Endogenously produced PGE$_2$ and PGI$_2$ (prostacyclin) and exogenous PGE$_1$ dilate the DA. Circulating levels of PGI$_2$ from the placenta are much higher (10 times) than PGE$_2$, although PGE$_2$ is a much more potent vasodilator than PGI$_2$. Inhibitors of prostaglandin synthesis, such as indomethacin and other nonsteroidal agents, produce constriction of the DA that can be reversed by PGE$_1$ infusion. Prostaglandins are metabolized in the lung, which for the fetus means significantly higher circulating levels compared with the neonatal counterpart with perfusion of the lungs.

Fetal and Neonatal Regulation of Thyroid Hormone

The ontogenic changes in the thyroid hormones thyroid-releasing hormone (TRH), thyroid-stimulating hormone (TSH), T$_4$ (thyroxine), reverse triiodothyronine (rT$_3$), and triiodothyronine (T$_3$) are demonstrated in Figure 1.11. During fetal life there is a progressive

increase in hypothalamic release of TRH, but TSH levels fall slightly during late gestation because of negative feedback from rising T3 levels. The placenta is instrumental in converting T4 into rT3 during fetal life (inner ring deiodinase) rather than T3 (outer ring deiodinase found in the fetal liver) in order to minimize thermogenesis and thus oxygen consumption while also minimizing respiratory drive. In late gestation, an increase in glucocorticoid synthesis within the fetus upregulates outer ring deiodinase found in fetal liver, leading to the rising T3 levels. At birth, with the removal of the placenta and stress response from delivery, there is a logarithmic increase in TSH, T$_4$, and T$_3$ levels, while rT$_3$ levels fall. This is the basis for all neonatal thyroid screening tests. The increase in T$_3$ drives many metabolic processes, including the conversion of myosin heavy chain transformation into the V1 adult form and increasing β-receptors, as described earlier [42–46].

Conclusion

This chapter reviewed the current state of knowledge regarding the important changes that occur in cardiovascular physiology during fetal life through the complex birthing process into neonatal life and beyond into childhood and adulthood. This information is important to the practicing pediatric cardiac intensivist who must make critical decisions about stabilizing premature infants and neonates in the pediatric intensive care unit. These strategies are different from those utilized for the older child and adult. Once patients are stable, timing of surgical procedures must be made with knowledge of these developmental transitions in cardiac function. Finally, future research will be aimed at developing new strategies to either transition the neonatal myocardium to a more advantageous state or employ novel therapies to maximize fetal/neonatal physiology.

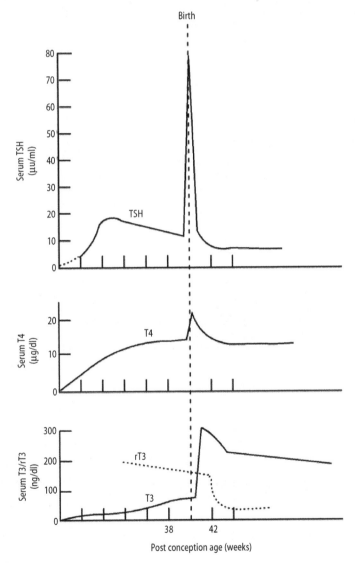

FIGURE 1.11. The ontogenic changes in the thyroid hormones: thyroid-releasing hormone (TRH), thyroid-stimulating hormone (TSH), T4 (thyroxine), reverse triiodothyronine (rT3), and triiodothyronine (T3). Note the logarithmic increase in TSH, T4, and T3 levels, while rT3 levels fall.

References

1. Moore KL. The Developing Human: Clinically Oriented Embryology, 6th ed. Philadelphia: WB Saunders; 1998.
2. Sadler TW. Langman's Medical Embryology, 9th ed. Chapel Hill, NC: Lippincott Williams & Wilkins; 2003.
3. Katz AM. Physiology of the Heart, 3rd ed. Philadelphia: Lippincott Williams & Wilkins; 2001.
4. Severs NJ. The cardiac muscle cell. Bioessays 2000;22(2):188–199.
5. Angst BD, Khan LU, Severs NJ, et al. Dissociated spatial patterning of gap junctions and cell adhesion junctions during postnatal differentiation of ventricular myocardium. Circ Res 1997;80(1):88–94.
6. Yeager M. Structure of cardiac gap junction intercellular channels. J Struct Biol 1998;121(2):231–245.
7. Gillette P, Garson A. Pediatric Arrhythmias: Electrophysiology and Pacing. Philadelphia: WB Saunders; 1990.
8. Barton PJ, Robert B, Fiszman MY, Leader DP, Buckingham ME. The same myosin alkali light chain gene is expressed in adult cardiac atria and in fetal skeletal muscle. J Muscle Res Cell Motil 1985;6(4):461–475.
9. Hirzel H, Tuchschmid C, Schneider J, Krayenbuehl H, Schaub M. Relationship between myosin isoenzyme composition, hemodynamics, and myocardial structure in various forms of human cardiac hypertrophy. Circ Res 1985;57(5):729–740.
10. Miyata S, Minobe W, Bristow MR, Leinwand LA. Myosin heavy chain isoform expression in the failing and nonfailing human heart. Circ Res 2000;86(4):386–390.
11. Morano M, Zacharzowski U, Maier M, et al. Regulation of human heart contractility by essential myosin light chain isoforms. J Clin Invest 1996;98(2):467–473.

12. Reiser PJ, Portman MA, Ning XH, Schomisch Moravec C. Human cardiac myosin heavy chain isoforms in fetal and failing adult atria and ventricles. Am J Physiol Heart Circ Physiol 2001;280(4): H1814–H1820.

13. Schaub MC, Hefti MA, Zuellig RA, Morano I. Modulation of contractility in human cardiac hypertrophy by myosin essential light chain isoforms. Cardiovasc Res 1998;37(2):381–404.

14. Sutsch G, Brunner UT, von Schulthess C, et al. Hemodynamic performance and myosin light chain-1 expression of the hypertrophied left ventricle in aortic valve disease before and after valve replacement. Circ Res 1992;70(5):1035–1043.

15. Yamashita H. Myosin light chain isoforms modify force generating ability of cardiac myosin by changing the kinetics of actin-myosin interaction. Cardiovasc Res 2003.

16. Molloy J. Movement and force produced by a single myosin head. Nature 1995.

17. Rayment I. Three dimensional structure of myosin subfragment-1: a molecular motor. Science 1993.

18. Uyeda T. The neck region of the myosin motor domain acts as a lever arm to generate movement. Proc Natl Acad Sci USA 1996.

19. Hernandez O. Plasticity in skeletal cardiac and smooth muscle: invited review: pathophysiology of cardiac muscle contraction and relaxation as a result of alterations in thin filament regulation. J Appl Physiol 2001.

20. Al-Hillawi E. The effects of phosphorylation of cardiac troponin-I on its interactions with actin and cardiac troponin C. Eur J Biochem 1995.

21. Farah C. The troponin complex and regulation of muscle contraction. FASEB J 1995.

22. Parmacek M. Biology of the troponin complex in cardiac myocytes. Prog Cardiovasc Dis 2004.

23. Michele D. Physiological consequences of tropomyosin mutations associated with cardiac and skeletal myopathies. J Mol Med 2000.

24. Solaro RJ, Rarick HM. Troponin and tropomyosin: proteins that switch on and tune in the activity of cardiac myofilaments. Circ Res 1998; 83(5):471–480.

25. Gordon A. Skeletal and cardiac muscle contractile activation: tropomyosin "rocks and rolls". New Physiol Sci 2001.

26. Cummins P, Lambert SJ. Myosin transitions in the bovine and human heart. A developmental and anatomical study of heavy and light chain subunits in the atrium and ventricle. Circ Res 1986;58(6):846–858.

27. Price KM, Littler WA, Cummins P. Human atrial and ventricular myosin light-chains subunits in the adult and during development. Biochem J 1980;191(2):571–580.

28. VanBuren P, Harris DE, Alpert NR, Warshaw DM. Cardiac V1 and V3 myosins differ in their hydrolytic and mechanical activities in vitro. Circ Res 1995;77(2):439–444.

29. Sanbe A, Gulick J, Hayes E, et al. Myosin light chain replacement in the heart. Am J Physiol Heart Circ Physiol 2000;279(3):H1355–H1364.

30. Humphreys JE, Cummins P. Regulatory proteins of the myocardium. Atrial and ventricular tropomyosin and troponin-I in the developing and adult bovine and human heart. J Mol Cell Cardiol 1984; 16(7):643–657.

31. Venkatraman G, Gomes AV, Kerrick WG, Potter JD. Characterization of troponin T dilated cardiomyopathy mutations in the fetal troponin isoform. J Biol Chem 2005;280(18):17584–17592.

32. Anderson PA, Malouf NN, Oakeley AE, Pagani ED, Allen PD. Troponin T isoform expression in humans. A comparison among normal and failing adult heart, fetal heart, and adult and fetal skeletal muscle. Circ Res 1991;69(5):1226–1233.

33. Anderson PA, Greig A, Mark TM, et al. Molecular basis of human cardiac troponin T isoforms expressed in the developing, adult, and failing heart. Circ Res 1995;76(4):681–686.

34. Hastings KE, Koppe RI, Marmor E, Bader D, Shimada Y, Toyota N. Structure and developmental expression of troponin I isoforms. cDNA clone analysis of avian cardiac troponin I mRNA. J Biol Chem 1991;266(29):19659–19665.

35. Bodor GS, Oakeley AE, Allen PD, Crimmins DL, Ladenson JH, Anderson PA. Troponin I phosphorylation in the normal and failing adult human heart. Circulation 1997;96(5):1495–1500.

36. Hunkeler NM, Kullman J, Murphy AM. Troponin I isoform expression in human heart. Circ Res 1991;69(5):1409–1414.

37. Bhavsar PK, Dhoot GK, Cumming DV, Butler-Browne GS, Yacoub MH, Barton PJ. Developmental expression of troponin I isoforms in fetal human heart. FEBS Lett 1991;292(1–2):5–8.

38. Corrado D, Basso C, Thiene G, et al. Spectrum of clinicopathologic manifestations of arrhythmogenic right ventricular cardiomyopathy/ dysplasia: a multicenter study. J Am Coll Cardiol 1997;30(6):1512–1520.

39. Swan H, Piippo K, Viitasalo M, et al. Arrhythmic disorder mapped to chromosome 1q42-q43 causes malignant polymorphic ventricular tachycardia in structurally normal hearts. J Am Coll Cardiol 1999; 34(7):2035–2042.

40. Yamashita H, Tyska MJ, Warshaw DM, Lowey S, Trybus KM. Functional consequences of mutations in the smooth muscle myosin heavy chain at sites implicated in familial hypertrophic cardiomyopathy. J Biol Chem 2000;275(36):28045–28052.

41. Hoh J, McGrath P, Hale P. Electrophoretic analysis of multiple forms of rat cardiac myosin: effects of hypophysectomy and thyroxine replacement. J Mol Cell Cardiol 1978;10(11):1053–1076.

42. Bottinelli R, Canepari M, Cappelli V, Reggiani C. Maximum speed of shortening and ATPase activity in atrial and ventricular myocardia of hyperthyroid rats. Am J Physiol 1995;269(3 Pt 1):C785–C790.

43. Gluckman P. The transition from fetus to neonate-an endocrine perspective. Acta Paediatr 1999.

44. Hoh J. Electrophoretic analysis of multiple forms of rat cardiac myosin: effects of hypophysectomy and thyroxine replacement. J Mol Cell Cardiol 1978.

45. Izumo S. Myosin heavy chain messenger RNA and protein isoform transitions during cardiac hypertrophy. Interaction between hemodynamic and thyroid hormone induced signals. J Clin Invest 1987.

46. Fisher D. Ontogenesis of hypothalamic-pituitary-thyroid function and metabolism in man, sheep, and rat. Recent Prog Hormone Res 1976.

47. Stern MD. Theory of excitation-contraction coupling in cardiac muscle. Biophys J 1992;63(2):497–517.

48. Tibbits GF, Xu L, Sedarat F. Ontogeny of excitation-contraction coupling in the mammalian heart. Comp Biochem Physiol A Mol Integr Physiol 2002;132(4):691–698.

49. Cheng H, Lederer WJ, Cannell MB. Calcium sparks: elementary events underlying excitation-contraction coupling in heart muscle. Science 1993;262(5134):740–744.

50. Fabiato A. Calcium-induced release of calcium from the cardiac sarcoplasmic reticulum. Am J Physiol 1983;245(1):C1–C14.

51. Frank JS, Mottino G, Reid D, Molday RS, Philipson KD. Distribution of the Na(+)-Ca2+ exchange protein in mammalian cardiac myocytes: an immunofluorescence and immunocolloidal gold-labeling study. J Cell Biol 1992;117(2):337–345.

52. Haddock PS, Coetzee WA, Artman M. Na+/Ca2+ exchange current and contractions measured under Cl(-)-free conditions in developing rabbit hearts. Am J Physiol 1997;273(2 Pt 2):H837–H846.

53. Kaufman TM, Horton JW, White DJ, Mahony L. Age-related changes in myocardial relaxation and sarcoplasmic reticulum function. Am J Physiol 1990;259(2 Pt 2):H309–H316.

54. Sauer H, Theben T, Hescheler J, Lindner M, Brandt MC, Wartenberg M. Characteristics of calcium sparks in cardiomyocytes derived from embryonic stem cells. Am J Physiol Heart Circ Physiol 2001;281(1): H411–H421.

55. Sham JS, Cleemann L, Morad M. Functional coupling of Ca2+ channels and ryanodine receptors in cardiac myocytes. Proc Natl Acad Sci USA 1995;92(1):121–125.

56. Friedman WF. The intrinsic physiologic properties of the developing heart. Prog Cardiovasc Dis 1972;15(1):87–111.

57. Covell JW. Factors influencing diastolic function. Possible role of the extracellular matrix. Circulation 1990;81(2 Suppl):III155–III158.

58. Nassar R, Reedy MC, Anderson PA. Developmental changes in the ultrastructure and sarcomere shortening of the isolated rabbit ventricular myocyte. Circ Res 1987;61(3):465–483.

59. Cullen S, Shore D, Redington A. Characterization of right ventricular diastolic performance after complete repair of tetralogy of Fallot. Restrictive physiology predicts slow postoperative recovery. Circulation 1995;91(6):1782–1789.

60. McMahon C, Nagueh S, Pignatelli R, et al. Characterization of left ventricular diastolic function by tissue Doppler imaging and clinical status in children with hypertrophic cardiomyopathy. Circulation 2004;109(14):1756–1762.

61. Oh J, Appleton C, Hatle L, Nishimura R, Seward J, Tajik A. The non-invasive assessment of left ventricular diastolic function with two-dimensional and Doppler echocardiography. J Am Soc Echocardiogr 1997;10(3):246–270.

62. Stokes DL, Wagenknecht T. Calcium transport across the sarcoplasmic reticulum: structure and function of Ca2+-ATPase and the ryanodine receptor. Eur J Biochem 2000;267(17):5274–5279.

63. Mattiazzi A, Mundina-Weilenmann C, Guoxiang C, Vittone L, Kranias E. Role of phospholamban phosphorylation on Thr17 in cardiac physiological and pathological conditions. Cardiovasc Res 2005;68(3):366–375.

64. Giordano FJ. Oxygen, oxidative stress, hypoxia, and heart failure. J Clin Invest 2005;115(3):500–508.

65. Jafri MS, Dudycha SJ, O'Rourke B. Cardiac energy metabolism: models of cellular respiration. Annu Rev Biomed Eng 2001;3:57–81.

66. Lopaschuk GD, Spafford MA, Marsh DR. Glycolysis is predominant source of myocardial ATP production immediately after birth. Am J Physiol 1991;261(6 Pt 2):H1698–H1705.

67. Teitel DF, Klautz R, Steendijk P, van der Velde ET, van Bel F, Baan J. The end-systolic pressure–volume relationship in the newborn lamb: effects of loading and inotropic interventions. Pediatr Res 1991;29(5):473–482.

68. Coughlin SR. Expanding horizons for receptors coupled to G proteins: diversity and disease. Curr Opin Cell Biol 1994;6(2):191–197.

69. Birnbaumer L, Abramowitz J, Brown AM. Receptor-effector coupling by G proteins. Biochim Biophys Acta 1990;1031(2):163–224.

70. Cotecchia S, Kobilka BK, Daniel KW, et al. Multiple second messenger pathways of alpha-adrenergic receptor subtypes expressed in eukaryotic cells. J Biol Chem 1990;265(1):63–69.

71. Stiles GL, Caron MG, Lefkowitz RJ. Beta-adrenergic receptors: biochemical mechanisms of physiological regulation. Physiol Rev 1984; 64(2):661–743.

72. Kobilka B. Adrenergic receptors as models for G protein-coupled receptors. Annu Rev Neurosci 1992;15:87–114.

73. Oakley RH, Laporte SA, Holt JA, Barak LS, Caron MG. Molecular determinants underlying the formation of stable intracellular G protein-coupled receptor-beta-arrestin complexes after receptor endocytosis. J Biol Chem 2001;276(22):19452–19460.

74. Lefkowitz RJ, Hausdorff WP, Caron MG. Role of phosphorylation in desensitization of the beta-adrenoceptor. Trends Pharmacol Sci 1990; 11(5):190–194.

75. Benovic JL. Purification and characterization of beta-adrenergic receptor kinase. Methods Enzymol 1991;200:351–362.

76. Bristow MR, Ginsburg R, Minobe W, et al. Decreased catecholamine sensitivity and beta-adrenergic-receptor density in failing human hearts. N Engl J Med 1982;307(4):205–211.

77. White M, Roden R, Minobe W, et al. Age-related changes in beta-adrenergic neuroeffector systems in the human heart. Circulation 1994; 90(3):1225–1238.

78. Shaul PW, Farrar MA, Zellers TM. Oxygen modulates endothelium-derived relaxing factor production in fetal pulmonary arteries. Am J Physiol 1992;262(2 Pt 2):H355–H364.

79. Friedman AH, Fahey JT. The transition from fetal to neonatal circulation: normal responses and implications for infants with heart disease. Semin Perinatol 1993;17(2):106–121.

80. Rudolph AM. Congenital Diseases of the Heart. Chicago: Year Book Medical Publishers; 1974.

81. Heymann MA. Regulation of the pulmonary circulation in the perinatal period and in children. Intensive Care Med 1989;15(Suppl 1): S9–S12.

82. Agata Y, Hiraishi S, Misawa H, et al. Regional blood flow distribution and left ventricular output during early neonatal life: a quantitative ultrasonographic assessment. Pediatr Res 1994;36(6):805–810.

83. Adams FH, Latta H, el-Salawy A, Nozaki M. The expanded lung of the term fetus. J Pediatr 1969;75(1):59–66.

84. Heymann MA, Rudolph AM, Nies AS, Melmon KL. Bradykinin production associated with oxygenation of the fetal lamb. Circ Res 1969; 25(5):521–534.

85. Rudolph AM. Fetal and neonatal pulmonary circulation. Am Rev Respir Dis 1977;115(6 Pt 2):11–18.

86. Long W. Fetal and Neonatal Cardiology. Philadelphia: WB Saunders; 1990.

87. Coceani F, Kelsey L. Endothelin-1 release from lamb ductus arteriosus: relevance to postnatal closure of the vessel. Can J Physiol Pharmacol 1991;69(2):218–221.

88. Quinn D, Cooper B, Clyman RI. Factors associated with permanent closure of the ductus arteriosus: a role for prolonged indomethacin therapy. Pediatrics 2002;110(1 Pt 1):e10.

89. Reller MD, Colasurdo MA, Rice MJ, McDonald RW. The timing of spontaneous closure of the ductus arteriosus in infants with respiratory distress syndrome. Am J Cardiol 1990;66(1):75–78.

90. Shaffer CL, Gal P, Ransom JL, et al. Effect of age and birth weight on indomethacin pharmacodynamics in neonates treated for patent ductus arteriosus. Crit Care Med 2002;30(2):343–348.

91. Silver MM, Freedom RM, Silver MD, Olley PM. The morphology of the human newborn ductus arteriosus: a reappraisal of its structure and closure with special reference to prostaglandin E1 therapy. Hum Pathol 1981;12(12):1123–1136.

92. Seidner SR, Chen YQ, Oprysko PR, et al. Combined prostaglandin and nitric oxide inhibition produces anatomic remodeling and closure of the ductus arteriosus in the premature newborn baboon. Pediatr Res 2001;50(3):365–373.

93. Patent ductus arteriosus. In: Moss, Adams, eds. Heart Disease in Infants, Children, and Adolescents Including the Fetus and Young Adult, 6th ed. Baltimore: Lippincott Williams & Wilkins; 2000.

2
Hemodynamic Monitoring

Shane M. Tibby

Introduction

Hemodynamic monitoring encompasses all pressure and flow measurements in relation to the cardiovascular system. The science of hemodynamics has its origins in the 17th and 18th centuries, from the pioneering work of William Harvey and the Reverend Stephen Hales. Hemodynamics incorporates monitoring within the wider consideration of the theoretical aspects of the forces responsible for the development and propagation of the pressure and flow pulses. Appreciation of hemodynamic monitoring requires an understanding of the structure of the heart and blood vessels, cardiovascular physiology, and fluid mechanics [1].

Vascular Pressure Measurement

Maintaining an adequate perfusion pressure is a vital adjunct to ensuring adequate oxygen delivery [2]. The two common invasive pressure measurements undertaken in the pediatric intensive care unit (PICU) are arterial and central venous pressures. Pressure measurement typically involves an indwelling catheter; fluid-filled, noncompliant tubing; and a pressure chamber containing a diaphragm, which is connected to a pressure transducer. Pulsatile pressure transmitted from the blood vessel displaces the diaphragm; this movement is sensed by a transducer, which relays an electric signal to a visual monitor via a preamplifier. Blood sampling and zeroing to atmosphere are possible via a three-way tap within the tubing, and the system is kept patent via a continuous infusion of saline [1,3].

The relationship between signal input and output is known as the *transfer function*; in a system measuring vascular pressures the transfer function has two components—one relating to the steady-state response and the other to the transient response [4]. Here the steady-state response relates to the regular, periodic signals produced by an unchanging or minimally changing blood pressure and heart rate; such a signal can be represented by Fourier analysis [5]. The transient response refers to the how the system attempts to re-achieve a steady state when the input is rapidly altered in terms of both frequency (heart rate) and amplitude (blood pressure). Two interacting components affect the transient response, the natural frequency of the system and the damping constant [6]. For each natural frequency there is a range of optimal dampening. If the system is overdamped, systolic pressure will be underestimated and diastolic pressure overestimated (however, mean pressures will be relatively accurate); conversely, an underdamped system will overestimate systolic pressure and give a distorted waveform overall [6]. Dampening can be estimated crudely at the bedside by observation of the waveform and a *fast-flush* test in which 1–2 mL of saline is flushed rapidly through the system at a pressure in excess of the systolic pressure and the ensuing signal observed. In an overdamped system, the pressure trace will be slow to return to the pulsatile waveform after the flush, and there will be no oscillation as it reequilibrates with the blood pressure signal. The pressure trace in an underdamped system will return rapidly toward the blood pressure wave but will show a series of rapid oscillations around the blood pressure as it reequilibrates [6,7]. The transient response can be optimized by utilizing tubing that is noncompliant and not of excessive length, monitoring for kinks in the tubing and the intravascular catheter, and avoiding small air bubbles and clots within the system [8,9].

The arterial pressure pulse waveform is a function of a number of factors, including stroke volume, arterial compliance, arterial impedance, peripheral resistance, inertia, and wave reflection (see Arterial Pulse Contour Analysis, later) [10,11]. As these properties change along the arterial tree, so does the pulse pressure waveform; these changes are more marked in children than in adults [12]. This means that a centrally measured pressure will have a lower systolic and higher diastolic pressure but an approximately equal mean arterial blood pressure to that from a peripherally measured site.

Cardiac Output

Cardiac output is the volume of blood ejected by the heart per minute. It is usually expressed relative to body surface area, which means that the normal range of 3.5–5.5 L/min/m² is applicable throughout the entire pediatric age range. Cardiac output is the net result of interrelating factors affecting both myocardial systolic

D.S. Wheeler et al. (eds.), *Cardiovascular Pediatric Critical Illness and Injury*,
DOI 10.1007/978-1-84800-923-3_2, © Springer-Verlag London Limited 2009

(heart rate, preload, contractility, and afterload) and diastolic function [13]. Measurement of cardiac output is uncommon in pediatrics because of a variety of factors, including perceived worth and technical difficulty [2]. However, the relevance of cardiac output monitoring for selected patients is underlined by the facts that (1) the heart is one of the most common organs to fail during critical illness [14]; (2) other failing organs and supportive therapies aimed at these organs can impact on cardiac function (e.g., mechanical ventilation) [15]; (3) it cannot be estimated clinically [16]; and (4) low-flow states carry a higher mortality in certain diseases [17]. Traditionally, cardiac output has been difficult to measure in small children. However, a variety of less invasive methods are now available. Nonetheless, the decision to measure cardiac output represents a balance between the risks involved with the technique and the potential benefits gained from the additional hemodynamic information. The latter point requires a thorough understanding of both the modality used and the basic principles of cardiovascular physiology. If both of these criteria are not fulfilled, there is potential for iatrogenic harm to the patient. Cardiac output monitoring is unnecessary in all PICU patients but may be indicated for patients in the following categories: shock states, multiple organ failure, cardiopulmonary interactions during mechanical ventilation, congenital and acquired heart disease, assessment of selected new therapies, and during clinical research that leads to a greater understanding of a disease process [18].

Measurement of Cardiac Output: Indicator Dilution Techniques

Techniques for measurement of cardiac output can be categorized as utilizing indicator dilution, the Fick principle, Doppler ultrasound, impedance, and pulse contour analysis. In addition, these can also be categorized as intermittent versus continuous, invasive versus noninvasive (or minimally invasive), and so forth. When considering which modality to use for a particular patient, it is worth considering the eight desirable monitoring characteristics defined by Shephard: accuracy, reproducibility, rapid response time, operator independence, ease of application, no morbidity, continuous use, and cost effectiveness [19].

Stewart published the first indicator dilution method for measurement of blood volume flow in 1897, based upon Hering's earlier work on blood velocity measurement [20]. Between 1928 and 1932, Hamilton applied this principle to the measurement of cardiac output [21]. A number of dilution techniques are now available; however, all follow the same principle regardless of the indicator used (temperature, dye, charge) [22]. Blood flow can be calculated following a central venous injection of an indicator by measuring the change in indicator concentration over time at a point downstream of the injection. This can be expressed mathematically as

$$\text{cardiac output} = \frac{\text{amount of indicator injected}}{\int_0^\infty \text{conc indicator (t) dt}}$$

The denominator refers to the integral of the indicator concentration with time, in other words, the area under the curve for indicator concentration versus time measured between time of injection and infinity. High-flow situations produce small, peaked curves, whereas low-flow situations produce curves that are larger, less peaked, and with a longer tail (Figure 2.1).

One problem inherent in dilution methods is that of recirculation. Recirculation refers to the phenomenon whereby the indicator within the initial portion of the concentration-time curve traverses the body and arrives back at the measurement site before the terminal portion of the concentration-time curve has passed the measurement site, the net effect being a secondary (and sometimes tertiary) curve superimposed on the primary curve (Figure 2.2). This may occur in states of low cardiac output. Calculation of cardiac output thus requires the *separation* of the primary curve from the composite. Several methods are available for this. The most widely used is that offered by Stewart and Hamilton, which

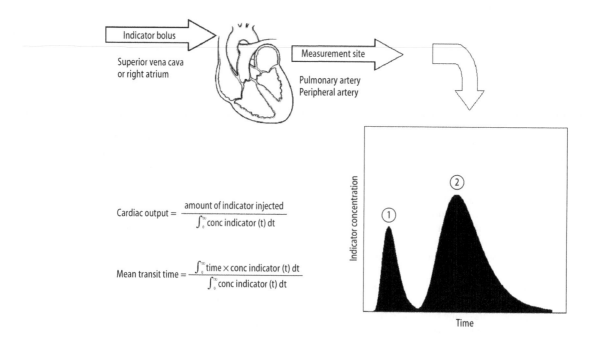

$$\text{Cardiac output} = \frac{\text{amount of indicator injected}}{\int_0^\infty \text{conc indicator (t) dt}}$$

$$\text{Mean transit time} = \frac{\int_0^\infty \text{time} \times \text{conc indicator (t) dt}}{\int_0^\infty \text{conc indicator (t) dt}}$$

FIGURE 2.1. Generalized schema for an indicator dilution method. Curve 1 shows a typical curve with a high cardiac output; curve 2, occurring with a low cardiac output, is larger with an accentuated tail secondary to recirculation.

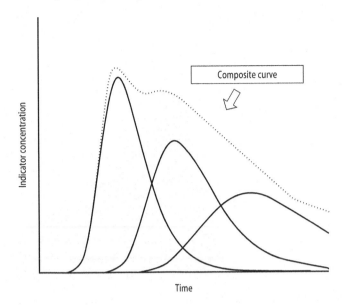

FIGURE 2.2. Early recirculation, as in the case of an intracardiac shunt, may produce a composite curve with several peaks and a prolonged delay phase. Here the composite curve results from superposition of the primary, secondary, and tertiary curves. Note the double peak, which may be seen with an anatomic shunt.

assumes a monoexponential decay of the primary curve after a given time point [23]. Other methods include deconvolution [24] and fitting the declining part of the primary curve with log normal, gamma, and local density random walk probability distributions [25]. A possible source of extreme recirculation pertinent to pediatric practice is that which occurs in the presence of an anatomic shunt, both left to right and right to left, depending on where the indicator is measured. In the presence of a large shunt, it may be impossible to identify the primary curve. Conversely, other authors have suggested methods for quantifying the shunt in relation to the appearance of the second peak [26–32]. Indicator dilution is accurate provided a series of conditions are met. These include rapid and even indicator injection, complete mixing of the indicator and

blood, no loss of indicator between injection and measurement, no anatomic shunt, minimal valve regurgitation, and steady-state flow [33]. Another useful property of indicator dilution curves is that they also allow for calculation of vascular volumes via the mean transit and exponential down slope times (see Figure 2.1) [34]. Various vascular volumes have been used as measures of preload (see Transpulmonary Thermodilution, later). Indeed, other calculations relating to tissue volumes and liver function are also possible, depending on the indicator used.

The hemodynamic calculations discussed in this chapter are summarized in Table 2.1.

Pulmonary Thermodilution

Pulmonary thermodilution utilizes temperature as the indicator and involves injection of a cooled solution into the right atrium (typically normal saline or 5% dextrose), with temperature change sensed by thermistors at the injection site and in the pulmonary artery. This technique was first used in dogs by Fegler in 1954 [35] and subsequently in humans by Branthwaite and Bradley in 1968 [36]; it was introduced clinically with the development of the Swan-Ganz, or pulmonary artery, catheter in 1970 [37]. Over the next 30 years this became the most widely used method for measurement of cardiac output in adults, although use in children remained limited, mainly because of technical constraints [18,38–41]. Over the past 10 years the use of the pulmonary artery catheter has declined, possibly as a consequence of other, less-invasive methods becoming available, lack of benefit (and perhaps even harm) from several large studies, and also several authors questioning the value of cardiac output measurement, particularly via this technique [42–48]. This last point is supported by two large, trans-Atlantic surveys that showed that many intensive care unit clinicians lack the rudimentary skills to perform safe pulmonary artery catheter insertion and interpretation of readings [49,50].

The Swan-Ganz catheter is typically inserted percutaneously through a sheath introducer (of a size larger than the catheter itself, e.g., 8.5 French introducer for a 7 French catheter) using the Seldinger technique. The left subclavian or right internal jugular route is the preferred access point to encourage proper placement,

TABLE 2.1. Summary of hemodynamic variables.

Parameter	Formula	Normal range	Units
Cardiac index	$CI = CO/\text{body surface area}$	3.5–5.5	$L/min/m^2$
Stroke index	$SI = CI/\text{heart rate}$	30–60	mL/m^2
Arterial oxygen content	$CaO_2 = (1.34 \times Hg \times SaO_2) + (PaO_2 \times 0.003)$		mL/L
Oxygen delivery	$DO_2 = CI \times CaO_2$	570–670	$mL/min/m^2$
Fick principle	$CI = VO_2/(CaO_2 - CvO_2)$	160–180 (infant VO_2)	$mL/min/m^2$
		100–130 (child VO_2)	$mL/min/m^2$
Mixed venous oxygen saturation		65%–75%	
Oxygen extraction ratio*	$OER = (SaO_2 - SvO_2)/SaO_2$	0.24–0.28	
Oxygen excess factor*	$\Omega = SaO_2/(SaO_2 - SvO_2)$	3.6–4.2	
Systemic vascular resistance index	$SVRI = 79.9 \times (MAP - CVP)/CI$	800–1,600	$dyn\text{-}sec/cm^5/m^2$
Pulmonary vascular resistance index	$PVRI = 79.9 \times (MPAP - LAP)/CI$	80–240	$dyn\text{-}sec/cm^5/m^2$
Left ventricular stroke work index	$LVSWI = SI \times MAP \times 0.0136$	50–62 (adult)	$g\text{-}m/m^2$

Note: CO, cardiac output; CI, cardiac index; CVP, central venous pressure (mm Hg); CaO_2, arterial oxygen content; CvO_2, mixed venous oxygen content; DO_2, oxygen delivery; Hgb, hemoglobin concentration (g/L); LVSWI, left ventricular stroke work index; MAP, mean systemic arterial pressure (mm Hg); MPAP, mean pulmonary arterial pressure; LAP, left atrial pressure; OER, oxygen extraction ratio; PaO_2, partial pressure of dissolved oxygen; SaO_2, arterial oxygen saturation; SvO_2, mixed venous oxygen saturation; SI, stroke index; SVRI, systemic vascular resistance index; PVRI, pulmonary vascular resistance index; VO_2, oxygen consumption; Ω, oxygen excess factor.
*The equations given for OER and Ω are only valid if the contribution from dissolved oxygen is minimal. If this is not the case, oxygen content (CaO_2, CvO_2) must be substituted for saturation (SaO_2, SvO_2).
Source: Compiled from data in Perloff [264] and Shann [265].

although any of the major upper limb veins are appropriate. The catheter is advanced until the tip lies within a branch pulmonary artery in a position suitable for measuring pulmonary artery occlusion pressure (PAOP) or pulmonary wedge pressure (PWP) (see later). A variety of sizes are available, including 7 French (suitable for use in older children), 5 French (suitable for use in children 10–18 kg), and 3 French (suitable for use in children less than 10 kg) [51]. The larger catheters are typically four or five channel, including (1) a proximal lumen that sits in the right atrium for measurement of right atrial pressure and injection of the indicator, (2) a thermistor channel for measuring temperature of the injectate and blood within the pulmonary artery following injection, (3) an inflatable balloon to allow acquisition of occlusion pressure, (4) a distal lumen for measurement of pulmonary artery and occlusion pressures and mixed venous blood sampling, and (5) a fiberoptic line for continuous measurement of mixed venous oxygen saturation (SvO_2). Smaller catheters may contain fewer channels and are typically inserted under direct vision during cardiac surgery. Percutaneous insertion and placement is difficult in small children and carries the risk of several potential complications, including pneumothorax, hemothorax, catheter malposition, catheter knotting, ventricular arrhythmias, balloon rupture, embolization, pulmonary artery occlusion, pulmonary infarction, and sepsis [53–55]. Interestingly, several studies have suggested that the subclavian route may be associated with a lower complication rate [55,56].

Because of its long history of clinical use, pulmonary thermodilution is often regarded as the benchmark against which newer modalities are tested. However, it must be stressed that pulmonary thermodilution is not a gold standard and has many potential sources of inaccuracy [33,57–59]. These include technical errors, variation in blood temperature within the pulmonary artery that is unrelated to indicator injection, and fluctuations in cardiac output. Perhaps the most common source of fluctuation in cardiac output pertinent to the PICU is that seen with mechanical ventilation. Positive pressure ventilation causes a transient drop in venous return and hence preload to the right ventricle, which produces a transient fall in right heart stroke volume. Because the time between injection and temperature sensing in the pulmonary artery is very short, the apparent cardiac output may vary, depending on when the measurement is taken in relation to the ventilatory cycle. To account for this, three to four measurements should be taken at systematic intervals throughout the ventilatory cycle and then averaged; this will produce an estimate within ±10% of the true cardiac output in adults (provided all other sources of accuracy are dealt with) [60]. Stetz et al. have concluded that there must be a minimal change of 12%–15% between serial averaged thermodilution measurements to represent a true change in cardiac output [61]. It is possible that this figure may be higher in children, however, as thermodilution is thought to be less accurate and more variable [62]. Over the last decade, intermittent bolus thermodilution has been incorporated into a semicontinuous mode using a thermal filament [63]. Although commercially available devices perform comparatively in adults [64] with reasonable accuracy at high- and low-flow states [65], they have yet to be evaluated in children.

In addition to measuring cardiac output, the pulmonary artery catheter can provide a measure of right ventricular function (ejection fraction), PAOP, pulmonary and right atrial pressures, and SvO_2 (via either direct intermittent measurement or continuous oximetry). Right ventricular ejection fraction requires a thermistor with a rapid response time [66]. This reveals a characteristic series of temperature plateaus in the pulmonary artery after indicator

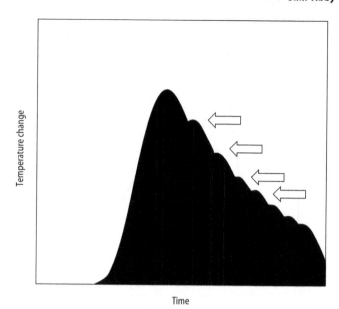

FIGURE 2.3. Temperature plateaus (arrows) seen with a rapid response thermistor in the pulmonary artery. Plateaus reflect intraventricular temperature during the previous heartbeat. From these, right ventricular end diastolic volume and ejection fraction can be calculated.

injection into the right ventricle during diastole (Figure 2.3). These plateaus reflect intraventricular temperature during the previous heartbeat and can be used to calculate ejection fraction via an algorithm and, hence, end diastolic volume (because stroke volume is known from the thermodilution measurement and end diastolic volume = stroke volume/ejection fraction).

Pulmonary Artery Occlusion Pressure

When the balloon near the tip of the pulmonary artery catheter is inflated so as to occlude upstream flow, a continuous column of nonflowing blood is then present between the catheter tip and the point of pulmonary venous convergence just behind the left atrium (referred to as the *J-1 point*) [37,67]. This is known as the *occlusion pressure* or *wedge pressure* and is thought to approximate left atrial pressure. Occlusion pressure is sometimes erroneously referred to as *pulmonary capillary pressure*; however, the latter entity, as the name suggests, refers to pressure within the pulmonary capillaries, which will be greater than the venous pressure by an amount influenced by both flow and pulmonary venous resistance (pulmonary vascular resistance has both an arterial and a venous component, which can be differentiated by a logarithmic plot of the pulmonary artery pressure decay after balloon occlusion) [68,69]. Occlusion pressure is traditionally measured at end expiration. This is important because occlusion pressure will vary throughout the respiratory cycle because of the influence of alveolar pressure. In situations where alveolar pressure greatly exceeds occlusion pressure, pulmonary vasculature distal to the catheter tip may collapse, and the pressure reading will reflect alveolar pressure rather than left atrial pressure. This may occur in West zones 1 and 2 of the lung or in situations where high positive end-expiratory pressure (PEEP) is used during mechanical ventilation [67]. This situation should be readily discernible from inspection of the pressure trace during occlusion, as large pressure swings will be seen in synchrony with the mechanical ventilator. Occlusion pressure can be used in the calculation of pulmonary vascular resistance and has been suggested as a measure of both left ventricular preload and performance. Unfortunately, this is often not the case in clinical practice for a variety of factors, including technical problems, lack of user understanding, and difficulties in extrapolating a volume from a pressure reading [70,71].

Transpulmonary Thermodilution

The principle of transpulmonary thermodilution is similar to that of pulmonary thermodilution; however, here the temperature change is measured in a large artery, typically the femoral artery. Thus the journey from injection to measurement traverses the right atrium, right ventricle, pulmonary vascular bed, left atrium, left ventricle, and aorta [72]. At first glance this appears to violate one of the fundamental requirements of indicator measurement—no loss of indicator between injection and measurement. In fact, it has been shown that, provided the injectate is cooled sufficiently (to less than 10°C), the loss of heat is small and relatively constant and does not affect the accuracy of cardiac output measurement [73–76]. In addition, the loss of heat has been utilized to calculate extravascular lung water, which may be a marker of disease severity in certain states (e.g., acute respiratory distress syndrome) [77,78]. Transpulmonary thermodilution via a commercial system utilizes the theory of Newman to calculate a series of vascular volumes via the mean transit and exponential downslope times of the primary thermodilution curve [79]. These include intrathoracic blood volume and global end diastolic volume, which may be markers of preload, and cardiac function index (stroke volume divided by the global end diastolic volume in the heart), which may provide a measure of contractility. To date little work has been performed in pediatrics validating the usefulness of these parameters, although preliminary adult and animal work is encouraging [71,80–82].

Transpulmonary thermodilution offers two main advantages over pulmonary thermodilution: (1) the need to access the pulmonary artery is obviated (all that is required is a central venous and arterial catheters) and (2) a commercially available device (PiCCO™, Pulsion Medical Systems, Munich, Germany) combines this modality with pulse contour analysis (calibration occurs via thermodilution), thereby representing an application of this technique to the provision of continuous cardiac output.

Dye Dilution

Several dyes have been utilized as the indicator; however, indocyanine green is the most common. Injection is via a central vein, with measurement from a systemic artery traditionally utilizing a photometric technique. Two main limitations with this method have restricted its clinical application at the bedside. First, the concentration-time curve is measured using a densitometer, which requires calibration with samples of the patient's blood containing known concentrations of the dye—this can be time consuming. Second, measurement typically occurs extracorporeally, meaning that further blood must be withdrawn with each measurement. These two limitations have largely been overcome through the use of fiberoptic sensors utilizing the technique of pulse dye densitometry, a principle similar to pulse oximetry. Unfortunately, the accuracy of this technique is questionable at low cardiac output and also within certain patients [83,84]. Finally, because indocyanine green is removed by the liver, recirculation is guaranteed, which restricts the time between successive measurements; obviously, this is exacerbated in the face of significant hepatic impairment. For these reasons, use of dye dilution has been restricted chiefly to benchmarking newer modalities of cardiac output measurement.

Lithium Dilution

Use of lithium dilution is a relatively recent innovation with ionic concentration as the indicator [85,86]. The ion used is lithium (injected as lithium chloride). Measurement occurs via a blood pump attached to the patient's arterial line, which transports the blood through a flow-through cell containing a lithium-selective electrode. The electrode contains a membrane that is selectively permeable to lithium ions, with change in voltage across the membrane being related to change in lithium ion concentration via the Nernst equation. Limitations are similar to those with dye dilution in that blood sampling is required with every measurement and rapid repeated measurements are not possible (however, the time between injections is much less than that for the dye method). It is also thought that several drugs may interfere with readings, on the basis of their charge. Although this has proven accurate in pediatric patients [87], it is not currently licensed for patients weighing less than 40 kg.

The Fick Principle

Originally described in 1870, the Fick principle calculates flow by measuring the amount of indicator added (or removed) from a system divided by the change in indicator concentration upstream and downstream of where the indicator is added (or removed) (Figure 2.4) [88]. Calculation of systemic cardiac output may utilize one of two indicators: either O_2 (systemic oxygen consumption) or CO_2 (systemic carbon dioxide production), with upstream and downstream representing the systemic arterial and mixed venous sites, respectively. When these variables are measured directly, this is known as the direct Fick technique. Although accurate, the Fick principle has several sources of error and limitations, which are elaborated later. The following discussion refers primarily to the Fick calculation utilizing oxygen consumption rather than carbon dioxide production.

Oxygen Consumption Measurement

Oxygen consumption measurement relies on the assumption that oxygen consumption by the body is in equilibrium with oxygen uptake in the lung [89]. Traditionally, the Douglas bag or spirome-

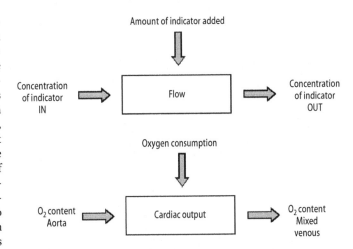

FIGURE 2.4. Generalized representation of the Fick principle. It is assumed that the system is in steady state. Flow = amount of indicator added/change in indicator concentration; in the case of cardiac output, this equation becomes Cardiac output = oxygen consumption/change in oxygen content between aorta and mixed venous blood.

try has been used to measure oxygen uptake; however, both are impractical in the PICU environment. Now, portable metabolic monitors exist that utilize a gas dilution principle to measure flow, a fast-response paramagnetic differential O_2 sensor to measure change in oxygen concentration, and an infrared CO_2 sensor [90,91]. If flow and differential concentrations are known, content can be calculated via the Haldane transformation. Newer metabolic monitors are accurate within the pediatric range of oxygen consumption, CO_2 production, and gas flow, provided four conditions are met [91–94]:

1. There must be no loss of expired gas. This means that the technique is invalid in the face of a pneumothorax with a chest drain or if air leak occurs around the tracheal tube [95]. Several authors have suggested that the error may be acceptable in the absence of an audible leak [96], although this is controversial [97]. Others have claimed that the error may be acceptable if the measured leak is less than 5% of expiratory tidal volume. However, significant air leak is common [98] and may be difficult to quantify in an infant, given the inaccuracy of tidal volume measurement in most mechanical ventilators [99]. Thus, a cuffed tracheal tube is recommended.

2. The partial pressure of water vapor within the system must be carefully controlled. Newer metabolic monitors use specialized tubing (e.g., Nafion) that equalizes the water vapor concentration of gas inside and outside the machine.

3. Conversion of gas volumes to standard conditions. Again, this occurs in all modern monitors.

4. Limitation of the fraction of inspired oxygen. When the FiO_2 is very high, for example, in the face of significant lung disease, the difference between the fraction of inspired and expired oxygen may be very small. This creates an error in the denominator of the Haldane algorithm. Ideally the FiO_2 should be less than 0.60; at levels greater than 0.85, the error is likely to be large [100,101].

A final source of error relates to oxygen consumption by the lung itself, which may occur with significant lung pathology. The numerator in the Fick equation is *systemic* oxygen consumption; however, the metabolic monitor measures *total* oxygen consumption, that is, consumption by both the body and the lungs. In health, the majority of the pulmonary oxygen consumption occurs via the bronchial vessels, which can be regarded as being of systemic origin. However, in disease states, significant pulmonary oxygen consumption can occur within the lung from the blood supplied by the pulmonary (right-sided) circulation as well. This means that oxygen consumption as measured by the metabolic monitor will overestimate systemic oxygen consumption and hence cardiac output. An animal model using pneumococcal pneumonia has estimated this error to be of the order of 13%–15% [102]. A similar finding has been demonstrated in ventilated premature neonates at risk for chronic lung disease [103]; however, this is not seen in adults with pneumonia [104].

Arterial and Mixed Venous Oxygen Content

Oxygen content is a function of hemoglobin and dissolved oxygen and is calculated via the formula:

$$\text{O}_2 \text{ content (mL O}_2 \text{ per L blood)} = \frac{[1.34 \times \text{Hg (g/L)} \times \%\text{saturation}/100]}{+ [\text{PaO}_2 \text{ (mmHg)} \times 0.003]}$$

Normally, the contribution from dissolved O_2 is minimal and can be ignored without producing significant error. However, this is not

the case when the PaO_2 is very high (e.g., a patient without significant lung disease who is receiving an FiO_2 >0.30). Mixed venous sampling requires accessing the pulmonary artery, as blood taken from within the right atrium may inadvertently sample desaturated coronary sinus blood. Finally, oxygen saturation must be measured via a co-oximeter and not calculated from the blood gas PO_2 value.

Presence of Anatomic Shunt

The Fick equation can potentially allow for cardiac output estimation in the setting of an anatomic shunt [105]. This may be unrealistic at the bedside, however, for two reasons: shunting is often bi-directional, and calculation may require blood sampling pre- and post-shunt. To understand these concepts, it is necessary to apply the Fick equation to both the systemic (Qs) and pulmonary (Qp) blood flows. The formulas are the following:

$$Q_S = \frac{VO_2}{C_{aorta} - C_{mixed\ venous}} \qquad Q_P = \frac{VO_2}{C_{pulm\ vein} - C_{pulm\ artery}}$$

where C refers to the oxygen content in the respective sites. Thus, in the absence of anatomic shunt, Qs = Qp. This means that the formulas are essentially interchangeable, as mixed venous blood is sampled from the pulmonary artery, and oxygen content in the pulmonary veins and systemic arteries are the same (ignoring the small right-to-left shunt that occurs from bronchial venous and thebesian drainage). However, in the setting of left-to-right shunt (e.g., with a large ventricular septal defect), blood in the pulmonary artery is highly saturated; thus, mixed venous sampling must occur proximal to the site of mixing. Options include right atrial sampling or a weighted average of superior and inferior vena caval blood (weighting to reflect the assumed proportion of total venous return from each caval vessel, which is age dependent) [106]. In reality, both methods may be inaccurate. Conversely in the setting of a right-to-left shunt, systemic arterial blood is less saturated than pulmonary venous, and so Qp can only be calculated if pulmonary venous blood is sampled. Finally, these two formulas can be combined to provide a ratio of pulmonary to systemic blood flow:

$$Q_P : Q_S = \frac{C_{aorta} - C_{mixed\ venous}}{C_{pulm\ vein} - C_{pulm\ artery}}$$

Indirect Fick Principle

If the Fick principle is applied to CO_2 production, it may be possible to estimate the Fick parameters indirectly from the inspired and expired gases using a CO_2 rebreathing technique, whereby the patient rebreathes exhaled CO_2 for a short period of time while mechanically ventilated [107,108]. Here the Fick equation relates to pulmonary capillary blood flow (in essence, effective or nonshunt blood flow) rather than total pulmonary blow. By measuring change in the parameters before and at the end of the CO_2 rebreathing period, pulmonary capillary blood flow is calculated from the following formula:

$$Q_{pcbf} = \frac{\Delta VCO_2}{\Delta C_{mixed\ venous} - \Delta C_{pulmonary\ end\ capillary}}$$

In this equation, (1) ΔVCO_2 is measured; (2) it is assumed that a brief rebreathing period does not change mixed venous CO_2, hence

ΔVCO_2 is zero; and (3) $\Delta C_{pulmonary\ end\ capillary}$ is estimated from alveolar CO_2 content, which is in turn estimated from end-tidal PCO_2 via a correction factor. Intrapulmonary shunt flow is calculated from Nunn's iso-shunt diagrams [109] and added to pulmonary capillary blood flow, giving total pulmonary blood flow. As can be seen, this technique relies on a series of assumptions, which may limit its validity in the PICU setting [110–112].

Doppler Ultrasound

In 1961, Franklin applied the Doppler principle to measurement of blood flow [113]. The principle states that the frequency shift of reflected ultrasound will be proportional to the velocity of the reflecting blood cells, and is related by the following formula:

$$Blood\ velocity = \frac{\Delta frequency \times c}{2 \times f_t \times \cos \theta}$$

where $\Delta frequency$ is the frequency shift between transmitted and reflected signal, c is the sound velocity in blood, f_t is the transmitting frequency, and θ is the angle of insonation (i.e., between the beam and blood flow). Doppler ultrasound signals may be continuous or pulsed. Continuous signals react to all flow within their path so that the point at which blood velocity is measured is unknown; this is known as *range ambiguity*. Pulsed signals allow for adjustment of the sampling depth and volume but may be prone to errors in calculation of velocity because of the relationship between the frequency (and hence wavelength) of the transmitted signal and the velocity being measured (this phenomenon is called *aliasing*). In essence, the chosen frequency represents a trade-off between velocity measurement and image resolution [114].

Doppler ultrasound can be applied to any pulsatile blood vessel, although measurement of cardiac output is typically performed in the aorta via either the transthoracic or the transesophageal approach (the latter allowing for continuous measurement) [115]. Spectral representation of the velocity-time signal characteristically shows a triangular shape from which a variety of flow-related variables can be derived (Figure 2.5) [116,117]. The integral of velocity-time (area under the triangle) represents stroke distance, the distance that a column of blood will travel along the aorta in one cardiac cycle. Stroke distance is not stroke volume; conversion of the former to the latter requires multiplication by left heart outflow area. This can be achieved in two ways—either echocardiography [118] or a nomogram [117,119,120]. Both methods carry advantages and disadvantages.

Echocardiography, either two dimensional or M mode, can be used to calculate outflow tract area at a variety of sites, including aortic valve annulus, aortic root, and ascending aorta. Of these, measurement at the valve annulus in systole via two-dimensional mode appears the most accurate, producing a variation coefficient of approximately 6% [121,122]. Echocardiography in children can often be performed transthoracically, which is obviously less invasive than via the transesophageal route. In addition to providing a means of acquiring cardiac output, echocardiography, in the hands of a skilled operator, also supplies a vast amount of functional and morphologic information, including indices of diastolic dysfunction, regional wall abnormalities, valve regurgitation, pericardial effusion, chamber dilatation, and cardiac chamber interdependence. The main disadvantage of echocardiography is the requirement for significant user expertise.

Conversely, Doppler ultrasound requires little in the way of user training and thus can be performed by any trained intensive care

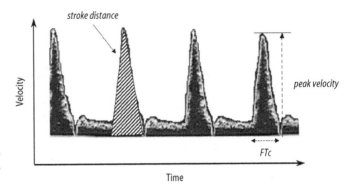

Hemodynamic state	Effect on doppler parameter	
↓ contractility	↓↑ FTc +/–	↓ peak velocity ++
↑ afterload	↓ FTc ++	↓ peak velocity +
hypovolemia	↓ FTc ++	↓ peak velocity +/–

FIGURE 2.5. Spectral representation of a Doppler velocity-time signal, showing effects of differing hemodynamic states. The area under the triangular waveform is stroke distance, which represents the distance a column of blood will travel down the descending aorta in one cardiac cycle. Peak velocity is affected predominantly by changes in contractility and to a lesser extent by changes in preload and afterload. Corrected flow time (FTc) represents the systolic time corrected to a heart rate of 60 beats per minute. This parameter may be reduced in the face of diminished preload (e.g., hypovolemia) or an increased afterload. Both states can also decrease the peak velocity; they may be differentiated, however, on the basis of response to a fluid challenge.

unit practitioner [123]. Here, left heart outflow area is estimated via a nomogram. Not surprisingly, the assumptions inherent in the nomogram produce an error in cardiac output unique to each patient, although changes in cardiac output are tracked accurately [119,124]. Of the two modes, transesophageal Doppler has greater intra- and interuser agreement [125] because the aorta lies approximately parallel to the esophagus, allowing the angle of insonation to be fixed at 45° and adjusted for. Unfortunately, probe fixation is a significant problem in pediatrics; both probe rotation and vertical movement can occur, resulting in signal alteration. For this reason, this modality cannot be considered as truly continuous. Transthoracic Doppler allows both the aortic and pulmonary outflows to be estimated via separate nomograms; however, the angle of insonation is unknown, and the coefficient of variation is generally higher than that for transoesophageal Doppler [125]. More recently, a Doppler-based technique known as *surface integration of velocity vectors*, has been reported in animals with encouraging results [126]. This technique utilizes multiplanar Doppler sampling, which is reconstructed to a three-dimensional flow field [127]. Measurements take between 2 and 8 minutes to perform.

Impedance/Conductance Methods

Impedance is the opposition to the flow of an alternating current and can be defined using Ohm's law in the same manner as resistance for direct current:

$$Impedance\ (Z) = \frac{potential\ difference\ (V)}{alternating\ current\ (I)}$$

$$Resistnace\ (R) = \frac{potential\ difference\ (V)}{direct\ current\ (I)}$$

Admittance is the reciprocal of impedance; conductance is the reciprocal of resistance. Although described in relation to the cardiac cycle in 1953 [128]. In 1966, Kubicek et al. were the first to apply this principle to the measurement of cardiac output [129]. Here, the chest is regarded as a conductor whose impedance is altered by the changes in blood volume and velocity that occur with each heartbeat; from this, stroke volume is calculated. Impedance is measured via a series of voltage-sensing and current-transmitting electrodes. Alternating rather than direct current is used to achieve charge balancing and thus avoid any residual polarization at the interface between electrode and tissue, which would result in an increase in measured impedance [130]. The site of electrode placement defines the type of impedance measurement, from the noninvasive (thoracic bioimpedance, where electrodes are placed on the chest) to the highly invasive (intracardiac requiring electrode placement within the left ventricle).

Thoracic Impedance

A series of electrodes are placed at fixed intervals around the chest wall, and stroke volume is calculated with the following formula:

$$\text{stroke volume} = \frac{L^3 \times VET \times dZ/dt_{max}}{4.25 \times Z_0}$$

where L is thoracic segment length, VET is ventricular ejection time, dZ/dt_{max} is maximum rate of impedance change, and Zo is transthoracic baseline impedance. It is now known that the volume change sensed by thoracic bioimpedance is almost exclusively extracardiac, as the myocardium tends to shield the electrodes from the impedance changes occurring within the ventricle. Thus, the change in impedance signal, and hence stroke volume estimation, comes predominantly from blood volume alterations within the systemic and pulmonary vessels inside the chest [131,132]. Thoracic bioimpedance is not widely used in the clinical setting; indeed, several authors have expressed concern at the accuracy of this method in the intensive care unit environment, particularly at states of low cardiac output, hypotension, and chest wall edema [133–136].

Intracardiac Impedance

Stroke volume is measured from catheters placed directly into the left ventricle. Accuracy is increased by utilizing multipolar catheters, which partition the ventricle into a series of cylindrical segments [137]. Several studies have reported a small but consistent underestimation of stroke volume, perhaps because of simultaneous conductance into surrounding tissues (atria, myocardium); this may be improved via a correction factor [138–140]. The invasiveness of this technique means that use in the intensive care unit is effectively impossible, apart from when catheters are placed during cardiac surgery. Nonetheless, this technique can also provide valuable information concerning myocardial systolic function via either end systolic elastance calculation or preload recruitable stroke work [141–144]. The latter technique involves plotting the pressure–volume curves after manipulation of preload (typically reducing preload via progressive caval snaring). The area within the pressure–volume loop represents stroke work; when this is plotted against end diastolic volume, the slope of this relationship is termed *preload recruitable stroke work* and is a load-independent measure of contractility [143]. These techniques have provided insight into previously unsuspected degrees of cardiac

dysfunction after relatively short periods on cardiopulmonary bypass [145]. Recently, a less invasive modification of this technique, known as *transcardiac conductance*, has been described [146]. Here, the current transmitting electrodes are placed in the superior vena cava just above the right atrium and in an epithoracic position just lateral to the xyphisternal joint. Voltage sensing electrodes are placed epithoracically, in the position of standard electrocardiographic electrodes. A correction factor is applied to account for parallel conductance outside the heart. Several methodologic problems exist, such as interindividual and cardiac phase variabilities, along with the need to calibrate absolute stroke volume with another invasive method; however, this may be a promising new technique. To date this method has not been evaluated in children.

Arterial Pulse Contour Analysis

A century ago, Erlanger and Hooker suggested a relationship between stroke volume and arterial pulse contour [147]. The advent of fast computer microprocessors has meant that a variety of pulse contour systems are now commercially available that estimate beat-to-beat changes in stroke volume. Interestingly, all utilize different techniques for pulse contour analysis; this is in part because of differing theories concerning both the relationship between flow and pressure within the arterial system and the mechanism of pulse wave transmission along the arterial tree [1,148–150]. In addition, the majority of commercial systems estimate only beat-to-beat *change* in cardiac output, thus requiring initial calibration via an alternative method of cardiac output measurement.

An appreciation of several basic concepts and terminology is a prerequisite for understanding pulse contour analysis—in essence, how a volume change supplied from the left ventricle translates into a pressure change within the arterial system [1]. Both flow and pressure are primarily pulsatile events in the proximal arterial system and do not achieve nonpulsatile or mean values until the level of the arterioles. Resistance to flow occurs in both the large and small arteries; in the vessels receiving pulsatile flow, this is called *impedance*; for those receiving nonpulsatile flow, this is designated as *resistance* (also known as *systemic peripheral resistance*). The largest pressure drop occurs across the arterioles. In addition, arteries contain variable amounts of elastic tissue; in the largest vessels, such as the aorta, this means that they can expand to store volume (compliance) and contract in relation to the downstream load (elastic recoil). The relationship between stress (force applied to the arterial wall) and strain (reaction of the arterial wall to the stress applied) has traditionally been represented using a proportionality constant known as *Young's modulus of elasticity*. This in turn affects wave velocity via the following formula:

$$\text{wave velocity} = \sqrt{\frac{E \times h}{2 \times \rho \times r}}$$

where E is Young's modulus, h is vessel wall thickness, ρ is fluid density, and r is radius. The phenomena of compliance and elastic recoil within the aorta partially explain the continuation of blood flow within small arteries after systole has terminated. In the aorta, compliance is nonlinear (as is impedance), meaning that the pressure change for a given volume ejected by the heart will vary according to both the diastolic arterial pressure (and hence peripheral resistance) and stroke volume. This relationship, as well as the pressure wave reflected from the periphery back to the aorta, influences the shape of the arterial waveform (Figure 2.6) [151]. Postmortem studies have shown that aortic compliance shows considerable interpatient variation [152,153]. Although the shape of the aortic cross-sectional area versus pressure curve is relatively constant, it demonstrates differing intercepts between individuals, meaning that the error in estimating cross-sectional area (and hence compliance) can be as high as 30% at maximal pressures (Figure 2.7) [153–155]. Furthermore, compliance is also affected by a variety of factors, including age, disease, and catecholamines. Finally, pressure waves are also influenced by wave reflection back from the periphery to the proximal arteries.

A variety of methods for continuous pulse contour analyses exist, all utilizing a combination of calculations for aortic impedance, aortic compliance, total or systemic peripheral resistance, pressure wave reflection, and transfer function between large and small arteries (although not all components are included in every method) [1,148–150,155–158]. Perhaps the best known of these is the modified Windkessel approach [159,160]. This was first described by Otto Frank in 1899, who adopted the term *Windkessel* (German for *wind kettle*) from Hales' 18th century description of the elastic arteries as being like a water pump [161]. The modified Windkessel approach describes the pressure response of the arterial system to an input of flow (stroke volume) as being a function of characteristic impedance of the proximal aorta, aortic compliance, and total systemic peripheral resistance; the latter two variables are described in parallel [159,160]. The accuracy of this approach may be improved by either ultrasonic measurement of aortic cross sectional area, which allows for a recalibration of the aortic compliance relationship for the individual patient (Modelflow™) [155], or a more sophisticated analysis of the pressure waveform taking into account the shape as well as the area of the

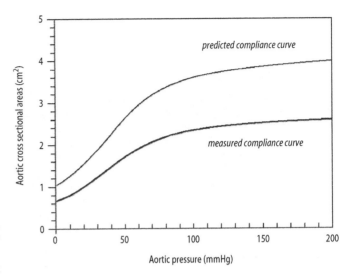

Figure 2.7. *Typical* aortic compliance has been estimated in vitro from cadaveric studies, as following an arctangent relationship [152,153]. In vivo, the shape of the aortic cross-sectional area versus arterial pressure relationship (similar to compliance vs. pressure) is relatively constant; however, the intercept may vary among patients. The diagram shows this relationship in a 59-year-old patient (adapted from [155]), highlighting how aortic compliance may be overestimated using the in vitro formula.

pressure wave (PiCCO™) [158]. An alternative method (LiDCO™-plus) involves arterial pulse power analysis, and, because it does not rely on waveform morphology, it is not strictly speaking a pulse contour method [148]. To date, only preliminary evaluations of beat-to-beat analysis have appeared in the pediatric literature [162,163].

Other Methods

Several other methods exist for measurement of cardiac output. These include radionuclide techniques [164], magnetic resonance imaging [165,166], and transluminal Doppler flow probes; all are as yet impractical for intensive care unit use.

Measuring the Adequacy of Flow

Shock occurs when oxygen consumption is inadequate to meet the metabolic needs of the body [167]. This may occur for a variety of reasons, including inadequate global oxygen delivery, inadequate local oxygen delivery, excessive oxygen consumption, and inability of cells to consume oxygen (e.g., mitochondrial dysfunction) [167,168]. The three components of oxygen delivery are cardiac output, hemoglobin concentration, and hemoglobin oxygen saturation [168], that is, oxygen delivery (DO_2) is equal to cardiac output (CO) × arterial oxygen content (CaO_2):

$$DO_2 = CO \times CaO_2$$
$$CO = HR \times SV$$
$$CaO_2 = [1.34 \times Hg\ (g/L) \times \%saturation/100] + (0.003 \times PaO_2)$$
$$DO2 = HR \times SV\ [1.34 \times Hg\ (g/L) \times \%saturation/100 + 0.003 \times PaO_2]$$

For many reasons, it is more important to decide whether flow is adequate to allow for required oxygen consumption, on both a global and a regional basis, than to merely derive an absolute value

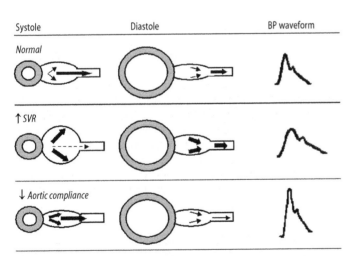

Figure 2.6. Pulse pressure diagram. A simplified, two-element Windkessel approach, utilizing aortic compliance and systemic vascular (peripheral) resistance, illustrates influences on the blood pressure waveform. The effects of aortic impedance and wave reflection are ignored. In the top diagram, the normal situation is shown, whereby a proportion of flow and pressure is channeled into the compliant aorta during systole. During diastole, the elastic recoil of the aorta causes a pressure and flow pulse to be transmitted into the distal arterial system. When systemic vascular resistance is increased (middle), more pressure and flow are transmitted to the aorta during systole, producing a greater flow and pressure in diastole. The net result is a narrower pulse pressure (lower systolic, higher diastolic). When aortic compliance is reduced (lower diagram), flow and pressure are greater in the distal arterial tree during systole, producing a characteristic spiky waveform.

for flow [2]. Two global markers of adequacy are primarily used: mixed venous oxygen saturation (SvO_2) and whole blood lactate.

Mixed Venous Oxygen Saturation

Mixed venous blood refers to the sum total of systemic venous return, that is, that from the upper and lower body and the heart itself, which drain into the superior and inferior vena cavae and the coronary sinus, respectively. Provided there is no anatomic shunt, complete mixing occurs downstream of the right atrium, in either the right ventricle or pulmonary artery; it is customary to use the latter site for mixed venous sampling [169,170]. When the oxygen delivery/consumption balance becomes perturbed, various compensatory mechanisms are triggered; one of these is an increase in oxygen extraction, resulting in a fall in mixed venous oxygen saturation. This is best understood by referring back to the Fick equation:

$$Cardiac\ output = \frac{VO_2}{C_{aorta} - C_{mixed\ venous}}$$
$$\approx \frac{VO_2}{O_2\ sat_{aorta} - O_2\ sat_{mixed\ venous}}$$

Thus, when cardiac output falls or oxygen consumption rises (without a concomitant equivalent rise in cardiac output), the only way to balance this equation is for the denominator to increase. This can only be achieved by a fall in mixed venous oxygen saturation (i.e., an increase in oxygen extraction), as there is no mechanism for increasing arterial oxygen saturation acutely. It is important to appreciate that the relationship between cardiac output and mixed venous oxygen saturation is thus not linear and will vary according to the initial arterial oxygen saturation, oxygen consumption, and hemoglobin concentration (Figure 2.8).

The normal value for mixed venous oxygen saturation is approximately 73% (range 65%–75%) [169–172]. As the oxygen delivery/supply ratio becomes perturbed, compensatory oxygen extraction will occur, and the mixed venous saturation will decrease. If this is inadequate, anaerobic metabolism will commence, generating a subsequent lactic acidosis [168,173]. The exact point at which oxygen extraction becomes inadequate or exhausted varies from patient to patient and is affected by chronicity. For example, in the acute setting, lactic acidosis may occur when the mixed venous saturation falls below 50%; however, patients with long-standing hypoxia (e.g., congenital cyanotic cardiac disease) or a chronically failing myocardium (e.g., cardiomyopathy) may exhibit mixed venous saturations below 50% in the face of normal blood lactate levels [174]. Finally, it is important to appreciate that tissue hypoxia is not the only source of a raised blood lactate (see next section, Blood Lactate).

Hypoxia is common in pediatric practice (e.g., in the setting of congenital heart disease) and may affect the mixed venous saturation [175]. Thus, it may be preferable to monitor either the arteriovenous oxygen saturation difference or the oxygen extraction ratio. The latter is given by the following:

$$Oxygen\ extraction\ ratio = (SaO_2 - SvO_2)/SaO_2$$

Normal values are between 0.24 and 0.28 [2]. This equation is only valid if the contribution from dissolved oxygen is minimal; if no, then saturation should be substituted by content [105]. Other authors have suggested using the inverse of the oxygen extraction ratio; this is known as the *oxygen excess factor*, or omega (Ω) [176]:

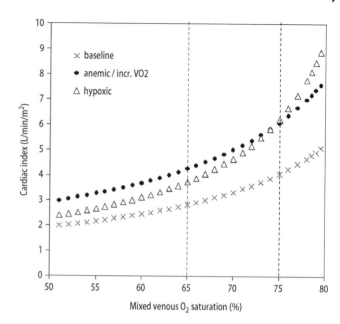

FIGURE 2.8. Theoretical relationship between mixed venous oxygen saturation and cardiac index. The baseline relationship assumes typical values for hemoglobin of 120 g/L, oxygen consumption (VO_2) of 120 mL/min/m², and arterial oxygen saturation of 98%. In situations of either increased VO_2 (220 mL/min/m²) or anemia (80 g/L), the curve is shifted upward. In all three situations, a fall in mixed venous saturation from 75% to 65% represents a relative decrease in cardiac index of approximately 40% (assuming all other variables remain constant). However, in the case of mild baseline hypoxia (arterial oxygen saturation 90%), the shape of the curve changes, such that the same drop in mixed venous saturation now represents a fall in cardiac index of 50%.

$$Oxygen\ excess\ factor\ (\Omega) = SaO_2/(SaO_2 - SvO_2)$$

The rationale for this is that Ω is mathematically equivalent to the ratio of oxygen delivery to oxygen consumption and is easier to assimilate clinically. It is also valid in states of hypoxia [177]. Normally this ratio is of the order of 4:1; it has also been shown that decompensation is more likely when Ω falls below 2:1 [178].

Unfortunately, obtaining access to true mixed venous blood is difficult in pediatric practice. However, placement of a central venous catheter is common in critically ill patients and may represent an alternative to mixed venous blood [179]. Because of the wide variation in the oxygen saturation of venous blood draining organs below the diaphragm (Table 2.2), central venous blood should ideally be sampled from the superior vena cava, just before it enters the right atrium. However, the right atrium may also represent a

TABLE 2.2. Typical venous oxygen saturation values from organs and tissue beds.

Site	Saturation
Brain	69
Heart	30–37
Liver	66
Gut	66
Kidney	92
Muscle	60–71
Skin	88

Source: Compiled from data in Bloos and Reinhart [174], Whyte [179], and Finch and Lenfant [263].

suitable site. There is a theoretical risk that sampling from the right atrium may selectively sample desaturated blood from the coronary sinus; in reality, the probability of this is likely to be low [170,179]. There are no large studies examining the relationship between central and mixed venous saturation in critically ill children; however, in the immediate period after cardiac surgery, central venous values are, on average, lower than mixed venous, by between 7% and 17% [180,181]. Data from adult patients in shock of varying etiology suggest that, on average, the central venous saturation is 7% higher than the mixed venous oxygen saturation [182,183], although much larger differences (up to 20%) may be found within individual patients [184]. Reassuringly, when sequential sampling is performed, both sites trend in the same direction in the majority (90%) of cases [182]. The validity of central venous saturation as a monitoring tool has been shown in a large randomized controlled trial of adult patients in shock. In this study of early goal-directed resuscitation, mortality was decreased in the group in which normalization of central venous saturation was one of the end points (30.5% vs. 46.5%) [185].

Application and interpretation of adult-derived values for central venous oxygen monitoring to children may be complicated by proportionate differences in superior vena caval flow between adults and children [186]. In adults, the superior vena cava carries approximately 35% of the total body venous return. In childhood, this is age dependent, typically being 50% in newborns, rising to a peak of 55% by 2.5 years, and decreasing to adult values by age 6.5 years (Figure 2.9). These represent average values in health, however, and there are major differences in these proportions within each age band. Furthermore, whether the same relationship holds in disease states is unknown [186].

Finally, it is worth considering causes of an elevated mixed/central venous saturation in a critically ill patient. Broadly speaking, there are five causes: (1) a very high cardiac output; (2)

functional arteriovenous shunting (typically occurring at the microcirculatory level); (3) impairment of cellular oxygen utilization, including mitochondrial dysfunction seen in sepsis, congenital defects of oxidative phosphorylation, and certain toxins, such as cyanide poisoning; (4) organ death; and (5) extreme reductions in basal metabolic rate (e.g., during hypothermia).

Blood Lactate

As discussed earlier, lactic acidosis may result from tissue hypoxia [187]. However, it is important to appreciate that a rise in blood lactate may occur in the critically ill patient for reasons other than inadequate oxygen delivery [188]. In sepsis, muscles may generate lactate under aerobic conditions [189,190]. This is probably caused by catecholamine-induced stimulation of sarcolemmal Na^+-K^+/ATPase [191]. The energy supply for this enzyme is linked to the glycolytic and glycogenolytic pathways; overstimulation produces pyruvate at a rate that outstrips the oxidative capacity of the mitochondria, resulting in lactate accumulation. It is also becoming increasingly apparent that lactate serves as a currency for maintaining the redox potential both within and between cells; this is known as the *lactate shuttle concept* [192]. Nonetheless, an elevated lactate level, or more importantly an elevated lactate level that does not fall, has prognostic implications, and the cause should always be vigorously sought [193–196].

Regional Perfusion

Both mixed/central venous oxygen saturation and blood lactate are global markers. Delivery and consumption abnormalities can occur at the regional level. Unfortunately, robust measures of regional perfusion at the bedside are lacking.

Tissue PCO₂ Monitoring Using Tonometry

Tonometry is a technique whereby a CO_2-permeable balloon is placed in proximity to a mucosal surface [197]. Hypoperfusion of the tissue bed in question causes tissue, and hence mucosal, intracellular CO_2 accumulation, and, as CO_2 diffuses freely across cell membranes, it will equilibrate within the tonometer balloon. The difference between tonometric and arterial PCO₂ (*PCO₂ gap*) is thought to quantify the degree of hypoperfusion; this has been corroborated in several studies measuring splanchnic mucosal perfusion with other methods (microspheres, laser Doppler, flow probes) [198–200]. Gastric tonometry as a surrogate for splanchnic perfusion was the first application of this principle in the critical care setting. A vast number of studies utilizing this technique were published in the 1990s; many appeared to show an adverse prognosis with the presence of an increased PCO₂ gap (particularly if this did not respond to resuscitation) [201–206]. Several suggested that early tonometric-guided therapy might improve outcome; however, the results were by no means uniform. With hindsight, the results of many of the earlier studies have been questioned on the basis of methodologic flaws [197]. These include the tonometer medium (air being more accurate than saline) [207,208], use of buffers [207], gastric acid blockade [209], influence of feeding [210], inaccuracy in blood gas analyzers for measuring PCO₂ in saline [211], and use of calculated mucosal pH (using the Henderson-Hasselbalch equation and assuming mucosal and arterial bicarbonate to be equal) in preference to PCO₂. To date, gastric tonometry has not been widely adopted as a routine monitoring tool in the intensive care

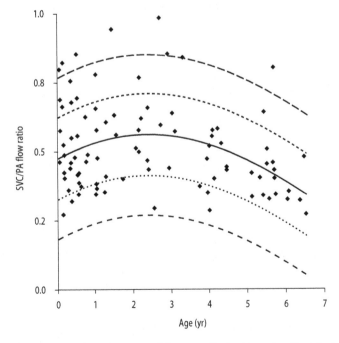

Figure 2.9. Ratio of superior vena caval flow to total body venous return throughout childhood. Lines represent mean, one and two standard deviations (From Salim et al. [186]. Copyright 1995 from American Heart Association, Inc. All right reserved. Reprinted with permission.)

unit. Recently, sublingual tonometry has been suggested as a more accessible alternative, particularly during the early phases of resuscitation [212,213].

Optical Monitoring Methods

A variety of optical methods for measuring tissue perfusion have recently become available, including laser Doppler flowmetry [214], near infrared spectroscopy [215], peripheral perfusion index [216,217], and orthogonal polarization spectral imaging [218].

Capillary Refill

Capillary refill figures prominently in the major resuscitation manuals and has been shown to be a marker of hypovolemia in the emergency room setting [219–221]. The significance of this variable in the PICU is less clear, perhaps because of the coexistence of confounding factors such as fever, hypothermia, and vasocative medication use [222]. In the PICU, capillary refill bears a weak relationship to stroke volume, with the optimal predictive value occurring with a capillary refill greater than 6 sec (well above the traditional upper limit of 2 sec) [222,223]. It bears no relationship to systemic vascular resistance [222].

Assessing the Components of Cardiac Output

If it appears that flow is inadequate, the next step is to attempt to isolate which component may be contributing: heart rate, preload, contractility, afterload, or diastolic function. One of the great problems is that all of these components are interdependent; thus, an apparent deficiency in one parameter may be caused by abnormalities in another or, indeed, in several of the others. For example, the combination of a moderate sinus tachycardia (secondary to fever) coexistent with diastolic dysfunction may result in a functional preload deficit; the solution thus may not be to administer volume but rather to slow the heart rate and give a lusitropic agent. It is also worth considering that many of the therapies aimed at increasing flow carry a cost; for example, increasing inotropy may also increase myocardial oxygen consumption, which may be undesirable in the setting of a failing myocardium. It may be preferable to decrease oxygen consumption (mechanical ventilation, increasing sedation, neuromuscular blockade, avoiding hyperthermia).

Heart Rate

Heart rate is the easiest component affecting cardiac function but is often the most overlooked. Extreme tachycardia may compromise diastolic filling time, particularly if diastolic dysfunction coexists. Loss of atrioventricular synchrony will also compromise forward flow.

Preload Versus Volume Responsiveness

Preload relates to the variety of factors influencing the amount of ventricular fiber stretch at the end of diastole (and hence end diastolic volume) [224,225]. Preload is difficult to both measure and interpret at the bedside; as a result, attention has recently focused on the clinical question of identifying when a patient is likely to increase stroke volume in response to fluid administration [226]. In reality, we may wish to address both issues simultaneously [227].

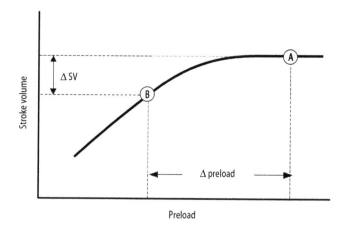

FIGURE 2.10. Cyclical changes in stroke volume and pulse pressure induced by positive pressure ventilation can be used to predict a patient's response to fluid administration. However, this can produce both false-positive and false-negative results. In position A, the patient is optimally filled and functioning at the top of the Starling curve. Ventilation with excessive tidal volumes produces a cyclical decrease in preload and hence stroke volume (to position B), suggesting that the patient may respond to volume administration. This is an example of a false-positive result.

Failure of a patient to increase stroke volume following a fluid bolus when predicted to do so may occur for three reasons: (1) the prediction tool is inaccurate, and the patient is already functioning at the top of the Starling curve (Figure 2.10); (2) contractility is severely impaired; and (3) the infusion volume is not sufficient to increase preload (this may be more common than we expect) [228]. In the first two scenarios, preload will increase, but the scenarios may be differentiated by a measure of contractility, whereas in the third scenario preload will not increase [227].

Traditionally, the two commonly used measures of preload have been central venous pressure (right heart) and pulmonary artery occlusion pressure (left heart); however, both perform poorly in this regard [71,229]. This is because many factors affect the ability of a pressure measurement to act as a marker of volume status, including venous capacitance, cardiac chamber compliance, valve competence, pulmonary artery pressures, and the ability of the lung to function as a Starling resistor with positive pressure ventilation [67,230]. Nonetheless, it is reasonable to assume that a low central venous pressure may represent underfilling, and this parameter may be useful for trending [231].

Three volume-based measures, intrathoracic blood volume, global end diastolic volume, and right ventricular end diastolic volume, have been evaluated favorably in adult practice [71,229,232]. The former two are calculated from transpulmonary thermodilution, the latter from pulmonary thermodilution via a rapid response thermistor. Corrected flow time is a Doppler-derived measurement that has been used successfully in adults to guide intraoperative volume replacement [233–235], although it is also affected by afterload and contractility. Two echocardiographic indicators of preload have been suggested. The functional preload index requires specialized software and a series of calculations, thus limiting its clinical utility [236], and interpretation of mitral inflow velocity profiles is frequently difficult because of confounding variables [237].

In contrast to the static measures of preload, predictors of fluid responsiveness are dynamic; all relate to the cyclical fluctuations in right heart preload induced by positive pressure mechanical ventilation [226,238]. These produce beat-to-beat variations in stroke volume, which are evident using any of the continuous measures of cardiac output described earlier. Fluid responsiveness can also be predicted from the arterial blood pressure trace [239]. Three measures have been suggested: pulse pressure variation, systolic pressure variation, and the downward portion of systolic pressure variation from baseline (delta down). All three show promise; however, pulse pressure variation may be the most predictive, as it is theoretically more closely related to stroke volume (pulse pressure is influenced by stroke volume and arterial compliance, while systolic pressure is also influenced by diastolic pressure) [240]. The majority of studies suggest fluid responsiveness (an increase in stroke volume of greater than 10%–15%) is likely when the pulse pressure variation exceeds approximately 15%.

One of the major difficulties in comparing any variability parameter based on preload changes induced from positive pressure ventilation is the lack of standardization of the stimulus inducing the variation. Changes in preload are affected primarily by swings in pleural pressure, which are affected by tidal volume and transmural pressure gradient across the lung (which is in turn affected by factors such as pulmonary edema, consolidation, etc.). Thus, there is a potential for inducing false-positive readings because of excessive ventilation as well as false-negative readings when low tidal volumes are used (see Figure 2.10) [241]; the latter may be avoided by using tidal volumes of at least 8 mL/kg [242].

Contractility

Of all the parameters affecting cardiac output, contractility is perhaps the most difficult to measure at the bedside. The echocardiographic stress velocity index plots stress velocity (contractility) against end systolic wall stress (afterload) and has provided pathophysiologic insight into several disease states [243–245]. This relationship changes in the failing heart in two ways: contractility is reduced for a given afterload, and the slope of the contractility-afterload relationship is steeper, meaning that afterload reduction may offer greater benefit (and conversely afterload may cause greater harm; Figure 2.11). Tissue Doppler is a relatively new modality that may provide information on diastolic function as well as contractility [246,247]. The cardiac function index, derived from transpulmonary thermodilution, is defined as stroke volume

divided by global end diastolic volume; this is said to be a load-independent measure of contractility. To date this has not been investigated in pediatric practice. The stroke work index represents the area enclosed by the ventricular pressure–volume loop; however, this may be estimated at the bedside from stroke index and arterial pressure measurements. Although not a true measure of contractility, it allows some insight into cardiac reserve, namely, how stoke index (volume) is adjusted in the face of changing afterload.

Afterload

Afterload is defined as the force opposing left ventricular fiber shortening during ventricular ejection, in other words, left ventricular wall stress [248,249]. Wall stress can be measured at various points throughout cardiac ejection, although it is thought that calculation at end systole provides the best measure of afterload [250]. Calculation of wall stress requires measurement of end systolic transmural ventricular pressure and echocardiographic measurement of left ventricular end systolic dimension and wall thickness. Here transmural pressure equals the difference between intra- and extraventricular (or intrathoracic) pressures. Although intraventricular pressure can be estimated from the mean arterial pressure [251], accurate estimation of extraventricular/intrathoracic pressure is difficult and may involve measurement of esophageal or pleural pressures [252]. Using this approach it is easy to understand how factors that increase intrathoracic pressure, such as positive pressure ventilation, result in a reduction in afterload [15].

Systemic vascular resistance is commonly used as a surrogate measure of afterload in the clinical situation, predominantly because it is easier to measure than wall stress. It is important to appreciate that vascular resistance is not synonymous with afterload; rather, it is one of several contributory factors. Systemic vascular resistance is analogous to Ohm's law, treating the heart as a DC (constant) rather than an AC (pulsatile) generator of flow by measuring the ratio of mean pressure drop across the systemic vascular bed to the flow (see preceding discussion in Arterial Pulse Contour Analysis):

$$SVR = \frac{79.9 \times (MAP - CVP)}{cardiac\ index}$$

where SVR is systemic vascular resistance; MAP is mean arterial pressure; CVP is central venous pressure, and the units of measurement are dyn-sec/cm^5/m^2. Seen in this light, the limitations of this calculation are obvious; however, it provides the clinician with a single figure that may have some prognostic value [253,254]. The importance of minimizing afterload in the failing myocardium is well documented. However, the clinical dilemma is usually one of balancing afterload reduction against maintaining perfusion pressure (blood pressure); in reality, this can only be optimized if cardiac output is measured.

Diastolic Function

The traditional definition of diastole covers the period from the end of aortic ejection (aortic valve closure) until the onset of ventricular tension occurring with the following beat [255]. Diastole is an energy-consuming process, which is influenced by both active and passive mechanisms. Active processes (relaxation) occur within the cardiomyocytes, whereas passive mechanisms (stiffness) involve external factors, including viscoelastic properties of the extracellular matrix, and changes in both diastolic load and after-

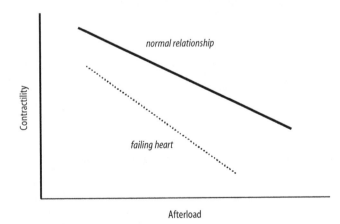

Figure 2.11. Contractility versus afterload. A negative correlation exists between contractility and afterload [243]. When the heart is failing, this relationship may change in two ways: the intercept decreases (downward shift), and the slope may become increasingly negative. Thus, a failing heart may manifest both a loss of contractility for a given afterload and a greater decline in contractility when afterload is increased.

load [256]. One of the primary active events concerns the regulation of cytosolic Ca^{2+} levels. Diastolic relaxation requires a drop in calcium concentration within the cytosol, thereby encouraging Ca^{2+} dissociation from troponin C and hence inhibition of actin-myosin cross-bridge activity [257]. Calcium concentration decreases in a variety of ways, the most important being reuptake into the sarcoplasmic reticulum via a Ca^{2+}-ATPase pump (SERCA), which is in turn regulated by phospholamban. In its dephosphorylated form, phospholamban inhibits Ca^{2+} reuptake [258]. However, when phosphorylated via a variety of agents, including β-adrenergic agents and phosphodiesterase inhibitors (e.g., milrinone), phospholamban increases Ca^{2+} uptake and hence diastolic relaxation (*lusitropy*) [259]. This same mechanism also improves systolic function by increasing the Ca^{2+} reservoir. Phosphodiesterase inhibitors appear to act via a second mechanism to increase lusitropy, namely, a direct action on phosphodiesterase III located on the outer membrane of the sarcoplasmic reticulum [260].

The contribution of diastolic function to myocardial performance is now well established. Intracardiac pressure and volume measurements allow quantification of the active and passive components of diastolic function. Active relaxation can be estimated by (1) the time constant of isovolumic pressure decline (the time for ventricular pressure to fall by approximately two thirds), (2) the isovolumic relaxation time, or (3) the maximum rate of pressure decay $(-dP/dt)$ [256,261]. Passive stiffness can be estimated by the diastolic slope of the pressure–volume curve. Unfortunately, the ability to measure diastolic function at the bedside is limited in pediatric practice. The most common technique is echocardiography. A variety of Doppler-derived parameters can be used to estimate the time constant of isovolumic pressure decline and the isovolumic relaxation time and also to examine patterns of mitral valve and pulmonary venous flow during left ventricular filling (including mitral E and A wave velocities). Unfortunately, the majority of these measures are affected by many factors, including age, heart rate, afterload, volume status, and ventricular filling [256,261,262]. Recently, attention has focused on tissue Doppler indices; however, their utility as monitoring tools is as yet unexplored.

References

1. Nichols WW, O'Rourke MF, eds. McDonald's Blood Flow in Arteries, 5th ed. London: Arnold; 2005.
2. Tibby SM, Murdoch IA. Monitoring cardiac function in intensive care. Arch Dis Child 2003;88:46–52.
3. Kaye W. Invasive monitoring techniques: arterial cannulation, bedside pulmonary artery catheterization, and arterial puncture. Heart Lung 1983;12:395–427.
4. Fry DL. Physiologic recording by modern instruments with particular reference to pressure recording. Physiol Rev 1960;40:753–788.
5. Patel DJ, Mason DT, Ross J Jr, Braunwald E. Harmonic analysis of pressure pulses obtained from the heart and great vessels of man. Am Heart J 1965;69:785–794.
6. Gardner RM, Hollingsworth KW. Optimizing the electrocardiogram and pressure monitoring. Crit Care Med 1986;14:651–658.
7. Kleinman B, Powell S, Kumar P, Gardner RM. The fast flush test measures the dynamic response of the entire blood pressure monitoring system. Anesthesiology 1992;77:1215–1220.
8. Gibbs NC, Gardner RM. Dynamics of invasive pressure monitoring systems: clinical and laboratory evaluation. Heart Lung 1988;17:43–51.
9. Heimann PA, Murray WB. Medical Construction and use of catheter-manometer systems. J Clin Monit 1993;9:45–53.
10. O'Rourke MF. What is blood pressure? Am J Hypertens 1990;3:803–810.
11. O'Rourke MF. What is the arterial pressure? Aust NZ J Med 1988;18:649–650.
12. O'Rourke MF, Blazek JV, Morreels CL Jr, Krovetz LJ. Pressure wave transmission along the human aorta. Changes with age and in arterial degenerative disease. Circ Res 1968;23:567–579.
13. Teitel DF. Cardiac Physiology. In: Chang AC, Hanley FL, Wernovsky G, Wessel DL, eds. Pediatric Cardiac Intensive Care. Philadelphia: Lippincott Williams & Wilkins; 1998:25–29.
14. Proulx F, Gauthier M, Nadeau D, Lacroix J, Farrell CA. Timing and predictors of death in pediatric patients with multiple organ system failure. Crit Care Med 1994;22:1025–1031.
15. Shekerdemian L, Bohn D. Cardiovascular effects of mechanical ventilation. Arch Dis Child 1999;80:475–480.
16. Tibby SM, Hatherill M, Marsh MJ, Murdoch IA. Clinicians' abilities to estimate cardiac index in ventilated children and infants. Arch Dis Child 1997;77:516–518.
17. Mercier JC, Beaufils F, Hartmann JF, Azema D. Hemodynamic patterns of meningococcal shock in children. Crit Care Med 1988;16:27–33.
18. Thompson AE. Pulmonary artery catheterization in children. New Horiz 1997;5:244–250.
19. Shephard JN, Brecker SJ, Evans TW. Bedside assessment of myocardial performance in the critically ill. Intensive Care Med 1994;20:513–521.
20. Stewart GN. Researches on the circulation time and on the influences which affect it. IV. The output of the heart. J Physiol 1897;22:159–183.
21. Hamilton WF, Moore JW, Kinsman JM, et al. Studies on the circulation. IV. Further analysis of the injection method, and changes in hemodynamics under physiological and pathological conditions. Am J Physiol 1932;99:534–542.
22. Zierler K. Indicator dilution methods for measuring blood flow, volume, and other properties of biological systems: a brief history and memoir. Ann Biomed Eng 2000;28:836–848.
23. Millard RK. Indicator-dilution dispersion models and cardiac output computing methods. Am J Physiol 1997;272:H2004–H2012.
24. Stephenson JL. Theory of measurement of blood flow by the dilution on an indicator. Bull Math Biophys 1948;10:117–121.
25. Wise ME. Tracer dilution curves in cardiology and random walk and lognormal distributions. Acta Physiol Pharmacol Neerl 1966;14:175–204.
26. Morady F, Brundage BH, Gelberg HJ. Rapid method for determination of shunt ratio using a thermodilution technique. Am Heart J 1983;106:369–373.
27. Hedvall G. The applicability of the thermodilution method for determination of pulmonary blood flow and pulmonary vascular resistance in infants and children with ventricular septal defects. Scand J Clin Lab Invest 1978;38:581–585.
28. Hedvall G, Kjellmer I, Olsson T. An experimental evaluation of the thermodilution method for determination of cardiac output and of intracardiac right-to-left shunts. Scand J Clin Lab Invest 1973;31:61–68.
29. Joji P, Werner O. Left-to-right shunt assessed by thermodilution during surgery for congenital heart disease. Scand J Thorac Cardiovasc Surg 1987;21:203–206.
30. Saitoh M, Sudoh M, Haneda N, Watanabe K, Kajino Y, Mori C. Determination of left to right shunt by thermodilution in patients with ventricular septal defect. Jpn Circ J 1989;53:1205–1214.
31. Boehrer JD, Lange RA, Willard JE, Grayburn PA, Hillis LD. Advantages and limitations of methods to detect, localize, and quantitate intracardiac right-to-left and bidirectional shunting. Am Heart J 1993;125:215–220.
32. Boehrer JD, Lange RA, Willard JE, Grayburn PA, Hillis LD. Advantages and limitations of methods to detect, localize, and quantitate intracardiac left-to-right shunting. Am Heart J 1992;124:448–455.
33. Nishikawa T, Dohi S. Errors in the measurement of cardiac output by thermodilution. Can J Anaesth 1993;40:142–153.

34. Zierler K. Equations for measuring blood flow by external monitoring of radioisotopes. Circ Res 1965;16:309–321.

35. Fegler G. Measurement of cardiac output in anaesthetized animals by a thermodilution method. Q J Exp Physiol 1954;39:153–164.

36. Branthwaite MA, Bradley RD. Measurement of cardiac output by thermal dilution in man. J Appl Physiol 1968;24:434–438.

37. Swan HJ, Ganz W, Forrester J, Marcus H, Diamond G, Chonette D. Catheterization of the heart in man with use of a flow-directed balloon-tipped catheter. N Engl J Med 1970;283:447–451.

38. Silove ED, Tynan MJ, Simcha AJ. Thermal dilution measurement of pulmonary and systemic blood flow in secundum atrial septal defect, and transposition of great arteries with intact interventricular septum. Br Heart J 1972;34:1142–1146.

39. Freed MD, Keane JF. Cardiac output measured by thermodilution in infants and children. J Pediatr 1978;92:39–42.

40. Colgan FJ, Stewart S. An assessment of cardiac output by thermodilution in infants and children following cardiac surgery. Crit Care Med 1977;5:220–225.

41. Pollack MM, Reed TP, Holbrook PR, Fields AI. Bedside pulmonary artery catheterization in pediatrics. J Pediatr 1980;96:274–276.

42. Connors AF Jr, Speroff T, Dawson NV, et al. The effectiveness of right heart catheterization in the initial care of critically ill patients. SUPPORT Investigators. JAMA 1996;276:889–897.

43. Robin ED. Death by pulmonary artery flow-directed catheter. Time for a moratorium? Chest 1987;92:727–731.

44. Sandham JD, Hull RD, Brant RF, et al, and the Canadian Critical Care Clinical Trials Group. A randomized, controlled trial of the use of pulmonary-artery catheters in high-risk surgical patients. N Engl J Med 2003;348:5–14.

45. Richard C, Warszawski J, Anguel N, et al, and French Pulmonary Artery Catheter Study Group. Early use of the pulmonary artery catheter and outcomes in patients with shock and acute respiratory distress syndrome: a randomized controlled trial. JAMA 2003; 290:2713–2720.

46. Yu DT, Platt R, Lanken PN, et al, and AMCC Sepsis Project Working Group. Relationship of pulmonary artery catheter use to mortality and resource utilization in patients with severe sepsis. Crit Care Med 2003;31:2734–2741.

47. Binanay C, Califf RM, Hasselblad V, et al, and ESCAPE Investigators and ESCAPE Study Coordinators. Evaluation study of congestive heart failure and pulmonary artery catheterization effectiveness: the ESCAPE trial. JAMA 2005;294:1625–1633.

48. Shah MR, Hasselblad V, Stevenson LW, Binanay C, O'Connor CM, Sopko G, Califf RM. Impact of the pulmonary artery catheter in critically ill patients: meta-analysis of randomized clinical trials. JAMA 2005;294:1664–1670.

49. Iberti TJ, Fischer EP, Leibowitz AB, et al. A multicenter study of physicians' knowledge of the pulmonary artery catheter. JAMA 1990;264:2928–2932.

50. Gnaegi A, Feihl F, Perret C. Intensive care physicians' insufficient knowledge of right-heart catheterization at the bedside: time to act? Crit Care Med 1997;25:213–220.

51. Mori Y, Nakanishi T, Satoh M, Kondoh C, Momma K. Catheterization of the pulmonary artery using a 3 French catheter in patients with congenital heart disease. Cathet Cardiovasc Diagn 1998;45:45–50.

52. Janik JE, Conlon SJ, Janik JS. Percutaneous central access in patients younger than 5 years: size does matter. J Pediatr Surg 2004;39:1252–1356.

53. Smith-Wright DL, Green TP, Lock JE, Egar MI, Fuhrman BP. Complications of vascular catheterization in critically ill children. Crit Care Med 1984;12:1015–1017.

54. Bagwell CE, Salzberg AM, Sonnino RE, Haynes JH. Potentially lethal complications of central venous catheter placement. J Pediatr Surg 2000;35:709–713.

55. Johnson EM, Saltzman DA, Suh G, Dahms RA, Leonard AS. Complications and risks of central venous catheter placement in children. Surgery 1998;124:911–916.

56. Finck C, Smith S, Jackson R, Wagner C. Percutaneous subclavian central venous catheterization in children younger than one year of age. Am Surg 2002;68:401–404.

57. Jansen JRC. The thermodilution method for the clinical assessment of cardiac output. Intensive Care Med 1995;21:691–697.

58. Levett JM, Replogle RL. Thermodilution cardiac output: a critical analysis and review of the literature. J Surg Res 1979;27:392–404.

59. Moodie DS, Feldt RH, Kaye MP, et al. Measurement of cardiac output by thermodilution: development of accurate measurements at flows applicable to the pediatric patient. J Surg Res 1978;25:305–311.

60. Jansen JRC, Schreuder JJ, Settels JJ, et al. An adequate strategy for the thermodilution technique in patients during mechanical ventilation. Intensive Care Med 1990;16:422–425.

61. Stetz CW, Miller RG, Kelly GE, Raffin TA. Reliability of the thermodilution method in the determination of cardiac output in clinical practice. Am Rev Respir Dis 1982;126:1001–1004.

62. van Grondelle A, Ditchey RV, Groves BM, Wagner WW Jr, Reeves JT. Thermodilution method overestimates low cardiac output in humans. Am J Physiol 1983;245:H690–H692.

63. Yelderman ML, Ramsay MA, Quinn MD, et al. Continuous thermodilution cardiac output measurement in intensive care unit patients. J Cardiothorac Vasc Anesth 1992;6:270–274.

64. Neto EP, Piriou V, Durand PG, et al. Comparison of two semicontinuous cardiac output pulmonary artery catheters after valvular surgery. Crit Care Med 1999;27:2694–2697.

65. Medin DL, Brown DT, Wesley R, et al. Validation of continuous thermodilution cardiac output in critically ill patients with analysis of systematic errors. J Crit Care 1998;13:184–189.

66. Nelson LD. The new pulmonary arterial catheters. Right ventricular ejection fraction and continuous cardiac output. Crit Care Clin 1996;12:795–818.

67. O'Quin R, Marini JJ. Pulmonary artery occlusion pressure: clinical physiology, measurement, and interpretation. Am Rev Respir Dis 1983;128:319–326.

68. Pinsky MR. Pulmonary artery occlusion pressure. Intensive Care Med 2003;29:19–22.

69. Collee GG, Lynch KE, Hill RD, Zapol WM. Bedside measurement of pulmonary capillary pressure in patients with acute respiratory failure. Anesthesiology 1987;66:614–620.

70. Pinsky MR. Clinical significance of pulmonary artery occlusion pressure. Intensive Care Med 2003;29:175–178.

71. Lichtwarck-Aschoff M, Beale R, Pfeiffer UJ. Central venous pressure, pulmonary artery occlusion pressure, intrathoracic blood volume, and right ventricular end-diastolic volume as indicators of cardiac preload. J Crit Care 1996;11:180–188.

72. von Spiegel T, Hoeft A. Transpulmonary indicator methods in intensive medicine. Anaesthesist 1998;47:220–228.

73. Arfors KE, Malmberg P, Pavek K. Conservation of thermal indicator in lung circulation. Cardiovasc Res 1971;5:530–534.

74. Tibby SM, Hatherill M, Marsh MJ, Morrison G, Anderson D, Murdoch IA. Clinical validation of cardiac output measurements using femoral artery thermodilution with direct Fick in ventilated children and infants. Intensive Care Med 1997;23:987–991.

75. Pauli C, Fakler U, Genz T, Hennig M, Lorenz HP, Hess J. Cardiac output determination in children: equivalence of the transpulmonary thermodilution method to the direct Fick principle. Intensive Care Med 2002;28:947–952.

76. von Spiegel T, Wietasch G, Bursch J, Hoeft A. Cardiac output determination with transpulmonary thermodilution. An alternative to pulmonary catheterization? Anaesthesist 1996;45:1045–1050.

77. Eisenberg PR, Hansbrough JR, Anderson D, Schuster DP. A prospective study of lung water measurements during patient management in an intensive care unit. Am Rev Respir Dis 1987;136:662–668.

78. Davey-Quinn A, Gedney JA, Whiteley SM, Bellamy MC. Extravascular lung water and acute respiratory distress syndrome—oxygenation and outcome. Anaesth Intensive Care 1999;27:357–362.

79. Newman EV, Merrell M, Genecin A, Monge C, Milnor WR, McKeever WP. The dye dilution method for describing the central circulation. An analysis of factors shaping the time-concentration curves. Circulation 1951;4:735–746.

80. Wiesenack C, Prasser C, Keyl C, et al. Assessment of intrathoracic blood volume as an indicator of cardiac preload: single transpulmonary thermodilution technique versus assessment of pressure preload parameters derived from a pulmonary artery catheter. J Cardiothorac Vasc Anesth 2001;15:584–588.

81. Nirmalan M, Willard TM, Edwards DJ, Little RA, Dark PM. Estimation of errors in determining intrathoracic blood volume using the single transpulmonary thermal dilution technique in hypovolemic shock. Anesthesiology 2005;103:805–812.

82. Hofer CK, Furrer L, Matter-Ensner S, Maloigne M, Klaghofer R, Genoni M, Zollinger A. Volumetric preload measurement by thermodilution: a comparison with transoesophageal echocardiography. Br J Anaesth 2005;94:748–755.

83. Imai T, Takahashi K, Fukura H, Morishita Y. Measurement of cardiac output by pulse dye densitometry using indocyanine green: a comparison with the thermodilution method. Anesthesiology 1997;87:816–822.

84. Hillis LD, Firth BG, Winniford MD. Analysis of factors affecting the variability of Fick versus indicator dilution measurements of cardiac output. Am J Cardiol 1985;56:764–768.

85. Linton RA, Band DM, Haire KM. A new method of measuring cardiac output in man using lithium dilution. Br J Anaesth 1993;71:262–266.

86. Linton RA, Linton NW, Band DM. A new method of analysing indicator dilution curves. Cardiovasc Res 1995;30:930–938.

87. Linton RA, Jonas MM, Tibby SM, et al. Cardiac output measured by lithium dilution and transpulmonary thermodilution in patients in a paediatric intensive care unit. Intensive Care Med 2000;26:1507–1511.

88. Fick A. Über die Messung des Blutquantums in den Herzventrikeln. Sitx der Physik-Med ges Wurzburg 1870;2:16.

89. Fishman AP. Respiratory gases in the regulation of the pulmonary circulation. Physiol Rev 1961;41:214–279.

90. Takala J, Keinanen O, Vaisanen P, Kari A. Measurement of gas exchange in intensive care: laboratory and clinical validation of a new device. Crit Care Med 1989;17:1041–1047.

91. Weyland W, Weyland A, Fritz U, Redecker K, Ensink FB, Braun U. A new paediatric metabolic monitor. Intensive Care Med 1994;20:51–57.

92. Chang AC, Kulik TJ, Hickey PR, Wessel DL. Real-time gas-exchange measurement of oxygen consumption in neonates and infants after cardiac surgery. Crit Care Med 1993;21:1369–1375.

93. Wippermann CF, Huth RG, Schmidt FX, Thul J, Betancor M, Schranz D. Continuous measurement of cardiac output by the Fick principle in infants and children: comparison with the thermodilution method. Intensive Care Med 1996;22:467–471.

94. Behrends M, Kernbach M, Brauer A, Braun U, Peters J, Weyland W. In vitro validation of a metabolic monitor for gas exchange measurements in ventilated neonates. Intensive Care Med 2001;27:228–235.

95. Rasanen J. Continuous breathing circuit flow and tracheal tube cuff leak: sources of error during pediatric indirect calorimetry. Crit Care Med 1992;20:1335–1340.

96. Chwals WJ, Lally KP, Woolley MM. Indirect calorimetry in mechanically ventilated infants and children: measurement accuracy with absence of audible airleak. Crit Care Med 1992;20:768–770.

97. Selby AM, McCauley JC, Schell DN, O'Connell A, Gillis J, Gaskin KJ. Indirect calorimetry in mechanically ventilated children: a new technique that overcomes the problem of endotracheal tube leak. Crit Care Med 1995;23:365–370.

98. Bernstein G, Knodel E, Heldt GP. Airway leak size in neonates and autocycling of three flow-triggered ventilators. Crit Care Med 1995;23:1739–1744.

99. Castle RA, Dunne CJ, Mok Q, Wade AM, Stocks J. Accuracy of displayed values of tidal volume in the pediatric intensive care unit. Crit Care Med 2002;30:2566–2574.

100. Ultman JS, Bursztein S. Analysis of error in the determination of respiratory gas exchange at varying FIO sub 2. J Appl Physiol 1981;350:210–216.

101. Kalhan SC, Denne SC. Energy consumption in infants with bronchopulmonary dysplasia. J Pediatr 1990 Apr;116(4):662–664.

102. Light RB. Intrapulmonary oxygen consumption in experimental pneumococcal pneumonia. J Appl Physiol 1988;64:2490–2495.

103. Schulze A, Abubakar K, Gill G, Way RC, Sinclair JC. Pulmonary oxygen consumption: a hypothesis to explain the increase in oxygen consumption of low birth weight infants with lung disease. Intensive Care Med 2001;27:1636–1642.

104. Weyland A, Weyland W, Sydow M, Weyland C, Kettler D. Inverse Fick's principle in comparison to measurements of oxygen consumption in respiratory gases. Does intrapulmonary oxygen uptake account for differences shown by different system methods? Anaesthesist 1994;43:658–666.

105. Wilkinson JL. Haemodynamic calculations in the catheter laboratory. Heart 2001;85:113–120.

106. Miller HC, Brown DJ, Miller GA. Comparison of formulae used to estimate oxygen saturation of mixed venous blood from caval samples. Br Heart J 1974;36:446–451.

107. Jaffe MB. Partial CO2 rebreathing cardiac output–operating principles of the NICO system. J Clin Monit Comput 1999;15:387–401.

108. Haryadi DG, Orr JA, Kuck K, McJames S, Westenskow DR. Partial CO_2 rebreathing indirect Fick technique for non-invasive measurement of cardiac output. J Clin Monit Comput 2000;16:361–374.

109. Lumb AB. Nunn's Applied Respiratory Physiology, 5th ed. Oxford: Butterworth-Heinemann; 2000.

110. Levy RJ, Chiavacci RM, Nicolson SC, Rome JJ, Lin RJ, Helfaer MA, Nadkarni VM. An evaluation of a noninvasive cardiac output measurement using partial carbon dioxide rebreathing in children. Anesth Analg 2004;99:1642–1647.

111. Tachibana K, Imanaka H, Takeuchi M, Takauchi Y, Miyano H, Nishimura M. Noninvasive cardiac output measurement using partial carbon dioxide rebreathing is less accurate at settings of reduced minute ventilation and when spontaneous breathing is present. Anesthesiology 2003;98:830–883.

112. Tibby SM. The indirect Fick principle: great idea, but can we use it in critical care? Pediatr Crit Care Med 2006;7(3):284–285.

113. Franklin DL, Schlegel WA, Rushmer RF. Blood flow measured by Doppler frequency shift of back-scattered ultrasound. Science 1961;134:564–565.

114. Colan SD. Echocardiography. In: Chang AC, Hanley FL, Wernovsky G, Wessel DL, eds. Pediatric Cardiac Intensive Care. Philadelphia: Lippincott Williams & Wilkins; 1998:431–433.

115. Side CD, Gosling RG. Non-surgical assessment of cardiac function. Nature 1971;232:335–336.

116. Cholley BP, Singer M. Esophageal Doppler: noninvasive cardiac output monitor. Echocardiography 2003;20:763–769.

117. Singer M, Clarke J, Bennett ED. Continuous hemodynamic monitoring by esophageal Doppler. Crit Care Med 1989;17:447–452.

118. Tibballs J. Doppler measurement of cardiac output—a critique. Anaesth Intensive Care 1988;16:475–477.

119. Tibby SM, Hatherill M, Murdoch IA. Use of transesophageal Doppler ultrasonography in ventilated pediatric patients: derivation of cardiac output. Crit Care Med 2000;28:2045–2050.

120. Wodey E, Senhadji L, Carre F, Ecoffey C. Extrapolation of cardiac index from analysis of the left ventricular outflow velocities in children: implication of the relationship between aortic size and body surface area. Paediatr Anaesth 2002;12:220–226.

121. Morrow WR, Murphy DJ Jr, Fisher DJ, Huhta JC, Jefferson LS, Smith EO. Continuous wave Doppler cardiac output: use in pediatric patients receiving inotropic support. Pediatr Cardiol 1988;9:131–136.

122. Rein AJ, Hsieh KS, Elixson M, Colan SD, Lang P, Sanders SP, Castaneda AR. Cardiac output estimates in the pediatric intensive care unit using a continuous-wave Doppler computer: validation and limitations of the technique. Am Heart J 1986;112:97–103.

123. Lefrant JY, Bruelle P, Aya AG, Saissi G, Dauzat M, de La Coussaye JE, Eledjam JJ. Training is required to improve the reliability of esophageal Doppler to measure cardiac output in critically ill patients. Intensive Care Med 1998;24:347–352.

124. Murdoch IA, Marsh MJ, Tibby SM, McLuckie A. Continuous haemodynamic monitoring in children: use of transoesophageal Doppler. Acta Paediatr 1995;84:761–764.

125. Chew MS, Poelaert J. Accuracy and repeatability of pediatric cardiac output measurement using Doppler: 20-year review of the literature. Intensive Care Med 2003;29:1889–1894.

126. Chew MS, Brandberg J, Bjarum S, et al. Pediatric cardiac output measurement using surface integration of velocity vectors: an in vivo validation study. Crit Care Med 2000;28:3664–3671.

127. Chew MS, Brandberg J, Canard P, Sloth E, Ask P, Hasenkam JM. Doppler flow measurement using surface integration of velocity vectors (SIVV): in vitro validation. Ultrasound Med Biol 2000;26: 255–262.

128. Rushmer RF, Crystal DK, Wagner C, Ellis RM. Intracardiac impedance plethysmography. Am J Physiol 1953;174:171–174.

129. Kubicek WG, Karnegis JN, Patterson RP, Witsoe DA, Mattson RH. Development and evaluation of an impedance cardiac output system. Aerosp Med 1966;37:1208–1212.

130. Stokes K, Bornzin G. The electrode interface: Stimulation. In: Barold SS, ed. Modern Cardiac Pacing. Mount Kisco, NY: Futura; 1985:33–77.

131. Bonjer FH, van den Berg J, Dirken MN. The origin of the variations of body impedance occurring during the cardiac cycle. Circulation 1952;6:415–420.

132. Patterson RP, Kubicek WG, Witsoe DA, From AH. Studies on the effect of controlled volume change on the thoracic electrical impedance. Med Biol Eng Comput 1978;16:531–536.

133. Ikegaki J, Goto R, Obara H. Bioimpedance measurement of cardiac output after open heart surgery. J Pediatr 1990;116:668–669.

134. Tibballs J. Bioimpedance measurement of cardiac output after open heart surgery. J Pediatr 1990;116:669.

135. Jensen L, Yakimets J, Teo KK A review of impedance cardiography. Heart Lung 1995;24:183–193.

136. Fuller HD. The validity of cardiac output measurement by thoracic impedance: a meta-analysis. Clin Invest Med 1992;15:103–112.

137. Geddes LA, Hoff HE, Mello A. The development and calibration of a method for the continuous measurement of stroke-volume in the experimental animal. Jpn Heart J 1966;7:556–565.

138. Baan J, van der Velde ET, de Bruin HG, et al. Continuous measurement of left ventricular volume in animals and humans by conductance catheter. Circulation 1984;70:812–823.

139. Salo RW, Wallner TG, Pederson BD. Measurement of ventricular volume by intracardiac impedance: theoretical and empirical approaches. IEEE Trans Biomed Eng 1986;33:189–195.

140. Salo RW. Improvement in intracardiac impedance volumes by field extrapolation. Eur Heart J 1992;13(Suppl E):35–39.

141. Grossman W, Braunwald E, Mann T, McLaurin LP, Green LH. Contractile state of the left ventricle in man as evaluated from end-systolic pressure–volume relations. Circulation 1977;56:845–852.

142. Sagawa K. The end-systolic pressure–volume relation of the ventricle: definition, modifications and clinical use. Circulation 1981;63:1223–1227.

143. Glower DD, Spratt JA, Snow ND, et al. Linearity of the Frank-Starling relationship in the intact heart: the concept of preload recruitable stroke work. Circulation 1985;71:994–1009.

144. Little WC, Cheng CP, Mumma M, Igarashi Y, Vinten-Johansen J, Johnston WE. Comparison of measures of left ventricular contractile performance derived from pressure-volume loops in conscious dogs. Circulation 1989;80:1378–1387.

145. Chaturvedi RR, Lincoln C, Gothard J, et al. Left ventricular dysfunction after open repair of simple congenital heart defects. J Thorac Cardiovasc Surg 1998;116:881–884.

146. Steendijk P, Lardenoye JW, van der Velde ET, Schaliji MJ, Baan J. Evaluation of a new transcardiac conductance method for continuous on-line measurement of left ventricular volume. Crit Care Med 2000;28:1599–1606.

147. Erlanger J, Hooker DR. An experimental study of blood pressure and of pulse pressure in man. Johns Hopkins Hosp Rec 1904;12:145–378.

148. Rhodes A, Sunderland R. Arterial pulse contour analysis: The LiDCO™ plus system. In: Pinsky MR, Payen D, eds. Functional Hemodynamic Monitoring. Berlin: Springer-Verlag, 2005:183–192.

149. Dart AM, Kingwell BA. Pulse pressure: a review of mechanisms and clinical relevance. J Am Coll Cardiol 2001;37:975–984 [update in Intensive Care and Emergency Medicine, vol 42].

150. Kouchoukos NT, Sheppard LC, McDonald DA. Estimation of stroke volume in the dog by a pulse contour method. Circ Res 1970;26:611–623.

151. Remington JW, Nobach CB, Hamilton WF, Gold JJ. Volume elasticity characteristics of the human aorta and the prediction of stroke volume from the pressure pulse. Am J Physiol 1948;153:198–308.

152. Langewouters GJ, Wesseling KH, Goedhard WJ. The pressure dependent dynamic elasticity of 35 thoracic and 16 abdominal human aortas in vitro described by a five component model. J Biomech 1985;18:613–620.

153. Langewouters GJ, Wesseling KH, Goedhard WJ. The static elastic properties of 45 human thoracic and 20 abdominal aortas in vitro and the parameters of a new model. J Biomech 1984;17:425–435.

154. Heerman JR, Segers P, Roosens CD, Gasthuys F, Verdonck PR, Poelaert JI. Echocardiographic assessment of aortic elastic properties with automated border detection in an ICU: in vivo application of the arc-tangent Langewouters model. Am J Physiol Heart Circ Physiol 2005;288:H2504–H2511.

155. de Vaal JB, de Wilde RB, van den Berg PC, Schreuder JJ, Jansen JR. Less invasive determination of cardiac output from the arterial pressure by aortic diameter-calibrated pulse contour. Br J Anaesth 2005;95:326–331.

156. Linton NWF, Linton RAF. Estimation of changes in cardiac output from the arterial blood pressure waveform in the upper limb. Br J Anaesth 2001;86:486–496.

157. Jansen JRC, Schreuder JJ, Mulier JP, et al. A comparison of cardiac output derived from the arterial pressure wave against thermodilution in cardiac surgery patients. Br J Anaesth 2001;87:212–222.

158. Godje O, Hoke K, Goetz AE, et al. Reliability of a new algorithm for continuous cardiac output determination by pulse-contour analysis during hemodynamic instability. Crit Care Med 2002;30:52–58.

159. Toorop GP, Westerhof N, Elzinga G. Beat-to-beat estimation of peripheral resistance and arterial compliance during pressure transients. Am J Physiol 1987;252:H1275–H1283.

160. Wesseling KH, Jansen JR, Settels JJ, Schreuder JJ. Computation of aortic flow from pressure in humans using a nonlinear, three-element model. J Appl Physiol 1993;74:2566–2573.

161. Frank O. Die Grundform des Arteriellen Pulses. Zeitschrift für Biologie 1899;37:483–526.

162. Mahajan A, Shabanie A, Turner J, Sopher MJ, Marijic J. Pulse contour analysis for cardiac output monitoring in cardiac surgery for congenital heart disease. Anesth Analg 2003;97:1283–1288.

163. Torgay A, Pirat A, Akpek E, Zeyneloglu P, Arslan G, Haberal M. Pulse contour cardiac output system use in pediatric orthotopic liver transplantation: preliminary report of nine patients. Transplant Proc 2005;37:3168–3170.

164. Petretta M, Storto G, Ferro A, Cuocolo A. Radionuclide monitoring of left ventricular function. J Nucl Cardiol 2001;8:606–615.

165. Kaji S, Yang PC, Kerr AB, et al. Rapid evaluation of left ventricular volume and mass without breath-holding using real-time interactive cardiac magnetic resonance imaging system. J Am Coll Cardiol 2001;38:527–533.

166. Muthurangu V, Taylor A, Andriantsimiavona R, et al. Novel method of quantifying pulmonary vascular resistance by use of simultaneous invasive pressure monitoring and phase-contrast magnetic resonance flow. Circulation 2004;110:826–834.

167. Shoemaker WC. Diagnosis and treatment of the shock syndromes. In: Shoemaker WC, Ayres SM, Grenvik A, Holbrook PR, eds. Textbook of Critical Care, 3rd ed. London: WB Saunders; 1995:85–102.

168. Leach RM, Treacher DF. The pulmonary physician in critical care 2: oxygen delivery and consumption in the critically ill. Thorax 2002;57:170–177.

169. Barratt-Boyes BG, Wood EH. The oxygen saturation of blood in the venae cavae, right-heart chambers, and pulmonary vessels of healthy subjects. J Lab Clin Med 1957;50:93–106.

170. Freed MD, Miettinen OS, Nadas AS. Oximetric detection of intracardiac left-to-right shunts. Br Heart J 1979;42:690–694.

171. Kandel G, Aberman A. Mixed venous oxygen saturation. Its role in the assessment of the critically ill patient. Arch Intern Med 1983;143:1400–1402.

172. Nelson LD. Continuous venous oximetry in surgical patients. Ann Surg 1986;203:329–333.

173. Schumacker PT, Cain SM. The concept of a critical oxygen delivery. Intensive Care Med 1987;13:223–229.

174. Bloos F, Reinhart K. Venous oximetry. Intensive Care Med 2005;31:911–913.

175. Schulze A, Whyte RK, Way RC, Sinclair JC. Effect of the arterial oxygenation level on cardiac output, oxygen extraction, and oxygen consumption in low birth weight infants receiving mechanical ventilation. J Pediatr 1995;126:777–784.

176. Buheitel G, Scharf J, Hofbeck M, Singer H. Estimation of cardiac index by means of the arterial and the mixed venous oxygen content and pulmonary oxygen uptake determination in the early post-operative period following surgery of congenital heart disease. Intensive Care Med 1994;20:500–503.

177. Barnea O, Santamore WP, Rossi A, Salloum E, Chien S, Austin EH. Estimation of oxygen delivery in newborns with a univentricular circulation. Circulation 1998;98:1407–1413.

178. Charpie JR, Dekeon MK, Goldberg CS, Mosca RS, Bove EL, Kulik TJ. Postoperative hemodynamics after Norwood palliation for hypoplastic left heart syndrome. Am J Cardiol 2001;87:198–202.

179. Whyte RK. Mixed venous oxygen saturation in the newborn. Can we and should we measure it? Scand J Clin Lab Invest 1990;50(Suppl 203):203–211.

180. Rasanen J, Peltola K, Leijala M. Superior vena caval and mixed venous oxyhemoglobin saturations in children recovering from open heart surgery. J Clin Monit 1992;8:44–49.

181. Tibby SM, Sykes K, Durward A, Austin C, Murdoch IA. Utility of mixed venous versus central venous oximetry following cardiac surgery in infants [abstr]. Crit Care 2002;6(Suppl 1):P205.

182. Reinhart K, Kuhn HJ, Hartog C, Bredle DL. Continuous central venous and pulmonary artery oxygen saturation monitoring in the critically ill. Intensive Care Med 2004;30:1572–1578.

183. Scheinman MM, Brown MA, Rapaport E. Critical assessment of use of central venous oxygen saturation as a mirror of mixed venous oxygen in severely ill cardiac patients. Circulation 1969;40:165–172.

184. Edwards JD, Mayall RM. Importance of the sampling site for measurement of mixed venous oxygen saturation in shock. Crit Care Med 1998;26:1356–1360.

185. Rivers E, Nguyen B, Havstad S, et al. Early goal-directed therapy in the treatment of severe sepsis and septic shock. N Engl J Med 2001;345:1368–1377.

186. Salim MA, DiSessa TG, Arheart KL, Alpert BS. Contribution of superior vena caval flow to total cardiac output in children. A Doppler echocardiographic study. Circulation 1995;92:1860–1865.

187. Mizock BA, Falk JL. Lactic acidosis in critical illness. Crit Care Med 1992;20:80–93.

188. James JH, Luchette FA, McCarter FD, Fischer JE. Lactate is an unreliable indicator of tissue hypoxia in injury or sepsis. Lancet 1999;354:505–508.

189. James JH, Fang CH, Schrantz SJ, Hasselgren PO, Paul RJ, Fischer JE. Linkage of aerobic glycolysis to sodium-potassium transport in rat skeletal muscle. Implications for increased muscle lactate production in sepsis. J Clin Invest 1996;98:2388–2397.

190. Bundgaard H, Kjeldsen K, Suarez Krabbe K, et al. Endotoxemia stimulates skeletal muscle Na+-K+-ATPase and raises blood lactate under aerobic conditions in humans. Am J Physiol Heart Circ Physiol 2003;284:H1028–H1034.

191. Levy B, Gibot S, Franck P, Cravoisy A, Bollaert PE. Relation between muscle Na+K+ ATPase activity and raised lactate concentrations in septic shock: a prospective study. Lancet 2005;365:871–875.

192. Gladden LB. Lactate metabolism: a new paradigm for the third millennium. J Physiol 2004;558:5–30.

193. Hatherill M, Waggie Z, Purves L, Reynolds L, Argent A. Mortality and the nature of metabolic acidosis in children with shock. Intensive Care Med 2003;29:286–291.

194. Hatherill M, McIntyre AG, Wattie M, Murdoch IA. Early hyperlactataemia in critically ill children. Intensive Care Med 2000;26:314–318.

195. Munoz R, Laussen PC, Palacio G, Zienko L, Piercey G, Wessel DL. Changes in whole blood lactate levels during cardiopulmonary bypass for surgery for congenital cardiac disease: an early indicator of morbidity and mortality. J Thorac Cardiovasc Surg 2000;119:155–162.

196. Nguyen HB, Rivers EP, Knoblich BP, et al. Early lactate clearance is associated with improved outcome in severe sepsis and septic shock. Crit Care Med. 2004;32(8):1637–1642.

197. Kolkman JJ, Otte JA, Groeneveld AB. Gastrointestinal luminal PCO_2 tonometry: an update on physiology, methodology and clinical applications. Br J Anaesth 2000;84:74–86.

198. Antonsson JB, Haglund UH. Gut intramucosal pH and intraluminal PO_2 in a porcine model of peritonitis or haemorrhage. Gut 1995;37:791–797.

199. Heino A, Hartikainen J, Merasto ME, Alhava E, Takala J. Systemic and regional pCO_2 gradients as markers of intestinal ischaemia. Intensive Care Med 1998;24:599–604.

200. Tang W, Weil MH, Sun S, Noc M, Gazmuri RJ, Bisera J. Gastric intramural PCO_2 as monitor of perfusion failure during hemorrhagic and anaphylactic shock. J Appl Physiol 1994;76:572–577.

201. Calvo C, Ruza F, Lopez-Herce J, Dorao P, Arribas N, Alvarado F. Usefulness of gastric intramucosal pH for monitoring hemodynamic complications in critically ill children. Intensive Care Med 1997;23:1268–1274.

202. Casado-Flores J, Mora E, Perez-Corral F, Martinez-Azagra A, Garcia-Teresa MA, Ruiz-Lopez MJ. Prognostic value of gastric intramucosal pH in critically ill children. Crit Care Med 1998;26:1123–1127.

203. Duke T, Butt W, South M, Shann F. The DCO_2 measured by gastric tonometry predicts survival in children receiving extracorporeal life support. Comparison with other hemodynamic and biochemical information. Chest 1997;111:174–179.

204. Hatherill M, Tibby SM, Evans R, Murdoch IA. Gastric tonometry in septic shock. Arch Dis Child 1998;78:155–158.

205. Krafte-Jacobs B, Carver J, Wilkinson JD. Comparison of gastric intramucosal pH and standard perfusional measurements in pediatric septic shock. Chest 1995;108:220–225.

206. Duke TD, Butt W, South M. Predictors of mortality and multiple organ failure in children with sepsis. Intensive Care Med 1997;23:684–692.

207. Thorburn K, Hatherill M, Roberts PC, Durward A, Tibby SM, Murdoch IA. Evaluation of the 5-French saline paediatric gastric tonometer. Intensive Care Med 2000;26:973–980.

208. Uusaro A, Lahtinen P, Parviainen I, Takala J. Gastric mucosal end-tidal PCO_2 difference as a continuous indicator of splanchnic perfusion. Br J Anaesth 2000;85:563–569.

209. Odes HS, Hogan DL, Steinbach JH, Ballesteros MA, Koss MA, Isenberg JI. Measurement of gastric bicarbonate secretion in the human

stomach: different methods produce discordant results. Scand J Gastroenterol 1992;27:829–836.

210. Thorburn K, Durward A, Tibby SM, Murdoch IA. Effects of feeding on gastric tonometric measurements in critically ill children. Crit Care Med 2004;32:246–249.

211. Groeneveld AB, Kolkman JJ. Splanchnic tonometry: a review of physiology, methodology, and clinical applications. J Crit Care 1994;9:198–210.

212. Marik PE, Bankov A. Sublingual capnometry versus traditional markers of tissue oxygenation in critically ill patients. Crit Care Med 2003;31:818–822.

213. Weil MH, Nakagawa Y, Tang W, et al. Sublingual capnometry: a new noninvasive measurement for diagnosis and quantitation of severity of circulatory shock. Crit Care Med 1999;27:1225–1229.

214. Schabauer AM, Rooke TW. Cutaneous laser Doppler flowmetry: applications and findings. Mayo Clin Proc 1994;69:564–574.

215. Taylor DE, Simonson SG. Use of near-infrared spectroscopy to monitor tissue oxygenation. New Horiz 1996;4:420–425.

216. Lima AP, Beelen P, Bakker J. Use of a peripheral perfusion index derived from the pulse oximetry signal as a noninvasive indicator of perfusion. Crit Care Med 2002;30:1210–1213.

217. De Felice C, Latini G, Vacca P, Kopotic RJ. The pulse oximeter perfusion index as a predictor for high illness severity in neonates. Eur J Pediatr 2002;161:561–562.

218. Groner W, Winkelman JW, Harris AG, Ince C, Bouma GJ, Messmer K, Nadeau RG. Orthogonal polarization spectral imaging: a new method for study of the microcirculation. Nat Med 1999;5:1209–1212.

219. Saavedra JM, Harris GD, Li S, Finberg L. Capillary refilling (skin turgor) in the assessment of dehydration. Am J Dis Child 1991;145:296–298.

220. Hoelzer DJ, Brian MB, Balsara VJ, Varner WD, Flynn TC, Miner ME. Selection and nonoperative management of pediatric blunt trauma patients: the role of quantitative crystalloid resuscitation and abdominal ultrasonography. J Trauma 1986;26:57–62.

221. Mackenzie A, Barnes G, Shann F. Clinical signs of dehydration in children. Lancet 1989;2:605–607.

222. Tibby SM, Hatherill M, Murdoch IA. Capillary refill and core-peripheral temperature gap as indicators of haemodynamic status in paediatric intensive care patients. Arch Dis Child 1999;80:163–166.

223. Schriger DL, Baraff L. Defining normal capillary refill: variation with age, sex and temperature. Ann Emerg Med 1988;17:932–935.

224. Braunwald E, Sonnenblick EH, Ross J. Mechanisms of cardiac contraction and relaxation. In: Braunwald E, ed. Heart Disease. Philadelphia: WB Saunders; 1988:389–425.

225. Guyton AC. Determination of cardiac output by equating venous return curves with cardiac response curves. Physiol Rev 1955;35:123–129.

226. Michard F, Teboul JL. Predicting fluid responsiveness in ICU patients: a critical analysis of the evidence. Chest 2002;121:2000–2008.

227. Michard F, Reuter DA. Assessing cardiac preload or fluid responsiveness? It depends on the question we want to answer. Intensive Care Med 2003;29:1396.

228. Axler O, Tousignant C, Thompson CR, et al. Small hemodynamic effect of typical rapid volume infusions in critically ill patients. Crit Care Med 1997;25:965–970.

229. Wiesenack C, Prasser C, Keyl C, Rodig G. Assessment of intrathoracic blood volume as an indicator of cardiac preload: single transpulmonary thermodilution technique versus assessment of pressure preload parameters derived from a pulmonary artery catheter. J Cardiothorac Vasc Anesth 2001;15:584–588.

230. Magder S. How to use central venous pressure measurements. Curr Opin Crit Care 2005;11:264–270.

231. Skinner JR, Milligan DW, Hunter S, Hey EN. Central venous pressure in the ventilated neonate. Arch Dis Child 1992;67:374–377.

232. Michard F, Alaya S, Zarka V, Bahloul M, Richard C, Teboul JL. Global end-diastolic volume as an indicator of cardiac preload in patients with septic shock. Chest 2003;124:1900–1908.

233. Sinclair S, James S, Singer M. Intraoperative intravascular volume optimisation and length of hospital stay after repair of proximal femoral fracture: randomised controlled trial. BMJ 1997;315:909–912.

234. Venn R, Steele A, Richardson P, Poloniecki J, Grounds M, Newman P. Randomized controlled trial to investigate influence of the fluid challenge on duration of hospital stay and perioperative morbidity in patients with hip fractures. Br J Anaesth 2002;88:65–71.

235. McKendry M, McGloin H, Saberi D, Caudwell L, Brady AR, Singer M. Randomised controlled trial assessing the impact of a nurse delivered, flow monitored protocol for optimisation of circulatory status after cardiac surgery. BMJ 2004;329(7460):258.

236. Colan SD, Trowitzsch E, Wernovsky G, Sholler GF, Sanders SP, Castaneda AR. Myocardial performance after arterial switch operation for transposition of the great arteries with intact ventricular septum. Circulation 1988;78:132–141.

237. Appleton CP, Hatle LK, Popp RL. Relation of transmitral flow velocity patterns to left ventricular diastolic function: new insights from a combined hemodynamic and Doppler echocardiographic study. J Am Coll Cardiol 1988;12:426–440.

238. Bendjelid K, Romand JA. Fluid responsiveness in mechanically ventilated patients: a review of indices used in intensive care. Intensive Care Med 2003;29:352–360.

239. Magder S. Clinical usefulness of respiratory variations in arterial pressure. Am J Respir Crit Care Med 2004;169:151–155.

240. Michard F, Boussat S, Chemla D, et al. Relation between respiratory changes in arterial pulse pressure and fluid responsiveness in septic patients with acute circulatory failure. Am J Respir Crit Care Med 2000;162:134–138.

241. Reuter DA, Bayerlein J, Goepfert MS, Weis FC, Kilger E, Lamm P, Goetz AE. Influence of tidal volume on left ventricular stroke volume variation measured by pulse contour analysis in mechanically ventilated patients. Intensive Care Med 2003;29:476–480.

242. De Backer D, Heenen S, Piagnerelli M, Koch M, Vincent JL. Pulse pressure variations to predict fluid responsiveness: influence of tidal volume. Intensive Care Med 2005;31:517–523.

243. Colan SD, Borow KM, Neumann A. Left ventricular end-systolic wall stress-velocity of fiber shortening relation: a load-independent index of myocardial contractility. J Am Coll Cardiol 1984;4:715–724.

244. Feltes TF, Pignatelli R, Kleinert S, Mariscalco MM. Quantitated left ventricular systolic mechanics in children with septic shock utilizing noninvasive wall-stress analysis. Crit Care Med 1994;22:1647–1658.

245. Bryant RM, Shirley RL, Ott DA, Feltes TF. Left ventricular performance following the arterial switch operation: use of noninvasive wall stress analysis in the postoperative period. Crit Care Med 1998;26:926–932.

246. Vogel M, Cheung MM, Li J, et al. Noninvasive assessment of left ventricular force-frequency relationships using tissue Doppler-derived isovolumic acceleration: validation in an animal model. Circulation 2003;107:1647–1652.

247. Oki T, Tabata T, Yamada H, et al. Clinical application of pulsed Doppler tissue imaging for assessing abnormal left ventricular relaxation. Am J Cardiol 1997;79:921–928.

248. Gould KL, Lipscomb K, Hamilton GW, Kennedy JW. Relation of left ventricular shape, function and wall stress in man. Am J Cardiol 1974;34:627–634.

249. Weber KT, Janicki JS. The dynamics of ventricular contraction: force, length, and shortening. Fed Proc 1980;39:188–195.

250. Lang RM, Borow KM, Neumann A, Janzen D. Systemic vascular resistance: an unreliable index of left ventricular afterload. Circulation 1986;74:1114–1123.

251. Rowland DG, Gutgesell HP. Use of mean arterial pressure for noninvasive determination of left ventricular end-systolic wall stress in infants and children. Am J Cardiol 1994;74:98–99.

252. Haney MF, Johansson G, Haggmark S, Biber B. Analysis of left ventricular systolic function during elevated external cardiac pressures: an

examination of measured transmural left ventricular pressure during pressure–volume analysis. Acta Anaesthesiol Scand 2001;45:868–874.

253. Groeneveld AB, Nauta JJ, Thijs LG. Peripheral vascular resistance in septic shock: its relation to outcome. Intensive Care Med 1988;14:141–147.

254. Ceneviva G, Paschall JA, Maffei F, Carcillo JA. Hemodynamic support in fluid-refractory pediatric septic shock. Pediatrics 1998;102:e19.

255. Wiggers CJ. Studies on the duration of the consecutive phases of the cardiac cycle. 1: The duration of the consecutive phases of the cardiac cycle and criteria for their precise determination. Am J Physiol 1921;56:415–438.

256. Zile MR, Brutsaert DL. New concepts in diastolic dysfunction and diastolic heart failure: Part I: diagnosis, prognosis, and measurements of diastolic function. Circulation 2002;105:1387–1393.

257. Villars PS, Hamlin SK, Shaw AD, Kanusky JT. Role of diastole in left ventricular function, I: biochemical and biomechanical events. Am J Crit Care 2004;13:394–403.

258. Bers DM. Calcium fluxes involved in control of cardiac myocyte contraction. Circ Res 2000;87:275–281.

259. Tanigawa T, Yano M, Kohno M, et al. Mechanism of preserved positive lusitropy by cAMP-dependent drugs in heart failure. Am J Physiol Heart Circ Physiol 2000;278:H313–H320.

260. Yano M, Kohno M, Ohkusa T, et al. Effect of milrinone on left ventricular relaxation and Ca(2+) uptake function of cardiac sarcoplasmic reticulum. Am J Physiol Heart Circ Physiol 2000;279:H1898–H1905.

261. Hamlin SK, Villars PS, Kanusky JT, Shaw AD. Role of diastole in left ventricular function, II: diagnosis and treatment. Am J Crit Care 2004;13:453–466.

262. Quinones MA. Assessment of diastolic function. Prog Cardiovasc Dis 2005;47:340–355.

263. Finch CA, Lenfant C. Oxygen transport in man. N Engl J Med 1972;286:407–415.

264. Perloff WH. Invasive measurements in the PICU. In Fuhrman BP, Zimmerman JJ, eds. Pediatric Critical Care, 2nd ed. St Louis: Mosby; 1998:70–86.

265. Shann F. Drug Doses, 8th ed. Melbourne: Collective Pty Ltd; 1994:61.

3
Cardiopulmonary Interactions

Desmond J. Bohn

Introduction

The development in our knowledge and understanding of both cardiovascular and respiratory physiology has tended to proceed along parallel lines. However, many of the texts on cardiac physiology have largely ignored or underestimated the major hemodynamic changes that occur during the transit of blood through the thoracic cavity from the venous to the arterial side of the circulation. Because the heart and lungs share the same body cavity, changes in pleural pressure associated with either spontaneous or mechanical ventilation have important effects on preload or afterload of both ventricles. With the development of intensive care and in particular positive pressure ventilation, we now have a greater appreciation that the heart and lungs are more than two independent but connected systems, and events that occur in either organ will impact on the other. These important interactions between the heart and lungs may be influenced by either a cardiac or a respiratory disease process or the therapies used in intensive care treatment. It is important, therefore, that we have a fundamental understanding of the normal physiology of cardiopulmonary interactions as a prelude to an explanation of how these may change because of therapeutic interventions in the critically ill patient.

The Cardiopulmonary Circulation

Perhaps the easiest way to begin to understand the fundamentals of the complex interaction between the systemic and pulmonary circulations is to use a model of two pumps connected in series enclosed within a chamber where the pressure is constantly changing. The reservoir for the filling of the right heart lies partly outside the thorax and is consequently subject to atmospheric or intra-abdominal pressure (inferior vena cava), whereas some of the large

venous connections (superior vena cava) are intrathoracic and subject to pleural pressure. On the other hand, the reservoir for left heart filling (the pulmonary circulation) and the systemic pumping chamber lie entirely within the thorax, although the pump ejects against high impedance, which is largely extrathoracic (systemic vascular resistance). Because pleural pressure is constantly changing during the respiratory cycle, it follows that the resulting fluctuations in intrathoracic pressure will affect the output from the pump by altering preload or filling on the right side and afterload or ejection on the left side. Two further factors influence the performance of the left and right ventricles; because there are cardiac muscle fibers that interconnect both ventricles and they share a common septum, changes in the contractile state of one ventricle will be reflected in the other, a phenomenon known as *ventricular interdependence* [1–3]. Both pumping chambers are also constrained within a viscoelastic membrane (the pericardium), which, although it does not normally have a significant influence on function, may inhibit contraction in situations where intrapericardial pressure increases. The interaction between respiratory and cardiac functions is a complex one with major differences occurring under conditions of spontaneous or positive pressure respiration. Finally, changes in lung volume, independent of any change in intrathoracic pressure, alter the caliber of the pulmonary vascular bed and thereby influence right ventricular afterload. These various changes and their point of impact are summarized in Figure 3.1. To better understand the complex cardiopulmonary interactions involved in the cohabitation of the thorax, the best approach is to describe the structure and functions of the two ventricles before describing the hemodynamic effects associated with changes in intrathoracic pressure.

The Right Heart Function: Structure Related to Function

The morphometry of the right ventricle shows that its structure is well adapted to its function in that it is a crescent-shaped, heavily trabeculated, thin-walled chamber that serves as a low-pressure, high-volume displacement pump. The right ventricle can be considered to be made up of four anatomically distinct components: (1) the right ventricle free wall; (2) the septal wall, anchored to the left ventricle; (3) the inflow portion of the cavity; and (4) the outflow portion. Contraction of the right ventricle is anything but homogeneous, and it functions like two different chambers connected in series. The heavily trabeculated inflow portion at the apex is

D.S. Wheeler et al. (eds.), *Cardiovascular Pediatric Critical Illness and Injury*,
DOI 10.1007/978-1-84800-923-3_3, © Springer-Verlag London Limited 2009

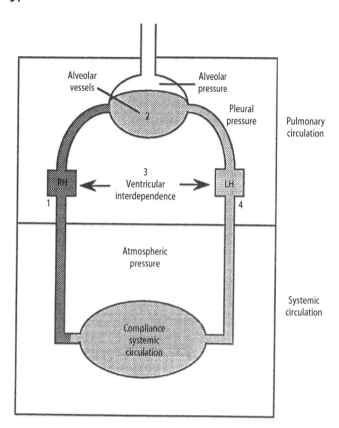

FIGURE 3.1. A summary of cardiopulmonary interactions in a two compartment model of the circulation. Both the right heart (RH) and left heart (LH) are subjected to pleural (intrathoracic) pressure while the systemic vasculature is subjected to atmospheric or, in the case of the inferior vena cava, intraabdominal pressure. (From Permutt S. How Changes in Pleural and Alveolar Pressure Cause Changes in Preload and Afterload in Heart Lung Interactions in Health and Disease. New York: Decker; 1989, with permission from Taylor & Francis Group.)

electrically activated and contracts before the outflow tract, giving rise to an almost peristaltic action when visualized angiographically. The geometry of the right ventricle is entirely different from that of the left as can be seen when comparing the two chambers in cross section. The right ventricle is crescent shaped, while the left ventricle in comparison has an entirely different configuration with a structure that conforms well to its function. It is thick walled and ellipsoid in shape, which allows for an efficient and homogeneous contraction capable of generating high pressures.

The function of the right ventricle is to pump venous blood through what is normally a low-resistance pulmonary vascular bed. Blood flow through the lung to the left atrium is sustained by the pressure differential between the pulmonary artery, the downstream pressure in the pulmonary resistance vessels, and the intracavity pressure in the left atrium. To accomplish this requires only 20 to 30 mm Hg at rest, although this may rise to 50 mm Hg with strenuous exercise when venous return may increase by three to four times normal. The fact that the right ventricle and pulmonary circulation are essentially a low-pressure system with the generation of modest systolic pressures has led some investigators to question its importance in the maintenance of normal circulatory homeostasis. Several animal studies have shown that experimental destruction of myocardium in the right ventricular free wall does not result in alteration in cardiac output or a rise in right atrial pressure as long as pulmonary vascular resistance remains low

[4–7]. The introduction of the Fontan procedure for the surgical correction of obstructive lesions of the right heart, whereby the right atrium is connected to the pulmonary artery, has also shown that effective pulmonary blood flow can be sustained in the absence of a right ventricle when the pulmonary vascular resistance is not elevated [8]. Acute rises in pulmonary vascular resistance result in ventricular dilatation rather than an increase in end diastolic pressure [9]. Although the degree of dilatation is limited by the constraints of the pericardium, it can result in leftward shift of the septum and encroachment on the left ventricular cavity. However, in diseases associated with sustained elevations in pulmonary vascular resistance, demanding an increase in driving pressure to sustain adequate pulmonary blood flow, the right ventricle hypertrophies and undergoes adaptation to a thick-walled pressure chamber capable of generating pressures up to and above systemic levels. In this situation pulmonary artery pressure may reach a level where ischemic injury to the right ventricle may occur [10].

The Pulmonary Vascular Bed

The pulmonary vasculature bridges the connection between the right and left heart and is the impedance for the right ventricle as well as being the preload for the left ventricle. Transpulmonary artery pressure can increase with or without an increase in vasomotor tone. Examples of the former include exercise and left ventricular failure because of a rise in outflow (pulmonary venous) pressure. Pulmonary vasomotor tone can be increased by pulmonary vascular and parenchymal disease, chronic hypoxia, and sustained elevations in pulmonary blood flow associated with left-to-right intracardiac shunts.

The pulmonary vascular bed has a great capacity to dilate in response to acute increases in pulmonary blood flow. The fact that pulmonary artery pressure rarely rises to greater than 50 mm Hg even during strenuous exercise is attributable to recruitment of previously nonperfused vessels. In situations with excessively high pulmonary blood flow associated with left-to-right intracardiac shunting, the pulmonary vasculature will become abnormally muscularized, and there will be a rise in pulmonary vascular resistance and increased right ventricular afterload. These will also be increased in situations where there is either a fixed arteriolar obstruction, as in primary pulmonary hypertension, or in acute and chronic hypoxia. When the PAO_2 in the alveolus falls below 60 mm Hg, local vasomotor tone shunts blood away from the affected area. This *hypoxic pulmonary vasoconstriction* is a prominent feature of patients with acute respiratory distress syndrome where reduced lung compliance and atelectasis results in loss of the traction mechanism that keeps pulmonary capillaries open.

The Left Heart: Structure Related to Function

The left ventricle differs from the right in its anatomic configuration, being a thick-walled, spherical chamber capable of supporting high systemic pressures. Systolic function of the left ventricle is governed by contractility, heart rate, and the afterload forces against which it contracts, defined as the systolic wall stress. This consists of aortic pressure and the forces acting across the chamber wall. In the normal situation, where there is no pressure gradient between left ventricle and aorta, the wall stress is the major component of left ventricular afterload and correlates well with left ventricular end systolic volume [11,12]. The preload for filling of the left ventricle comes from pulmonary venous return and left atrial filling, and, because this reservoir and the chamber itself lie within the thorax, both preload and afterload for the left ventricle can be said to be influenced by changes in intrathoracic pressure.

The Ventricular Septum and Ventricular Interdependence

Although the right and left ventricles function as circulations in series, the structure and function of one intimately affect the other. The two chambers differ in terms of their morphometry and the preload and afterload forces to which they are subjected. However, the function of one ventricle is related to another by muscle fibers that encircle both chambers, a common deformable septum, and the pericardium that surrounds them both. This symbiotic relationship has been termed *ventricular interdependence* [1] and affects both systolic and diastolic function.

The intraventricular septum can be considered to be functionally an extension of the left ventricular free wall as the muscle fiber alignment closely resembles that part of the heart [13] and makes an important contribution to ventricular systolic ejection. Any acute change in either the volume or pressure of the right ventricle can result in shift in septal position. This alters the distensibility of the left ventricle, thereby reducing its compliance. In extreme situations this can have an adverse effect on left ventricular function, leading to the erroneous assumption that the left heart is also abnormal. This may be particularly pronounced in advanced pulmonary vascular disease where it is not uncommon for pressures in the right ventricle to approach or even exceed systemic pressures. In this situation the septal muscle hypertrophies, and its motion is altered. Leftward deviation of the septum, especially at the base of the right ventricle, can result in encroachment on the left ventricular outflow tract and compromise its function. This may be part of the explanation for the acute falls in cardiac output and development of pulmonary edema occasionally seen with the use of vasodilator therapy in pulmonary hypertension. Similar distortions in ventricular geometry are seen in patients with cor pulmonale and right ventricular enlargement.

The presence of a common septum may further influence the function of one ventricle in conjunction with the other. The septum acts as a fixation point for the right ventricular free wall and, as it contracts, shifts in relation to the different diastolic pressures in either chamber. Depending on its radius of curvature this can either help or hinder right ventricular ejection. The conformation of the septum also aids systolic ejection of the right ventricle by anchoring the free wall and thereby creating a radial force that draws it toward the septum. The position and curvature of the septum is determined by the balance of forces between the two chambers, which create an axial force. Normally, high pressures within the left ventricular chamber result in an axial force that bows the septum toward the right ventricle during systole, whereas the radial forces produced by the alignment of muscle fibers within the septum predominate in the direction of the left ventricular free wall.

The right ventricle is integrated with the left ventricle by being directly attached to the septal wall and by an anatomic attachment of muscle fibers between the free walls of the left and right ventricles. The close anatomic arrangement of the right ventricle with the left in fact enhances the efficiency of its contraction. The continuity of muscle fibers between the two free walls means that they are pulling together toward a common center of gravity, thereby enhancing contraction [14]. Right ventricular ejection is also enhanced by left ventricular contraction. Isolated heart studies

have shown that an augmented left ventricular volume increases the pressure generated by the right ventricle [15–17]. In addition, there are angiographic studies that show rightward displacement of either a normal muscular or artificial septum associated with left ventricular contraction [13,18–21].

In addition to ventricular interdependence produced by a shared septum, common myocardial muscle fibers, and the intact pericardium, direct mechanical compression of the chambers from inflation and deflation of the lung (mechanical heart–lung interactions) will also affect left heart function. Santamore et al. [22] have shown a decrease in left ventricular diastolic volume and an increase in right ventricular volume during a spontaneous inspiration. In the isolated heart Janicki et al. [23] have demonstrated that, if left ventricular end diastolic volume is held constant while right ventricular end diastolic volume is increased, then left ventricular end diastolic pressure will rise. This diastolic interdependence is thought to be responsible for the decrease in left ventricular stroke volume seen during spontaneous respiration because of an acute change in left ventricular afterload [24]. Studies in intact humans and experimental animals, on the other hand, have shown that, although diastolic compliance of the left ventricle is altered by septal wall shift during right ventricular filling, this does not affect systolic function in the absence of cardiopulmonary disease [25]. The corollary of this is the finding of systolic interdependence. As the right ventricular volume rises the end systolic volume of the left ventricle decreases [26], indicating that the left ventricular stroke volume is maintained. Thus systolic interdependence is a compensatory mechanism for the reduction in left ventricular output caused by diastolic interdependence [27].

The Pericardium

Because it surrounds the heart and limits acute changes in chamber size, the pericardium will influence cardiac function both directly and indirectly through the mechanism of ventricular interdependence. The two ventricles have similar end diastolic volumes so there is little space for acute dilatation within the pericardial space. In the normal situation, the pericardium has some minor influence on both diastolic and systolic functions of the ventricles in that ventricular interaction is enhanced during diastole by transmission of pressures throughout the myocardium. Any influence that the pericardium may have on function of either ventricle is related to a change in transmural pressure across the wall of the myocardium, which in this instance is the difference between intracavity and intrapleural pressures. Therefore, changes in intrapericardial pressure cannot be examined in isolation without making reference to pressure changes in the thorax produced by respiration. In situations where there is an increase in intrapericardial pressure, as in the dilated failing heart or with the development of pericardial fluid accumulation, there can be major alterations in systolic and diastolic performance of both ventricles. However, constraint on ventricular function caused by changes in intrapericardial pressure will always be more pronounced in diastole than in systole. The development of a pericardial effusion will interfere with diastolic filling, and, the larger the effusion and the more rapidly it develops, the greater will be the compromise to ventricular function [28]. The intrapericardial pressure also contributes to ventricular interdependence, being increased in situations of cardiac tamponade [29] and reduced following pericardectomy [30]. As the majority of coronary blood flow occurs during diastole, the pericardial constraint on the right ventricular free wall may limit coronary perfusion in situations where the ventricle has hypertrophied [31,32]. This seems to be particularly important in situations of right heart failure where the dilated failing heart is constrained within the pericardial cavity, resulting in a rise in intrapericardial pressure and interference with diastolic filling. Goldstein et al. [33] have shown that, following right ventricular failure produced by infarction, intrapericardial pressure rises and left ventricular filling decreases. This impairment of diastolic function was confirmed to be caused by an alteration in the diastolic pressure–volume relationship of the ventricle, which could be relieved by pericardiotomy [34]. The effect of pericardial constraint on cardiac function has also been demonstrated after open heart surgery, particularly in situations where right ventricular failure is compromised by the development of pulmonary hypertension [35]. The mechanical constraint on diastolic function produced by intrathoracic pressure provides the rational basis for the practice of either delaying sternal closure or reopening the sternum in the postoperative period in situations of increased myocardial edema following cardiopulmonary bypass [36].

The Effect of Changes in Intrathoracic Pressure on Heart Function

During ventilation gas moves in and out of the lung under the influence of changes in intrathoracic pressure. This results in important changes in hemodynamics, which differ according to whether intrathoracic pressure is negative or positive during inspiration or alveolar pressure is zero or positive at end expiration (PEEP). These changes are also influenced by underlying cardiac or respiratory disease. Although the term *intrathoracic pressure* is used generically to cover all pressure changes within the mediastinum, sometimes a differentiation needs to be made between it, pleural, alveolar, and transpulmonary (alveolar minus pleural) pressures.

Right Heart Function: Spontaneous Versus Positive Pressure Ventilation

In the spontaneously breathing healthy human a fundamental principle of normal cardiovascular physiology is the ability to balance the outputs of the left and right heart, and that, in the event of a sudden change in either venous return or cardiac output, the balance is restored within a few heartbeats. Although the normal heart will pump all the blood returned to it from the venous side of the circulation, differing changes in venous return to the right atrium occur during the inspiratory and expiratory phases of respiration. The forces that govern venous return and how these are influenced by spontaneous respiration have been defined in the classic experiments of Guyton et al. [37–40].

The pressure generated for return of blood flow to the heart is the driving pressure (mean systemic pressure) minus the downstream pressure opposing venous return, which in this instance is the right atrial pressure. Acute elevations in right atrial pressure will result in a fall in cardiac output until compensated for by a change in compliance in the venous capacitance system. The pressure within the venous system is determined by the compliance and the volume of blood in the vascular bed, and, with total circulatory arrest, the mean systemic pressure is 7 mm Hg on both sides of the heart [40]. The negative pleural pressure that occurs during a normal spontaneous inspiration produces a fall in right atrial pres-

sure and hence the upstream pressure that the venous capacitance sees, resulting in increased atrial filling (Figure 3.2). The filling pressure gradient for venous return to the right atrium is usually around 5 mm Hg and is determined by the difference between the extrathoracic and intrathoracic venous pressures. As negative intrathoracic pressure increases the caliber of intrathoracic veins, one might suppose that a dramatic increase in venous return might occur during a reduction in right atrial pressure produced by a deep inspiration. In the normal human there is flow limitation,

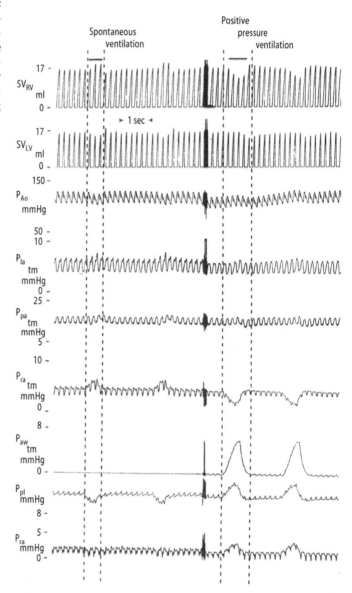

Figure 3.2. Changes in hemodynamics associated with spontaneous and positive pressure ventilation in the normal human. The area between the dashed lines represents the inspiratory phase. The reduction in pleural pressure (P$_{pl}$) during spontaneous inspiration increases right atrial filling and the right atrial pressure (P$_{ra}$) rises together with right ventricular stroke volume (SV$_{RV}$). There is a simultaneous fall in left ventricular stroke volume (SV$_{LV}$). During positive pressure ventilation right heart filling decreases as left ventricular stroke volume rises. For a more detailed explanation, see text. P$_{aw}$, alveolar pressure; tm, transmural; P$_{la}$, left atrial pressure; P$_{pa}$, pulmonary arterial pressure; P$_{Ao}$, pulmonary artery occluded pressure. (From Pinsky MR. In: Dantzker DR, ed. Cardiopulmonary Interactions in Cardiopulmonary Critical Care, 2nd ed. Philadelphia: Saunders; 1991. Copyright 1991 with permission.)

as this augmentation of venous return by negative intrathoracic pressure is limited by the fact that when pleural pressure becomes subatmospheric the extrathoracic veins collapse at the thoracic inlet, limiting flow, while the intrathoracic cavae are maintained patent by a series of valves.

The increase in venous return to the right atrium that occurs during the inspiratory phase of the respiratory cycle increases preload to the right ventricle and results in a transient increase in right ventricular stroke volume. At the same time the rise in right atrial pressure decreases this gradient, so, in effect, there are differing and opposite effects during a single inspiratory cycle. Coincident with the rise in right ventricular stroke volume there is an initial minor fall in left ventricular output, which is caused by the reduction in intrathoracic pressure producing an increase in afterload on the left side (see later) and a fall in preload due to lung expansion causing compression of the extraalveolar pulmonary capillaries.

With the introduction of positive pressure ventilation it was recognized from the outset that there were important effects on hemodynamics that were different from spontaneous respiration. Cournand et al. [41] were the first to show the association between the decreased cardiac output and increased airway pressure in normal humans with mask positive pressure ventilation experiments over 50 years ago. The explanation for this finding was that increased intrathoracic pressure is transmitted to the systemic venous system, which resulted in reduced caval blood flow. The rise in right atrial pressure reduced the gradient for right atrial filling, which in turn leads to a fall in right ventricular stroke volume (see Figure 3.2). This finding has been confirmed in numerous studies since then that have shown that in the absence of cardiopulmonary disease positive intrathoracic pressure will reduce cardiac output through the mechanism of decreased venous return [42–46], especially in situations of absolute or relative hypovolemia, while in the hypervolemic state pulmonary venous return to the left ventricle would be increased because of augmented antegrade flow. In human studies of a postoperative surgical population this was associated with a right atrial pressure of >10 mm Hg [47].

These same principles have also been shown to apply when the increase in pleural pressure occurs without a change in lung volume as in a Valsalva maneuver [48–50]. What has been less widely appreciated is that in the normal situation there is an initial increase in both aortic pressure and left ventricular output early in the inspiratory phase of positive pressure ventilation before falling toward the end of inspiration [45,51–53] and that this increase in aortic pressure is more pronounced at faster respiratory rates (Figure 3.3) [45]. In contrast, changes in respiratory rate have little effect on pulmonary artery flow, which declines during inspiration and rises during expiration. It therefore appears that increased pleural pressure will have different effects on the right and left heart output at different phases of the respiratory cycle where a fall in pulmonary artery flow and rise in pulmonary artery pressure are seen at the same time as there is a rise in both pressure and flow in the aorta early in the inspiratory phase of positive pressure ventilation.

These differing effects require more detailed analysis. Among the theories that have been advanced to account for these differences are a phase lag because of pulmonary blood transit time, reduction in left ventricular afterload associated with positive pleural pressure, increased left ventricular preload because of forward flow of pulmonary venous blood caused by lung expansion, and increased left ventricular compliance because of ventricular interdependence. The fact that pulmonary transit time has little or no bearing on the

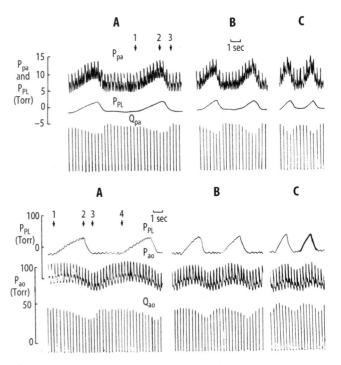

FIGURE 3.3. Pulmonary and aortic blood flow during increasing rates of positive pressure ventilation (**A–C**) measured at 1, beginning of inspiration; 2, end inhalation; and 3, end expiration. Aortic flow (Q_{ao}) begins to decrease shortly after the start of each inspiration, reaching a nadir at end expiration. Aortic pressure (P_{ao}), on the other hand, rises slightly to a peak that occurs closer to end inspiration at more rapid respiratory rates and reaches a nadir that is almost simultaneous with the nadir in Q_{ao}. P_{pa}, pulmonary arterial pressure; P_{PL}, pleural pressure. (From Scharf SM. Hemodynamic effects of positive-pressure ventilation. J Appl Physiol 1980;49:124. Reprinted with permission from the American Physiological Society.)

asynchrony between right and left heart has been demonstrated in the intact animal by Robotham et al. [54]. In their experiments in which right heart output was replaced by a roller pump to maintain a constant left-sided preload, aortic flow still increased during the early phase of inspiration despite the elimination of the variation in right ventricular output. In a further series of experiments in open chest animals, where pleural pressure is no longer a factor, and with the right heart decompressed, eliminating the ventricular interdependence factor, Robotham and Mintzner have also been able to show that the application of positive pressure to the lung still resulted in increased left ventricular output [55].

Many of the studies of the effect of positive pressure ventilation on the right heart have been done in steady-state conditions after increases in intrathoracic pressure rather than examining the instantaneous effects of increases in airway pressure [56]. Also, many of these studies did not take into account the potential impact of the changes in intravascular volume status that might occur in patients on the relationship between intrathoracic pressure and venous return. Important information on caval blood flow is now available using echocardiography and pulsed Doppler techniques [57]. Studies on changes in intrathoracic pressure in normal animals who are not hypovolemic have shown that mean systemic pressure is maintained even as intrathoracic pressure increases [58]. The explanation for this is as the diaphragm descends during inspiration the increase in intraabdominal pressure results in increased venous return by enhancing the splanchnic inferior vena cava flow [59,60]. Under relatively hypervolemic conditions, when right atrial

FIGURE 3.4. The effect of an inspiratory hold on (A) alveolar pressure (Paw), (B) right atrial pressure (P_{ra}), (C) arterial pressure (P_a), (D) pulmonary arterial pressure (P_{pa}), (E) abdominal pressure (P_{abd}), and (F) thermodilution cardiac output (T). With sustained increases in Paw and P_{ra} neither cardiac output nor right ventricular end diastolic pressure volume changed. (From van den Berg et al. [63]. Reprinted with permission from the American Physiological Society.)

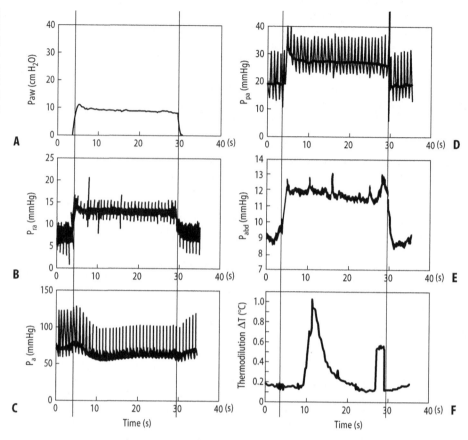

pressure exceeds intraabdominal pressure, the situation is analogous to zone III conditions described for pulmonary blood flow in the lung [61]. In situations of hypovolemia, however, intraabdominal pressure exceeds right atrial pressure (zone II) and the total inferior vena cava venous return is reduced [59,62]. These findings have been confirmed in humans. van Den Berg et al. [63] have shown that, in fluid resuscitated postoperative cardiac surgical patients, increases of airway pressure up to 20 cm H_2O resulted in no change in cardiac output or right ventricular end diastolic volume (Figure 3.4). This was ascribed to the fact that there were parallel increases in right atrial pressure as well as intraabdominal pressure, and therefore there was no effect on venous return. This study demonstrates that venous return can be maintained when intrathoracic pressure and right atrial pressure increase as long as mean systemic pressure increases by an equivalent amount. This happens because the rise in intraabdominal pressure compresses the liver and squeezes the lungs. The same does not apply if the patient is hypovolemic, when increased intrathoracic pressure results in zone II conditions and collapse of the thoracic portion of the vena cava. A summary of these studies would conclude that venous return and stroke volume of the right heart increase because of the negative intrathoracic pressure associated with spontaneous breathing, while positive intrathoracic pressure only significantly impacts on right heart filling when patients are hypovolemic.

Ventilation and Pulmonary Vascular Resistance

Ventilation influences pulmonary vascular resistance in a number of different ways (see Figure 3.1). Changes in alveolar pressure

during spontaneous and positive pressure ventilation alter pulmonary blood flow by changes in the caliber of pulmonary capillaries. Lung distention per se has significant neurohormonal effects on pulmonary vascular resistance and right ventricular function via the vagus nerve and the release of prostanoids, antidiuretic hormone (ADH), atrial natriuretic peptide, and catecholamines [64–69]. There is also the important effect of pH on pulmonary vascular resistance mediated by altering $PaCO_2$, independent of any change in lung volume.

For the purposes of examining the effect of the change in alveolar pressure on pulmonary vascular resistance it has been convenient to think of pulmonary vessels as being divided into two functional groups: the large pulmonary vessels and the heart, which sense changes in interstitial pressure in the lung, and those that are exposed to an extravascular pressure, which reflects alveolar pressure (intraalveolar vessels). The change in blood flow in the intraalveolar vessels depends on their position within the different zones of the lung as outlined by West et al. [61] and Permutt et al. [70], who defined the relationship between pressures in the alveolus (PA) and pulmonary artery (Pa) and left atrium (Pla). Where zone I (lung apex) conditions apply, the pressure within the arterial end of the vessel is less than alveolar pressure (PA > Pa > Pla) and is therefore insufficient to open the vessels, which remain collapsed and there is no flow [71]. These conditions exist in the uppermost parts of the lung in the upright human or in the superior part of the lung when lying supine. Where zone II conditions apply (Pa > PA > Pla), arterial pressure is higher than alveolar and the intraalveolar vessels behave like Starling resistors surrounded by alveolar pressure where flow depends on the difference between arterial and alveolar pressures and is independent of changes in left atrial pressure. These conditions predominate in the mid zone of the lung in the upright and supine human and can also be seen during the inspiratory phase of positive pressure ventilation [72]. In zone II conditions the back pressure to right ventricular ejection is alveolar rather than left atrial pressure, and the relevant resistance is only that between the pulmonary artery and the downstream end of the alveolar vessels. An increase in lung volume produces an increase in back pressure to right ventricular ejection compared with the pressure around the heart and increased afterload. This requires that an approximately equal increase in pressure be produced in the pulmonary artery and alveolus to maintain pulmonary blood flow, which translates into increased right ventricular wall stress. Thus, an increase in alveolar relative to pleural pressure increases right ventricular afterload, and it is this change in alveolar pressure relative to arterial pressure that can produce a marked degree of increased afterload seen in acute asthma [73]. In zone III conditions (Pa > Pla > PA), the pressure in the venous side of the capillary is higher than alveolar pressure and pulmonary blood flow behaves like a Starling resistor where flow is independent of alveolar pressure and is governed by the difference between pulmonary arterial and venous pressures. These conditions predominate in the dependent lung regions.

The effect of a change in lung volume on extraalveolar vessels is somewhat different. An increase in lung volume during inspiration increases radial traction on extraalveolar vessels, increasing their caliber and causing a fall in pulmonary vascular resistance and a decrease in right ventricular afterload. The net effect of these various changes is that pulmonary vascular resistance is lowest at functional residual capacity, is minimally changed at airway pressures of 5–10 cm H_2O, and rises in situations where vessels are compressed during lung collapse or where there is overdistention of the lung [74]. Loss of functional residual capacity, as seen with the development of pulmonary edema or atelectasis, will result in a rise in pulmonary vascular resistance, as will overdistention of the lung caused by airway obstruction or high peak airway pressure ventilation that puts the lung on the flat portion of the pressure volume curve. In this situation, zone I conditions would predominate throughout the lung (PA > Pa > Pla) and pulmonary vascular resistance would be increased. Changes in transpulmonary pressure will have the same effect on pulmonary vascular resistance, whether they are produced by positive or negative changes in pleural pressure.

Important new insights into the effect of positive intrathoracic pressure on right heart function have been gained from the use of echocardiography and pulsed Doppler in critical care medicine [57]. These show that when tidal volume is progressively increased the right ventricle has to generate an increasingly higher pressure to open the pulmonary valve [75]. Increases in transpulmonary pressure (airway pressure minus pleural pressure) and tidal volume during the inspiratory phase of positive pressure ventilation resulted in a sharp but transient reduction in flow acceleration in the pulmonary artery. However, when airway pressure was increased without a change in tidal volume there was no effect on right ventricular afterload.

The effects of PEEP on heart function have been a source of major interest in critical care medicine since the original description of its use in acute respiratory distress syndrome over 30 years ago. These include the potential for diminished myocardial contractility and ventricular compression by lung distention [3]. The application of PEEP in the normal human and animal heart results

in a fall in cardiac output because of a decreased preload (venous return) and increased afterload (pulmonary vascular resistance) [25]. In addition, Doppler flow studies have shown backward flow of blood through the tricuspid valve [76]. Positive end-expiratory pressure, in addition to increasing pleural pressure, will increase lung volume and functional residual capacity depending on lung and chest wall compliance. If application of PEEP overdistends the lung and increases pulmonary vascular resistance, an increase in right ventricular volume will occur that may adversely affect left ventricular compliance by leftward shift of the intraventricular septum. However, in the situation where the appropriate amount of PEEP is being used, lung volume will be recruited, the end-expiratory volume will be at functional residual capacity, and pulmonary vascular resistance will fall. This was confirmed in the classic paper by Suter et al. [77] where they described the "best PEEP" (8 ± 4 cm H_2O), which had no negative effect on pulmonary vascular resistance or impact on cardiac output. This topic is discussed in further detail later in the section on acute respiratory distress syndrome.

High levels of PEEP have been shown to compromise flow in a marginal right coronary circulation because of decreases in flow associated with the rise in right ventricular systolic pressure and intrapericardial pressure [78–80]. Similar observations on the differing effects of PEEP on right ventricular ejection fraction have been made in adults with ischemic heart disease after cardiopulmonary bypass [81]. Patients with pronounced right coronary artery stenosis had diminished right ventricular ejection fraction and increased right ventricular end diastolic volume, whereas there was no effect in patients with minor coronary artery stenosis. Paradoxically, in situations where severe right ventricular failure results in profoundly low cardiac output, ventilation with high peak inflation pressures at rapid rates may result in a rapid improvement in hemodynamics. Serra et al. [82] have reported a dramatic improvement in four children with profound right ventricular failure after corrective cardiac surgery when switching from conventional ventilator settings to higher frequency (50/min), high-volume (TV [tidal volume] 30 mL/kg) ventilation. The increased intrathoracic pressure in this situation probably acts as a right ventricular assist device in increasing forward flow from a dilated and noncontractile right ventricle in much the same way that it produces forward flow in simultaneous ventilation compression cardiopulmonary resuscitation.

The Effect of Changes in Intrathoracic Pressure on Left Heart Function

The changes in intrathoracic pressure produced by respiration have important and hitherto underappreciated effects on left ventricular function that assume greater importance in the failing heart. To evaluate the significance of these various forces and the effects of positive or negative intrathoracic pressure on left ventricular preload and afterload it is important to understand the changes in cardiac output and left heart function secondary to respiration. The most commonly observed change in left heart function that occurs with spontaneous respiration is an initial a fall in arterial pressure during inspiration because of a decrease in left ventricular stroke volume (see Figure 3.2). The reasons for this have been largely attributed to events occurring on the right side of the circulation and include (1) the pooling of blood in the pulmonary circulation because of lung expansion, (2) a phase lag between right and left ventricular output, (3) the stimulation of systemic baroreceptors or pulmonary stretch receptors, and (4) right heart filling causing a change in left ventricular diastolic compliance or ejection mediated through ventricular interdependence. Although studies of pulmonary transit time have shown that it takes one to two cardiac cycles for a change in right-sided output to be reflected in the left side [83,84], the phase lag theory is unlikely to fully explain the decrease in left ventricular ejection associated with a reduction in intrathoracic pressure.

Changes in right heart output must affect the left side as the two circulations are connected in series, which accounts for the observation that blood pressure and left ventricular stroke volume may rise after an initial fall. In this situation, the increase in venous return eventually overrides the other factors that tend to impede left ventricular output. Neural receptors that have been suggested to influence left ventricular function include stretch receptors in the lung mediated via the vagus nerve and intra- and extrathoracic baroreceptors that are mediated by the autonomic system. There is reliable experimental data to suggest that neither of these is likely to be a major mechanism in the fall in left-sided output.

Robotham et al. [85] found that there were still significant falls in left ventricular stroke volume in vagotomized animals during a Mueller maneuver (inspiratory effort against a closed glottis), where intrapleural pressure falls but lung volume remains unchanged. A decrease in left ventricular stroke volume during inspiration is still observed even after autonomic blockade of vagal and sympathetic efferent nerves. If left atrial and ventricular diastolic pressures were measured relative to atmosphere, then one could demonstrate a fall in these pressures during inspiration, which would support the concept that the principal cause of the decrease in left-sided output during inspiration was pooling of blood in the lungs secondary to lung expansion. However, it has been shown that, during inspiration in both the intact animal and the isolated lung preparation, pulmonary venous return actually increases at the same time that left ventricular stroke volume is

falling [86,87]. This apparent paradox is explained when these pressures are related to intrapleural pressure where it can be shown that transmural (intracavity minus intrapleural) filling pressures on the left side actually increase during inspiration. Thus it is more valid to define the afterload as being the left ventricular transmural pressure, which in this instance is the intracavity pressure minus the intrapleural pressure (Figure 3.5).

The observation that afterload increases with negative intrathoracic pressure has been confirmed by studies of left ventricular function during spontaneous breathing with increased inspiratory loads that demonstrated that both left ventricular end diastolic and end systolic volumes are increased [88,89]. However, this occurs independently of changes in lung volume as has been demonstrated in experiments that showed that afterload was found to increase during a Mueller maneuver. Both Brinker et al. [90] and Guzman et al. [91] have also confirmed septal wall displacement during the Mueller maneuver that was associated with decreased diastolic compliance and volume of the left ventricle. Sustained decreases in intrathoracic pressure have also been shown clinically to result in mild degrees of left ventricular dysfunction when associated with ischemic heart disease [92].

Various mechanisms have been invoked to explain the marked fall in left ventricular stroke volume and arterial blood pressure that occurs with large negative intrathoracic pressures during spontaneous respiration during severe airways obstruction. It has been difficult to determine whether this is caused by decreased left ventricular filling or increased afterload, because left ventricular filling and emptying may occur simultaneously with inspiration extending over several cardiac cycles. In a series of experiments, Peters et al. [93,94] have attempted to clarify this issue by synchronizing negative intrathoracic pressure with systole and diastole independently. The findings would suggest that negative intrathoracic pressure with the airway obstructed during systole reduces left ventricular stroke volume predominantly by increasing after-

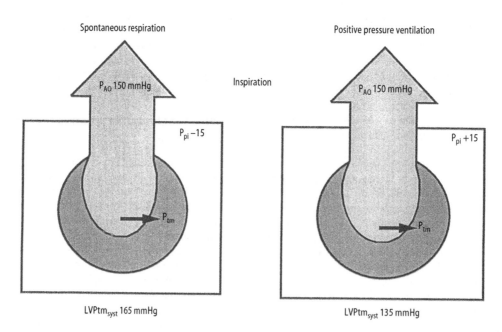

Spontaneous respiration

P_{AO} 150 mmHg

P_{pi} −15

P_{tm}

LVPtm$_{syst}$ 165 mmHg

Positive pressure ventilation

Inspiration

P_{AO} 150 mmHg

P_{pi} +15

P_{tm}

LVPtm$_{syst}$ 135 mmHg

FIGURE 3.5. Changes in afterload on the left ventricle associated with the inspiratory and expiratory phases of spontaneous ventilation. The numbers for pleural and intracavity pressures are arbitrary and chosen only to illustrate the point that afterload (end systolic pressure) increases during inspiration. LVtmsyst, left ventricular transmural systolic pressure; P_{AO}, pulmonary artery occluded pressure; P_{pl}, pleural pressure; P_{tm}, transmural pressure.

load and impedance to blood flow out of the thorax. When negative intrathoracic pressure was synchronized with diastole, left ventricular output fell because of ventricular interdependence.

Because the generation of large negative intrathoracic pressures can impede both diastolic and systolic performance of the left ventricle, it is not surprising that this will occasionally result in acute left ventricular failure and the development of pulmonary edema. This has been well documented during acute upper airway obstruction occurring with laryngospasm during anesthesia [95–97] and with croup and epiglottitis [98–100]. It may also occur following the relief of upper airway obstruction [101] and during status asthmaticus where at the peak of inspiration negative intrathoracic pressures of up to minus 40 cm H_2O can be produced [102]. The overall effect of a negative intrathoracic pressure on left ventricular function is therefore a balance between its effect on the preload and left ventricular systolic ejection (afterload). The increase in afterload caused by negative pleural pressure is one of the mechanisms responsible for the worsening of heart failure seen with obstructive sleep apnea [103,104]. It may become even more pronounced in situations of decreased lung compliance, such as pulmonary edema or lung disease, where there are increasingly negative swings in intrathoracic pressure [105].

The effect of positive pressure ventilation on the left heart is particularly relevant in critical care medicine. The following considerations need to be taken into account: (1) right heart preload and septal shift influence left ventricular end diastolic volume; (2) there is a phase lag before this is manifest in left heart output; (3) the effect is most pronounced at end inspiration; and (4) there is a difference between increased pleural pressure, which impedes venous return, and increased lung volume, which both compresses the heart and increases the pulmonary extraalveolar capacity at peak inspiration. Intrathoracic pressure affects systolic performance, and this is significantly influenced by the underlying function of the left ventricle. Attempts have been made to separate these different effects by examining ventricular function during apnea, by synchronizing ventilation with ventricular systole using a jet ventilator, by changing alveolar pressure independent of intrathoracic pressure with an abdominal binder, and by examining the effect of positive pressure ventilation in a heart failure model induced by β-blockade.

Positive pressure ventilation alters left ventricular function by both mechanical forces and changes in lung volume. An increase in intrathoracic pressure alters diastolic compliance and pericardial pressure. The net result is a decrease in left ventricular end diastolic volume because of decreased preload but no change in systolic right ventricular function. Several studies [85,106,107] have shown that left ventricular dimensions are altered by both intermittent positive pressure ventilation and PEEP in that the septal to free wall and anterior to posterior minor axis dimensions diminish, which is consistent with an overall decrease in left ventricular end diastolic volume. The effect is greater in the septal to free wall dimension, which suggests that ventricular interdependence is the important mechanism that contributes to the decreased left ventricular preload seen with the application of PEEP.

Positive pressure ventilation–induced changes in lung volume also affect left ventricular function independent of the change in intrathoracic pressure. Lung expansion changes the capacitance of the pulmonary venous system, thereby altering pulmonary blood flow depending on the underlying pulmonary blood volume and vascular tone [108]. Increasing lung volume will also restrict cardiac filling in a similar fashion to cardiac tamponade by encroachment

of the lung on the cardiac fossa [3]. This may have important implications in positive pressure ventilation in status asthmaticus where overinflation of the lung caused by rapid respiratory rates and inadequate expiratory time can result in low output and cardiac arrest.

Recently more sophisticated techniques for measuring left heart performance using cardiac echocardiography and conductance catheters have become available. These have allowed investigators to measure chamber size and display pressure–volume loops of the left ventricle while lung volume and intrathoracic pressure were altered [109]. These studies have shown that the influence of ventilation on left ventricular function is complex and influenced by pulmonary mechanics, circulating volume status, and the underlying contractile state of the ventricle. When ventricular function is normal and there is a normal circulating volume, the preload effect predominates and increases in intrathoracic pressure at end inspiration results in a decrease in left ventricular end diastolic volume, without a change in systolic performance. As this occurs at the same time that there is a rise in left ventricular end diastolic pressure, the purported mechanism is compression of the heart by the lungs. When contractility is impaired and ventricular volumes are increased, positive pressure inspiration reduces left ventricular end systolic volume by lowering ejection pressure, improving ejection [109]. This has important implications for the treatment of heart failure, as is discussed later.

Cardiorespiratory Function and Heart Disease

We have seen that in the normal individual a decrease in intrathoracic pressure tends to both augment cardiac output by increased systemic venous return and diminish it by increasing left ventricular afterload—the net result being a balance between these opposite effects. These changes assume greater significance in the setting of abnormal heart function cause by either congenital or acquired heart disease. Knowledge of these interactions is important in order to optimize cardiac performance particularly in ventilated patients in the postoperative period.

Congenital Heart Disease

The presence of congenital heart disease in children will frequently produce changes within the lung and result in respiratory symptoms that sometimes make it difficult to distinguish whether the primary disease process is within the pulmonary or cardiac system. Lesions that produce abnormal patterns of pulmonary blood flow through the lungs can produce changes in mechanics that can both mimic lung disease and, by increasing respiratory work and oxygen consumption, aggravate heart failure. The extent of these changes depends on whether pulmonary blood flow is increased, as in the situation of a left-to-right intracardiac shunt, or decreased, as in the situation of an obstructive right heart lesion. The combination of increased pulmonary blood flow and pulmonary hypertension is well recognized to produce severe respiratory symptoms [110].

Respiratory distress and atelectasis in the spontaneously breathing child can result from compression of the large bronchi by an enlarged left atrium or pulmonary artery dilatation. The left atrium lies immediately inferior to both main stem bronchi, and the left main stem bronchus, left upper lobe bronchus, and right middle lobe bronchus are the most common sites of obstruction [111].

Infantile lobar emphysema has also been described in association with pulmonary stenosis [110]. Rabinovitch et al. [111] have described compression of large bronchi by dilated main pulmonary arteries and compression of intrapulmonary bronchi by tufts of abnormal pulmonary vessels in the tetralogy of Fallot with absent pulmonary valve syndrome. Any of these abnormalities can result in lobar atelectasis, emphysema, intermittent attacks of wheezing, and blood gas abnormalities.

Single-Ventricle Lesions with Duct-Dependent Systemic Perfusion or Systemic-to-Pulmonary Artery Shunts

The management of mechanical ventilation in infants with functional single-ventricle lesions presents some unique challenges. Instead of two ventricles in series, these patients have parallel circulation supported by a single pumping chamber. The objective is to achieve a 1:1 distribution of systemic to pulmonary blood flow, which is consistent with an arterial saturation of 75%–80%, assuming that the pulmonary venous saturation is >95%. Reductions in pulmonary vascular resistance induced by hyperoxia or alkalosis will lead to pulmonary overcirculation and reduced oxygen delivery to other vital organs. This can result in end-organ damage such as cerebral ischemia and necrotizing enterocolitis. Methods to optimize systemic output and control pulmonary blood flow in this situation have included the induction of a moderate degree of hypercarbia with a respiratory acidosis via the addition of inspiratory CO_2 or alveolar hypoxia by decreased FiO_2 (<0.21) in the inspiratory gas mixture. The latter two strategies have been compared in infants with hypoplastic left heart syndrome [112,113]. These studies have shown that the use of an $FiCO_2$ of 3% compared with an FiO_2 of 17% resulted in better oxygen delivery and cerebral oxygen saturation.

These data would suggest that the use of respiratory acidosis is a better method of controlling pulmonary blood flow than using hypoxic gas mixtures. This has been highlighted by a recent study by Taeed et al. [114], who showed that there is a high incidence of pulmonary venous desaturation in infants after the Norwood procedure. Because a key part of the management strategy for limiting pulmonary blood flow in the postoperative period has been to limit the FiO_2 to 0.21 while assuming a saturation of >95% in pulmonary venous blood with an SaO_2 of 75%–80% indicating a 1:1 ratio of systemic to pulmonary blood flow, the assumptions behind this must now be questioned. Decreasing the FiO_2 in this situation may result in hypoxemia and reduced oxygen delivery. Therefore, the preferred strategy should be to use a respiratory acidosis (pH 7.3) to increase pulmonary vascular resistance while maintaining a PaO_2 of 35–40 mm Hg.

Left-to-Right Intracardiac Shunts

Children with congenital heart lesions associated with left-to-right shunts frequently have respiratory symptoms caused by increased pulmonary blood flow. The bronchiolar narrowing caused by the high flows and pulmonary venous pressure produces interstitial and alveolar edema. Hordof et al. [115] have described clinical and radiologic manifestations of peripheral airways obstruction in infants with ventricular septal defect associated with high pulmonary to systemic flow ratios, which regressed with closure of the defect. Schindler et al. [116] have demonstrated that rises in pulmonary artery pressure in the postoperative period are associated with increases in measured airways resistance and that there is increased smooth muscle in the airways of these children. These

observations may explain the finding of sudden episodes of bronchospasm commonly seen in patients who develop rapid rises in pulmonary artery pressure following corrective cardiac surgery for lesions such as ventricular septal defect and atrioventricular septal defect. It is likely that some of the bronchoconstrictor response seen in pulmonary hypertension may be mediated, at least in part, by the leukotriene products of arachidonic metabolism. Leukotrienes C4 and D4, known as mediators of bronchoconstriction in asthma, have been shown to be present in large quantities in the lung lavage fluid of infants with persistent pulmonary hypertension of the newborn [117].

There are also changes in lung compliance seen in congenital cardiac disease [118–120]. Bancalari et al. [118] have found that both total and specific lung compliance were significantly lower in children with congenital heart disease in situations where there was increased pulmonary blood flow compared with lesions with a normal or decreased pulmonary blood flow. When pulmonary blood flow was increased but pulmonary artery pressure was normal, compliance was unchanged, suggesting that it was the pressure level rather than the increased flow within the lung that actually caused the alteration in compliance. Decreased pulmonary compliance has also been described in newborn infants with persistent pulmonary hypertension [121]. It is these changes in compliance that are responsible for the increased respiratory rate and decreased tidal volume seen during spontaneous respiration in children with left-to-right intracardiac shunts [122]. In the infant and small child with a highly compliant chest wall this is frequently associated with chest wall retraction and intercostal recession. With increasing age, these become less prominent as pulmonary vascular resistance rises secondary to increased flow and left-to-right shunting diminishes. These respiratory symptoms are more likely to occur after the first 2 months of life, when the pulmonary vascular resistance drops and left-to-right shunting increases, and before the end of the first year, when the airways become more cartilaginous and less liable to compression [123].

The use of positive pressure ventilation in children with heart failure secondary to increased pulmonary blood flow is effective in reducing respiratory muscle work and oxygen consumption. However, hyperventilation-induced respiratory alkalosis, together with hyperoxia, may actually increase pulmonary blood flow and cause worsening pulmonary edema. Therefore, tidal volume and rate should be adjusted to produce a normal pH or mild respiratory acidosis together with a level of FiO_2 sufficient to produce a SaO_2 of 90%. The application of PEEP may also be effective in limiting pulmonary blood flow.

Obstructive Right Heart Lesions and Cavopulmonary Connections

Patients who undergo surgical reconstruction of obstructive right heart lesions constitute a group in whom changes in intrathoracic pressure have important effects on venous return and pulmonary blood flow. These would include patients with tetralogy of Fallot, tricuspid atresia, and pulmonary atresia, as well as post-Fontan and bidirectional cavopulmonary anastomosis. Diastolic right ventricular dysfunction is a common finding following surgical repair of severe right ventricular outflow tract obstruction and is characterized by a pulsed Doppler signal showing antegrade pulmonary artery flow during atrial systole accompanied by retrograde flow in the superior vena cava [124,125]. This is due to the fact that right ventricular end diastolic pressure exceeds pulmonary artery diastolic pressure because of the stiffness of the right ventricle. There is premature opening of the pulmonary valve and the right ventricle acts as a passive conduit between the right atrium and the pulmonary artery.

In a study by Cullen et al. [126] of postoperative tetralogy patients, half had this feature, and those who did had a higher incidence of ascites and pleural effusions and longer durations of intensive care unit stay. They also made the important observation that during the inspiratory phase of positive pressure ventilation the Doppler signal of antegrade flow in the pulmonary artery disappeared (Figure 3.6). Further important observations of this association between positive intrathoracic pressure and reduced pulmonary blood flow have been made in patients with the Fontan circulation. In this single ventricle type of reconstruction, pulmonary blood flow is dependent on systemic venous pressure. During spontane-

ous respiration, negative pleural pressure is associated with increased pulmonary blood flow [127]. The application of a Valsalva maneuver results in complete obliteration of the Doppler signal of pulmonary blood flow, whereas the Mueller maneuver gives rise to augmentation of the signal (Figure 3.7) [128].

The implication from these studies is that positive intrathoracic (pleural) pressure impedes pulmonary blood flow while negative pressure increases it. This theory was put to the test in a number of studies by Shekerdemian et al. in which positive pressure ventilation was compared with negative pressure delivered by a Hayek high-frequency oscillator in patients after repair of tetralogy and Fontan operation [129–133]. These studies showed that cardiac output and pulmonary blood flow increased by a factor between 40% and 60% during the periods of negative pressure ventilation

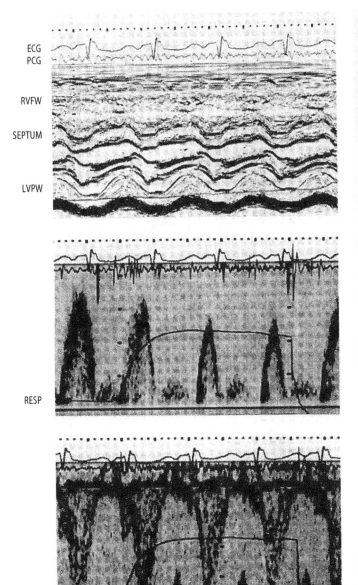

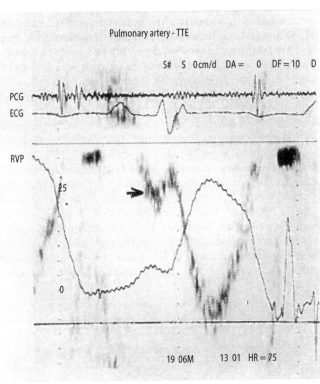

FIGURE 3.6. Transtricuspid **(A)** and pulmonary artery **(B)** Doppler flow in a patient with tetralogy of Fallot demonstrating the effect of positive intrathoracic pressure in restrictive right ventricular physiology. During the inspiratory phase of positive pressure ventilation there is diminution of peak velocity (middle trace) and antegrade pulmonary artery diastolic flow (B, arrow). ECG, electrocardiogram; PCG, phonocardiogram; RVFW, right ventricular free wall; LVPW, left ventricular posterior wall; RESP, respiration. (From Cullen et al. [126]. Copyright 1995 from American Heart Association, Inc. All rights reserved. Reprinted with permission from Lippincott Williams & Wilkins.)

(Figure 3.8). Although it is unlikely that negative pressure will be adopted as the standard for postoperative ventilation in these patients, these studies do demonstrate an important physiologic principle, that is, that all other things being equal, spontaneous breathing is the preferred option over positive pressure ventilation and the goal should be early extubation in this patient population [134]. With increased numbers of children with single-ventricle lesions surviving to the third stage reconstruction, there are important messages to be learned from these studies by practitioners administering anesthesia to patients with Fontan physiology, namely, the importance of maintaining adequate filling pressures and using low intrathoracic pressure ventilation.

A second group of patients with whom there have been important new insights into cardiopulmonary interactions are those following the bidirectional cavopulmonary anastomosis (BCPA) as a second stage reconstruction for single-ventricle lesions. In this operation, the superior vena cava is disconnected from the right atrium and anastomosed to the pulmonary artery. Pulmonary blood flow is dependent on venous return from the head and neck and upper limbs. Oxygenation depends on an adequate transpulmonary pressure gradient between the superior vena cava and the pulmonary capillaries. Typically, the postoperative systemic saturation is in the region of 80%. In patients who remain desaturated after the BCPS, the traditional approach, after ensuring an adequate filling pressure, has been to attempt to reduce the pulmonary vascular resistance with hyperventilation and/or inhaled nitric oxide, which has proved to be largely unsuccessful [135]. Indeed, in a study that measured cerebral blood flow velocity, hyperventilation has been shown to result in worse oxygen saturation in postoperative BCPA patients [136]. The proposed mechanism was an alkalosis induced cerebral vasoconstriction resulting in lower superior vena cava blood flow. This was confirmed in a second study where hypoventilation resulted in improved systemic saturation and increased cerebral blood flow velocity [137]. In both instances care was taken to keep intrathoracic pressure constant in

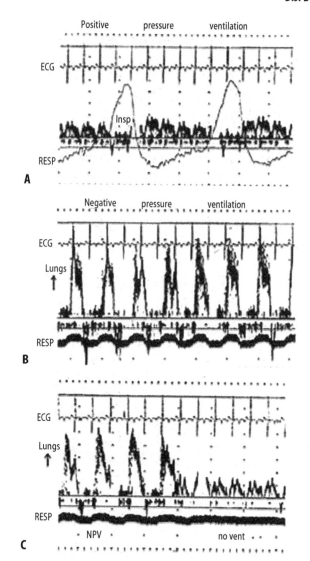

A

B

C

FIGURE 3.8. The effect of **(A)** positive and **(B)** negative pressure ventilation in a patient after the Fontan operation. During the positive pressure inspiration antegrade pulmonary artery flow is lost while there is a marked increase during negative pressure inspiration. The augmentation of pulmonary blood flow was lost when the negative pressure cuirass was removed **(C)**. ECG, electrocardiogram; NPV, negative pressure ventilation; RESP, respiration. (From Shekerdemian et al. [133]. Copyright 1996 from American Heart Association, Inc. All rights reserved. Reprinted with permission from Lippincott Williams & Wilkins.)

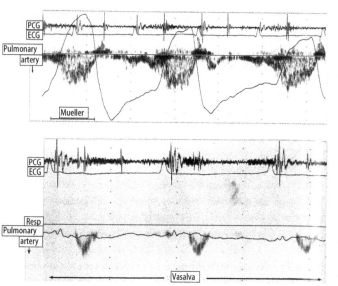

FIGURE 3.7. The effect of changes in intrathoracic pressure on pulmonary blood flow in patients following total cavopulmonary connection measured by Doppler. During the Mueller maneuver the flow signal is augmented, whereas during the Valsalva maneuver it decreases. PCG, phonocardiogram; ECG, electrocardiogram; RVP, right ventricular pressure. (From Redington et al. [128]. Reproduced with permission from the BMJ Publishing Group.)

order to minimize any impact on pulmonary blood flow. This suggestion that cerebral and therefore pulmonary blood flow is increased during hypercarbia was confirmed in a more recent study where cerebral oxygen saturation and systemic oxygen delivery increased at $PaCO_2$ levels of 45 and 55 mmHg compared with 35 mmHg [138,139]. These studies suggest that mild hypercarbia is the best ventilation strategy after the BCPA.

Acquired Heart Disease: Positive Pressure Ventilation and Heart Failure

The cardiac effects of the negative pleural pressure during spontaneous respiration have been discussed previously. Whether the increase in afterload on the left ventricle becomes hemodynamically significant depends on the underlying pump function. If ventricular function is normal, the negative intrathoracic pressure associated with spontaneous breathing will result in little or no significant hemodynamic change [140]. However, some of the studies that have examined the magnitude of the afterload effect produced by increased negative or positive intrathoracic pressure have tended to underestimate its significance because of different methods of measuring afterload. Considering the left ventricle in isolation, in situations where there is a major change in intrathoracic pressure associated with increasing negative intrapleural pressures secondary to lung disease or positive intrapleural pressures secondary to mechanical ventilation, aortic pressure does not reflect left ventricular afterload. Buda et al. [141], in a study of the effects of Valsalva and Mueller maneuvers on left ventricular function in humans, found that left ventricular ejection fraction decreased despite an increase in left ventricular volume and a decline in arterial pressure. When arterial pressures were corrected for changes in intrapleural pressure, they correlated better with left ventricular end systolic volumes than with uncorrected arterial pressures. These findings suggested that negative intrathoracic pressure affects left ventricular function by increasing left ventricular transmural pressures and thus afterload. Physiologically more consistent function curves for the left ventricle were obtained when transmural pressure was used for the pressure load for left ventricular ejection. If the left ventricular filling pressure is unchanged, similar changes in left ventricular afterload can result from either reducing aortic pressure by vasodilator therapy or increasing intrathoracic pressure if the net result is no change in transmural pressure.

Although acute impairment of left ventricular ejection associated with the generation of large negative intrathoracic pressures can be demonstrated when ventricular function is normal [88,89,92,142], it is only comparatively recently that the clinical significance of this has been realized in the presence of left ventricular failure. Rasanen et al. [143] showed that changing from spontaneous to positive pressure breathing in patients with myocardial infarction resulted in a decrease in the pattern of injury seen on the electrocardiogram and subsequently confirmed that the myocardial sparing occurred only when the negative swings in intrathoracic pressure were abolished [144,145]. Similarly, Beach et al. [146] have described a series of adult patients with left ventricular failure supported with positive pressure ventilation who could not tolerate weaning to spontaneous ventilation until left ventricular function was improved with inotropic support. However, raised intrathoracic pressure does have the potential to adversely affect contractility in the setting of marginal coronary blood flow. Positive end-expiratory pressure has been reported to cause a decrease in myocardial blood flow in experimental animals [147,148] and Tittley et al. [149] have shown that the application of 15 cm H_2O after coronary artery bypass surgery resulted in small but measurable amounts of markers of marginal coronary perfusion in half the patients studied without a change in ventricular function.

Based on these findings we can conclude that in patients with overt cardiac failure or borderline left ventricular function the increased afterload associated with the negative intrathoracic pressure generated during spontaneous respiration will result in worsening heart failure. Furthermore, in situations where pulmonary edema develops following myocardial infarction the pulmonary venous congestion and alveolar flooding that occur lead to a fall in lung compliance that translates into increased respiratory work and greater negative intrathoracic pressure [105]. In this situation respiratory muscle work may contribute significantly to inadequate oxygen delivery and lactic acidosis. Under these conditions positive intrathoracic pressure with the use continuous positive airway pressure may result in rapid improvement in the situation with interruption of the cycle of increasingly negative intrathoracic pressure producing an ever decreasing lung compliance. Therefore, increasing intrathoracic pressure, far from adversely affecting cardiac output, as has been widely assumed for many years, may in fact enhance cardiac performance as long as filling pressures are adequate [150,151]. The extreme example of this would be the discovery that during ventricular fibrillation, when there is no left ventricular function output, raising pleural pressure by coughing results in forward blood flow out of the thorax by a combination of the direct effect on the heart and great vessels and the decreased afterload. This phenomenon is commonly referred to as *cough CPR* [152].

Some of the most interesting insights into the effects of elevations in intrathoracic pressure in the setting of left ventricular failure come from the work of Pinsky and colleagues [153–159]. In their animal model, left ventricular failure was induced with large doses of β-adrenergic blockade while adequate venous return was maintained by volume infusion. In order to study the effects of large increases in intrathoracic pressure on cardiac function without overdistending the lung and causing increased pulmonary vascular resistance and pulmonary barotraumas, they reduced thoracic cage compliance by applying a thoracoabdominal binder [153]. Tidal volumes of 35 mL/kg were used to produce a *phasic high intrathoracic pressure support* (PHIPS) ventilation. This study showed that there was an improvement in both left and right ventricular function curves with increased intrathoracic pressure, a finding that they attributed to a decrease in left ventricular wall stress analogous to the use of vasodilator therapy in congestive heart failure. The same technique was applied to a group of patients with cardiogenic shock, and when conventional ventilator settings were changed to the PHIPS technique there was an improvement in cardiac output and mean arterial pressure [160]. Although it is clear that these large changes in intrathoracic pressure augment cardiac output in the failing heart, the mechanism responsible for this action is a balance between the effect on left ventricular preload and afterload. Large changes in lung volume will affect intra- and extraalveolar blood volume [108] and result in increased forward flow. At the same time increased intrathoracic pressure will reduce left ventricular afterload.

These differing mechanisms were studied in a further series of experiments by Pinsky et al. [44] where they varied respiratory frequency, percent inspiratory time, and swings in intrathoracic pressure using a jet ventilator under normal conditions and during acute left ventricular failure. They found that despite a decrease in transmural left atrial pressure, a rise in intrathoracic pressure resulted in an increase in left ventricular stroke volume. Furthermore, this increase in stroke volume continued until a lower limit of left atrial pressure was reached after which there was no further augmentation of left ventricular stroke volume. This demonstrates that when cardiac function is reduced and filling pressures are elevated, an increase in intrathoracic pressure can result in an increase in cardiac output despite a fall in filling pressures. However, this augmentation becomes limited once a critical value is reached when cardiac output becomes again dependent on filling pressures. A similar effect has been described when intrathoracic pressure is increased by the addition of PEEP in the setting of left ventricular dysfunction in humans. The application of PEEP in this situation does not result in a decrease in cardiac output until the filling pressure fell below 15 mm Hg [150].

These data and data from human studies that show enhanced cardiac performance with increased intrathoracic pressure in the setting of cardiogenic shock [143,144] would suggest that this aspect of the beneficial effect of increased intrathoracic pressure on left ventricular performance is influenced by preload, being least beneficial when left ventricular filling was reduced and most marked where left ventricular filling pressures were elevated. It has also become evident that hemodynamic changes that occur with increased intrathoracic pressure vary according to different phases in the cardiac cycle. This has been demonstrated in further studies by Pinsky et al. [161], where positive pressure ventilation was linked to the cardiac cycle by the use of a jet ventilator in animals with left ventricular failure. When positive pressure was timed to occur early in diastole in normal animals, left ventricular stroke volume was decreased, whereas when it was timed to coincide with early systole there was no effect. In addition, it was noted that positive pressure was phased with early diastole, the reduction in stroke volume of the right ventricle preceded that of the left ventricle by one to two heartbeats, suggesting that the cause of the reduction was due to a reduced venous return. In the animals with left ventricular failure, increased intrathoracic pressure in phase with systole increased left ventricular stroke volume compared with diastole, although the increased intrathoracic pressure in either phase was associated with increased stroke volume when compared with apnea. These investigators then compared the hemodynamic effects of increases in intrathoracic pressure synchronized to early and late systole. They found that while increased intrathoracic pressure in both phases of the systolic cycle was associated with an increase in stroke volume when compared to apnea, early systolic phase ventilation resulted in an increase in stroke volume without a change in aortic pressure, while late systolic ventilation increased both stroke volume and pressure. These findings would suggest that positive pressure ventilation synchronized with early cardiac systole allows for left ventricular ejection into a volume-depleted thoracic aorta. They have recently applied these principles in the clinical arena for the ventilatory management of patients with severe congestive cardiomyopathy who are undergoing heart transplantation [162] when they compared the effects of high-frequency jet ventilation (HFJV) synchronized with cardiac systole, HFJV

asynchronous with the cardiac cycle, and conventional ventilation at similar levels of intrathoracic pressure They found that changing to synchronous HFJV was associated with an increase in cardiac output compared with the other modes of ventilation.

The Use of Noninvasive Continuous Positive Airway Pressure in Heart Failure

One of the most important advances in the treatment of congestive heart failure in the past decade has been the use of non-invasive ventilation either in the form of continuous positive airway pressure (CPAP) or bilevel positive airway pressure (BiPAP) [103–105,163–171]. The predominant hemodynamic effect of increased intrathoracic pressure will be caused by changes in preload if contractility and circulating volume are normal, whereas in situations of reduced left ventricular function, where filling pressures are frequently elevated, the principal hemodynamic change will be changes in left ventricular wall stress (afterload). This has been confirmed in human studies where nasal CPAP has been used to treat adult patients with congestive heart failure. The application of 5 cm H_2O in patients with congestive cardiac failure and a pulmonary capillary wedge pressure greater than 12 mm Hg resulted in an increase in the measured cardiac output while it remained unchanged or fell in patients whose cardiac failure was associated with a normal filling pressure (Figure 3.9) [163]. In a further study, application of CPAP of 5, 7.5, and 10 cm H_2O showed a similar beneficial effect in that left ventricular systolic transmural pressure (afterload) fell [105]. The same group has been able to demonstrate improved left ventricular function and symptomology in a randomized controlled trial of nocturnal nasal CPAP in patients with heart failure associated with Cheyne-Stokes respiration and central sleep apnea [104]. Other randomized trials in adults have shown a reduction in the need for tracheal intubation [171], a reduction in the degree of mitral regurgitation and atrial natriuretic factor levels [168], decreases in respiratory muscle effort [172], improved left ventricular end systolic dimensions, and improved left ventricular ejection fraction, as well as reduced heart rate and blood pressure [167].

There are no equivalent studies in children. However, CPAP and BiPAP have become widely accepted in pediatric practice for the treatment of myocarditis and cardiomyopathy. These patients have

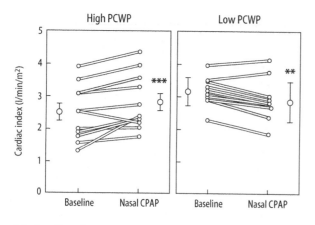
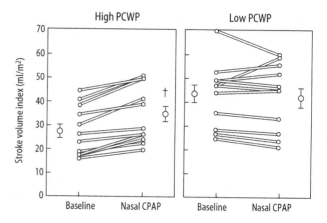

FIGURE 3.9. The effect of nasal continuous positive airway pressure (CPAP) on cardiac output in a series of adult patients with congestive heart failure. Individual data for patients with high and low capillary wedge pressures (PCWP) are shown together with the grouped data. With the application of CPAP, cardiac index rose in 10 of 11 high PCWP patients while it decreased in 9 of 11 in the low PCWP group. $**p < 0.025$, $***p < 0.001$ compared with baseline. (From Bradley et al. [163]. Copyright 1992 from American Lung Association. Reprinted with permission.)

severely reduced ventricular function and increased respiratory distress due to pulmonary edema. The use of noninvasive ventilation avoids the need to administer the sedative/anesthetic drugs that would be required for tracheal intubation with the precipitate drop in cardiac output that it would produce. The dual effect of decreasing respiratory work at the same time as decreasing the left ventricular afterload often leads to a dramatic symptomatic improvement.

Heart–Lung Interactions in Sepsis and Acute Respiratory Distress Syndrome

One of the most important areas where positive intrathoracic pressure potentially impacts on cardiac function is in patients with sepsis and the acute respiratory distress syndrome (ARDS). The current focus on lung recruitment strategies using high PEEP as part of the open lung approach, while improving oxygenation, pays scant attention to what impact this might have on cardiac function. If the only consideration were an improvement in oxygenation, then it would simply be a case of increasing PEEP until the best PaO_2 was achieved. However, the potential adverse effects of PEEP on cardiac function means that the most important therapeutic goal is the level of PEEP that gives the best combination of oxygenation and cardiac output, thereby achieving maximum oxygen delivery (oxygen content × cardiac output), a level frequently referred to as *best* or *optimal PEEP* [77]. Given that ARDS is a multisystem disease it is important that we focus our attention on how positive pressure ventilation, PEEP, and lung disease affect the other major organ that shares the chest cavity.

In the past, attempts to define the effects of PEEP on the cardiovascular system have relied on studies in intact animals and small studies in humans using intracardiac pressure measurements from pulmonary artery catheters in normal and disease states. These studies have shown that the magnitude of changes depend partly on factors that influence the underlying cardiovascular status (circulating volume, ventricular dysfunction, increased pulmonary vascular resistance) and on factors within the lung that may modulate the transmission of airway (alveolar) pressure to the pleural space and consequently to the heart and vascular structures. Decreased lung compliance will reduce pressure transmission, whereas increased thoracic compliance will enhance it [173,174]. Taking all these factors into consideration it is not unusual to see a fall in cardiac output and stroke volume with high levels of positive pressure ventilation with PEEP in ARDS. The mechanisms that have been invoked as a cause for this decrease include decreased venous return, increased right ventricular afterload, decreased left ventricular compliance, and decreased ventricular contractility. However, these studies are limited by the fact that pressure was measured rather than changes in volume.

The importance of right ventricular function in patients with ARDS has been the subject of increasing attention [10,72,75,175–179]. As is seen with positive pressure ventilation in the normal lung, the increase in pleural pressure with PEEP will reduce venous return to the right heart in ARDS [180–182], and this is frequently compensated for by increasing filling pressures. In patients with severe acute respiratory failure, levels of PEEP above 10 cm H_2O have also been associated with an increase in right ventricular afterload [180,182–184]. In the setting of severely depressed baseline right ventricular ejection in humans, the application of PEEP

has been shown to result in the depression of contractile function [185]. Following right coronary artery ligation in animals, application of PEEP caused right ventricular ejection fraction to decline, which was associated with an increase in end systolic volume [186]. Even in the absence of overt ischemia acute right heart dysfunction has been identified as a cause of morbidity and mortality in ARDS [187]. This is not only because of the effects of ventilation and PEEP but also a result of the underlying lung disease. The alveolar collapse and microvascular obstruction cause an increase in pulmonary vascular resistance and pulmonary artery pressure [188], and there is an association between this increase in pulmonary vascular resistance and mortality [189].

The more widespread use of echocardiography and pulse Doppler has improved our understanding of the effect of PEEP on right heart function or cor pulmonale in ARDS. Before the advent of reduced tidal volume ventilation a 61% incidence of acute cor pulmonale, defined as paradoxical septal motion with acute right ventricle enlargement, was reported in adults with ARDS (Figure 3.10) [177]. More recently the same investigators reported a 25% incidence in a study where tidal volume was limited to 8 mL/kg [179]. Another study compared the effect on pulmonary blood flow of zero PEEP with two other levels of PEEP, one determined by the level of PEEP that resulted in the highest value of lung compliance, and the second by the coordinates for the lower inflection point on the lung pressure–volume curve [190]. These investigators found that the PEEP level that had the least effect on right ventricle impedance was that associated with highest compliance (6 ± 3 cm H_2O), a number remarkably similar to that found in the best PEEP study by Suter et al. 30 years ago (8 cm H_2O) [77]. In a landmark study in 1981, Jardin et al. [191] measured right and left heart pressures together with measurements of chamber size with echocardiography while PEEP levels of up to 25 cm H_2O were applied. They found that increasing levels of PEEP were associated with a gradual decrease in left ventricular end systolic and end diastolic dimensions as lung hyperinflation-induced increases in right ventricular afterload led to leftward shift of the septum, which encroached on the left ventricular cavity (Figure 3.11). The thin-walled right ventricle dilates as afterload increases, but the free wall is constrained by the pericardium and therefore it can only dilate leftward as the end diastolic volume increases. In previous studies the reduction in cardiac output was frequently compensated for by expansion of circulating volume, which increased right ventricular preload and right ventricular myocardial segment length [180,182, 183,191–193]. In this study, however, the fall in cardiac output could be compensated for by infusing volume only in patients who were on low levels of PEEP. Left ventricular contractility was unaltered by any level of PEEP.

Echocardiography has also been a very useful tool in helping us understand more ventilation-induced changes in intrathoracic pressure and intravascular volume in patients with sepsis and ARDS. Investigators have used echocardiography, pulsed Doppler, and interrogation of the arterial pulse pressure to evaluate changes in chamber dimensions, collapsibility of the great veins, and the response to volume loading [2,53,57,175,178,179,194–206]. It has long been recognized that arterial pressure rises during positive pressure lung inflation, a phenomenon sometimes referred to as *reversed pulsus paradoxus* [207,208]. The changes in pulse pressure can be described as a succession of inspiratory increases followed by expiratory decreases [53]. Studies in humans with sepsis and respiratory failure have shown that at peak inflation the left ventricular stroke volume increases while that of the right ventricle

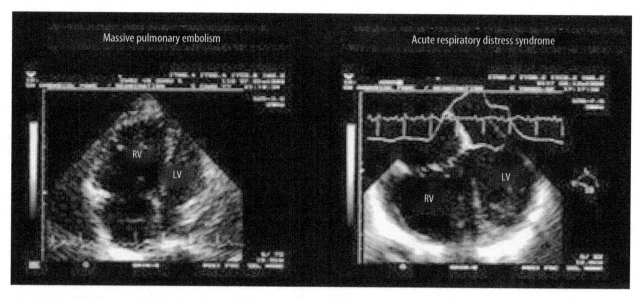

FIGURE 3.10. Two examples of acute right heart dilatation affecting left heart compliance in acute pulmonary embolism and acute respiratory distress syndrome. The septum is shifted leftward and encroaches on the left ventricular (LV) cavity RV, right ventricular. (From Jardin [2]. With kind permission of Springer Science+Bussiness Media.)

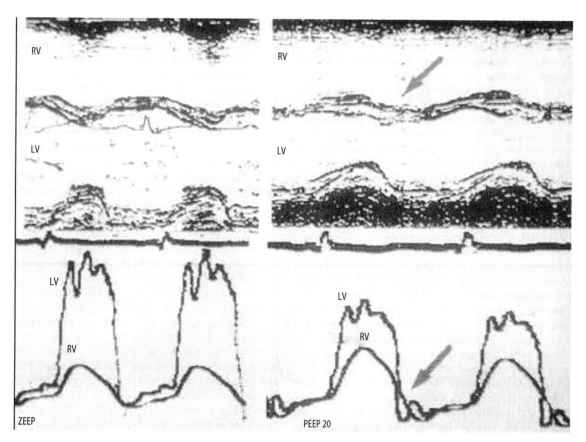

FIGURE 3.11. (Top) Cardiac M-mode echo recording of septal wall motion before and after the application of 20 cm H$_2$O positive end-expiratory pressure (PEEP). This produces paradoxical septal motion with leftward displacement at end systole (arrow). **(Bottom)** Simultaneous right ventricular (RV) and left ventricular (LV) pressure recordings that show reversal of the transeptal pressure gradient at end systole (arrow) and diastolic pressure equalization, maintaining the ventricular septum in a shifted position. (From Jardin et al. [195]. Reprinted with permission from American College of Chest Physicians.)

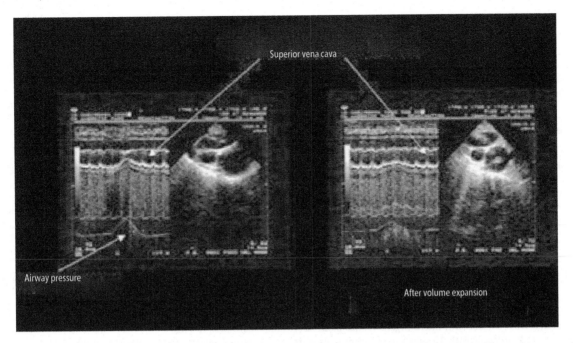

FIGURE 3.12. Illustration of the effect of positive intrathoracic pressure on superior vena cava flow in a patient before and after volume expansion. The superior vena cava demonstrates "collapsibility" at peak inspiration before volume expansion. (From Jardin [2]. With kind permission of Springer Science+Business Media.)

falls. The increase in alveolar pressure is associated with an increase in left atrium size and an augmented Doppler flow signal in the pulmonary veins as the capillaries are squeezed [198]. At the same instant right ventricular stroke volume falls because of an increase in impedance [202], while the delay in refilling of the capillary bed results in a drop in arterial pulse pressure back to the preinspiratory level as the filling reserve of the left ventricle falls in the next few cardiac cycles [198,209]. In patients who are hypovolemic there is a pronounced fall in arterial pulse pressure reflecting predominantly a reduction in RV preload that results in reduced left ventricular stroke volume. The amplitude of the expiratory decrease has been used to detect fluid responsiveness [210,211]. Vieillard-Baron and co-workers have also used echocardiography measurements of inferior vena cava and superior vena cava sizes during inspiration and expiration to diagnose hypovolemia [199,212], as well as a *collapsibility index*, to help guide fluid administration in ventilated patients with sepsis (Figure 3.12) [57,197].

Similar principles that govern the increased intrathoracic pressure associated with positive pressure ventilation govern the use of noninvasive ventilation in ARDS. Depending on the underlying lung compliance, patients who are capable of maintaining adequate spontaneous ventilation in ARDS with use of CPAP may achieve better oxygenation for the same level of PEEP with less adverse hemodynamic effect and therefore better oxygen delivery because of the lower mean airway pressures [213–215]. Dhainaut et al. [180] have observed that when patients were changed from spontaneous respiration to CPAP in ARDS there is a decrease in right ventricular end systolic and end diastolic volumes, suggesting a fall in right ventricular afterload. Jardin et al. [184] have observed the opposite effects in normal subjects without lung disease. The explanation for this discrepancy lies in the fact that when functional residual capacity is normal, pulmonary vascular resistance is at its lowest and right ventricular afterload is minimal. The application of CPAP in normal individuals will increase lung volume above functional residual capacity and compress the extraalveolar vessels, thereby

increasing right ventricular afterload. In ARDS, functional residual capacity is considerably reduced and pulmonary vascular resistance is increased at these low lung volumes, a situation that can be reversed by the application of CPAP. Dhainaut et al. [180] have also been able to demonstrate during CPAP both cardiac output and oxygen consumption decrease, but, with volume expansion, cardiac output increases while oxygen consumption remains low, suggesting decreased oxygen demand. They have suggested that the explanation for the reduced demand is the reduction in oxygen consumed by the work of breathing following the application of CPAP.

Conclusion

The interactions between the cardiac and respiratory systems as the blood flows through the thorax are complex and become increasingly important in the presence of cardiorespiratory disease. Spontaneous and positive pressure ventilation modes have differing and often opposite effects on cardiac function. The alteration in cardiac output that occurs with respiration is caused by changes in both pleural pressure and lung volume, the former affecting right heart filling and left heart afterload while changes in lung volume affect pulmonary vascular resistance and right ventricular afterload. Changes in preload and afterload in either ventricle can affect the opposite chamber by the mechanism of ventricular interdependence. In left heart failure the positive intrathoracic pressure generated by mechanical ventilation may cause a reduction in stroke volume because of inhibition of right heart filling. This is frequently more than compensated for by the decrease in afterload.

Children with obstructive right heart lesions and single-ventricle physiology present some unique challenges in managing their pulmonary blood flow. In patients with ARDS the combination of pulmonary vascular changes and the effect of positive intrathoracic pressure have important effects on cardiac function. However, in a new era of ventilation in ARDS where permissive hypercapnia together with an open lung strategy has become the standard of care we may have to redirect our attention to their affects on heart function rather than simply assuming that what is good for the lungs is good for all other organs.

References

1. Bove AA, Santamore WP. Ventricular interdependence. Prog Cardiovasc Dis 1981;23:365–388.
2. Jardin F. Ventricular interdependence: how does it impact on hemodynamic evaluation in clinical practice? Intensive Care Med 2003;29:361–363.
3. Lloyd TC, Jr. Mechanical cardiopulmonary interdependence. J Appl Physiol 1982;52:333–339.
4. Donald DE, Essex HE. Pressure studies after inactivation of the major portion of the canine right ventricle. Am J Physiol 1954;176:155–161.
5. Kagan A. Dynamic responses of the right ventricle following extensive damage by cauterization. Circulation 1952;5:816–823.
6. Sawatani S, Mandell G, Kusaba E, et al. Ventricular performance following ablation and prosthetic replacement of right ventricular myocardium. Trans Am Soc Artif Intern Organs 1974;20 B:629–636.
7. Starr I, Jeffers WA, Meade RHJ. The absence of conspicuous increments of venous pressure after severe damage to the right ventricle of the dog, with a discussion of the relationship between clinical congestive failure and heart disease. Am Heart J 1943;26:291.
8. Fontan F, Baudet E. Surgical repair of tricuspid atresia. Thorax 1971;26:240–248.
9. Hurford W, Barlai-Kovach M, Strauss H, et al. Canine biventricular performance during acute progressive pulmonary microembolisation. J Crit Care 1987;2:270.
10. Hurford WE, Zapol WM. The right ventricle and critical illness: a review of anatomy, physiology, and clinical evaluation of its function. Intensive Care Med 1988;14(Suppl 2):448–457.
11. Grossman W, Braunwald E, Mann T, et al. Contractile state of the left ventricle in man as evaluated from end-systolic pressure-volume relations. Circulation 1977;56:845–852.
12. Suga H, Sagawa K. Instantaneous pressure–volume relationships and their ratio in the excised, supported canine left ventricle. Circ Res 1974;35:117–126.
13. Pearlman AS, Clark CE, Henry WL, et al. Determinants of ventricular septal motion. Influence of relative right and left ventricular size. Circulation 1976;54:83–91.
14. Robotham JL, Scharf SM. Effects of positive and negative pressure ventilation on cardiac performance. Clin Chest Med 1983;4:161–187.
15. Oboler AA, Keefe JF, Gaasch WH, et al. Influence of left ventricular isovolumic pressure upon right ventricular pressure transients. Cardiology 1973;58:32–44.
16. Santamore WP, Lynch PR, Heckman JL, et al. Left ventricular effects on right ventricular developed pressure. J Appl Physiol 1976;41:925–930.
17. Santamore WP, Lynch PR, Meier G, et al. Myocardial interaction between the ventricles. J Appl Physiol 1976;41:362–368.
18. Badke FR, Boinay P, Covell JW. Effects of ventricular pacing on regional left ventricular performance in the dog. Am J Physiol 1980;238:H858–H867.
19. Little WC, Barr WK, Crawford MH. Altered effect of the Valsalva maneuver on left ventricular volume in patients with cardiomyopathy. Circulation 1985;71:227–233.
20. Shimazaki Y, Kawashima Y, Mori T, et al. Ventricular function of single ventricle after ventricular septation. Circulation 1980;61:653–660.
21. Weyman AE, Wann S, Feigenbaum H, et al. Mechanism of abnormal septal motion in patients with right ventricular volume overload: a cross-sectional echocardiographic study. Circulation 1976;54:179–186.
22. Santamore WP, Heckman JL, Bove AA. Right and left ventricular pressure–volume response to respiratory maneuvers. J Appl Physiol 1984;57:1520–1527.
23. Janicki JS, Reeves RC, Weber KT, et al. Application of a pressure servo system developed to study ventricular dynamics. J Appl Physiol 1974;37:736–741.
24. Robotham JL. Cardiovascular disturbances in chronic respiratory insufficiency. Am J Cardiol 1981;47:941–949.
25. Rankin JS, Olsen CO, Arentzen CE, et al. The effects of airway pressure on cardiac function in intact dogs and man. Circulation 1982;66:108–120.
26. Weber KT, Janicki JS, Shroff SG, et al. The right ventricle: physiologic and pathophysiological considerations. Crit Care Med 1983;11:323–328.
27. Slinker BK, Glantz SA. End-systolic and end-diastolic ventricular interaction. Am J Physiol 1986;251:H1062–H1075.
28. Janicki JS. Influence of the pericardium and ventricular interdependence on left ventricular diastolic and systolic function in patients with heart failure. Circulation 1990;81:III15–III20.
29. Reddy PS, Curtiss EI, O'Toole JD, et al. Cardiac tamponade: hemodynamic observations in man. Circulation 1978;58:265–272.
30. Taylor RR, Covell JW, Sonnenblick EH, et al. Dependence of ventricular distensibility on filling of the opposite ventricle. Am J Physiol 1967;213:711–718.
31. Jarmakani JM, McHale PA, Greenfield JC Jr. The effect of cardiac tamponade on coronary haemodynamics in the awake dog. Cardiovasc Res 1975;9:112–117.
32. O'Rourke RA, Fischer DP, Escobar EE, et al. Effect of acute pericardial tamponade on coronary blood flow. Am J Physiol 1967;212:549–552.
33. Goldstein JA, Vlahakes GJ, Verrier ED, et al. The role of right ventricular systolic dysfunction and elevated intrapericardial pressure in the genesis of low output in experimental right ventricular infarction. Circulation 1982;65:513–522.
34. Goto Y, Yamamoto J, Saito M, et al. Effects of right ventricular ischemia on left ventricular geometry and the end-diastolic pressure-volume relationship in the dog. Circulation 1985;72:1104–1114.
35. del Nido PJ, Williams WG, Villamater J, et al. Changes in pericardial surface pressure during pulmonary hypertensive crises after cardiac surgery. Circulation 1987;76:III93–III96.
36. Shore DF, Capuani A, Lincoln C. Atypical tamponade after cardiac operation in infants and children. J Thorac Cardiovasc Surg 1982;83:449–452.
37. Guyton AC, Lindsey AW, Abernathy B, et al. Mechanism of the increased venous return and cardiac output caused by epinephrine. Am J Physiol 1958;192:126–130.
38. Guyton AC, Lindsey AW, Abernathy B, et al. Venous return at various right atrial pressures and the normal venous return curve. Am J Physiol 1957;189:609–615.
39. Guyton AC, Lindsey AW, Gilluly JJ. The limits of right ventricular compensation following acute increase in pulmonary circulatory resistance. Circ Res 1954;2:326–332.
40. Guyton AC, Lindsey AW, Kaufmann BN. Effect of mean circulatory filling pressure and other peripheral circulatory factors on cardiac output. Am J Physiol 1955;180:463–468.
41. Cournand A, Motley H, Werko L, et al. Physiological studies of the effect of intermittent positive pressure breathing on cardiac output in man. Am J Physiol 1948;152:162–174.
42. Brecher GA, Hubay CA. Pulmonary blood flow and venous return during spontaneous respiration. Circ Res 1955;3:210–214.
43. Charlier AA, Jaumin PM, Pouleur H. Circulatory effects of deep inspirations, blocked expirations and positive pressure inflations at equal transpulmonary pressures in conscious dogs. J Physiol 1974;241:589–605.
44. Pinsky MR, Matuschak GM, Klain M. Determinants of cardiac augmentation by elevations in intrathoracic pressure. J Appl Physiol 1985;58:1189–1198.

45. Scharf SM, Brown R, Saunders N, et al. Hemodynamic effects of positive-pressure inflation. J Appl Physiol 1980;49:124–131.

46. Scharf SM, Caldini P, Ingram RH Jr. Cardiovascular effects of increasing airway pressure in the dog. Am J Physiol 1977;232:H35–H43.

47. Jellinek H, Krafft P, Fitzgerald RD, et al. Right atrial pressure predicts hemodynamic response to apneic positive airway pressure. Crit Care Med 2000;28:672–678.

48. Brooker JZ, Alderman EL, Harrison DC. Alterations in left ventricular volumes induced by Valsalva manoeuvre. Br Heart J 1974;36:713–718.

49. Korner PI, Tonkin AM, Uther JB. Reflex and mechanical circulatory effects of graded Valsalva maneuvers in normal man. J Appl Physiol 1976;40:434–440.

50. Parisi AF, Harrington JJ, Askenazi J, et al. Echocardiographic evaluation of the Valsalva maneuver in healthy subjects and patients with and without heart failure. Circulation 1976;54:921–927.

51. Morgan BC, Crawford EW, Guntheroth WG. The hemodynamic effects of changes in blood volume during intermittent positive-pressure ventilation. Anesthesiology 1969;30:297–305.

52. Morgan BC, Martin WE, Hornbein TF, et al. Hemodynamic effects of intermittent positive pressure respiration. Anesthesiology 1966;27:584–590.

53. Jardin F. Cyclic changes in arterial pressure during mechanical ventilation. Intensive Care Med 2004;30:1047–1050.

54. Robotham JL, Cherry D, Mitzner W, et al. A re-evaluation of the hemodynamic consequences of intermittent positive pressure ventilation. Crit Care Med 1983;11:783–793.

55. Robotham JL, Mintzner W. A model of the effects of respiration on left ventricular performance. J Appl Physiol 1979;46:411–418.

56. Pinsky MR. Instantaneous venous return curves in an intact canine preparation. J Appl Physiol 1984;56:765–771.

57. Vieillard-Baron A, Augarde R, Prin S, et al. Influence of superior vena caval zone condition on cyclic changes in right ventricular outflow during respiratory support. Anesthesiology 2001;95:1083–1088.

58. Fessler HE, Brower RG, Wise RA, et al. Effects of positive end-expiratory pressure on the gradient for venous return. Am Rev Respir Dis 1991;143:19–24.

59. Takata M, Robotham JL. Effects of inspiratory diaphragmatic descent on inferior vena caval venous return. J Appl Physiol 1992;72:597–607.

60. Takata M, Wise RA, Robotham JL. Effects of abdominal pressure on venous return: abdominal vascular zone conditions. J Appl Physiol 1990;69:1961–1972.

61. West JB, Dollery CT, Naimark A. Distribution of blood flow in isolated lung; relation to vascular and alveolar pressures. J Appl Physiol 1964;19:713–724.

62. Kitano Y, Takata M, Sasaki N, et al. Influence of increased abdominal pressure on steady-state cardiac performance. J Appl Physiol 1999;86:1651–1656.

63. van den Berg PC, Jansen JR, Pinsky MR. Effect of positive pressure on venous return in volume-loaded cardiac surgical patients. J Appl Physiol 2002;92:1223–1231.

64. Farge D, De la Coussaye JE, Beloucif S, et al. Interactions between hemodynamic and hormonal modifications during PEEP-induced antidiuresis and antinatriuresis. Chest 1995;107:1095–1100.

65. Berry EM, Edmonds JF, Wyllie H. Release of prostaglandin E_2 and unidentified factors from ventilated lungs. Br J Surg 1971;58:189–192.

66. Edmonds JF, Berry E, Wyllie JH. Release of prostaglandins caused by distension of the lungs. Br J Surg 1969;56:622–623.

67. Frass M, Watschinger B, Traindl O, et al. Atrial natriuretic peptide release in response to different positive end-expiratory pressure levels. Crit Care Med 1993;21:343–347.

68. Glick G, Wechsler AS, Epstein SE. Reflex cardiovascular depression produced by stimulation of pulmonary stretch receptors in the dog. J Clin Invest 1969;48:467–473.

69. Payen DM, Brun-Buisson CJ, Carli PA, et al. Hemodynamic, gas exchange, and hormonal consequences of LBPP during PEEP ventilation. J Appl Physiol 1987;62:61–70.

70. Permutt S, Bromberger-Barnea B, Bane HN. Alveolar pressure, pulmonary venous pressure, and the vascular waterfall. Med Thorac 1962;19:239–260.

71. Hughes JM, Glazier JB, Maloney JE, et al. Effect of lung volume on the distribution of pulmonary blood flow in man. Respir Physiol 1968;4:58–72.

72. Jardin F, Vieillard-Baron A. Right ventricular function and positive pressure ventilation in clinical practice: from hemodynamic subsets to respirator settings. Intensive Care Med 2003;29:1426–1434.

73. Permutt S. Relation between pulmonary arterial pressure and pleural pressure during the acute asthmatic attack. Chest 1973;63:Suppl:25S–28S.

74. Nunn JF. Applied Respiratory Physiology, 3rd ed. London: Butterworths; 1987.

75. Jardin F, Brun-Ney D, Cazaux P, et al. Relation between transpulmonary pressure and right ventricular isovolumetric pressure change during respiratory support. Cathet Cardiovasc Diagn 1989;16:215–220.

76. Jullien T, Valtier B, Hongnat JM, et al. Incidence of tricuspid regurgitation and vena caval backward flow in mechanically ventilated patients. A color Doppler and contrast echocardiographic study. Chest 1995;107:488–493.

77. Suter PM, Fairley B, Isenberg MD. Optimum end-expiratory airway pressure in patients with acute pulmonary failure. N Engl J Med 1975;292:284–289.

78. Bishop SP, White FC, Bloor CM. Regional myocardial blood flow during acute myocardial infarction in the conscious dog. Circ Res 1976;38:429–438.

79. Brooks H, Kirk ES, Vokonas PS, et al. Performance of the right ventricle under stress: relation to right coronary flow. J Clin Invest 1971;50:2176–2183.

80. Fessler HE, Brower RG, Wise RA, et al. Mechanism of reduced LV afterload by systolic and diastolic positive pleural pressure. J Appl Physiol 1988;65:1244–1250.

81. Boldt J, Kling D, von Bormann B, et al. Influence of PEEP ventilation immediately after cardiopulmonary bypass on right ventricular function. Chest 1988;94:566–571.

82. Serra J, McNicholas KW, Moore R, et al. High frequency, high volume ventilation for right ventricular assist. Chest 1988;93:1035–1037.

83. Franklin DL, Van Citters RL, Rushmer RF. Balance between right and left ventricular output. Circ Res 1962;10:17–26.

84. Maloney JE, Bergel DH, Glazier JB, et al. Transmission of pulsatile blood pressure and flow through the isolated lung. Circ Res 1968;23:11–24.

85. Robotham JL, Rabson J, Permutt S, et al. Left ventricular hemodynamics during respiration. J Appl Physiol 1979;47:1295–1303.

86. Guntheroth WG, Morgan BC, Mullins GL. Effect of respiration on venous return and stroke volume in cardiac tamponade. Mechanism of pulsus paradoxus. Circ Res 1967;20:381–390.

87. Howell JB, Permutt S, Proctor DF, et al. Effect of inflation of the lung on different parts of pulmonary vascular bed. J Appl Physiol 1961;16:71–76.

88. Scharf SM, Brown R, Saunders N, et al. Effects of normal and loaded spontaneous inspiration on cardiovascular function. J Appl Physiol 1979;47:582–590.

89. Scharf SM, Brown R, Tow DE, et al. Cardiac effects of increased lung volume and decreased pleural pressure in man. J Appl Physiol 1979;47:257–262.

90. Brinker JA, Weiss JL, Lappe DL, et al. Leftward septal displacement during right ventricular loading in man. Circulation 1980;61:626–633.

91. Guzman PA, Maughan WL, Yin FC, et al. Transseptal pressure gradient with leftward septal displacement during the Mueller manoeuvre in man. Br Heart J 1981;46:657–662.

92. Scharf SM, Bianco JA, Tow DE, et al. The effects of large negative intrathoracic pressure on left ventricular function in patients with coronary artery disease. Circulation 1981;63:871–875.

93. Peters J, Kindred MK, Robotham JL. Transient analysis of cardiopulmonary interactions. II. Systolic events. J Appl Physiol 1988;64:1518–1526.

94. Peters J, Kindred MK, Robotham JL. Transient analysis of cardiopulmonary interactions. I. Diastolic events. J Appl Physiol 1988;64:1506–1517.

95. Cozanitis DA, Leijala M, Pesonen E, et al. Acute pulmonary oedema due to laryngeal spasm. Anaesthesia 1982;37:1198–1199.

96. Jackson FN, Rowland V, Corssen G. Laryngospasm-induced pulmonary edema. Chest 1980;78:819–821.

97. Lee KW, Downes JJ. Pulmonary edema secondary to laryngospasm in children. Anesthesiology 1983;59:347–349.

98. Oswalt CE, Gates GA, Holmstrom MG. Pulmonary edema as a complication of acute airway obstruction. JAMA 1977;238:1833–1835.

99. Stradling JR, Bolton P. Upper airways obstruction as cause of pulmonary oedema. Lancet 1982;1:1353–1354.

100. Travis KW, Todres ID, Shannon DC. Pulmonary edema associated with croup and epiglottitis. Pediatrics 1977;59:695–698.

101. Sofer S, Bar-Ziv J, Scharf SM. Pulmonary edema following relief of upper airway obstruction. Chest 1984;86:401–403.

102. Stalcup SA, Mellins RB. Mechanical forces producing pulmonary edema in acute asthma. N Engl J Med 1977;297:592–596.

103. Naughton MT, Benard DC, Rutherford R, et al. Effect of continuous positive airway pressure on central sleep apnea and nocturnal PCO_2 in heart failure. Am J Respir Crit Care Med 1994;150:1598–1604.

104. Naughton MT, Liu PP, Bernard DC, et al. Treatment of congestive heart failure and Cheyne-Stokes respiration during sleep by continuous positive airway pressure. Am J Respir Crit Care Med 1995;151:92–97.

105. Naughton MT, Rahman MA, Hara K, et al. Effect of continuous positive airway pressure on intrathoracic and left ventricular transmural pressures in patients with congestive heart failure. Circulation 1995;91:1725–1731.

106. Robotham JL, Bell RC, Badke FR, et al. Left ventricular geometry during positive end-expiratory pressure in dogs. Crit Care Med 1985;13:617–624.

107. Visner MC, Arentzen CE, O'Connor MJ, et al. Alterations in left ventricular three-dimensional dynamic geometry and systolic function during acute right ventricular hypertension in the conscious dog. Circulation 1983;67:353–365.

108. Brower R, Wise RA, Hassapoyannes C, et al. Effect of lung inflation on lung blood volume and pulmonary venous flow. J Appl Physiol 1985;58:954–963.

109. Denault AY, Gorcsan J, 3rd, Pinsky MR. Dynamic effects of positive-pressure ventilation on canine left ventricular pressure–volume relations. J Appl Physiol 2001;91:298–308.

110. Stanger P, Lucas RV, Jr., Edwards JE. Anatomic factors causing respiratory distress in acyanotic congenital cardiac disease. Special reference to bronchial obstruction. Pediatrics 1969;43:760–769.

111. Rabinovitch M, Grady S, David I, et al. Compression of intrapulmonary bronchi by abnormally branching pulmonary arteries associated with absent pulmonary valves. Am J Cardiol 1982;50:804–813.

112. Ramamoorthy C, Tabbutt S, Dean Kurth C, et al. Effects of inspired hypoxic and hypercapnic gas mixtures on cerebral oxygen saturation in neonates with univentricular heart defects. Anesthesiology 2002;96:283–288.

113. Tabbutt S, Ramamoorthy C, Montenegro LM, et al. Impact of inspired gas mixtures on preoperative infants with hypoplastic left heart syndrome during controlled ventilation. Circulation 2001;104:I159–I164.

114. Taeed R, Schwartz SM, Pearl JM, et al. Unrecognized pulmonary venous desaturation early after Norwood palliation confounds Gp:Gs assessment and compromises oxygen delivery. Circulation 2001;103:2699–2704.

115. Hordof AJ, Mellins RB, Gersony WM, et al. Reversibility of chronic obstructive lung disease in infants following repair of ventricular septal defect. J Pediatr 1977;90:187–191.

116. Schindler MB, Bohn DJ, Bryan AC, et al. Increased respiratory system resistance and bronchial smooth muscle hypertrophy in children with acute postoperative pulmonary hypertension. Am J Respir Crit Care Med 1995;152:1347–1352.

117. Stenmark KR, James SL, Voelkel NF, et al. Leukotriene C4 and D4 in neonates with hypoxemia and pulmonary hypertension. N Engl J Med 1983;309:77–80.

118. Bancalari E, Jesse MJ, Gelband H, et al. Lung mechanics in congenital heart disease with increased and decreased pulmonary blood flow. J Pediatr 1977;90:192–195.

119. Howlett G. Lung mechanics in normal infants and infants with congenital heart disease. Arch Dis Child 1972;47:707–715.

120. Wallgren G, Geubelle F, Koch G. Studies of the mechanics of breathing in children with congenital heart lesions. Acta Paediatr 1960;49:415–425.

121. Yeh TF, Lilien LD. Altered lung mechanics in neonates with persistent fetal circulation syndrome. Crit Care Med 1981;9:83–84.

122. Lees MH, Burnell RH, Morgan CL, et al. Ventilation–perfusion relationships in children with heart disease and diminished pulmonary blood flow. Pediatrics 1968;42:778–785.

123. Lister G, Pitt BR. Cardiopulmonary interactions in the infant with congenital cardiac disease. Clin Chest Med 1983;4:219–232.

124. Kisanuki A, Tei C, Otsuji Y, et al. Doppler echocardiographic documentation of diastolic pulmonary artery forward flow. Am J Cardiol 1987;59:711–713.

125. Redington A, Penny D, Rigby M, et al. Antegrade diastolic pulmonary arterial flow as a marker of right ventricular restriction after complete repair of pulmonary atresia with intact ventricular septum and critical pulmonary valve stenosis. Cardiol Young 1992;2:382–386.

126. Cullen S, Shore D, Redington A. Characterization of right ventricular diastolic performance after complete repair of tetralogy of Fallot. Restrictive physiology predicts slow postoperative recovery. Circulation 1995;91:1782–1789.

127. Penny DJ, Redington AN. Doppler echocardiographic evaluation of pulmonary blood flow after the Fontan operation: the role of the lungs. Br Heart J 1991;66:372–374.

128. Redington AN, Penny D, Shinebourne EA. Pulmonary blood flow after total cavopulmonary shunt. Br Heart J 1991;65:213–217.

129. Shekerdemian LS, Bush A, Lincoln C, et al. Cardiopulmonary interactions in healthy children and children after simple cardiac surgery: the effects of positive and negative pressure ventilation. Heart 1997;78:587–593.

130. Shekerdemian LS, Bush A, Shore DF, et al. Cardiopulmonary interactions after Fontan operations: augmentation of cardiac output using negative pressure ventilation. Circulation 1997;96:3934–3942.

131. Shekerdemian LS, Bush A, Shore DF, et al. Cardiorespiratory responses to negative pressure ventilation after tetralogy of Fallot repair: a hemodynamic tool for patients with a low-output state. J Am Coll Cardiol 1999;33:549–555.

132. Shekerdemian LS, Schulze-Neick I, Redington AN, et al. Negative pressure ventilation as haemodynamic rescue following surgery for congenital heart disease. Intensive Care Med 2000;26:93–96.

133. Shekerdemian LS, Shore DF, Lincoln C, et al. Negative-pressure ventilation improves cardiac output after right heart surgery. Circulation 1996;94:II49–II55.

134. Shekerdemian LS, Penny DJ, Novick W. Early extubation after surgical repair of tetralogy of Fallot. Cardiol Young 2000;10:636–637.

135. Adatia I, Atz AM, Wessel DL. Inhaled nitric oxide does not improve systemic oxygenation after bidirectional superior cavopulmonary anastomosis. J Thorac Cardiovasc Surg 2005;129:217–219.

136. Bradley SM, Simsic JM, Mulvihill DM. Hyperventilation impairs oxygenation after bidirectional superior cavopulmonary connection. Circulation 1998;98:II372–II377.

137. Bradley SM, Simsic JM, Mulvihill DM. Hypoventilation improves oxygenation after bidirectional superior cavopulmonary connection. J Thorac Cardiovasc Surg 2003;126:1033–1039.

138. Hoskote A, Li J, Hickey C, et al. The effects of carbon dioxide on oxygenation and systemic, cerebral, and pulmonary vascular hemodynamics after the bidirectional superior cavopulmonary anastomosis. J Am Coll Cardiol 2004;44:1501–1509.

139. Li J, Hoskote A, Hickey C, et al. Effect of carbon dioxide on systemic oxygenation, oxygen consumption, and blood lactate levels after bidirectional superior cavopulmonary anastomosis. Crit Care Med 2005;33:984–989.

140. Polianski JM, Huchon GJ, Gaudebout CC, et al. Pulmonary and systemic effects of increased negative inspiratory intrathoracic pressure in dogs. Am Rev Respir Dis 1986;133:49–54.

141. Buda AJ, Pinsky MR, Ingels NB Jr, et al. Effect of intrathoracic pressure on left ventricular performance. N Engl J Med 1979;301:453–459.

142. Scharf SM, Woods BO, Brown R, et al. Effects of the Mueller maneuver on global and regional left ventricular function in angina pectoris with or without previous myocardial infarction. Am J Cardiol 1987;59:1305–1309.

143. Rasanen J, Nikki P, Heikkila J. Acute myocardial infarction complicated by respiratory failure. The effects of mechanical ventilation. Chest 1984;85:21–28.

144. Rasanen J, Heikkila J, Downs J, et al. Continuous positive airway pressure by face mask in acute cardiogenic pulmonary edema. Am J Cardiol 1985;55:296–300.

145. Rasanen J, Vaisanen IT, Heikkila J, et al. Acute myocardial infarction complicated by left ventricular dysfunction and respiratory failure. The effects of continuous positive airway pressure. Chest 1985;87:158–162.

146. Beach T, Millen E, Grenvik A. Hemodynamic response to discontinuance of mechanical ventilation. Crit Care Med 1973;1:85–90.

147. Cassidy SS, Mitchell JH, Johnson RL, Jr. Dimensional analysis of right and left ventricles during positive-pressure ventilation in dogs. Am J Physiol 1982;242:H549–H556.

148. Manny J, Patten MT, Liebman PR, et al. The association of lung distention, PEEP and biventricular failure. Ann Surg 1978;187:151–157.

149. Tittley JG, Fremes SE, Weisel RD, et al. Hemodynamic and myocardial metabolic consequences of PEEP. Chest 1985;88:496–502.

150. Grace MP, Greenbaum DM. Cardiac performance in response to PEEP in patients with cardiac dysfunction. Crit Care Med 1982;10:358–360.

151. Mathru M, Rao TL, El-Etr AA, et al. Hemodynamic response to changes in ventilatory patterns in patients with normal and poor left ventricular reserve. Crit Care Med 1982;10:423–426.

152. Criley JM, Blaufuss AH, Kissel GL. Cough-induced cardiac compression. Self-administered from of cardiopulmonary resuscitation. JAMA 1976;236:1246–1250.

153. Pinsky MR, Summer WR, Wise RA, et al. Augmentation of cardiac function by elevation of intrathoracic pressure. J Appl Physiol 1983;54:950–955.

154. Pinsky MR. The influence of positive-pressure ventilation on cardiovascular function in the critically ill. Crit Care Clin 1985;1:699–717.

155. Pinsky MR. The effects of mechanical ventilation on the cardiovascular system. Crit Care Clin 1990;6:663–678.

156. Pinsky MR. Ventricular support by synchronized jet ventilation. Appl Cardiopulm Pathophysiol 1990;3:235–245.

157. Pinsky MR. Cardiovascular effects of ventilatory support and withdrawal. Anesth Analg 1994;79:567–576.

158. Pinsky MR. Heart–lung interactions during positive-pressure ventilation. New Horiz 1994;2:443–456.

159. Pinsky MR. Clinical applications of cardiopulmonary interactions. J Physiol Pharmacol 1997;48:587–603.

160. Pinsky MR, Summer WR. Cardiac augmentation by phasic high intrathoracic pressure support in man. Chest 1983;84:370–375.

161. Pinsky MR, Matuschak GM, Bernardi L, et al. Hemodynamic effects of cardiac cycle-specific increases in intrathoracic pressure. J Appl Physiol 1986;60:604–612.

162. Pinsky MR, Marquez J, Martin D, et al. Ventricular assist by cardiac cycle-specific increases in intrathoracic pressure. Chest 1987;91:709–715.

163. Bradley TD, Holloway RM, McLaughlin PR, et al. Cardiac output response to continuous positive airway pressure in congestive heart failure. Am Rev Respir Dis 1992;145:377–382.

164. Mehta S, Jay GD, Woolard RH, et al. Randomized, prospective trial of bilevel versus continuous positive airway pressure in acute pulmonary edema. Crit Care Med 1997;25:620–628.

165. Mehta S, Liu PP, Fitzgerald FS, et al. Effects of continuous positive airway pressure on cardiac volumes in patients with ischemic and dilated cardiomyopathy. Am J Respir Crit Care Med 2000;161:128–134.

166. Naughton MT, Benard DC, Liu PP, et al. Effects of nasal CPAP on sympathetic activity in patients with heart failure and central sleep apnea. Am J Respir Crit Care Med 1995;152:473–479.

167. Kaneko Y, Floras JS, Usui K, et al. Cardiovascular effects of continuous positive airway pressure in patients with heart failure and obstructive sleep apnea. N Engl J Med 2003;348:1233–1241.

168. Tkacova R, Liu PP, Naughton MT, et al. Effect of continuous positive airway pressure on mitral regurgitant fraction and atrial natriuretic peptide in patients with heart failure. J Am Coll Cardiol 1997;30:739–745.

169. Sin DD, Logan AG, Fitzgerald FS, et al. Effects of continuous positive airway pressure on cardiovascular outcomes in heart failure patients with and without Cheyne-Stokes respiration. Circulation 2000;102:61–66.

170. Faccenda JF, Mackay TW, Boon NA, et al. Randomized placebo-controlled trial of continuous positive airway pressure on blood pressure in the sleep apnea–hypopnea syndrome. Am J Respir Crit Care Med 2001;163:344–348.

171. Bersten AD, Holt AW, Vedig AE, et al. Treatment of severe cardiogenic pulmonary edema with continuous positive airway pressure delivered by face mask. N Engl J Med 1991;325:1825–1830.

172. Lenique F, Habis M, Lofaso F, et al. Ventilatory and hemodynamic effects of continuous positive airway pressure in left heart failure. Am J Respir Crit Care Med 1997;155:500–505.

173. Jardin F, Genevray B, Brun-Ney D, et al. Influence of lung and chest wall compliances on transmission of airway pressure to the pleural space in critically ill patients. Chest 1985;88:653–658.

174. Pontoppidan H, Wilson RS, Rie MA, et al. Respiratory intensive care. Anesthesiology 1977;47:96–116.

175. Jardin F, Bourdarias JP. Right ventricular myocardial function in ARF patients: PEEP as a challenge for right heart. Intensive Care Med 1997;23:237–239.

176. Jardin F, Gueret P, Dubourg O, et al. Right ventricular volumes by thermodilution in the adult respiratory distress syndrome. A comparative study using two-dimensional echocardiography as a reference method. Chest 1985;88:34–39.

177. Jardin F, Gueret P, Dubourg O, et al. Two-dimensional echocardiographic evaluation of right ventricular size and contractility in acute respiratory failure. Crit Care Med 1985;13:952–956.

178. Vieillard-Baron A, Jardin F. Why protect the right ventricle in patients with acute respiratory distress syndrome? Curr Opin Crit Care 2003;9:15–21.

179. Vieillard-Baron A, Schmitt JM, Augarde R, et al. Acute cor pulmonale in acute respiratory distress syndrome submitted to protective ventilation: incidence, clinical implications, and prognosis. Crit Care Med 2001;29:1551–1555.

180. Dhainaut JF, Devaux JY, Monsallier JF, et al. Mechanisms of decreased left ventricular preload during continuous positive pressure ventilation in ARDS. Chest 1986;90:74–80.

181. Potkin RT, Hudson LD, Weaver LJ, et al. Effect of positive end-expiratory pressure on right and left ventricular function in patients

with the adult respiratory distress syndrome. Am Rev Respir Dis 1987;135:307–311.

182. Viquerat CE, Righetti A, Suter PM. Biventricular volumes and function in patients with adult respiratory distress syndrome ventilated with PEEP. Chest 1983;83:509–514.

183. Calvin JE, Driedger AA, Sibbald WJ. Positive end-expiratory pressure (PEEP) does not depress left ventricular function in patients with pulmonary edema. Am Rev Respir Dis 1981;124:121–128.

184. Jardin F, Farcot JC, Gueret P, et al. Echocardiographic evaluation of ventricles during continuous positive airway pressure breathing. J Appl Physiol 1984;56:619–627.

185. Schulman DS, Biondi JW, Matthay RA, et al. Effect of positive end-expiratory pressure on right ventricular performance. Importance of baseline right ventricular function. Am J Med 1988;84:57–67.

186. Schulman DS, Biondi JW, Zohgbi S, et al. Coronary flow limits right ventricular performance during positive end-expiratory pressure. Am Rev Respir Dis 1990;141:1531–1537.

187. Monchi M, Bellenfant F, Cariou A, et al. Early predictive factors of survival in the acute respiratory distress syndrome. A multivariate analysis. Am J Respir Crit Care Med 1998;158:1076–1081.

188. Zapol WM, Snider MT. Pulmonary hypertension in severe acute respiratory failure. N Engl J Med 1977;296:476–480.

189. Squara P, Dhainaut JF, Artigas A, et al. Hemodynamic profile in severe ARDS: results of the European Collaborative ARDS Study. Intensive Care Med 1998;24:1018–1028.

190. Schmitt JM, Vieillard-Baron A, Augarde R, et al. Positive end-expiratory pressure titration in acute respiratory distress syndrome patients: impact on right ventricular outflow impedance evaluated by pulmonary artery Doppler flow velocity measurements. Crit Care Med 2001;29:1154–1158.

191. Jardin F, Farcot JC, Boisante L, et al. Influence of positive end-expiratory pressure on left ventricular performance. N Engl J Med 1981;304:387–392.

192. Qvist J, Pontoppidan H, Wilson RS, et al. Hemodynamic responses to mechanical ventilation with PEEP: the effect of hypervolemia. Anesthesiology 1975;42:45–55.

193. Prewitt RM, Oppenheimer L, Sutherland JB, et al. Effect of positive end-expiratory pressure on left ventricular mechanics in patients with hypoxemic respiratory failure. Anesthesiology 1981;55:409–415.

194. Jardin F. The hemodynamic consequences of mechanical ventilation. Intensive Care Med 1997;23:1100–1101.

195. Jardin F, Dubourg O, Bourdarias JP. Echocardiographic pattern of acute cor pulmonale. Chest 1997;111:209–217.

196. Jardin F. Hemodynamic profile in severe ARDS. Intensive Care Med 1999;25:246–247.

197. Vieillard Baron A, Schmitt JM, Beauchet A, et al. Early preload adaptation in septic shock? A transesophageal echocardiographic study. Anesthesiology 2001;94:400–406.

198. Vieillard-Baron A, Chergui K, Augarde R, et al. Cyclic changes in arterial pulse during respiratory support revisited by Doppler echocardiography. Am J Respir Crit Care Med 2003;168:671–676.

199. Vieillard-Baron A, Chergui K, Rabiller A, et al. Superior vena caval collapsibility as a gauge of volume status in ventilated septic patients. Intensive Care Med 2004;30:1734–1739.

200. Vieillard-Baron A, Jardin F. Right level of positive end-expiratory pressure in acute respiratory distress syndrome. Am J Respir Crit Care Med 2003;167:1576; author reply 1576–1577.

201. Vieillard-Baron A, Prin S, Chergui K, et al. Early patterns of static pressure–volume loops in ARDS and their relations with PEEP-induced recruitment. Intensive Care Med 2003;29:1929–1935.

202. Vieillard-Baron A, Loubieres Y, Schmitt JM, et al. Cyclic changes in right ventricular output impedance during mechanical ventilation. J Appl Physiol 1999;87:1644–1650.

203. Vieillard-Baron A, Prin S, Chergui K, et al. Echo-Doppler demonstration of acute cor pulmonale at the bedside in the medical intensive care unit. Am J Respir Crit Care Med 2002;166:1310–1319.

204. Vieillard-Baron A, Prin S, Chergui K, et al. Hemodynamic instability in sepsis: bedside assessment by Doppler echocardiography. Am J Respir Crit Care Med 2003;168:1270–1276.

205. Vieillard-Baron A, Prin S, Schmitt JM, et al. Pressure–volume curves in acute respiratory distress syndrome: clinical demonstration of the influence of expiratory flow limitation on the initial slope. Am J Respir Crit Care Med 2002;165:1107–1112.

206. Vieillard-Baron A, Qanadli SD, Antakly Y, et al. Transesophageal echocardiography for the diagnosis of pulmonary embolism with acute cor pulmonale: a comparison with radiological procedures. Intensive Care Med 1998;24:429–433.

207. Jardin F, Farcot JC, Gueret P, et al. Cyclic changes in arterial pulse during respiratory support. Circulation 1983;68:266–274.

208. Massumi RA, Mason DT, Vera Z, et al. Reversed pulsus paradoxus. N Engl J Med 1973;289:1272–1275.

209. Preisman S, Pfeiffer U, Lieberman N, et al. New monitors of intravascular volume: a comparison of arterial pressure waveform analysis and the intrathoracic blood volume. Intensive Care Med 1997;23:651–657.

210. Michard F, Boussat S, Chemla D, et al. Relation between respiratory changes in arterial pulse pressure and fluid responsiveness in septic patients with acute circulatory failure. Am J Respir Crit Care Med 2000;162:134–138.

211. Tavernier B, Makhotine O, Lebuffe G, et al. Systolic pressure variation as a guide to fluid therapy in patients with sepsis-induced hypotension. Anesthesiology 1998;89:1313–1321.

212. Barbier C, Loubieres Y, Schmit C, et al. Respiratory changes in inferior vena cava diameter are helpful in predicting fluid responsiveness in ventilated septic patients. Intensive Care Med 2004;30:1740–1746.

213. Schlobohm RM, Falltrick RT, Quan SF, et al. Lung volumes, mechanics, and oxygenation during spontaneous positive-pressure ventilation: the advantage of CPAP over EPAP. Anesthesiology 1981;55:416–422.

214. Shah DM, Newell JC, Dutton RE, et al. Continuous positive airway pressure versus positive end-expiratory pressure in respiratory distress syndrome. J Thorac Cardiovasc Surg 1977;74:557–562.

215. Simonneau G, Lemaire F, Harf A, et al. A comparative study of the cardiorespiratory effects of continuous positive airway pressure breathing and continuous positive pressure ventilation in acute respiratory failure. Intensive Care Med 1982;8:61–67.

4
Echocardiography in the Pediatric Critical Care Setting

William L. Border, Erik C. Michelfelder, Kan Hor, and Dianna S. Meredith

Introduction

Echocardiography has an important role to perform in the pediatric intensive care unit (PICU), as it is an efficient, accurate, noninvasive diagnostic modality that can aid the pediatric intensivist in the management of a variety of cardiovascular conditions. The main objective of this chapter is to describe how echocardiography can answer 10 of the more commonly asked questions that arise in the PICU setting. Its purpose is not to give an in-depth discussion of the physics and foundations of ultrasound, nor is it meant to be a comprehensive text of echocardiography in congenital heart disease. The interested reader is referred to several excellent chapters and textbooks for additional information pertaining to these areas [1–11]. Rather, the intent of this chapter is to serve as a concise and useful reference for the clinician caring for patients in the PICU.

Is There Pericardial Tamponade?

Two-dimensional echocardiography is well suited to diagnosing pericardial fluid [12]. Pericardial fluid collections appear as echo-free spaces between the epicardium and the parietal pericardium. Pericardial effusions should be examined from all echocardiographic windows, and the echocardiographer will usually describe whether the fluid is predominantly anterior, posterior, or circumferential. The actual volume of pericardial fluid cannot be determined accurately from the echocardiogram, although many echocardiog-

raphers routinely use rather subjective and arbitrary terms such as *small*, *moderate*, or *large* to describe them [13]. However, the measurement of the dimension of the effusion can be helpful for serial follow-up studies and is usually measured at end diastole.

Pericardial tamponade is not an echocardiographic diagnosis but rather a clinical one. However, there are some echocardiographic indicators that can suggest tamponade. One such sign on the two-dimensional echocardiogram is collapse of the right atrial free wall in late diastole (Figure 4.1). This occurs because the pressure within the pericardial sac exceeds the pressure in the right atrium at end diastole. In general, the more hemodynamically severe the tamponade, the longer the duration of right atrial collapse extends into systole. In even more severe cases, right ventricular free wall collapse can occur in diastole. Another indicator of tamponade physiology is a marked increase in respiratory variation of flow velocities across the atrioventricular valves. Mitral valve variation is most useful, as tricuspid valve variations can be observed with respiration in normal individuals. Diminished diastolic flow velo-cities in the superior vena cava can also suggest tamponade phy-siology but are infrequently used in clinical practice.

Is There Systolic Dysfunction?

This is one of the most common questions asked of the echocardiography laboratory and is frequently asked in the context of a variety of clinical conditions. The most widely utilized measure in pediatrics is the shortening fraction, which is derived from M-mode images typically analyzed in the parasternal long axis or short axis. The shortening fraction is calculated by subtracting the left ventricular internal diameter in systole (D_{es}) from the left ventricular internal diameter in diastole (D_{ed}), dividing this by the left ventricular internal diameter in diastole, and multiplying by 100:

$$\text{Shortening fraction} = \frac{(D_{ed} - D_{es}) \times 100}{D_{ed}}$$

The normal range for the shortening fraction is generally greater than or equal to 28%. One limitation to this method occurs when a child has postoperative chest dressings and the echocardiographer is not able to obtain a parasternal long- or short-axis acoustic window. In this case, or in the case of patients with single-ventricle anatomy, a qualitative assessment of ventricular function is usually provided by the echocardiographer.

D.S. Wheeler et al. (eds.), *Cardiovascular Pediatric Critical Illness and Injury*,
DOI 10.1007/978-1-84800-923-3_4, © Springer-Verlag London Limited 2009

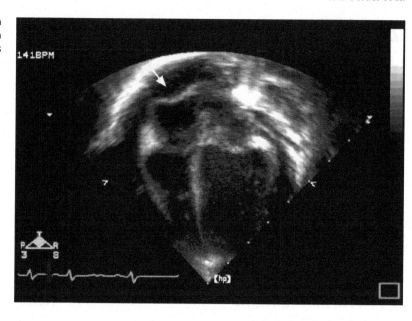

FIGURE 4.1. Two-dimensional apical four-chamber view of the heart of a patient with a significant pericardial effusion. Note the echodense area around the heart, representing pericardial fluid. The arrow highlights collapse of the right atrial free wall in diastole.

Another method of assessing ventricular contractility is to measure end systolic wall stress and the rate-corrected velocity of circumferential shortening (VCFc). The VCFc is a preload-independent index of left ventricular contractility that has an inverse, linear relationship with afterload, expressed as end systolic wall stress. One can then plot the wall stress–velocity relationship and come up with a load-independent index of contractility (Figure 4.2). This method depends on good technical tracings and can be more labor intensive. Another index of global myocardial function is the myocardial performance (or Tei) index (Figure 4.3). This index measures the ratio of isovolumic time intervals (isovolumic contraction and relaxation) to ventricular ejection time. This has been shown to be relatively independent of changes in preload. In normal children, the right ventricle Tei index is 0.32 ± 0.03 and the left ventricle Tei index is 0.35 ± 0.03. Its advantage is that it can usually be obtained even in the setting of poor acoustic two-dimensional windows [14–23].

Is There Diastolic Dysfunction?

The importance of left ventricular diastolic function has become increasingly apparent in critically ill children. However, this has been hampered by the complexities of evaluating ventricular filling. A variety of Doppler methods have been used, including (1) Doppler evaluation of transmitral inflow, with evaluation of peak E and peak A velocities, and the E:A ratio; (2) pulmonary vein Doppler with evaluation of peak S and D velocities, as well as A-wave reversals; (3) tissue Doppler evaluation of the mitral valve annulus with measurement of peak E and peak A myocardial velocities (Figure 4.4), as well as isovolumic relaxation time; and (4) evaluation of color M-mode Doppler of left ventricular inflow and measurement of the velocity of flow propagation. Investigators have validated these methods in the pediatric population and highlighted the strengths and weaknesses of the individual indices. However, rather than relying on a single index, we utilize all of these modali-

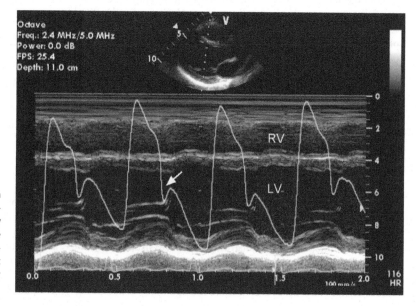

FIGURE 4.2. M-mode image of the ventricles (right, RV; and left, LV) with a simultaneous superimposed carotid artery pulse tracing. Blood pressure is measured at the same time, and the pulse trace is calibrated by linear interpolation so that the end systolic pressure (the pressure at the dicrotic notch, indicated by the arrow) can be obtained. The heart rate–corrected velocity of circumferential fiber shortening and end systolic wall stress can then be calculated and the left ventricular stress–velocity relationship obtained.

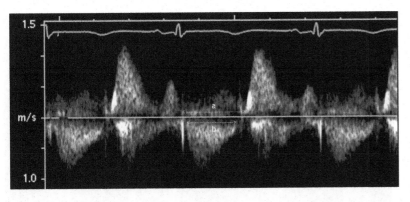

Figure 4.3. Doppler tracing showing mitral valve inflow (above the baseline) and aortic outflow (below the baseline). The myocardial performance (Tei) index is solved for as follows: $(a - b)/b$, where a is the mitral closing to opening time, and b is the aortic ejection time. This represents the isovolumic contraction time added to the isovolumic relaxation time, divided by the ejection time.

ties to give an overall impression of the diastolic function of the patient.

Right ventricular diastolic functional assessment can be more problematic. However, myocardial tissue Doppler assessment has been employed with some success. One helpful finding suggestive of restrictive physiology of the right ventricle is antegrade flow in the pulmonary artery in late diastole (during atrial systole) throughout the respiratory cycle. This has been shown to have some predictive role in postoperative patients who have undergone tetralogy of Fallot repair [24–26].

Does the Patient Have Pulmonary Hypertension?

This is a frequently asked question in a variety of different underlying conditions, ranging from congenital diaphragmatic hernia repair to patients with primary pulmonary hypertension. Echocardiography can estimate right ventricular systolic pressure from a tricuspid regurgitation jet (Figure 4.5). We measure the peak velocity and derive a gradient between the right ventricular and right atrium using the Bernoulli equation. If there is not a direct measure

of right atrial pressure, we assume a right atrial pressure of 10 mm Hg and add this number to the measured gradient to solve for right ventricular pressure. However, we cannot utilize this method in the absence of tricuspid regurgitation.

Another method, if the patient has pulmonary insufficiency, is to measure the velocity of the pulmonary regurgitation jet at end diastole (Figure 4.6). We can then derive a gradient between the pulmonary artery and right ventricle at end diastole and this represents pulmonary artery diastolic pressure. We can estimate right ventricular pressure if there is a shunt at the ventricular level, and we can also estimate it if there is shunting at the ductal level. Quantitative information can then be provided, which is helpful for clinicians following these patients. In the absence of shunts or regurgitation jets, the shape of the left ventricle and the interventricular septum can be assessed. In significant pulmonary hypertension and right ventricular pressure elevation, the interventricular septum will usually flatten in systole. A final indicator of pulmonary hypertension can be the profile of the pulmonary artery Doppler. The acceleration time is usually shortened in the setting of pulmonary hypertension [27].

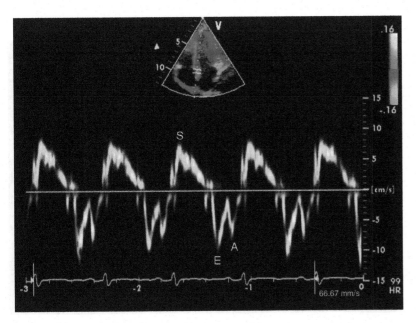

Figure 4.4. Representative tissue Doppler tracing of left ventricular myocardial velocities recorded at the septal mitral annulus. Systolic (S) and early (E) and late (A) diastolic annular velocities are indicated.

FIGURE 4.5. Doppler examination in the apical four-chamber view in a patient with pulmonary hypertension. A tricuspid regurgitation jet is seen also with a high peak velocity (asterisk), from which the right ventricular pressure can be derived using the simplified Bernoulli equation and an estimate of right atrial pressure.

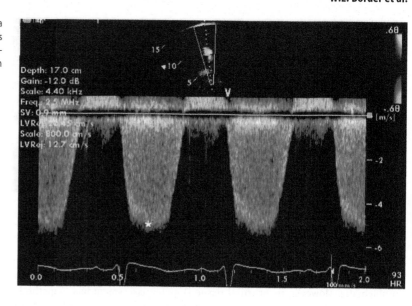

What Is the Volume Status of the Patient?

Both transthoracic (TTE) and transesophageal (TEE) echocardiography have been used in adults to evaluate hemodynamic status and help direct fluid management. Pediatric research studies have looked at the utility of a variety of different Doppler measures to calculate both cardiac output and stroke volume. However, their reproducibility and feasibility in routine PICU patient care remain questionable, especially in patients with congenital heart disease. We feel that its role in day-to-day volume assessment of the patient in the PICU is limited. However, we are able to provide some guidance with measurement of left ventricular systolic and diastolic dimensions and also a qualitative assessment of left ventricular volume.

Does the Patient Have a Significant Residual Postoperative Lesion?

Residual heart lesions in patients who have undergone cardiac surgical operations can hamper postoperative care and limit medical management. The practice at most cardiac centers is to perform pre- and postoperative TEEs in the operating room. This can provide very helpful information to the intensivist receiving the patient. Grading of atrioventricular valve regurgitation, the presence of residual intracardiac shunts, and assessment of cardiac function are critical in guiding postoperative medical management. Frequently, we are asked to reevaluate patients in the PICU if residual lesions are suspected. The images from standard transthoracic echo images can be limited by postoperative dressings,

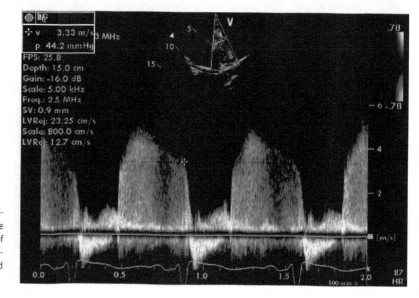

FIGURE 4.6. Continuous wave Doppler tracing in a patient with pulmonary vascular obstructive disease and pulmonary insufficiency. The velocity of the pulmonary regurgitation jet remains high at the end of diastole (asterisk). This indicates a significant gradient between the pulmonary artery and right ventricle at end diastole secondary to elevated pulmonary artery diastolic pressure.

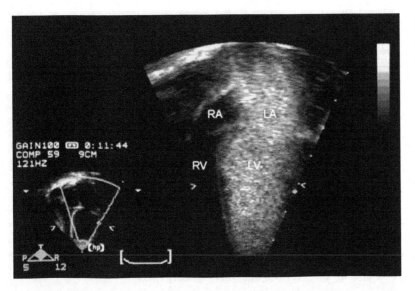

Figure 4.7. Apical four-chamber view of a patient with multiple pulmonary arteriovenous malformations three cardiac cycles after the injection of agitated saline in an antecubital vein. Note the dense contrast opacification in the left atrium (LA) and left ventricle (LV). RA, right atrium; RV, right ventricle.

and sonographers are often restricted to apical and subcostal windows only. Here, TEE can be useful in the PICU, especially when looking for residual intracardiac shunts and evaluating the atrioventricular valves. In addition, valvar gradients and the degree of regurgitation can be underestimated in the operating room because of altered loading conditions and anesthesia, and a repeated TEE in the PICU may reveal this [28].

Does the Patient Have Pulmonary Arteriovenous Malformations?

The question of whether the patient has pulmonary arteriovenous malformations (AVMs) arises for a child with unexplained cyanosis, for infants and children with liver failure, and for patients who have undergone single-ventricle palliation. This can be a very helpful study and is quite easy to do. At our center, we will place a peripheral intravenous line (preferably in an antecubital vein). We then agitate normal saline (usually with the use of two syringes) and inject it while simultaneously obtaining two-dimensional echocardiographic images. The apical four-chamber view is preferred (Figure 4.7). Contrast bubbles should not cross the pulmonary capillary bed. In the patient with pulmonary AVMs, there is rapid return (within three to five cardiac cycles) of contrast bubbles to the left atrium (because the pulmonary bed is bypassed). In general, this has been found to be more sensitive in detecting pulmonary AVMs than pulmonary angiography. However, the presence of intracardiac shunts (particularly atrial septal defects) will confound this test [29–31].

Does the Patient Have a Cardiac Contusion?

Cardiac and great vessel injury can occur after blunt trauma in children. The incidence of cardiac injury is fairly rare; however, it can be detected on TTE. Occasionally traumatic ventricular septal defects have been reported as well as pericardial effusions and right ventricular dysfunction. In addition, aortic injury can occur with both intimal tears and even aortic transection. An initial assessment by TTE in children is usually sufficient. If, however, images are suboptimal or an injury of the ascending aorta is suspected, a TEE can provide additional information [32–34].

Does the Patient Have an Intracardiac Thrombus?

This question is usually asked in the setting of patients admitted with chronic atrial arrhythmias (before cardioversion), those with prosthetic valves, those with central lines, and those with severe cardiac dysfunction. Echocardiography is sensitive at detecting the presence of intracardiac thrombi, but not that specific. In addition, it is usually not possible to make an accurate distinction between fresh and organized thrombus. Transthoracic echocardiography can be helpful with the serial assessment of thrombi in the setting of fibrinolytic therapy. Transesophageal echocardiography can provide improved sensitivity in the detection of intracavitary thrombi, especially those in the left atrium and left atrial appendage. An omniplane TEE probe is ideal for allowing clear visualization of the left atrial appendage. For older patients who have undergone Fontan palliation surgery and present with chronic atrial arrhythmias, TEE is crucial to allow for accurate clot assessment before cardioversion [35,36].

Are There Intracardiac Vegetations?

We are frequently asked to evaluate for the presence of intracardiac vegetations when clinicians suspect infective endocarditis. This is often in the setting of patients with central lines. The overall yield rate of echocardiographically diagnosed infective endocarditis in children suspected to have it clinically is quite low (12%). Thus, our usual practice is to obtain a TTE, because accurate imaging of the valves is possible in most pediatric subjects (Figure 4.8). If there is a strong clinical suspicion and transthoracic imaging is suboptimal, we will proceed to the performance of a TEE. This can allow for accurate visualization of the atrioventricular and semilunar valves. However, the potential morbidity associated with general anesthesia and TEE leads us to restrict TEE for these selected cases [37].

FIGURE 4.8. Apical four-chamber view of a patient with subacute bacterial endocarditis. A large vegetation (arrow) is seen also attached to the anterior leaflet of the tricuspid valve (TV). MV, mitral valve.

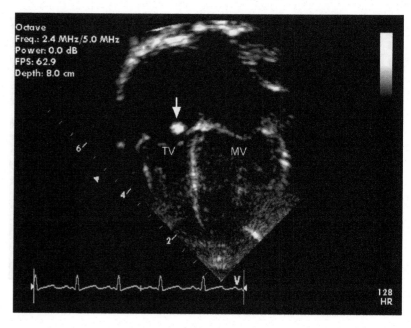

Conclusion

In the modern era, there has been an increasing demand for echocardiography in the care of the critically ill pediatric patient. Echocardiography fulfills more than just a diagnostic role in the PICU, where it can directly impact clinical care and management decisions. Intensivists need to have some understanding of its strengths and limitations in answering clinical questions and know in which settings to best utilize it.

References

1. Rice MJ, McDonald RW, Reller MD, Sahn DJ. Pediatric echocardiography: current role and a review of technical advances. J Pediatr 1996;128:1–14.
2. Colan SD. Echocardiography. In: Chang AC, Hanley FL, Wernovsky G, Wessel DL, eds. Pediatric Cardiac Intensive Care. Philadelphia: Lippincott Williams & Wilkins; 1998:425–446.
3. Orie JD, Pieroni DR, Roland J-MA, Gingell RL. Echocardiography. In: Fuhrman BP, Zimmerman JJ, eds. Pediatric Critical Care, 2nd ed. St Louis: Mosby; 1998:371–376.
4. Phoon CK, Divekar A, Rutkowski M. Pediatric echocardiography: applications and limitations. Curr Probl Pediatr 1999;29:157–185.
5. Kimball TR, Meyer RA. Echocardiography. In: Allen HD, Gutgesell HP, Clark EB, Driscoll DJ, eds. Moss and Adams' Heart Disease in Infants, Children, and Adolescents, 6th ed. Philadelphia: Lippincott Williams & Wilkins; 2001:204–233.
6. Snider AR, Ritter SB. Doppler echocardiography. In: Allen HD, Gutgesell HP, Clark EB, Driscoll DJ, eds. Moss and Adams' Heart Disease in Infants, Children, and Adolescents, 6th ed. Philadelphia: Lippincott Williams & Wilkins; 2001:234–263.
7. DeGroff CG. Doppler echocardiography. Pediatr Cardiol 2002;23: 307–333.
8. Ciccone TJ, Grossman SA. Cardiac ultrasound. Emerg Med Clin North Am 2004;22:621–640.
9. Frommelt PC. Update on pediatric echocardiography. Curr Opin Pediatr 2005;17:579–585.
10. Beaulieu Y, Marik PE. Bedside ultrasonography in the ICU: Part 1. Chest 2005;128:881–895.
11. Beaulieu Y, Marik PE. Bedside ultrasonography in the ICU: Part 2. Chest 2005;128:1766–1781.
12. Merce J, Sagrista-Sauleda J, Permanyer-Miralda G, Evangelista A, Soler-Soler J. Correlation between clinical and Doppler echocardiographic findings in patients with moderate and large pericardial effusion: implications for the diagnosis of cardiac tamponade. Am Heart J 1999;138:759–764.
13. D'Cruz II, Rehman AU, Hancock HL. Quantitative echocardiographic assessment in pericardial disease. Echocardiography 1997;14: 207–214.
14. Kimball TR, Daniels SR, Khoury P, Meyer RA. Age-related variation in contractility estimate in patients less than or equal to 20 years of age. Am J Cardiol 1991;68:1383–1387.
15. Wolfe LT, Rossi A, Ritter SB. Transesophageal echocardiography in infants and children: use and importance in the cardiac intensive care unit. J Am Soc Echocardiogr 1993;6:286–289.
16. Eidem BW, Tei C, O'Leary PW, Cetta F, Seward JB. Nongeometric quantitative assessment of right and left ventricular function: myocardial performance index in normal children and patients with Ebstein anomaly. J Am Soc Echocardiogr 1998;11:849–856.
17. Tibby SM, Hatherill M, Murdoch IA. Use of transesophageal Doppler ultrasonography in ventilated pediatric patients: derivation of cardiac output. Crit Care Med 2000;28:2045–2050.
18. Tibby SM, Hatherill M, Durward A, Murdoch IA. Are transoesophageal Doppler parameters a reliable guide to paediatric haemodynamic status and fluid management? Intensive Care Med 2001;27:201–205.
19. Courand JA, Marshall J, Chang Y, King ME. Clinical applications of wall-stress analysis in the pediatric intensive care unit. Crit Care Med 2001;29:526–533.
20. Mohan UR, Britto J, Habibi P, de MC, Nadel S. Noninvasive measurement of cardiac output in critically ill children. Pediatr Cardiol 2002;23:58–61.
21. Border WL, Michelfelder EC, Glascock BJ, et al. Color M-mode and Doppler tissue evaluation of diastolic function in children: simultaneous correlation with invasive indices. J Am Soc Echocardiogr 2003;16: 988–994.
22. Hruda J, Rothuis EG, van Elburg RM, Sobotka-Plojhar MA, Fetter WP. Echocardiographic assessment of preload conditions does not help at the neonatal intensive care unit. Am J Perinatol 2003;20:297–303.
23. Di Salvo G, Pacileo G, Caso P, et al. Strain rate imaging is a superior method for the assessment of regional myocardial function compared with Doppler tissue imaging: a study on patients with transcatheter device closure of atrial septal defect. J Am Soc Echocardiogr 2005;18: 398–400.

24. Norgard G, Gatzoulis MA, Josen M, Cullen S, Redington AN. Does restrictive right ventricular physiology in the early postoperative period predict subsequent right ventricular restriction after repair of tetralogy of Fallot? Heart 1998;79:481–484.

25. Galderisi M, Severino S, Cicala S, Caso P. The usefulness of pulsed tissue Doppler for the clinical assessment of right ventricular function. Ital Heart J 2002;3:241–247.

26. Friedberg MK, Rosenthal DN. New developments in echocardiographic methods to assess right ventricular function in congenital heart disease. Curr Opin Cardiol 2005;20:84–88.

27. Nishimura RA, Tajik A. Measurement of intracardiac pressures. State of the art—1986. Herz 1986;11:283–290.

28. Chin AJ, Vetter JM, Seliem M, Jones AA, Andrews BA. Role of early postoperative surface echocardiography in the pediatric cardiac intensive care unit. Chest 1994;105:10–16.

29. Chang RK, Alejos JC, Atkinson D, et al. Bubble contrast echocardiography in detecting pulmonary arteriovenous shunting in children with univentricular heart after cavopulmonary anastomosis. J Am Coll Cardiol. 1999;33:2052–2058.

30. Larsson ES, Solymar L, Eriksson BO, de Wahl Granelli A, Mellander M. Bubble contrast echocardiography in detecting pulmonary arteriovenous malformations after modified Fontan operations. Cardiol Young 2001;11:505–511.

31. Feinstein JA, Moore P, Rosenthal DN, Puchalski M, Brook MM. Comparison of contrast echocardiography versus cardiac catheterization for detection of pulmonary arteriovenous malformations. Am J Cardiol 2002;89:281–285.

32. Paone RF, Peacock JB, Smith DL. Diagnosis of myocardial contusion. South Med J 1993;86:867–870.

33. Karalis DG, Victor MF, Davis GA, McAllister MP, Covalesky VA, Ross JJ, Jr., Foley RV, Kerstein MD, Chandrasekaran K. The role of echocardiography in blunt chest trauma: a transthoracic and transesophageal echocardiographic study. J Trauma 1994;36:53–58.

34. Tiao GM, Griffith PM, Szmuszkovicz JR, Mahour GH. Cardiac and great vessel injuries in children after blunt trauma: an institutional review. J Pediatr Surg 2000;35:1656–1660.

35. Ozimek W, Wroblewska-Kaluzewska M, Gadomski A, et al. Echocardiographic assessment of right atrial thrombus related to the implanted port device in patient receiving chemotherapy for non-Hodgkin's lymphoma. Med Sci Monit 2000;6:1013–1017.

36. Ayres NA, Miller-Hance W, Fyfe DA, et al. Indications and guidelines for performance of transesophageal echocardiography in the patient with pediatric acquired or congenital heart disease: report from the task force of the Pediatric Council of the American Society of Echocardiography. J Am Soc Echocardiogr 2005;18:91–98.

37. Michelfelder EC, Ochsner JE, Khoury P, Kimball TR. Does assessment of pretest probability of disease improve the utility of echocardiography in suspected endocarditis in children? J Pediatr 2003;142:263–267.

5
Cardiac Catheterization in the Pediatric Critical Care Setting

Russell Hirsch and Robert H. Beekman III

Introduction

This chapter provides an overview of the principles involved with the performance of cardiac catheterization in high-risk patients. It is not intended to review cardiac catheterization in patients with specific congenital cardiac lesions, topics to be covered elsewhere in this text. Although the safety of cardiac catheterization has improved dramatically in recent decades with the advent of improved materials and smaller catheters, this risk amelioration has been offset by a marked increase in the complexity and acuity of children brought to the catheterization laboratory for diagnostic or therapeutic procedures. It is obviously incumbent on all providers of medical care to these patients to be familiar with the practice and potential risks surrounding these procedures.

Indications

The indications for cardiac catheterization have changed considerably in recent years. Improvements in noninvasive imaging with echocardiography, computerized tomography (CT), and magnetic resonance angiography have obviated the need for invasive cardiac catheterization in many cases. Nevertheless, there remain instances in which direct hemodynamic measurements are vital to guide medical or surgical management. Furthermore, the advent of transcatheter techniques and devices for intra- and extracardiac repair of congenital cardiovascular defects is rapidly expanding the indications for therapeutic catheterization.

Diagnostic Catheterization

Diagnostic catheterization is required for either hemodynamic assessment or specific anatomic definition if other less-invasive methods leave important questions unanswered. The most common single indication for a diagnostic catheterization is assessment of pulmonary artery pressure and resistance. The single-ventricle patient population, before ongoing surgical palliation, still has the greatest need for diagnostic catheterization. Measurement of pulmonary vascular resistance and assessment of pulmonary artery anatomy before the Glenn and Fontan procedures are usually required for these patients. However, some centers are relying increasingly on noninvasive testing alone in univentricular patients thought to be at low risk for findings that would prove to be contraindications for further palliative surgical intervention.

Diagnostic cardiac catheterization is rarely indicated for the two-ventricle patient population with shunt lesions (such as ventricular septal defects and atrioventricular canal defects). However, if such patients present beyond infancy, or substantial questions remain regarding pulmonary vascular resistance after noninvasive testing, then catheterization would be indicated to determine pulmonary vascular responsiveness (to agents such as inhaled oxygen or nitric oxide) and to further stratify risk before surgical correction. Finally, a large role for diagnostic cardiac catheterization remains for patients with pulmonary vascular occlusive disease. With the advent of newer and relatively effective palliative medications for this disease process, assessments of vascular responsiveness are important before long-term vasodilator therapy is instituted and response to treatment is evaluated.

Interventional or Therapeutic Catheterization

After the first balloon atrial septostomy was performed by Rashkind in 1966, the role of therapeutic cardiovascular interventions for children has expanded dramatically. The Rashkind procedure was followed later by the development of balloon pulmonary and aortic valvuloplasty and balloon angioplasty for pulmonary artery stenosis and coarctation of the aorta. These procedures are now generally considered standard therapies for congenital valvar and great artery stenoses. Much work has also been completed in the field of device development for closure of anatomically uncomplicated defects (such as patent ductus arteriosus and secundum atrial septal defect), culminating in U.S. Food and Drug Administration

D.S. Wheeler et al. (eds.), *Cardiovascular Pediatric Critical Illness and Injury*,
DOI 10.1007/978-1-84800-923-3_5, © Springer-Verlag London Limited 2009

TABLE 5.1. Indications for interventional or therapeutic cardiac catheterization.

I. Valvuloplasty procedures
    A. Aortic and pulmonary balloon valvuloplasty (see Figure 5.1)
    B. Tricuspid and mitral valvuloplasty (rare in the pediatric population)
II. Atrial septostomy procedures
    A. Dynamic atrial septostomy (Rashkind)
    B. Blade atrial septostomy (Park blade)
III. Angioplasty procedures
    A. Primary balloon dilation or stenting
        i.   Aortic coarctation dilation or stenting
        ii. Pulmonary artery dilation or stenting
        iii. Pulmonary venous dilation or stenting
        iv. Superior or inferior vena cava (SVC or IVC) dilation or stenting
    B. Secondary arterioplasty or venoplasty procedures (after prior surgical
        intervention)
        i.   Recoarctation dilation or stenting
        ii. Pulmonary artery rehabilitation after tetralogy of Fallot repair (with or
             without collateral unifocalization)
        iii. Pulmonary venous dilation or stenting when focal and discrete
        iv. SVC or IVC dilation or stenting after previous atrial switch surgery
IV. Vessel embolization (with coil or device placement)
    A. Aortopulmonary collateral embolization (during intermediate single ventricle
        palliation, and in some complex tetralogy of Fallot cases) (see Figure 5.2)
    B. Veno-venous collateral embolization (to address desaturation after single
        ventricle palliation)
    C. Patent ductus arteriosus closure
    D. Coronary artery fistula closure
    E. Intrapulmonary arteriovenous malformation closure
V. Septal defect closure
    A. Secundum atrial septal defect and patent foramen ovale closure
    B. Muscular or membranous ventricular septal defect closure
    C. Fenestration closure after the Fontan procedure

(FDA) approval for various devices for closure of these defects. Clinical trials are also actively underway evaluating other devices for the transcatheter closure of muscular and membranous ventricular septal defects. Currently, indications for therapeutic catheterization in children fall into the categories listed in Table 5.1.

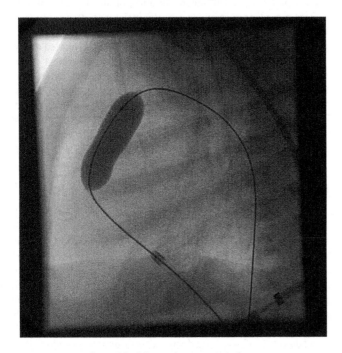

FIGURE 5.1. Balloon pulmonary valvuloplasty.

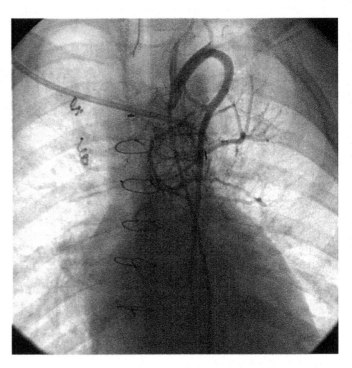

FIGURE 5.2. Aortopulmonary collateral vessels.

The specific indications for each of the described procedures are not specifically addressed here; in some cases will be covered elsewhere in this text. The specific urgency for each intervention is predicated upon the clinical scenario.

Practical Considerations

Given the complexity and high acuity of this patient population, the practice of cardiac catheterization should carefully balance the risk of the procedure against the potential benefits of hemodynamic or anatomic information obtained and/or transcatheter therapies provided. If the outstanding clinical questions relate purely to anatomy, every practical effort should be made to obtain the information with noninvasive imaging. Nevertheless, standardized catheterization protocols should be employed at all times (before, during, and after catheterization) to ensure that all physiologic and biochemical parameters are identified, monitored, and corrected as necessary, diminishing the overall risk to the patient.

Before Catheterization

General Status

For patients undergoing elective catheterization, assessment should be performed within 24 hr of the procedure to ensure the absence of any signs of infection (such as viral upper respiratory tract infection or pneumonia). The patient's chest x-ray should be reviewed to exclude any parenchymal infiltrates. In addition, the side of the aortic arch can be determined in most cases, as well as other ancillary information such as rib notching in older patients with coarctation of the aorta. The patient should be carefully assessed for dental caries; if the procedure is purely elective, and especially if interventions and device placement are likely, the procedure should be postponed until after dental reconstruction. Particular attention should be paid to the superficial skin areas overlying the points of arterial and venous access. The presence of any yeast infection in the groin area should necessitate postponement or a decision to use alternative access sites if catheterization is mandatory at that time.

Basic hematologic parameters (hemoglobin/hematocrit, white blood cell and platelet counts) should be assessed before proceeding. Catheterization is generally safe with platelet counts above 50,000. Blood type and cross should be arranged for newborns and for patients undergoing high-risk interventions. If the patient has previously been on anticoagulant therapy, or hepatic synthetic dysfunction is suspected to be abnormal in the setting of critical illness, a full coagulation profile should be obtained. Depending on the anticipated site of access and the urgency for the catheterization, correction of any abnormalities may be necessary. Airway and possible sedation problems should be considered in advance of the precatheterization assessment. This topic is discussed later in this chapter.

Cardiac Status

All cardiac related studies should be rigorously reviewed, including all previous catheterizations. Previous vascular access sites and the positions of all current indwelling central lines (and their functions) should be identified. Knowledge of previously documented vascular occlusions will also help guide access planning. The specific underlying anatomic diagnosis should be determined as clearly as possible, and the nature of the outstanding questions, or the intended intervention, should be clearly defined. At a minimum, the most recent electrocardiogram (ECG) and echocardiogram (echo) should be studied. Patients at risk for rhythm disturbances or conduction abnormalities should be identified (such as L-transposition of the great arteries ("congenitally corrected transposition"), postoperative tetralogy of Fallot with right bundle branch block and left axis deviation, or patients with preexcitation on their surface ECG). The status of ventricular function should be obtained from the echo; the presence of systemic ventricular outlet obstruction should be carefully assessed. It is in patients with impaired ventricular function or severe systemic outlet obstruction that changes in systemic vascular resistance or blunting of intrinsic catecholamine drive may have the most profound adverse effect with commencement of sedation or induction of anesthesia.

During Cardiac Catheterization

Basic physiologic parameters (heart rate, respiratory rate, arterial pressure, oxygen saturation [pulse oximetry], temperature) should be continuously monitored in an age-appropriate manner throughout the catheterization. Isothermic temperature control should be maintained at all times. This is most vital in neonates and small infants with smaller body surface area to weight ratios. This can be achieved with increasing the room temperature, exposing as little of the skin surface to the open environment as practically possible, and making use of commercially available surface body warmers. Skin temperature (and central temperature when appropriate) should be continuously monitored. Glucose-containing maintenance fluids should be infused through a peripheral intravenous line (IV). This is also most relevant in the newborn population with

immature homeostatic mechanisms and in those patients in whom parenteral nutrition has been interrupted before the catheterization. Blood glucose levels should be monitored on a regular basis during the procedure to avoid hypoglycemia.

The amount of blood loss should be determined frequently during the procedure. Fluid replacement in the form of crystalloid, colloid, or packed red blood cells will depend on the initial hemoglobin/hematocrit, the nature of the underlying heart disease (generally more critical in cyanotic than in acyanotic lesions), and the estimation of the patient's cardiac index. The risks associated with transfusion should be carefully weighed against the potential physiologic benefits; this is particularly relevant in patients who could later require heart transplantation (and who might be immunosensitized by blood product transfusion).

A stable acid–base balance should be maintained and abnormalities corrected accordingly. Arterial blood gas (ABG) analysis should be obtained at initiation of each catheterization at a minimum and intermittently during the catheterization as indicated or if repeated measures are obtained under different conditions. In the critical care population, a final ABG should be obtained immediately before transfer from the cardiac catheterization laboratory to the intensive care unit. Although respiratory acidosis is often noted with respiratory depression during sedation, tolerance for this abnormality should be balanced according to the underlying defect and the acuity of the situation; respiratory acidosis is never acceptable in patients with pulmonary hypertension and elevated pulmonary vascular resistance. Base deficits associated with metabolic acidosis should be corrected with sodium bicarbonate.

Standard clinical observation and electronic monitoring is expected in all patients undergoing cardiac catheterization. Apart from temperature monitoring previously discussed, every patient should have continuous heart rate and rhythm, pulse oximetry, noninvasive blood pressure (NIBP) and end-tidal carbon dioxide (etCO$_2$) monitoring. Commercially available nasal cannula based etCO$_2$ detectors are available and allow for supplemental oxygen administration by the same cannula if necessary.

After Catheterization

The decision regarding patient disposition after cardiac catheterization should in all cases take patient safety as the primary objective. Admission to an intensive care unit (or placement on a stepdown unit) is dependent on the underlying congenital defect, the acuity of the clinical situation, the nature of the intervention (if any was performed), and any complications that may have arisen during the procedure. In general, the patients with the highest risk for hemodynamic deterioration after cardiac catheterization include those with severe myocardial dysfunction, severe systemic ventricular outflow obstruction, or elevated pulmonary vascular resistance. The pathophysiologic changes that may occur with cardiac catheterization in pediatric patients may only manifest some hours after the procedure, and appropriate patient placement should take those potential changes into account. Those changes may result from simple alterations during patient transfer (such as temperature and position changes and variations in ventilation) or may be more complex (such as the impact of contrast administration on ventricular loading, myocardial function, or pulmonary resistance; rhythm and conduction disturbances, etc.). The necessary observation required can be categorized as follows.

General Status

After admission to the intensive care unit the patient should undergo a full assessment. Stability during the cardiac catheterization is not a reliable predictor of postprocedural stability, and continuous monitoring and reevaluation are required. Adjustments should be made as necessary to all physiologic parameters monitored during the procedure, such as temperature, blood glucose level, and maintenance fluid administration. The extremities distal to the vascular entry site should be carefully assessed at regular intervals. Venous stasis is manifest as a warm, plethoric limb that may become acutely edematous. The limb should be elevated and pressure dressings loosened. Expectant therapy is required and the extremity protected from inadvertent trauma. Arterial occlusion, on the other hand, usually results in a cool, pulseless extremity with delayed capillary refill. The most common cause is transient arterial spasm, which generally resolves in several hours and rarely threatens the viability of the limb. If the limb appears acutely ischemic (pale, pulseless, cold, and painful), then an etiology other than arterial spasm should be suspected (such as a thrombotic occlusion, an intimal flap, or dissection). Recommended treatment for arterial spasm with a pulseless extremity is detailed in Table 5.2.

Cardiac Status

The main factors pertaining to cardiovascular stability after catheterization relate to rhythm and conduction, intra-vascular volume status and anemia, myocardial function, and how these may have changed or been impacted by the catheterization.

Rhythm and Conduction

Physicians caring for patients after catheterization should be fully aware of any conduction or rhythm disturbances that occurred during the procedure. Hemodynamically significant or life-threatening arrhythmias should be well described. Other than specific catheter-induced disturbances (e.g., ventricular fibrillation associated with right coronary artery cannulation or narrow complex tachycardia caused by atrial catheter manipulation), there should be an expectation that the same abnormalities may occur in the immediate convalescent period after catheterization. Defibrillation pads should be applied if indicated, and appropriate antiarrhythmic drugs should be on hand.

Intravascular Volume Status and Anemia

Blood loss during catheterization may be difficult to estimate. In addition, some degree of hemodilution may occur with crystalloid or colloid administration in response to the systemic vascular resistance changes with anesthetic induction. The impact of contrast administration should also not be underestimated. Nonionic contrast will alter ventricular filling characteristics and elevate end diastolic pressures. The final hemodynamic parameters should be noted and appropriate alterations made in the convalescent period, such as fluid administration, blood transfusion, or diuretic administration.

Myocardial Function

Contractility may be profoundly altered during catheterization, especially in the face of interventions that may obstruct left ventricular outflow, or result in substantial aortic or atrioventricular valve insufficiency. Complex device placement that may require arteriovenous wire loops will often temporarily stent open cardiac valves and can thereby cause a significant, usually transient, decline in cardiac output. These changes may take some time to resolve, and temporary use of appropriate inotropic agents, often commenced during the catheterization, should be employed until myocardial function and cardiac output have returned to baseline.

Sedation and Anesthesia

The choice of sedation or anesthetic drugs should take into account their impacts on myocardial function and systemic and pulmonary vascular resistances. This is most germane in those patients with severely depressed myocardial function who have reliance on intrinsic catecholamine drive to maintain cardiac output or those patients with obstructed systemic ventricles. The former group is susceptible to sudden cardiac arrest with suppression of their intrinsic catecholamine support, whereas the latter are subject to myocardial ischemia related to the sudden decrease in systemic vascular resistance, both occurring after anesthetic induction or sedation administration. Use of sedation or general anesthesia can be categorized as follows.

Diagnostic Catheterization

The majority of diagnostic cardiac catheterizations can be safely performed under conscious sedation. An example of such a protocol is outlined in Table 5.3. However, general anesthesia for diagnostic procedures should be considered whenever there is a suspicion that the airway may become compromised with sedation (such as in patients with Down syndrome) or if there will be a need for airway positioning for purposes of intravenous access (e.g., via the subclavian or internal jugular veins). Patients with elevated pulmonary artery pressures with elevated pulmonary vascular resistance, especially in the absence of any intracardiac shunt, are at significant risk of pulmonary hypertensive crises if respiratory acidosis occurs, and for this reason general anesthesia is a safer option for these patients. Finally, general anesthesia should be considered for patients with underlying neurologic disorders or a history of difficult sedation.

TABLE 5.2. Guidelines for anticoagulation after cardiac catheterization in the absence of a palpable pulse.

Clinical setting	Medication	Notes
No pulse palpable within 2 hr of sheath removal	Heparin, continuous intravenous (IV) infusion (25 units/ kg/hr)	Maintain partial thromboplastin time at twice normal reference range
At 24 hr: pulse present	Discontinue heparin	
At 24 hr: pulse absent	Continue heparin IV infusion (at 15 units/ kg/hr); commence tissue plasminogen activator (tPA) IV infusion (0.3 mg/kg/hr)	Monitor blood pressure before and after infusion; monitor fibrinogen level before and after infusion. May repeat tPA IV infusion once if pulse does not return

TABLE 5.3. Example protocol for cardiac catheterization sedation.

Premedication	
Age	Medication and dosage
Birth to 6 months	None
6–12 months	Acyanotic patients: midazolam 0.5 mg/kg by mouth (PO)
	Cyanotic patients: none
>1 year old	Midazolam 0.5–0.75 mg/kg PO (maximum dose 20 mg)
>15 years old	Valium 5 mg PO 1 hr before catheterization; or midazolam
	0.75 mg/kg PO (20 mg max dose) on call to catheterization

Intraprocedural sedation*	
Medication	Dosage
Fentanyl	0.5–1.0 μg/kg intravenously (IV) for children <20 kg; 1 μg/kg for children >20 kg (up to 50 μg max dose)
Midazolam	0.05 mg/kg IV for children <20 kg; 1 mg IV dose for children >20 kg
Ketamine	0.5–1.0 mg/kg IV increments; or 2–4 mg/kg dose (intramuscularly) IM when unable to start IV (Note: atropine 0.01 mg/kg IM should be administered simultaneously at a different site when ketamine is given IM)
Glycopyrrolate	5 μg/kg IV, given before ketamine (not to exceed 20 μg/min IV)

*Sedation during cardiac catheterization consists of intravenous midazolam or fentanyl. Ketamine may be used for those children who require increased sedation or who have a history of difficult sedation with midazolam and fentanyl.

Therapeutic or Interventional Catheterization

The threshold for general anesthesia usage should be low for any patient undergoing a transcatheter intervention, with the common exceptions being coil or device closure of a patent ductus arteriosus and most cases of pulmonary and aortic balloon valvuloplasty in patients out of the neonatal age group. When any intervention requires absolute control of patient movement (such as aortic or pulmonary artery stent placement) or when there exists a potential risk of a major-life threatening mechanical complication (such as arterial or venous rupture), general anesthesia should also be employed.

Vascular Access

The purpose of this section is not to serve as a resource guide on how to obtain vascular access; that is covered elsewhere in this text. The smallest sheath size necessary for the given procedure or intervention should be used. Large vascular sheaths expose the vessels to additional risk of spasm or thrombosis and permanent occlusion. The majority of diagnostic and therapeutic catheterizations can be performed from the femoral sites (vein and/or artery, on the left or right). Nevertheless, there are occasions when alternative sites of entry are necessary or more convenient (Table 5.4). For example, in a typical bidirectional Glenn shunt (superior cavopulmonary anastomosis without antegrade flow), access to the pulmonary arteries can only be obtained from the subclavian or internal jugular approach (Figure 5.3). Catheter manipulation is not impossible, but it may be difficult from the femoral approach in patients with complex heterotaxy syndromes (Figure 5.4). The subclavian or jugular approach may allow for more complete studies with easier approach to the areas of interest.

TABLE 5.4. Scenarios when alternative vascular access may be necessary.

Glenn shunt anatomy
Inferior vena cava interruption with azygous or hemiazygous continuation in heterotaxy syndromes
Neonatal catheterization (umbilical artery or venous access available)
Absence of venous sites for cannulation
Device closure of ventricular septal defect
Arterial or venous cut-down

The umbilical venous and arterial vessels are generally adequate for cannulation and catheterization in neonates with this type of readily available vascular access. Bedside dynamic atrial septostomies are commonly performed through the umbilical vein. In addition, neonatal pulmonary and aortic valvuloplasty can also be performed safely through the umbilical vessels. However, owing to the tortuosity of this approach, intracardiac catheter manipulation may be somewhat limited; if excessive time is being expended, or if rhythm disturbances are excessive with complex intracardiac maneuvers, one should consider abandoning the umbilical route in favor of a femoral approach. Antibiotic coverage (typically vancomycin) should be provided to newborns with structural heart disease if the umbilical vessels are manipulated during the procedure.

Critically ill patients who have had previous catheterizations or multiple indwelling lines may have thrombosis and permanent occlusion of the usual peripheral sites of vascular access (Figure 5.5). Under these circumstances, the transhepatic approach (with direct stick or ultrasound guide) provides an effective means to catheterize the heart and great vessels (Figure 5.6). This approach may also be used electively in smaller infants when larger sheaths are required in an attempt to avoid damage to femoral or other vessels.

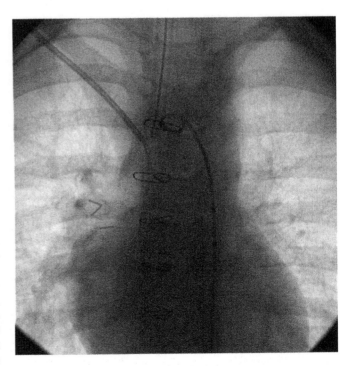

FIGURE 5.3. Subclavian vein access.

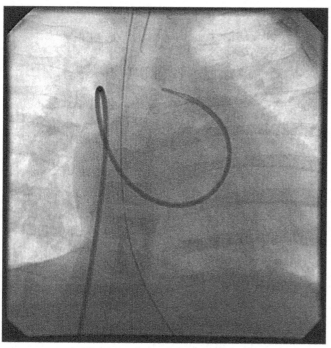

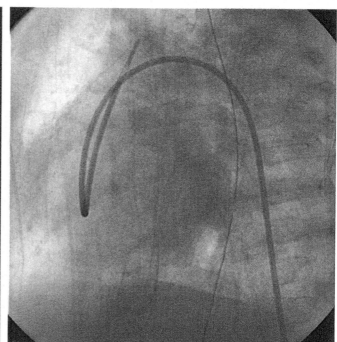

A

FIGURE 5.4. Interrupted inferior vena cava with azygous continuation. **(A)** Anterior-posterior view. **(B)** Lateral view.

During device closure of a ventricular septal defect, complexities of sheath positioning before placement of the device necessitates an arteriovenous wire loop, most often entering through the femoral artery and exiting the right internal jugular vein. Finally, there are occasions when it may be necessary for direct surgical cut-down to obtain access. The main indications for this is when large sheaths are required in small infants for completion of an intervention (such as aortic stent placement in an infant) or when aortic interventions are required but both femoral arteries are documented occluded. Surgical cut-down and vessel repair also provide a safer means of catheterization than the percutaneous approach in patients on extracorporeal membrane oxygen support who are aggressively anticoagulated.

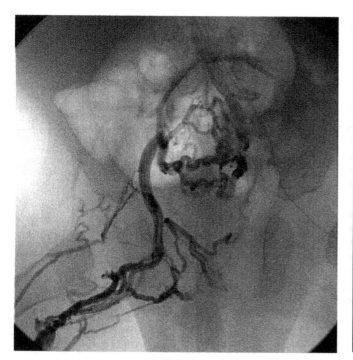

FIGURE 5.5. Right femoral venous occlusion.

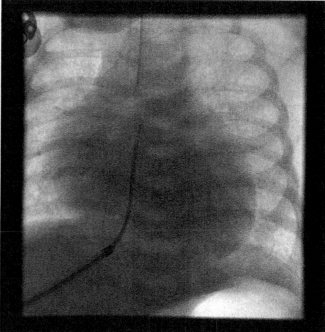

FIGURE 5.6. Transhepatic access.

Course of Catheterization

A standardized approach is utilized with every patient, and, although congenital cardiac defects vary greatly from patient to patient, the principles remain the same irrespective of the anatomy. During the data collection process, continual data analysis should occur; this promotes more meaningful, focused data collection and ensures that all viable hemodynamic and oximetric data points are obtained. The planned catheterization goals should be adjusted appropriately in response to data collected and the evolving understanding of each patient's anatomy and physiology. The focus of this section is not to describe actual catheter manipulations, as that topic is covered extensively in other texts dealing primarily with cardiac catheterization.

After adequate sedation or anesthesia has been instituted and central access has been obtained, the standard approach to data collection should be as follows (for the purposes of this discussion, access is assumed to be obtained from the femoral approach):

I. Initial catheter placement in the superior vena cava (SVC) and descending aorta
   A. Simultaneous blood samples from the descending aorta and SVC for
      i. Saturation from the SVC
      ii. Saturation and blood gas analysis from the aorta
      iii. Estimation of cardiac output
   B. Simultaneous pressure measurements from the descending aorta and SVC
II. Repositioning of the venous catheter into the mid right atrium (RA)
   A. Blood sampling from the RA for saturation
   B. Simultaneous pressure measurement from the descending aorta and the RA
III. Advancement of the venous catheter into the mid right ventricle (RV)
   A. Blood sampling from the RV for saturation
   B. Simultaneous pressure measurement from the descending aorta and the RV
IV. Advancement of the venous catheter into one of the pulmonary arteries (PAs) in preparation for a wedge pressure measurement and advancement of the arterial catheter retrograde into the body of the left ventricle (LV)
   A. Blood sampling from the PA for saturation
   B. Inflation of the balloon tip of the venous catheter and simultaneous pressure measurement from the PA catheter (now in the wedge position) and the LV
V. Deflation of the balloon on the venous catheter in the PA
   Simultaneous pressure measurement from the PA and the LV
VI. Advancement of the venous catheter into the contralateral PA in preparation of a wedge pressure measurement
   A. Blood sampling from the PA for saturation
   B. Inflation of the balloon tip of the venous catheter and simultaneous pressure measurement from the PA catheter (now in the wedge position) and the LV
VII. Deflation of the balloon on the venous catheter in the PA
   Simultaneous pressure measurement from the PA and the LV
VIII. Retraction of the venous catheter into the main pulmonary artery (MPA)
   Simultaneous pressure measurement from the MPA and the LV
IX. Retraction of the venous catheter from the MPA into the body of the RV and retraction of the arterial catheter into the ascending aorta
   Simultaneous pressure measurement from the RV and the ascending aorta
X. Retraction of the venous catheter into the RA and retraction of the arterial catheter into the descending aorta
   Simultaneous pressure measurement from the RA and the descending aorta

In patients with abnormal extra- or intracardiac connections, the catheter course is adjusted as necessary, but the principles of data collection remain the same. As an example, a patient who has undergone a Glenn shunt (superior cavopulmonary anastomosis) will have their catheterization commenced with a venous catheter in the superior vena cava, introduced from an internal jugular or subclavian access site. Simultaneously, arterial and venous catheters placed typically from the femoral site will allow for saturation and pressure data to be obtained from the right atrium, the aorta, and systemic ventricle as required. The superior vena cava catheter, when advanced, will pass into the pulmonary arteries, where saturation and pressure data are collected.

Angiography

The purpose of angiography is to define anatomy, provide a graphic assessment of ventricular function, and determine the degree of valve incompetence. Additionally, angiography is used as a direct guide to map the course for many different interventions. The site (atrial, ventricular, arterial, or venous) and the manner of injection (hand, power, or balloon occlusion) will depend on the particular indication for the angiogram. Typically, the volume of an injection is no more than 1 mL/kg (usually up to a maximum of 40 mL in an adult-sized patient) but may be increased in the presence of shunt lesions. Because of nephrotoxicity, the total volume of contrast is limited to no more than 6 mL/kg but should be decreased in the face of renal dysfunction. Table 5.5 outlines the most commonly performed angiograms and their indications.

Nonionic iodinated contrast with viscosity similar to that of plasma is most commonly used for angiography in the congenital cardiac population. This provides outstanding anatomic definition, with a low risk for adverse events. Nevertheless, several adverse events may occur in patients undergoing angiography. Although rare in children, acute anaphylaxis has been documented even in the absence of previous exposure. Skin reactions with urticaria are more common and respond to therapy with diphenhydramine and hydrocortisone. Contrast will alter ventricular filling conditions and may result in changes in ventricular compliance. This applies most acutely in ventricles that have preexisting diastolic abnormalities. If there is clinical indication (such as elevated atrial pressures after contrast administration in the presence of poor cardiac reserve), additional diuretics should be administered. An acute increase in pulmonary vascular resistance may occur particularly after direct pulmonary artery angiography. An acute elevation in pulmonary resistance may be very poorly tolerated in patients with pulmonary vascular obstructive disease or primary pulmonary hypertension, especially in the absence of an intracardiac shunt. Myocardial or vascular staining occurs when the

TABLE 5.5. Commonly performed angiograms and their indications.

Left and right ventriculography
Outline the ventricular septum and profile ventricular septal defects (left ventricle predominantly) (Figure 5.7)
Determine the degree of dilation and assess function (Figure 5.8)
Assess midcavitary or outflow tract obstruction
Quantify the degree of atrioventricular valve regurgitation
Aortography
Assess aortic valve competence
Define the aortic arch and brachiocephalic vessel anatomy
Diagnose the presence of patent ductus arteriosus and provide a map for placement of closure devices or coils
Provide a gross assessment of coronary artery origin and proximal course
Evaluate aortopulmonary collateral vessels
Pulmonary angiography (within the main or either branch pulmonary artery)
Define the pulmonary artery anatomy (Figure 5.9)
Define the angiographic degree of stenosis and provide a map for intervention (balloon dilation or stent placement)
Define pulmonary venous return during the levo phase of the contrast course
Diagnose the presence of pulmonary embolus
Coronary artery angiography
Define the origin and course in the presence of anomalies
Define the origin and course of any fistulae and serve as a map for intervention
Diagnose the presence of aneurysm or stenosis
Superior vena cava angiography
Evaluate pulmonary arteries and exclude stenosis after anastomosis with the pulmonary arteries (Glenn shunt)
Determine presence of stenosis or leak into the pulmonary venous baffle after Senning or Mustard surgery
Innominate vein angiography
Exclude persistent left superior vena cava (left common cardinal vein) before surgery requiring cardiopulmonary bypass or before a Glenn shunt
Selective pulmonary venography
Determine the course and presence of any stenosis within the particular vessel (Figure 5.10)
Selective angiography within aortopulmonary or venovenous collateral vessels
Determine the course and terminus of abnormal vasculature; serve as a map for possible coil or device occlusion if indicated

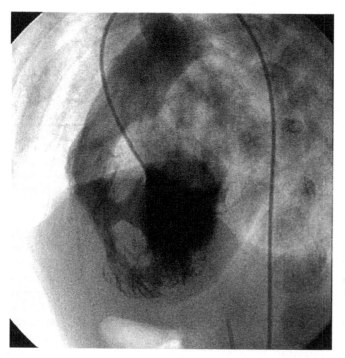

FIGURE 5.7. Ventricular septal defect.

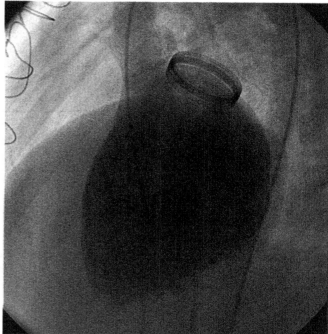

FIGURE 5.8. Left ventricular angiogram.

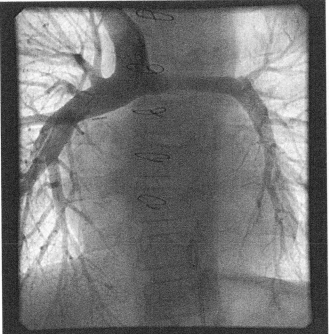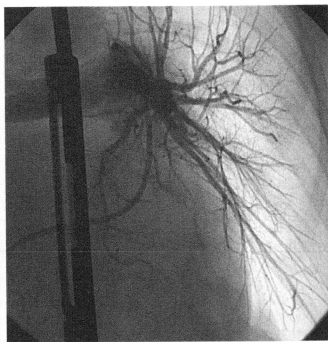

A **B**

FIGURE 5.9. Pulmonary angiogram. **(A)** Anterior-posterior view. **(B)** Lateral view.

angiographic catheter tip is lodged within ventricular trabecula-tions or the vascular endothelium. The power of the injection forces contrast to be lodged in extravascular and extracellular spaces, where it may remain until reabsorbed. Vascular staining may cause arterial spasm, and large myocardial staining may depress ventricular function.

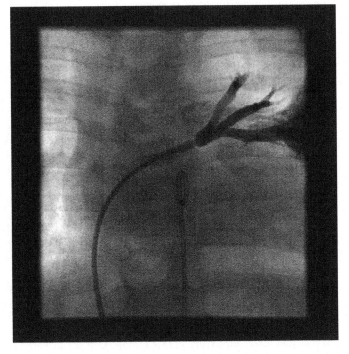

FIGURE 5.10. Pulmonary vein angiogram.

Hemodynamic Determinations

Measurement of cardiac output, determination of intracardiac shunts, and assessment of pulmonary and systemic vascular resistance are fundamental objectives of cardiac catheterization in patients with congenital cardiac defects. Accuracy in these measurements is imperative, as further palliation or corrective intervention (transcatheter or surgical) may depend on the results. In congenital cardiac catheterization, the following principles apply when assessing individual patient measurements:

Mixed venous saturation (MVS): In the presence of left-to-right shunt lesions, the superior vena cava saturation is utilized as the MVS. When the shunt is right to left, or if no shunt is present (intact atrial and ventricular septa and no supraventricular arterial connections, such as patent ductus arteriosus, aortopulmonary window, or aortopulmonary collateral vessels), the pulmonary artery saturation provides the most accurate measure of the MVS.

Cardiac output/index: In children, cardiac output measurements are typically indexed to body surface area to provide the cardiac index. The cardiac output can be measured directly by thermodilution technique or calculated on the basis of the Fick principle. The latter calculation requires a hemodynamic steady state, near simultaneous measurement of arterial and venous O_2 saturation, accurate measurement of circulating hemoglobin (for O_2 content calculation), and accurate measurement of oxygen consumption (VO_2). The VO_2 estimates can be found using standard La Farge tables. Calculation of cardiac index depends on accurate measures of the patient's weight and height (for body surface area).

Arteriovenous oxygen (AVO$_2$) saturation difference: The normal difference in saturations between the aorta and MVS is approximately 25% ($\pm$3%–5%), which represents normal tissue O_2 extraction when other co-morbidities, such as abnormalities in hemoglobin concentration, cardiac output, or systemic sepsis, are not present.

Pulmonary and systemic blood flow: In the absence of shunts (left to right or right to left), the pulmonary-to-systemic shunt ratio (Qp:Qs) is 1.0. With a net left-to-right shunt, the Qp:Qs ratio exceeds 1.0. With intracardiac shunts the flows can only be measured using the Fick principle (thermodilution is not accurate in patients with shunts). However, pulmonary blood flow cannot be accurately determined even by the Fick principle if accessory sources of pulmonary blood flow are present and the O_2 saturations within each pulmonary artery differ from one another. Examples of this include patent ductus arteriosus, where the left pulmonary artery saturation may be higher than the right pulmonary artery, or when multiple aortopulmonary collateral vessels are present. Under these clinical circumstances, there is no practical manner with which to calculate pulmonary blood flow.

Pulmonary and systemic vascular resistance: Determination of pulmonary vascular resistance (Rp) presumes equal blood flow to both lung fields. If a pulmonary artery stenosis (or multiple stenoses) is present, or lung volume on one side is decreased for any other reason, relative lung perfusion should be measured by a nuclear medicine scan and be taken into account when calculating Rp. Similarly, systemic vascular resistance (Rs) cannot be accurately calculated if any aortic narrowing occurs distal to the origin of the first brachiocephalic vessels.

Based on the measurements obtained during the cardiac catheterization, and the general principles outlined above, the following calculations can be completed to determine the following hemodynamic parameters.

Cardiac Index

Systemic (Qs) and pulmonary (Qp) blood flow measurements based on the Fick principle rely on calculating the oxygen extraction across a vascular bed (systemic or pulmonary) in the presence of steady-state tissue oxygen consumption. In the case of systemic blood flow, the oxygen content of blood returning from the systemic vascular bed (MVS) is subtracted from the oxygen content of blood (aortic) flowing toward the systemic vascular bed. Hence:

Arterial oxygen content = (AoSAT/100) $\times$ hemoglobin $\times$ 1.36
Venous oxygen content = (MVS/100) $\times$ hemoglobin $\times$ 1.36

where AOSat is aortic saturation, MVS is mixed venous saturation, hemoglobin is measured as g/100 mL of blood, and 1.36 is the mL of oxygen bound to 1 g of hemoglobin when fully saturated. As cardiac index is expressed in liters, the denominator should be multiplied by a factor 10.

The Fick equation for cardiac index is thus as follows:

$$Qs(1/min/m^2) = \frac{VO_2}{(AoSat/100 - MVS/100) \times Hb \times 1.36 \times 10}$$

where VO_2 is oxygen consumption (indexed to body surface area).

Similarly, pulmonary blood flow is calculated by subtracting the oxygen content of blood flowing toward the lungs (pulmonary artery) from the oxygen content of the blood returning from the lungs (pulmonary vein) using the following equation:

$$Qp(1/min/m^2) = \frac{VO_2}{(PVSat/100 - PASat/100) \times Hb \times 1.36 \times 10}$$

where PVSat is pulmonary vein saturation and PASat is pulmonary artery saturation.

The impact of dissolved oxygen on the cardiac index measurement can be ignored if the partial pressure of oxygen in the particular sample (aortic or pulmonary venous) is less than 150 mm Hg. However, if greater than this, then it should be taken into account by altering the Fick equation by adding the amount of dissolved oxygen based on 0.003 mL of oxygen dissolved per every 1 mm Hg partial pressure of oxygen in the blood sample:

$$Qs(1/min/m^2) = \frac{VO_2}{\substack{(AoSat/100 \times Hb \times 1.36 \times 10) - \\ (MVS/100 \times Hb \times 1.36 \times 10) + (0.003 \times AoPO_2)}}$$

where $AoPO_2$ is partial pressure of oxygen in the arterial sample.

When calculating Qp, and the partial pressure of oxygen is again greater than 150 mm Hg in the pulmonary venous sample, the calculation is as follows:

$$Qs(1/min/m^2) = \frac{VO_2}{\substack{(PVSat/100 \times Hb \times 1.36 \times 10) - \\ (PASat/100 \times Hb \times 1.36 \times 10) + (0.003 \times PVPO_2)}}$$

where $PVPO_2$ is partial pressure of oxygen in the pulmonary venous sample.

Systemic-to-Pulmonary Shunt Calculation

The systemic-to-pulmonary flow ratio (Qp:Qs) is based on the presence of increased saturation across the right heart structures (from the superior vena cava to the pulmonary arteries; i.e., a left-to-right shunt) or a decrease in saturations across the left heart structures (from the pulmonary veins to the aorta; i.e., a right-to-left shunt). Resolution of the Fick equations for Qs and Qp allow the flow ratio to be simplified as follows:

$$Qp/Qs = \frac{AoSat - SVCSat}{PVSat - PASat}$$

In the absence of any shunt (left to right or right to left), the aortic and pulmonary venous saturations are identical (AoSat = PVSat); and the true mixed venous saturation is the pulmonary artery saturation (SVCSat = PASat). Under these circumstances, Qs is equal to Qp, and thus the Qp:Qs ratio is 1.0. The Qp:Qs flow ratio is >1 when net shunting is left to right (e.g., atrial septal and ventricular septal defects) and <1 in the presence of a net right-to-left shunt (e.g. Blalock-Taussig shunt or Eisenmenger syndrome).

The concept of effective pulmonary blood flow (Qeff) refers to that portion of the pulmonary artery blood flow that has not already been oxygenated (i.e., the Qp subtracting any volume of blood that has already been oxygenated and that is recirculating to the lungs because of an intracardiac left-to-right shunt). Determination of Qeff allows for the calculation of the volume of intracardiac shunting even in complex bidirectional shunt lesions. The venous blood saturation used for calculation of Qeff is that measured in the superior vena cava; other than the rare occurrence of anomalous pulmonary venous return to the superior vena cava, there is no oxygenated blood admixture in this sample. Qeff is calculated in the following manner:

$$Qeff \left(1/\min/m^2 \right) = \frac{VO_2}{\left(PVSat/100 - SVCSat/100 \right) \times Hb \times 1.36 \times 10}$$

Intracardiac shunts can thus be calculated:

$$Left\text{-}to\text{-}right\ shunt = Qp - Qeff$$

$$Right\text{-}to\text{-}left\ shunt = Qs - Qeff$$

Vascular Resistances

Resistance calculation is based on Ohm's law that determines voltage (or potential difference) to be the product of current and a constant resistance:

$$V = I \times R$$

where V is voltage, I is current, and R is resistance.

This equation can be reworked to:

$$R = \frac{V}{I}$$

The hemodynamic equivalent of the Ohm's resistance calculation is modified with potential difference replaced by the transpulmonary or transsystemic gradient and current replaced by the flow across the particular vascular bed (systemic or pulmonary). Hence:

$$Systemic\ vascular\ resistnace\ (Rs) = \frac{AoPressure - RAPressure}{Qs}$$

where AoPressure and RAPressure are mean aortic and right atrial pressures, respectively.

Normal Rs is approximately 15–25 Wood units $\times m^2$ (the calculation is indexed to body surface area, when Qs used is the cardiac index).

$$Pulmonary\ vascular\ resistance\ (Rp) = \frac{PAPressure - LAPressure}{Qp}$$

where PAPressure and LAPressure are mean pulmonary artery and left atrial pressures, respectively. Pulmonary venous wedge pressures are used if the left atrial pressure is not measured directly.

Normal Rp is ≤ 3 Wood units $\times m^2$ (the calculation is indexed to body surface area, when the Qp used is the indexed pulmonary blood flow).

Emergency Cardiac Catheterization

The indications for emergency cardiac catheterization most frequently occur in the newborn period. Transposition physiology with inadequate mixing at the atrial or ductal level, and critical aortic and pulmonary valve obstruction account for the most common congenital lesions requiring acute intervention (Figure 5.11). All of these lesions require patency of the ductus arteriosus for the provision of systemic or pulmonary blood flow, respectively. These infants may often have their procedures performed solely with umbilical venous or arterial access, but alternative peripheral or central intravenous access should be obtained for the infusion of prostaglandin E_1 or other medications and for fluid and glucose administration. If indwelling umbilical lines are exchanged for arterial or venous sheaths and/or utilized for interventions, antibiotic prophylaxis for omphalitis and possible bacterial endocarditis is indicated (typically vancomycin for staph coverage). Given acute

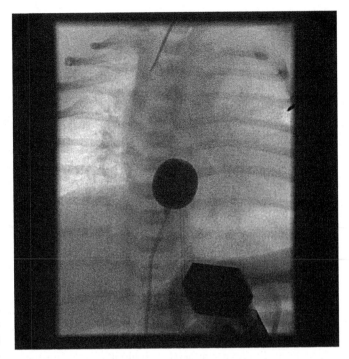

Figure 5.11. Dynamic atrial septostomy.

changes in physiology that may occur around interventions at this age (such as balloon atrial septostomy or valve dilation), these newborns should be managed in a critical care setting during the periprocedural period.

Complications

Careful preparation and planning and precise execution are instrumental in performing catheterization with low risk and few complications. Nevertheless, complications are intrinsic given the nature of these procedures. Thus, every attempt should be made to prepare for such complications as may arise, to respond to the adverse pathologic changes as expeditiously as possible when complications do occur, and to return the patient to a stable state for the continuation of the catheterization. If life-threatening complications do arise, the procedure should be discontinued and the patient stabilized before continuing. Exceptions to this principle should only occur when the procedure itself is of vital importance for survival (e.g., an atrial septal defect creation in a patient with transposition of the great arteries and severe cyanosis).

The following categories outline the broad types of complications associated with cardiac catheterization.

Rhythm and Conduction Disturbances

The expectation of rhythm and conduction abnormalities is germane to pediatric cardiac catheterization. The cardiac structures are small, and the onset of tachy- or bradyarrhythmias may result from only minor catheter movements. Drugs for immediate administration (such as adenosine, atropine, and epinephrine), pacing catheters and temporary pacemakers, and a DC defibrillator/cardioverter should be immediately available. The majority of the rhythm disturbances can be corrected rapidly and the catheterization continued; however, complete heart block, when catheter induced, may persist for some time before resolving and may interfere sufficiently with the hemodynamic assessment that the procedure may need to be deferred.

Hemorrhage

Substantial blood loss is unusual during diagnostic cardiac catheterization, but it is more likely in the course of prolonged interventions that may require multiple wire and catheter replacements. Generally, hemodilution is a more likely cause of an acute decrease in hematocrit. Careful attention should be paid to vascular entry sites after the procedure, as pressure dressings may mask substantial rebleeding. A high index of suspicion for retroperitoneal hemorrhage should be maintained for any patient complaining of low back pain after the procedure (Figure 5.12).

Vessel Perforation

Any patient who has undergone vascular balloon dilation or stent placement should be carefully assessed for vessel perforation after the procedure. To this end, routine chest radiography is performed during the immediate convalescent period. Changes in the diameter of the mediastinum, any new lung infiltrates, or the presence of a hemothorax should be regarded as an indication of this complication until proven otherwise.

Vascular Injury

This topic has been partially discussed in the section After Catheterization, General Status. Generally, the smallest arterial and venous sheath sizes required for the procedure should be used. Furthermore, the sheath (or sheaths) should be removed as soon as possible after completion of the procedure and only left in place in the event of extreme emergencies and the absence of other reliable central

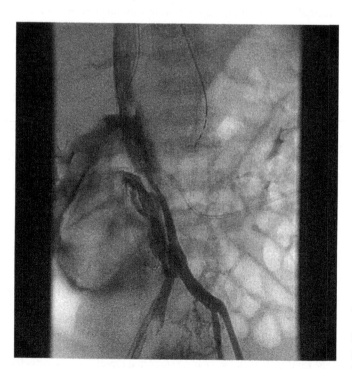

FIGURE 5.12. Retroperitoneal hematoma.

venous access. After sheath removal, sufficient pressure to stop bleeding, but not to completely compress the vessel, should be used to obtain hemostasis. These principles apply to all vascular sites, not only those in the femoral region. Chest radiography may not be necessary after subclavian or jugular venous entry if initial access was uncomplicated, and chest fluoroscopy at completion of the procedure did not reveal a new pleural effusion suggesting hemothorax.

Cardiac Perforation

Passage of catheters, wires, or other devices into extracardiac spaces may have negligible pathologic impact at one extreme or may result in immediate collapse of the patient with tamponade and cardiac arrest at the other extreme. As examples, inadvertent passage of an atrial transseptal (Brockenbrough) needle through the posterior wall of the left atrium may have no effect, whereas perforation of the right atrial appendage with a 5 French catheter may result in immediate tamponade. Perforation can almost always be avoided. Use of balloon tipped catheters and flexible or tip-deflectable guidewires should be utilized for catheter manipulation in the small structures of the infant heart. Catheters should never be manipulated unless under fluoroscopic guidance (and occasionally ultrasound); furthermore, the judicious use of small contrast injections assists greatly when exact catheter position is uncertain. All pediatric catheterization laboratories should have readily available kits for pericardiocentesis. Most often, a pigtail catheter of variable size is introduced into the pericardial space and left in situ for continuous aspiration if necessary. Equipment for autotransfusion should also be accessible.

Valve Injury

Damage to valve structures is rare during diagnostic procedures and most often occurs after balloon valvuloplasty procedures. Of these, aortic insufficiency is the most important. Depending on the severity, long-term medical management may need to be instituted, whereas immediate operation for valve repair or replacement may be required if aortic insufficiency is severe and symptomatic. Pulmonary insufficiency after pulmonary valvuloplasty, although more common, is well tolerated and does not generally require treatment. Damage to tricuspid valve chordal structures and resultant tricuspid regurgitation during right ventricular myocardial biopsy is well described. This is also typically well tolerated, even in the acute phase, but may need medical management or surgical intervention if associated pulmonary insufficiency and/or right ventricular dysfunction is present.

Cardiac Catheterization in Specific Circumstances

As outlined earlier, careful planning and cautious execution are essential for all cardiac catheterizations. There are specific clinical situations, however, that mandate unique planning or alternative approaches. Although not comprehensive, this section deals with some of these situations.

The Neonatal Patient

Special attention should be paid to temperature control and blood glucose management. Mechanical ventilation is mandatory, especially when the patient is receiving intravenous prostaglandin therapy for ductal maintenance, as administration of opioid sedatives will have a high likelihood of inducing apnea. Given the size of the cardiac structures, meticulous catheter manipulation is vital. Damage to valve tissues, potential for perforation, and the incidence of catheter-induced rhythm disturbances are all more likely in the neonatal patient.

Acute Myocarditis and Low Cardiac Output States

These patients, by definition, have low cardiac reserve and are unlikely to tolerate major changes in their physiologic status. Acute manipulation of systemic vascular resistance (such as occurs with anesthetic induction), rhythm disturbances, and depression of intrinsic catecholamine drive with administration of sedation may result in acute collapse. If cardiac catheterization is necessary, then preparation for such eventualities is required before commencement. Sedation or anesthetic techniques should be adapted to avoid rapid changes in systemic resistance, with pre- and afterload maintained with fluid administration and pharmacologically if necessary. Noninvasive monitoring should be continuous, but invasive arterial pressure monitoring should be obtained as soon as practically possible. Sinus node dysfunction with diminished heart rate variability and inappropriate heart rate response to hypotension (i.e., relative bradycardia) are particularly ominous signs and should result in immediate action.

Before and After Heart Transplantation Evaluations

Many of the issues outlined earlier for low cardiac output states apply to the pretransplant catheterization in patients with chronic heart failure, and the same precautions apply. Patients with acute graft failure or hemodynamically significant rejection will also behave in a similar manner. Post-transplant catheterization, for either rejection surveillance with biopsy or coronary evaluation, typically follows the course of routine diagnostic procedures. However, the presence of angiographically evident coronary stenoses should raise the concern for ventricular fibrillation, especially during coronary artery cannulation.

Pulmonary Hypertension

Cardiac catheterization in this population of patients is of particular high risk. Preload dependence and low cardiac reserve, especially in patients without intra- or extracardiac shunts, should be accommodated as described earlier for any patient with low cardiac output. Ventricular–ventricular interaction, with left ventricular compression by a hypertensive right ventricle, further contributes to impairment of cardiac output. In the periprocedure period, impaired coronary artery perfusion may result in a further acute decrease in cardiac ejection, myocardial ischemia, and arrhythmia genesis. During catheterization, consideration should be given to the creation of an atrial septal defect in these patients if right atrial pressures are excessively elevated and measured cardiac output is markedly decreased. This would allow cardiac output to be maintained but at the expense of lower arterial saturations.

Applying Catheterization Principles at the Bedside

Much hemodynamic information can be obtained at the bedside with minimally invasive and noninvasive monitoring. The determination of cardiac output and resistance may at times be based on some assumptions (depending on the extent of invasive monitoring available), but, with appropriate use of data, an overall impression can easily be obtained. Depending on the clinical status, more invasive monitoring may be required. For example, a central venous line with catheter tip in the superior vena cava can be used to measure mean superior vena cava pressure and oxygen saturation (via co-oximetry). Apart from the absolute pressure measurement (indicating the right ventricular filling pressure), the hemoglobin and measured or estimated oxygen consumption allow for determination of the cardiac index (using the peripheral pulse oximetry as an estimate of the arterial saturation) and the systemic vascular resistance (using the estimate of cardiac index and the mean blood pressure measured noninvasively). The accuracy of these estimates can be improved with invasive blood pressure and arterial saturation measurements. Simultaneous arterial and superior vena cava pressures can be measured, as well as blood for superior vena cava and arterial blood gas analysis. Central lines placed in the inferior vena cava, while providing important pressure monitoring data, are of little use in estimating mixed venous saturation. Depending on the location of the sampling tip, renal, splanchnic, or hepatic venous admixture may substantially alter the O_2 saturation of inferior vena cava blood in unpredictable ways.

Pulmonary artery and pulmonary artery wedge pressures can be obtained with an indwelling pulmonary artery catheter, and blood can be sampled for a true mixed venous saturation. With use of the hemoglobin and measured or estimated oxygen consumption, calculation of the cardiac index (using the peripheral pulse oximetry saturation, or a directly measured sample from an arterial blood gas for arterial oxygen saturation, and the mixed venous oxygen saturation from the pulmonary artery catheter) and the shunt fraction (using a superior vena cava oxygen saturation from the proximal tip of the pulmonary artery catheter, the pulmonary artery saturation from the distal tip in the pulmonary artery, and the arterial saturation) is possible. In patients with left-to-right shunts, both Qp and Qs can be calculated. In the absence of any shunt, the MVS is the pulmonary artery saturation, and the Qp will equal the Qs. In addition, the pulmonary and systemic vascular resistances (using the mean pulmonary artery and mean wedge pressure to calculate the transpulmonary gradient and the mean arterial and mean superior vena cava pressure to calculate the transsystemic gradient) can be determined.

Summary of Hemodynamic Calculations

1. Cardiac Index and pulmonary blood flow (taking arterial pO_2 into account):

$$Qs(1/min/m^2) = \frac{VO_2}{(AoSat/100 \times Hb \times 1.36 \times 10) - (MVS/100 \times Hb \times 1.36 \times 10) + (0.003 \times AoPO_2)}$$

$$Qs(1/min/m^2) = \frac{VO_2}{(PVSat/100 \times Hb \times 1.36 \times 10) - (PASat/100 \times Hb \times 1.36 \times 10) + (0.003 \times PVPO_2)}$$

2. Cardiac index and pulmonary blood flow (ignoring the contribution of dissolved oxygen [i.e., arterial PO_2 less than 150 mm Hg]):

$$Qs(1/min/m^2) = \frac{VO_2}{(AoSat/100 - MVS/100) \times Hb \times 1.36 \times 10}$$

$$Qp(1/min/m^2) = \frac{VO_2}{(PVSat/100 - PASat/100) \times Hb \times 1.36 \times 10}$$

3. Systemic-to-pulmonary shunt ratio:

$$Qp/Qs = \frac{AoSat - SVCSat}{PVSat - PASat}$$

4. Systemic and pulmonary vascular resistances:

$$Rs = \frac{AoPressure - RAPressure}{Qs}$$

$$Rp = \frac{PAPressure - LAPressure}{Qp}$$

where Qs is cardiac index (L/min/m^2); Qp, pulmonary blood flow (L/min/m^2); Rs, systemic vascular resistance (Wood units $\times$ m^2); Rp, pulmonary vascular resistance (Wood units $\times$ m^2); VO$_2$, oxygen consumption (mL/min/m^2); AoSat, arterial oxygen saturation; Hb, hemoglobin (g/dL); MVS, mixed venous oxygen saturation; AoPo$_2$, aortic partial pressure of oxygen (mm Hg); PVSat, pulmonary vein oxygen saturation; PASat, pulmonary artery oxygen saturation; PVPO$_2$, pulmonary vein partial pressure of oxygen (mm Hg); SVCSat, superior vena cava oxygen saturation; AoPressure, mean aortic pressure (mm Hg), RAPressure, mean right atrial pressure (mm Hg); PAPressure, mean pulmonary artery pressure (mm Hg); LAPressure, mean left atrial pressure (mm Hg).

Further Readings

Book WM, Raviele AA, Vincent RN. Transhepatic vascular access in pediatric cardiology patients with occlusion of traditional central venous sites. J Invasive Cardiol 1999;11(6):341–344.

Kanter JP, Hellenbrand WE. Recent advances in non-interventional pediatric cardiac catheterization. Curr Opin Cardiol 2005;20(2): 75–79.

Mullins CE. History of pediatric interventional catheterization: pediatric therapeutic cardiac catheterizations. Pediatr Cardiol 1998;19: 3–7.

Rome JJ, Kreutzer J. Pediatric interventional catheterization: reasonable expectations and outcomes. Pediatr Clin North Am 2004;51(6):1589–1610, viii.

Schneider DJ, Levi DS, Serwacki MJ, et al. Overview of interventional pediatric cardiology in 2004. Minerva Pediatr 2004;56(1):1–28.

Schroeder VA, Shim D, Spicer RL, et al. Surgical emergencies during pediatric interventional catheterization. J Pediatr 2002;140(5):570–575.

Toyono M, Harada K, Tamura M, et al. The efficacy of using pulmonary vein wedge pressure for the estimation of pulmonary artery pressure in children with congenital heart disease. Cathet Cardiovasc Intervent 2003;58:232–237.

Vitiello R, McCrindle B, Nykanen D, et al. Complications associated with pediatric cardiac catheterization. JACC 1998;1433–1440.

Zeevi B, Berant M, Fogelman R, et al. Acute complications in the current era of therapeutic cardiac catheterization for congenital heart disease. Cardiol Young 1999;266–272.

6
Introduction to Congenital Heart Disease: Nomenclature and Classification

James D. St. Louis

Introduction

Webster's dictionary defines the term *nomenclature* as *a system or process of naming*. Congenital defects of the heart present a unique challenge in establishing an accurate and consistent nomenclature. The challenge is secondary to an incomplete understanding of the embryology of the heart and the vast complexity of the science. In any attempt to describe a complex system, several lines of reasoning may evolve that foster not only controversy but also confusion. A system to describe congenital lesions of the heart is certainly no exception. Several giants in our field have been credited with the elucidation of specific theories that have provided a better understanding of these cardiac lesions. A brief review of the nomenclature and classification systems commonly used to describe congenital lesions of the heart is presented here as a general introduction to congenital heart disease.

Van Praagh's Segmental Approach to the Classification of Congenital Heart Disease

The heart is normally positioned in the left hemithorax with the apex pointing toward the left; this configuration is commonly referred to as *levocardia* (although, because this is the usual configuration, few physicians actually use this term). *Dextrocardia* refers to the anatomic configuration when the heart is in the right hemithorax and the apex points toward the right. *Mesocardia* describes an anatomic configuration with the heart in the midline. Dextrocardia and mesocardia are commonly associated with other congenital heart defects that are described in subsequent chapters.

Richard Van Praagh has presented a classification scheme based on the segmental anatomy of the developing heart [1–5]. The theory states that by understanding the anatomic cardiac segments, the majority of human hearts with congenital defects may be described. The three segments that Van Praagh described in turn consist of the atria, the ventricles, and the great vessels. The two determining factors that result from this understanding are the visceroatrial situs, which dictates where the atria are located, and the bulboventricular loop, which does the same for the ventricles and the great vessels. These segments are referenced in sequence, with each being designated by a letter. The term *situs* means *position* or *location*. The connection of the visceral venous vessels (the superior vena cava and inferior vena cava) and the atrial body is termed the *visceroatrial situs* and is described by the letters *S* (*situs solitus*), *I* (*situs inversus*), or *A* (*situs ambiguous*).

When the visceroatrial situs is normal (*situs solitus*), the morphologic right atrium (i.e., blunt atrial appendage with a broad junction or connection to the body of the right atrium [6]) is located on the right side of the body and connected to a right-sided superior and inferior vena cava. The inferior vena cava courses to the right of the descending aorta. The morphologic left atrium (i.e., narrow atrial appendage with a crenellated edge and narrow connection to the body of the left atrium [6]) is located on the left side of the body. The stomach and spleen lie to the left, the right lobe of the liver is larger than the left, the appendix is right sided, the right lung is trilobed, and the left lung is bilobed. Note that the embryologic development of the proximal inferior vena cava is closely associated with the embryologic development of the liver such that the right atrium and liver are almost invariably located on the same side.

In *situs inversus*, the position of the abdominal organs is reversed, with the stomach and spleen lying on the right and the dominant lobe of the liver to the left. The appendix and inferior vena cava are to the left, with the left lung being trilobed. The morphologic right atrium is on the left side of the chest, with the superior and inferior vena cava also entering the chest on the left side.

Situs ambiguous describes a group of anomalies in which the dominant characteristic is a lack of visceral sidedness. The abdominal organs may be positioned to the anatomic left or right, often with the liver lying in the midline. A unique characteristic of these individuals is the abnormal existence or lack of existence of the spleen (Ivemark syndrome). Polysplenic patients tend to have all atrial and pulmonary structures consistent with left-sided morphology, whereas asplenic patients tend to be right-sided dominate [7]. When two atria exist, both are of either the left or right

D.S. Wheeler et al. (eds.), *Cardiovascular Pediatric Critical Illness and Injury*,
DOI 10.1007/978-1-84800-923-3_6, © Springer-Verlag London Limited 2009

morphology. As such, Anderson and colleagues prefer to use the terms *right atrial isomerism* and *left atrial isomerism*, depending on the morphology of the atria [6–9]. In a majority of patients, a single atrium is present. Some authors use the term *heterotaxy* to describe the anatomic relationship when the position of the heart and viscera is discordant (e.g., situs inversus with normal cardiac position in the left hemithorax—this unique anatomy is usually accompanied by complex cardiac defects, and the inferior vena cava is usually interrupted).

The orientation of the ventricular mass is described by how the embryonic cardiac tube loops during its development. The terms *right* and *left* should be used to refer to the specific morphology of the ventricular mass and not their spatial arrangements. The anatomic right ventricle has a very trabeculated endocardium, and the left ventricular endocardium is smooth with fine trabeculation. The rightward (normal) orientation is given the term *D* for *D-looping*. This indicates that the morphologic right ventricle is oriented to the right and anterior to the morphologic left ventricle. If the cardiac tube undergoes looping in the leftward direction, the segment is given the reference letter *L* for *L-looping*. In this situation, the morphologic right ventricle lies posterior and to the left of the morphologic left ventricle.

The final segmental orientation described by Van Praagh deals with the relationship of the great vessels and semilunar valves to the ventricles. The aorta is normally committed to the morphologic left ventricle with the aortic valve located posterior and leftward to the pulmonary valve. This *normal* relationship is given the reference letter *S*. When the great vessels are transposed, with the aortic valve being rightward and anterior to the pulmonary valve, the convention used is *D*. With D-transposed great vessels, the aorta is committed to the morphologic right ventricle and the pulmonary artery to the morphologic left ventricle. When the orientation of the great vessels and semilunar valves are normal but the aorta is committed to the right ventricle and the pulmonary artery to the left ventricle, the term L-transposed great vessels is used. Thus, a normal heart would be classified as [S, D, S] using the Van Praagh classification.

An Alternative Approach to the Classification of Congenital Heart Disease

Although the segmental description put forth by Van Praagh is correct, it is how these segments are or are not aligned that is of greater significance. Robert Anderson devised a theory that places primary importance on the path that blood will take through the heart and major vessels as opposed to where the blood is at any moment in time [9]. This system describes an embryonic five-chamber heart tube and attributes all subsequent cardiac defects to their morphology, their connection, and the relationships of these segments. These two opposing theories have at times fostered controversy and confusion but established a strong foundation for our understanding of congenital heart defects. This approach has been applied utilizing the following terminology:

1. *Visceroatrial situs* is described as above with the following terms: situs solitus (morphologic right atrium on the right), situs inversus (morphologic right atrium on the left), left isomerism (bilateral left atria), and right isomerism (bilateral right atria). Bronchopulmonary anatomy is usually consistent with atrial situs,

which may provide an important diagnostic clue as to the visceroatrial situs. Right isomerism again is usually (but not always) associated with asplenia, and left isomerism is usually associated with polysplenia.

2. *Atrioventricular connection* is described by six types and four modes of connection. *Types* include concordant (morphologic right atrium connected to right ventricle and vice versa), discordant (morphologic right atrium connected to left ventricle and vice versa), ambiguous (atrial isomerism or situs ambiguous), double inlet (both atria connect to one ventricle), absent right connection, or absent left connection (the latter two describing the situation when one atrioventricular connection is absent). *Modes* include two perforate valves, single perforate valve, one perforate and one imperforate, and common valve.

3. *Ventriculoarterial connection* describes both the type of connection between the ventricle and great arteries (or artery, e.g., truncus arteriosus) as well as the mode of connection. *Types* include concordant (right ventricle connected to the pulmonary artery, left ventricle connected to the aorta), discordant (i.e., transposition), double outlet (both great arteries arise predominantly from a single ventricle), and single outlet (only one great artery is connected to the ventricle). The latter is further described as single outlet–common arterial trunk, single outlet–solitary aortic trunk with pulmonary atresia, single outlet–solitary pulmonary trunk with aortic atresia, and single outlet–solitary arterial trunk. *Modes* include two perforate valves, a single perforate valve, one perforate and one imperforate valve, and a common or truncal valve.

Although Anderson never described the side of the aortic arch in the sequential segmental analysis, many clinicians have added this description to the sequential segmental approach: aortic arch side [L = left aortic arch, R = right aortic arch]. Thus, while the *Andersonian* approach never advocated an alphabetical shorthand, many clinicians would describe a normal heart as SCCL or situs solitus, concordant atrioventricular connection, concordant ventriculoarterial connection, left aortic arch.

International Congenital Heart Surgery Nomenclature and Database

The idea of an International Congenital Heart Surgery Nomenclature and Database was developed to address the confusion and controversy that has perpetuated with diverging theories and conventions regarding the classification of congenital heart defects. Published in 2000, the Proceedings of the International Nomenclature and Database Conferences for Pediatric Cardiac Surgery set forth a standardized classification system and nomenclature conceived and supported by the international community of congenital heart surgeons [10]. The recommendations of these proceedings are presented in a manner consistent with the organization of this textbook. The grouping of individual defects is based on both anatomic and physiologic characteristics (Table 6.1). Cardiac defects with shunts that result in pulmonary overcirculation often present with congestive heart failure. Mixing lesions with increased pulmonary blood flow can present with cyanosis and are presented in a separate section. Obstructive lesions, both right and left sided, can present with either acute hemodynamic compromise requiring emergent intervention or without symptoms and minimal physical findings.

TABLE 6.1. Functional classification of congenital heart lesions.

Acyanotic congenital heart disease
Left-to-right shunts
    Atrial septal defects
    Ventricular septal defects
    Atrioventricular septal defects
    Aortopulmonary window
    Patent ductus arteriosus
Left-sided obstructive lesions
    Coarctation of the aorta
    Congenital aortic stenosis
    Interrupted aortic arch
    Mitral stenosis
Cyanotic congenital heart disease
Lesions associated with *decreased* pulmonary blood flow (right-to-left shunts)
    Tetralogy of Fallot
    Pulmonary stenosis
    Pulmonary atresia
        With intact ventricular septum (PA/IVS)
        With ventricular septal defect (PA/VSD)
    Tricuspid atresia
    Ebstein's anomaly
Lesions associated with *increased* pulmonary blood flow (complete mixing lesions)
    Transposition of the great vessels
        With intact ventricular septum (TGA/IVS, simple TGA)
        With ventricular septa defect (TGA/VSD)
    Double-outlet right ventricle (DORV)
    Total anomalous pulmonary venous connection
    Truncus arteriosus
Single-ventricle physiology
    Hypoplastic left heart syndrome
    Double-inlet left ventricle (DILV)

References

1. Van Praagh R. Terminology of congenital heart disease: glossary and commentary. Circulation 1977;56:139.
2. Van Praagh R. The segmental approach to diagnosis in congenital heart disease. Birth Defects 1972;8:4–23.
3. Van Praagh R, Vlad P. Dextrocardia, mesocardia, and levocardia. The segmental approach to diagnosis in congenital heart disease. In: Keith JD, Rowe RD, Vlad P, eds. Heart Disease in Infancy and Childhood. New York: MacMillan; 1978:638–695.
4. Van Praagh R. The segmental approach to understanding complex cardiac lesions. In: Eldredge WJ, Goldberg H, Lemole GM, eds. Current Problems in Congenital Heart Disease. New York: SP Medical and Scientific Books; 1979:1–18.
5. Van Praagh R. Diagnosis of complex congenital heart disease: morphologic–anatomic method and terminology. Cardiovasc Intervent Radiol 1984;7:115–120.
6. Anderson RH. Terminology. In: Anderson R, Shinebourne EA, Macartney FJ, Tynan M, eds. Paediatric Cardiology. Edinburgh: Churchill Livingstone; 1987:65–82.
7. Seo JW, Brown NA, Ho SY, Anderson RH. Abnormal laterality and congenital cardiac anomalies. Relations of visceral and cardiac morphologies in the mouse. Circulation 1992;86:642–650.
8. Becker AE, Anderson RH. Isomerism of the atrial appendages—goodbye to asplenia and all that. In: Clark EB, Takao A, eds. Developmental Cardiology: Morphogenesis and Function. Mount Kisco, NY: Futura; 1990:659–670.
9. Anderson RH. Normal and abnormal development of the heart. In: Baue A, Geha A, Hammond G, Laks H, Naunheim K, eds. Glenn's Thoracic and Cardiovascular Surgery. Stamford, CT: Appleton & Lange; 1996:5;955–970.
10. Society of Thoracic Surgeons National Congenital Heart Surgery Database Committee. Proceedings of the International Nomenclature and Database Conference for Pediatric Cardiac Surgery, 1998–1999. Ann Thorac Surg 2000;69:1–372.

7
Palliative Procedures

Mark A. Scheurer and Andrew M. Atz

Palliate: to alleviate a symptom without curing the underlying medical condition

> [From the past participle stem of palliare meaning *to cover or hide*; from pallium meaning *a covering*]
> (Merriam-Webster's Collegiate Dictionary, 11th edition)

Historical Perspective

As the definition of palliate suggests, palliations are performed on those patients who can never be completely cured or those patients who cannot be cured safely at the time of their initial presentation. Historically, all initial attempts to intervene in children with congenital heart disease were palliative in nature. The first surgical palliation for congenital heart disease was the now famous right subclavian artery to right pulmonary artery shunt performed on Eileen Saxon by Blalock and Thomas in 1944 [1]. Rashkind and Miller's development of the catheter-based atrial septostomy in 1966 opened the door to revolutionary invasive catheterization-based procedures that now often blur the distinction between surgeon and interventional cardiologist [2]. These procedures are not limited to the operating suite or to the catheterization laboratory, as a balloon atrial septostomy can now often be performed at the bedside [3]. Current techniques and procedures are varied and reflect the rapidly advancing technological achievements of designers and operators.

Indications for Palliation

Palliative procedures are performed on those children in whom an eventual biventricular circulation is possible or those with single-ventricle physiology in whom other future procedures will be required. Initial complete repairs are sometimes unfeasible or unwise to attempt in the neonatal period because of anatomic or co-morbid conditions. Stabilization of the physiology with a shunt or pulmonary artery band can result in adequate somatic growth that might allow for eventual complete biventricular repair [4,5].

Surgical Palliation to Supply Pulmonary Blood Flow

The most common palliative procedure to supply pulmonary blood flow is the systemic-to-pulmonary arterial shunt (Figure 7.1). The classic Blalock-Taussig shunt, as originally described [1], anastomosed the subclavian artery directly to the pulmonary artery. The modified Blalock-Taussig shunt (Gore-Tex interposition graft between the innominate artery and pulmonary artery) is the most commonly performed procedure to secure adequate pulmonary blood flow in children with cyanotic lesions [6,7]. This method has been shown to supply a more predictable shunt volume than previous techniques, and its thrombosis rate is less than or comparable to other techniques [8,9]. The classic Blalock-Taussig shunt (anastomosis of the subclavian artery to the ipsilateral branch pulmonary artery) has been associated with long-term limb growth deficiency and diminished arm strength [10,11]. Both the Waterston shunt (ascending aorta–right pulmonary artery) and Potts (descending aorta–left pulmonary artery) shunt have been largely abandoned, as they were associated with significant distortion of the branch pulmonary arteries and higher mortality because of either excessive or diminutive pulmonary blood flow [12–14]. However, complex aortic arch or pulmonary artery anatomy occasionally necessitates the use of one of these direct central shunts or the placement of a central Gore-Tex interposition graft between the aorta and central pulmonary arteries [15,16].

Surgical Palliation to Control Pulmonary Blood Flow

Banding of some portion of the pulmonary artery has traditionally been employed to limit pulmonary blood flow in those patients whose anatomy is not amenable to complete initial repair and who are at risk for pulmonary overcirculation [17–20]. As complete repairs are more commonly performed in the neonatal period and infancy, these techniques are becoming less frequent. However, there is a population of patients in whom initial complete repairs are unfeasible. This population includes a growing number of complex infants with multiorgan system dysfunction who are surviving because of aggressive intervention in the neonatal period. Banding procedures can sometimes be employed in these patients to allow for an evaluation of the extent and prognosis of their other organ system involvement. When performed, banding procedures are often done in infancy before the predictable drop in pulmonary arterial pressure by 2–3 months of age.

D.S. Wheeler et al. (eds.), *Cardiovascular Pediatric Critical Illness and Injury*,
DOI 10.1007/978-1-84800-923-3_7, © Springer-Verlag London Limited 2009

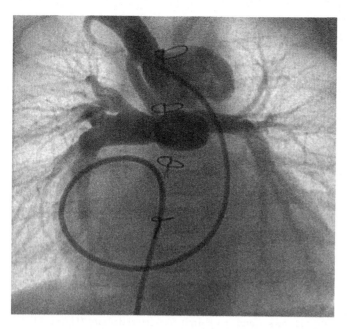

FIGURE 7.1. Modified Blalock-Taussig shunt as part of a Norwood procedure for hypoplastic left heart syndrome. The shunt provides a controlled source of pulmonary blood flow.

Several techniques of banding have evolved. However, there can be several complications of pulmonary artery banding. The band can migrate to the bifurcation of the branch arteries or disrupt pulmonary valvar structure [21]. They have been known to occasionally loosen and can be difficult to manipulate during placement to allow for the optimal balance of pulmonary blood flow. Even the well-placed pulmonary artery band that does not disturb pulmonary valve function or encroach on pulmonary artery branches may lead to inequitable pulmonary artery growth (Figure 7.2). It is

therefore essential to evaluate the pulmonary artery architecture before proceeding with additional future surgery.

There have been multiple attempts to develop surgically placed pulmonary arterial bands that can be later tightened or loosened externally depending on the clinical circumstance [22,23]. These methods have yet to reach widespread use. Recently, groups have developed the use of fenestrated patches placed within the right ventricular outflow tract or main pulmonary artery to limit pulmonary blood flow, although these techniques have the disadvantage of requiring cardiopulmonary bypass for placement [24]. Historically, surgical banding of individual pulmonary arterial branches has been attempted in few lesions. It was employed in early attempts to palliate children with truncus arteriosus but was thought to be a difficult technique to provide a predictable supply of pulmonary blood flow [25,26].

Catheter-Based Palliative Procedures

The technique to limit pulmonary arterial blood flow through placement of branch pulmonary artery flow limiters has recently been developed. This procedure, performed through catheter-based techniques, is undertaken either in the catheterization laboratory or in a modified operating room suite with adequate fluoroscopy equipment. It has been specifically developed for use in the initial palliation of children with single-ventricle physiology and is usually performed at the same time that a ductus arteriosus stent is placed to ensure adequate systemic blood flow. Children who undergo this procedure ultimately either undergo transplantation or proceed down the Fontan pathway to a combined surgical aortic arch reconstruction and bidirectional cavopulmonary anastomosis [27]. Alternatively, several groups have developed a technique of surgically placed branch pulmonary artery bands at the time of or after ductus arteriosus stenting [28–31]. These procedures have yet to gain widespread use, as only selected centers have primarily adopted delayed transplantation or this hybrid approach to single ventricle palliation.

Occasionally, a controlled source of blood flow is required in a cyanotic child with dynamic right ventricular outflow obstruction (such as in tetralogy of Fallot) who is an unfavorable surgical candidate because of extreme prematurity or other co-morbid factors. Stents have been placed in the ductus arteriosus in some cyanotic patients with limited success [32–35]. A stent has not been developed to this point that reliably holds the curve of the ductus architecture and is manufactured in a variety of sizes and arch angles. Additionally, care must be taken to not impede flow to the branch pulmonary arteries and to cover all aspects of ductal tissue, leaving no future substrate for coarctation of the aorta [36]. In selected patients, the right ventricular outflow tract can be balloon dilated or stented to allow for somatic growth and hopeful eventual complete repair [37].

Balloon atrial septostomy has been employed for many years as the initial palliative procedure in patients with transposition of the great arteries with an inadequate atrial level communication and no other significant source of mixing (multiple or large ventral septal defects and/or patent ductus arteriosus) [38,39]. Occasionally, this technique has been employed in children with in an intact or restrictive atrial communication in hypoplastic left heart syndrome [40]. In these children, this procedure may also involve the placement of an atrial septal stent, as the septum can be thick and resistant to balloon disruption [41].

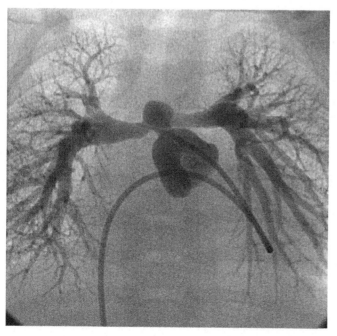

FIGURE 7.2. Pulmonary artery band. This is placed distal to the pulmonary valve and proximal to the branch pulmonary arteries and limits excessive pulmonary blood flow.

Intraoperative Assessment of Palliative Procedures

Experimental models have predicted that an ideal surgical systemic to pulmonary shunt is approximately 0.9–1.0 mm/kg body weight. In this model, a shunt of this size allows for predictable pulmonary to systemic blood flow and the ability to effectively manipulate this ratio with ventilatory and acid–base changes [42]. Reliable means do not exist in vivo, however, to evaluate the placement of a shunt that delivers the ideal shunt volume. Direct pressure measurement of the central pulmonary arteries and the ascending aorta provide a comparison of distal pulmonary arterial pressure to systemic pressure. Elevated pulmonary artery pressure in conjunction with low systemic diastolic pressure could signal that the shunt is too large. Elevated pulmonary arterial pressure with a normal pulse pressure would typically suggest intrinsic pulmonary arterial hypertension and/or left atrial hypertension. By directly sampling mixed venous saturation in the venous cannula, obtaining central or peripheral arterial saturation, and assuming pulmonary venous saturation, the systemic-to-pulmonary shunt flow rate can be determined intraoperatively. In the case of additional sources of pulmonary blood flow, such as a patent but diminutive right ventricular outflow tract, either the shunt or main pulmonary artery can be temporarily clamped and these measurements repeated to evaluate whether the additional source of pulmonary blood flow should be retained or modified.

The physiologic effects of main pulmonary arterial banding can be similarly evaluated intraoperatively. The surgeon can quickly obtain direct pressure measurement of right ventricular pressure and pulmonary arterial pressure distal to the band. This allows for modification of the band, if necessary. The systemic-to-pulmonary shunt flow rate can be determined intraoperatively. In the case of additional sources of pulmonary blood, flow can be determined as previously described. Intraoperative imaging with transesophageal echocardiogram also allows for both objective and subjective assessment of the operative procedure while still in the operative suite.

Postprocedure Management

Postoperative care of children with either a systemic-to-pulmonary arterial shunt or pulmonary artery band centers on the appraisal and maintenance of optimal pulmonary to systemic blood flow. Elevated systemic saturation together with evidence of poor peripheral perfusion and a metabolic acidosis signal an elevated systemic-to-pulmonary shunt flow rate. In this case, efforts should be made to elevate pulmonary vascular resistance by minimizing inspired oxygen concentration and allowing for a mild respiratory acidosis. Additionally, a consideration of systemic afterload reduction with an agent such as milrinone should be made. Conversely, cyanosis and warm extremities signal diminished pulmonary blood flow. This can be caused by elevated pulmonary vascular resistance or partial shunt occlusion or kinking that can occur after chest closure. Regardless, efforts can be made to encourage pulmonary blood flow by employing measures to drop pulmonary vascular resistance. These measures include increasing inspired oxygen content, elevating pH to 7.45–7.50 through ventilatory manipulations and bicarbonate infusions, and the considering use of inhaled nitric oxide. In the shunted patient, if bedside echocardiographic imaging cannot unequivocally confirm shunt patency in the face of profound cyanosis, shunt occlusion with thrombosis should be strongly considered. Extracorporeal membrane oxygenation can be used as a bridge to surgical revision or a clotted and/or kinked shunt or in the case of intrinsic but presumed time-limited pulmonary arterial hypertension with an adequate, functioning shunt [43].

If effective pulmonary blood flow is diminished because of obstruction of the shunt at the aortic or pulmonary arterial anastomosis or kinking along its length, urgent surgical revision is required. If thrombosis of a systemic-to-pulmonary arterial shunt is confirmed or highly suspected, infusion of tissue plasminogen activator or a similar fibrinolytic agent should be considered. There have been documented dramatic results of this therapy via systemic and directly guided tissue plasminogen activator routes [44–47]. If the patient has co-morbidities that make systemic anticoagulation exceedingly dangerous (such as with an intraventricular hemorrhage), consideration of emergent surgical shunt revision with thrombectomy should be made.

References

1. Blalock A, Taussig HB. The surgical treatment of malformations of the heart in which there is pulmonary stenosis or pulmonary atresia. JAMA 1945;128:189–202.
2. Rashkind WJ, Miller WW. Creation of an atrial septal defect without thoracotomy. A palliative approach to complete transposition of the great arteries. JAMA 1966;196:991–992.
3. Zellers TM, Dixon K, Moake L, Wright J, Ramaciotti C. Bedside balloon atrial septostomy is safe, efficacious, and cost-effective compared with septostomy performed in the cardiac catheterization laboratory. Am J Cardiol 2002;89:613–615.
4. Brouwer RMHJ, Cromme-Dijkhuis AH, Erasmus ME, et al. Decision making for the surgical management of aortic coarctation associated with ventricular septal defect. J Thorac Cardiovasc Surg 1996;111:168–175.
5. Park JK, Dell RB, Ellis K, Gersony WM. Surgical management of the infant with coarctation of the aorta and ventricular septal defect. J Am Coll Cardiol 1992;20:176–180.
6. Fenton KN, Siewers RD, Rebovich B, Pigula FA. Interim mortality in infants with systemic-to-pulmonary artery shunts. Ann Thorac Surg 2003;76:152–156.
7. Alkhulaifi AM, Lacour-Gayet F, Serraf A, Belli E, Planche C. Systemic pulmonary shunts in neonates: early clinical outcome and choice of surgical approach. Ann Thorac Surg 2000;69:499–504.
8. Gold JP, Violaris K, Engle MA, Klein AA, Ehlers KH, Lang SJ, et al. A five-year clinical experience with 112 Blalock-Taussig shunts. J Card Surg 1993;8:9–17.
9. Al Jubair KA, Al Fagih MR, Al Jarallah AS, Al Yousef S, Ali Khan MA, Ashmeg A, et al. Results of 546 Blalock-Taussig shunts performed in 478 patients. Cardiol Young 1998;8:486–490.
10. Skovranek J, Goetzova J, Samanek M. Changes in muscle blood flow and development of the arm following the Blalock-Taussig anastomosis. Cardiology 1976;61:131–137.
11. Zahka KG, Manolio TA, Rykiel MJ, Abel DL, Neill CA, Kidd L. Handgrip strength after the Blalock-Taussig shunt: 14 to 34 year follow-up. Clin Cardiol 1988;11:627–629.
12. Potts WJ, Smith s, Gibson S. Anastomosis of the aorta to a pulmonary artery. JAMA 1946;132:627–631.
13. Arciniegas E, Farooki ZQ, Hakimi M, Perry BL, Green EW. Classic shunting operations for congenital cyanotic heart defects. J Thorac Cardiovasc Surg 1982;84:88–96.
14. Parenzan L, Alfieri O, Vanini V, Bianchi T, Villani M, Tiraboschi R, et al. Waterston anastomosis for initial palliation of tetralogy of Fallot. J Thorac Cardiovasc Surg 1981;82:176–181.
15. Amato JJ, Marbey ML, Bush C, Galdieri RJ, Cotroneo JV, Bushong J. Systemic-pulmonary polytetrafluoroethylene shunts in palliative

operations for congenital heart disease. Revival of the central shunt. J Thorac Cardiovasc Surg 1988;95:62–69.

16. Barragry TP, Ring WS, Blatchford JW, Foker JE. Central aorta-pulmonary artery shunts in neonates with complex cyanotic congenital heart disease. J Thorac Cardiovasc Surg 1987;93:767–774.

17. Albert HM, Fowler RL, Craighead CC, Glass BA, Atik M. Pulmonary artery banding. A treatment for infants with intractable cardiac failure due to interventricular septal defects. Circulation 1961;23:16–20.

18. Van Nooten G, Deuvaert FE, De Paepe J, Primo G. Pulmonary artery banding. Experience with 69 patients. J Cardiovasc Surg (Torino) 1989; 30:334–337.

19. Horowitz MD, Culpepper WS III, Williams LC III, Sundgaard-Riise K, Ochsner JL. Pulmonary artery banding: analysis of a 25-year experience. Ann Thorac Surg 1989;48:444–450.

20. Pinho P, Von Oppell UO, Brink J, Hewitson J. Pulmonary artery banding: adequacy and long-term outcome. Eur J Cardiothorac Surg 1997;11:105–111.

21. Verel D, Taylor DG, Emery JL. Failure of pulmonary artery banding due to migration of the band. Thorax 1970;25:126–128.

22. Leeuwenburgh BP, Schoof PH, Steendijk P, Baan J, Mooi WJ, Helbing WA. Chronic and adjustable pulmonary artery banding. J Thorac Cardiovasc Surg 2003;125:231–237.

23. Ahmadi A, Rein J, Hellberg K, Bastanier C. Percutaneously adjustable pulmonary artery band. Ann Thorac Surg 1995;60:S520–S522.

24. Piluiko VV, Poynter JA, Nemeh H, Thomas RL, Forbes TJ, Delius RE, et al. Efficacy of intraluminal pulmonary artery banding. J Thorac Cardiovasc Surg 2005;129:544–550.

25. Smith GW, Thompson WM Jr, Dammmann JF Jr, Muller WH Jr. Use of the pulmonary artery banding procedure in treating type II truncus arteriosus. Circulation 1964;29:13.

26. McFaul RC, Mair DD, Feldt RH, Ritter DG, McGoon DC. Truncus arteriosus and previous pulmonary arterial banding: clinical and hemodynamic assessment. Am J Cardiol 1976;38:626–632.

27. Mitchell MB, Campbell DN, Boucek MM, Sondheimer HM, Chan KC, Ivy DD, et al. Mechanical limitation of pulmonary blood flow facilitates heart transplantation in older infants with hypoplastic left heart syndrome. Eur J Cardiothorac Surg 2003;23:735–742.

28. Gibbs JL, Wren C, Watterson KG, Hunter S, Hamilton JR. Stenting of the arterial duct combined with banding of the pulmonary arteries and atrial septectomy or septostomy: a new approach to palliation for the hypoplastic left heart syndrome. Br Heart J 1993;69:551–555.

29. Galantowicz M, Cheatham JP. Lessons learned from the development of a new hybrid strategy for the management of hypoplastic left heart syndrome. Pediatr Cardiol 2005;26:190–199.

30. Akintuerk H, Michel-Behnke I, Valeske K, Mueller M, Thul J, Bauer J, et al. Stenting of the arterial duct and banding of the pulmonary arteries: basis for combined Norwood stage I and II repair in hypoplastic left heart. Circulation 2002;105:1099–1103.

31. Michel-Behnke I, Akintuerk H, Marquardt I, Mueller M, Thul J, Bauer J, et al. Stenting of the ductus arteriosus and banding of the pulmonary arteries: basis for various surgical strategies in newborns with multiple left heart obstructive lesions. Heart 2003;89:645–650.

32. Coe JY, Olley PM. A novel method to maintain ductus arteriosus patency. J Am Coll Cardiol 1991;18:837–841.

33. Alwi M, Choo KK, Latiff HA, Kandavello G, Samion H, Mulyadi MD. Initial results and medium-term follow-up of stent implantation of patent ductus arteriosus in duct-dependent pulmonary circulation. J Am Coll Cardiol 2004;44:438–445.

34. Michel-Behnke I, Akintuerk H, Thul J, Bauer J, Hagel KJ, Schranz D. Stent implantation in the ductus arteriosus for pulmonary blood supply in congenital heart disease. Catheter Cardiovasc Intervent 2004;61:242–252.

35. Tyagi S, Dwivedi G, Gupta MD, Kaul UA. Stent implantation in right-sided patent ductus arteriosus to relieve severe cyanosis in adult patient with pulmonary atresia and ventricular septal defect. Catheter Cardiovasc Intervent 2004;61:271–274.

36. Gewillig M, Boshoff DE, Dens J, Mertens L, Benson LN. Stenting the neonatal arterial duct in duct-dependent pulmonary circulation: new techniques, better results. J Am Coll Cardiol 2004;43:107–112.

37. Godart F, Rey C, Prat A, Muilwijk C, Francart C, Vaksmann G, et al. Early and late results and the effects on pulmonary arteries of balloon dilatation of the right ventricular outflow tract in tetralogy of Fallot. Eur Heart J 1998;19:595–600.

38. Rashkind WJ, Miller WW. Transposition of the great arteries. Results of palliation by balloon atrioseptostomy in thirty-one infants. Circulation 1968;38:453–462.

39. Baylen BG, Grzeszczak M, Gleason ME, Cyran SE, Weber HS, Myers J, et al. Role of balloon atrial septostomy before early arterial switch repair of transposition of the great arteries. J Am Coll Cardiol 1992;19:1025–1031.

40. Atz AM, Feinstein JA, Jonas RA, Perry SB, Wessel DL. Preoperative management of pulmonary venous hypertension in hypoplastic left heart syndrome with restrictive atrial septal defect. Am J Cardiol 1999;83:1224–1228.

41. Vlahos AP, Lock JE, McElhinney DB, van der Velde ME. Hypoplastic left heart syndrome with intact or highly restrictive atrial septum: outcome after neonatal transcatheter atrial septostomy. Circulation 2004;109:2326–2330.

42. Kitaichi T, Chikugo F, Kawahito T, Hori T, Masuda Y, Kitagawa T. Suitable shunt size for regulation of pulmonary blood flow in a canine model of univentricular parallel circulations. J Thorac Cardiovasc Surg 2003;125(1):71–78.

43. Booth KL, Roth SJ, Perry SB, del Nido PJ, Wessel DL, Laussen PC. Cardiac catheterization of patients supported by extracorporeal membrane oxygenation. J Am Coll Cardiol 2002;40(9):1681–1686.

44. Singh V, Pillai S, Kulkarni S, Murthy KS, Coelho R, Ninan B, et al. Thrombolysis with percutaneous transluminal balloon angioplasty of a blocked modified Blalock-Taussig shunt. Indian Heart J 2004;56: 673–676.

45. Klinge J, Hofbeck M, Ries M, Schaf J, Singer H, von der EJ. [Thrombolysis of modified Blalock-Taussig shunts in childhood with recombinant tissue-type plasminogen activator.] Z Kardiol 1995;84:476–480.

46. Malm TK, Holmqvist C, Olsson CG, Johansson J, Olsson AK, Sandstrom S, et al. Successful thrombolysis of an occluded modified Blalock shunt three days after operation. Ann Thorac Surg 1998;65: 1453–1455.

47. Ries M, Singer H, Hofbeck M. Thrombolysis of a modified Blalock-Taussig shunt with recombinant tissue plasminogen activator in a newborn infant with pulmonary atresia and ventricular septal defect. Br Heart J 1994 Aug;72(2):201–202.

8

Congenital Heart Disease: Left-to-Right Shunt Lesions

Derek S. Wheeler, James D. St. Louis, and Catherine L. Dent

Introduction

A left-to-right shunt lesion is defined as a lesion wherein blood from the left atrium, left ventricle, or aorta crosses to the right atrium, the right ventricle, or the pulmonary artery. Because, in the absence of lung disease, the blood in the left atrium, left ventricle, and aorta is fully oxygenated, left-to-right shunt lesions do not present with cyanosis. Instead, the lungs receive both deoxygenated blood from the normal systemic venous return—the amount of which is equal to the cardiac output—as well as the fully oxygenated shunted blood via the left-to-right shunt defect. The presence of a left-to-right shunt therefore imposes a volume load on one or more chambers of the heart.

Under normal conditions, blood flow to the pulmonary circulation (Qp, i.e., 1 × cardiac output) is equal to the blood flow to the systemic circulation (Qs, i.e., 1 × cardiac output); therefore, Qp = Qs. The ratio of Qp to Qs is >1 in the presence of a left-to-right shunt. By convention, a Qp:Qs of 1.0 to 1.5 denotes a small shunt, a Qp:Qs of 1.5 to 2.0 denotes a moderate shunt, and a Qp:Qs of >2.0 denotes a large shunt. Calculation of the Qp:Qs ratio is discussed in Chapter 5.

Patent Ductus Arteriosus

Anatomy

The ductus arteriosus is derived from the sixth embryologic aortic arch and normally connects the main pulmonary artery or proximal left pulmonary artery to the upper descending thoracic aorta just distal to the origin of the left subclavian artery, although the origin and insertion of the ductus arteriosus may vary. The normal transition from fetal circulation to neonatal circulation is discussed in Chapters 1. In the vast majority of cases, the ductus arteriosus closes within a few days of birth (although, in most cases, functional

closure occurs within a few hours after birth). The ductus arteriosus remains patent in approximately 1 in 1,600 term births, although the incidence in infants born prematurely is much higher—on the order of 8 per 1,000 live births [1,2]. Maternal rubella virus infection during the first trimester of pregnancy and female sex are additional risk factors for a patent ductus arteriosus (PDA). A PDA in preterm infants may contribute to the pathophysiology of necrotizing enterocolitis, respiratory distress syndrome, and chronic lung disease [2].

Pathophysiology and Clinical Presentation

In the absence of other cardiac lesions, a PDA is often hemodynamically insignificant and may be detected only by echocardiography (usually obtained during a murmur evaluation). A large PDA, however, produces a left-to-right shunt, especially after pulmonary vascular resistance falls during the first few weeks of life, thereby imposing a volume load on the left ventricle and leading to signs and symptoms of congestive heart failure (CHF). If the PDA is left untreated, the child will eventually develop pulmonary hypertension with the eventual development of a right-to-left shunt (Eisenmenger syndrome). These children may also be at risk for bacterial endocarditis.

A small PDA usually produces minimal symptoms and is typically suspected on routine physical examination with a continuous machinery type of murmur at the left upper sternal border. A moderate-to-large sized PDA produces typical signs and symptoms of CHF, often resulting in failure to thrive and recurrent pulmonary infections. The pulses are classically described as bounding (which often may be detected as palmar pulses, especially in neonates and small infants) with a hyperdynamic precordium and widened pulse pressure. The electrocardiogram is usually normal (although left or even biventricular hypertrophy may be present with a large PDA). Chest x-ray is usually normal as well but may occasionally demonstrate an enlarged cardiothymic silhouette and increased pulmonary vascular markings (i.e., evidence of CHF). Echocardiography is diagnostic, and cardiac catheterization is most commonly used for treatment rather than diagnosis.

Surgical or Transcatheter Intervention

Any PDA that is apparent on physical examination should be closed, either surgically or in the cardiac catheterization labora-

D.S. Wheeler et al. (eds.), *Cardiovascular Pediatric Critical Illness and Injury*,
DOI 10.1007/978-1-84800-923-3_8, © Springer-Verlag London Limited 2009

tory. *Medical closure* (e.g., indomethacin) is often used in preterm infants and is not discussed further here. The first successful congenital heart repair was in fact a surgical ligation of a PDA in a 7-year-old child by Robert E. Gross at Boston Children's Hospital in 1938 [3]. There are now several described surgical approaches to PDA ligation, including left thoracotomy with simple ligation and division between vascular clamps (Figure 8.1) and hemoclip occlusion via video-assisted thoracoscopy (VATS) (reviewed elsewhere [1,2]).

Surgical complications are usually rare but include inadvertent ligation of the left pulmonary artery or damage to the recurrent laryngeal nerve (with subsequent vocal cord paralysis). Device closure in the cardiac catheterization is now commonly employed using a single Gianturco coil for small PDAs and multiple Gianturco coils for larger PDAs [1,2,4–7]. Complications of transcatheter closure include coil embolization to the pulmonary vessels or aorta, pulmonary artery stenosis, damage to the femoral artery (i.e., during catheter placement), hemolysis, or device failure or recanalization with residual PDA [1,2,4–7]. Wheeler et al. described surgical closure of a residual PDA following multiple, unsuccessful attempts at transcatheter closure with the coils left in situ [5]. Recent experience with the use of the Amplatzer ductal occluder device for transcatheter closure of large PDAs is encouraging and may obviate the need for placement of multiple coils, which is generally associated with a higher rate of complications [8–10]. Postoperative management of these patients is usually straightforward, and early tracheal extubation in the catheterization suite is usually performed.

Atrial Septal Defect

Anatomy

An atrial septal defect (ASD) arises from a defect in the embryonic separation of the atria. The normal atrial septum is made up of the septum primum (the thin, inferior portion) and the septum secundum (the thick, superior portion). The inferior edge of the septum primum fuses with the endocardial cushions to complete septation of the atrial septum during embryogenesis. There are four types commonly described: (1) ASD secundum, (2) ASD primum, (3) sinus venosus, and (4) ASD of the inferior vena cava (also called an *unroofed coronary sinus*).

A patent foramen ovale (PFO) is considered a small interatrial communication (and is closely related to secundum ASD) that does not result from a defect in the septum primum (distinguishing it from the secundum ASD). An aneurysm of the atrial septum is a bulging of the septum primum that usually resolves with age. A common atrium is described as a virtual complete absence of the atrial septum and is usually associated with complex congenital heart disease only. A secundum-type ASD occurs from a deficiency, perforation, or absence of the septum primum. The defect may be large or exist as multiple fenestrations or holes. A primum type of ASD is a type of endocardial cushion defect (and is therefore also known as a *partial* or *incomplete* atrioventricular septal defect or atrioventricular canal) that results when the septum primum fails to close. Primum ASDs are typically associated with a cleft in the anterior leaflet of the mitral valve; this may or may not result in mitral insufficiency. An ASD in the region of the sinus venosus, usually superiorly near the junction of the superior vena cava and atrium, is classified as a sinus venosus type of ASD. These defects are commonly associated with partial anomalous pulmonary venous return, typically of the right upper pulmonary veins [6]. A coronary sinus ASD or unroofed coronary sinus defect (*ASD of the inferior vena cava*) results from a deficiency in all or part of the wall separating the left atrium from the coronary sinus. When this deficiency is complete the coronary sinus is absent, and a communication exists in the posteroinferior region of the atrial septum. A left superior vena cava is often associated with this type of defect, entering the upper corner of the left atrium [11].

Pathophysiology and Clinical Presentation

An ASD in a patient without associated defects generally results in a left-to-right shunt. The degree of shunting is determined by both the size of the ASD as well as the compliance of the right and left ventricles. For example, left ventricular compliance is normally less than that of the right ventricle—this leads to a left-to-right shunt, which subsequently leads to excessive pulmonary blood flow (Qp:Qs may be as high as 4:1). Blood flow across the ASD primarily occurs during diastole. Most children with ASD are asymptomatic and come to attention for evaluation of a murmur noted on routine physical examination. Children with an unroofed coronary sinus

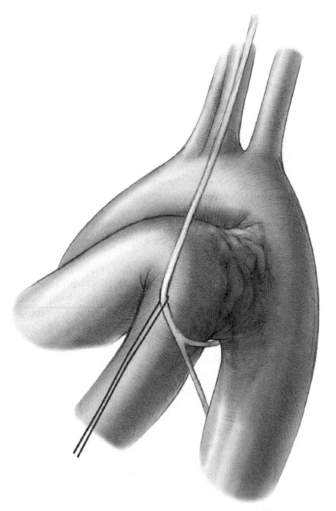

FIGURE 8.1. The patent ductus arteriosus has been exposed through a left thoracotomy. The vagus nerve is identified and retracted medially before ligation of the ductus arteriosus. (Courtesy of James D. St. Louis, MD, Medical College of Georgia.)

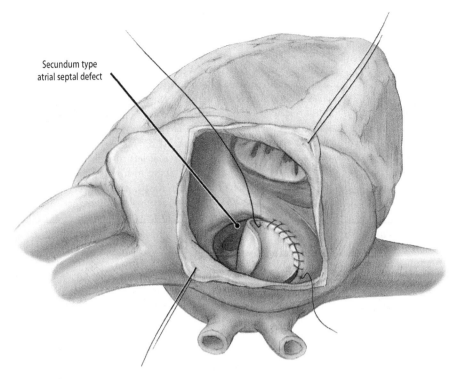

Figure 8.2. Secundum atrial septal defect repair. The right atrium has been opened and the defect is being closed with a patch—autologous pericardium or polytetrafluoroethylene (PTFE) patches are usually used. (Courtesy of James D. St. Louis, MD, Medical College of Georgia.)

Secundum type
atrial septal defect

and left superior vena cava may also have cyanosis. Physical examination classically demonstrates a widely split, fixed second heart sound and a systolic ejection murmur heard best at the upper left sternal border (because of excess blood flow across the pulmonary valve). Children with a primum-type ASD may also have a murmur of mitral insufficiency.

Preoperative Evaluation

The electrocardiogram may be normal if the left-to-right shunt is small. However, an RSR in the right precordial leads is classic for ASD (although it may also be found in normal individuals). If the left-to-right shunt is large, the electrocardiogram may show right atrial enlargement, right ventricular hypertrophy, and right axis deviation. Patients with a primum defect often have left axis deviation, as is typical for atrioventricular septal defects. Chest x-ray is frequently normal, but may show an enlarged cardiothymic silhouette with increased pulmonary vascular markings. Echocardiography is diagnostic.

Surgical or Transcatheter Intervention and Postoperative Care

Typically, ASDs do not undergo spontaneous closure with the exception of the secundum type, in which 15% or less may close by age 4 years [12,13]. Left untreated, patients with ASDs are at risk for atrial arrhythmias (e.g., atrial flutter, atrial fibrillation), pulmonary hypertension (Eisenmenger syndrome), paradoxic emboli, right ventricular dysfunction, and CHF. Bacterial endocarditis does not occur in children with an isolated secundum ASD. We generally recommend closure before children reach school age, usually between 2 and 5 years of age. The preferred surgical approach to ASD repair is via median sternotomy (usually a partial

sternotomy is adequate) with either stitch closure or patch (autologous pericardium) closure under cardiopulmonary bypass (Figure 8.2). Repair of the anomalous pulmonary veins is performed by placing the patch in such a manner that the pulmonary veins baffle to the left atrium.

Several transcatheter techniques have been described for ASD closure. The Amplatzer device (AGA Medical, Golden Valley, MN) was recently approved by the FDA, and other devices are likely to be approved in the near future (e.g., CardioSEAL, NMT Medical, Boston, MA; Helex septal occluders, WL Gore, Flagstaff, AZ). Transcatheter closure of small- to medium-sized ASDs is widely considered the treatment of choice.

Most children can be tracheally extubated in the operating room following surgical closure of an ASD and are usually monitored in the intensive care unit for 12–24 hr for postoperative bleeding and arrhythmias (especially sinus node dysfunction). Transcatheter device closure appears to be as effective as surgical closure, with a shorter length of stay in the hospital and decreased costs [14–18]. In most centers, surgical closure is reserved for those defects that are either too large or have insufficient superior or inferior rims for successful device placement, or following unsuccessful attempts at device closure.

Ventricular Septal Defect

Anatomy

A ventricular septal defect (VSD) is defined as a deficiency in the interventricular septum and is the most commonly recognized congenital heart defect [1,19,20]. A VSD can either be an isolated defect or occur in association with either simple defects (e.g., ASD, PDA, coarctation of the aorta) or complex defects (e.g., tetralogy of

Fallot, D-transposition of the great arteries). The ventricular septum is commonly divided into four parts—the membranous septum and the inlet, trabecular, and outlet portions of the muscular septum [1,20–23]. The terminology and management of specific types of VSDs are based on these anatomic regions (Figure 8.3).

Type I VSDs (less than 10% of isolated VSD) are located in the infundibular region—these defects are also known as subpulmonary, supracristal, subarterial, conal, infundibular, or outlet muscular VSDs. This particular type of VSD may be associated with aortic insufficiency (caused by prolapse of aortic valve leaflet through the defect) and is more common in individuals of Asian descent [1,20–23]. Type II VSDs (most common, accounting for approximately 30% of surgically repaired VSDs) exist in or near the membranous portion of the septum and are termed *perimembranous* or *paramembranous* VSDs (also called *conoventricular, subaortic, infracristal,* or *membranous*). The defect may be confined to this immediate region or extend into the infundibular or inlet portions of the septum.

Type III VSDs are also known as *atrioventricular canal type* or *inlet* VSDs. Type IV VSDs (also called *muscular* VSDs) exist in a portion of the trabecular (muscular) septum. These defects can be further described based on their relative position in the muscular septum. The defect is completely surrounded by muscle and removed from all conduction tissue. The defect may also exist as multiple coalescing holes, termed *Swiss cheese* VSD [24]. Malalignment VSDs are associated with other lesions (such as tetralogy of Fallot or interrupted aortic arch) and result from malalignment between the infundibular septum and the trabecular muscular septum, creating a large, usually nonrestrictive defect.

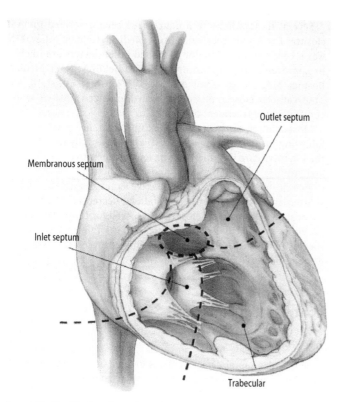

FIGURE 8.3. Classification of ventral septal defects. (Courtesy of James D. St. Louis, MD, Medical College of Georgia.)

Pathophysiology and Clinical Presentation

The size of the VSD and the relative pulmonary and systemic vascular resistances determine the degree of left-to-right shunt. For example, with a restrictive VSD (by convention, smaller than the aortic root diameter), the magnitude of the left-to-right shunt is largely determined by the size of the defect itself. Conversely, with a nonrestrictive VSD (no pressure gradient between the right and left ventricle), the magnitude of the shunt depends largely on the pulmonary vascular resistance. At birth the pulmonary vascular resistance is high, and the degree of left-to-right shunting across the VSD is relatively low, producing minimal symptoms. As the pulmonary vascular resistance drops, the degree of shunting increases, leading to left ventricular volume overload, increased pulmonary blood flow, and the clinical manifestations of CHF.

Preoperative Evaluation

Shunting occurs largely during systole—a loud, holosystolic murmur heard best at the left sternal border is usually noted on physical examination. Hepatomegaly and jugular venous distension may be present. The intensity of the murmur itself is inversely proportional to the size of the defect (i.e., larger defects are usually associated with a softer murmur). Chest x-ray shows cardiomegaly with increased pulmonary vascular markings. The electrocardiogram may show evidence of either left or biventricular hypertrophy and left atrial enlargement. Echocardiography is diagnostic, and cardiac catheterization is rarely required (unless there are significant concerns for pulmonary hypertension).

Surgical or Transcatheter Intervention and Postoperative Care

Infants with large VSDs are generally managed medically (with diuretics, afterload reduction, or digoxin), and repair is deferred until approximately 6 months of age, if possible. With perimembranous and muscular VSDs, medical management of CHF and poor weight gain with close follow up may be feasible, as many of these defects will undergo spontaneous closure during the first year of life. The probability of spontaneous closure falls precipitously thereafter, while the incidence of pulmonary vascular disease increases markedly. Older children occasionally present with large VSDs with varying degrees of elevated pulmonary vascular resistance—these children frequently improve from a symptomatic standpoint, as the elevation in pulmonary vascular resistance will necessarily decrease the magnitude of the left-to-right shunt. If elevated pulmonary vascular resistance is suspected, cardiac catheterization is frequently performed; surgery is then indicated if the shunt (Qp:Qs) is greater than 2:1 or if pulmonary vascular resistance is high (≥4 units/m^2). Surgical correction is controversial if the pulmonary vascular resistance is >8 units/m^2 without response to pulmonary vasodilators [25]. If aortic insufficiency is present (e.g., type I VSD), surgery is indicated to prevent further progression of valve insufficiency.

There are several described operative approaches for VSD closure (reviewed by Mavroudis [20]), although exposure through a median sternotomy and right atriotomy is the most commonly used approach in the majority of cases, especially for muscular and perimembranous VSDs (Figure 8.4). Complications of VSD closure, although rare, include residual VSD, pulmonary hypertension, heart block, junctional ectopic tachycardia, and complications attributed to

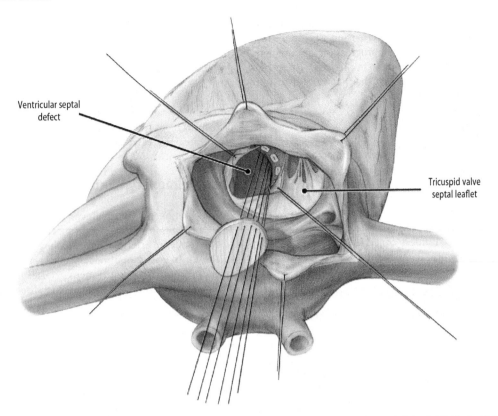

Ventricular septal defect

Tricuspid valve septal leaflet

Figure 8.4. Ventricular septal defect repair. Right atrial approach for ventricular septal defect closure. (Courtesy of James D. St. Louis, MD, Medical College of Georgia.)

cardiopulmonary bypass. However, these children usually do very well, and early tracheal extubation is frequently performed in the operating room. In addition, transcatheter closure of small VSDs may obviate the need for some surgeries in the future [26–28].

Atrioventricular Canal Defects

Anatomy

Atrioventricular (AV) septal defects, also commonly referred to as *endocardial cushion defects* or *atrioventricular canal defects*, are characterized by a common atrioventricular junction [29]. The defect is primarily caused by the absence of the membranous atrioventricular septum with a deficiency in the overlying region of the atrial and ventricular musculatures [30]. Atrioventricular septal defects may be placed into three separate categories based on the complexity of their anatomy. The spectrum of anomalies is divided into partial AV canal defects, transitional AV canal defects, and complete AV canal defects.

Partial (incomplete) AV canal defects have an ostium primum atrial septal defect and a cleft in the anterior leaflet of the mitral valve. The important characteristic of this defect is that there are two distinct atrioventricular valves with separate annuli. Complete AV canal defects, representing the opposite extreme in the spectrum of these anomalies, consist not only of a defect in the atrial (primum ASD) and ventricular septum (large, nonrestrictive VSD) but also a single atrioventricular valve with varying number of leaflets. Two dominant leaflets, the superior (anterior) and inferior (posterior), form the basis by which complete AV canal defects are classified. Transitional AV canal have two distinct atrioventricular annuli with septal defects at both the atrial and ventricular levels [31].

The Rastelli classification describes three types of complete AV septal defects based on the morphology of the superior (anterior) bridging leaflet and its chordal attachments to the ventricular septum [32]. In Rastelli type A defects, the superior bridging leaflet is split equally over the septum, with the left portion of the leaflet completely committed to the left ventricle and the right side committed to the right ventricle. This division is the result of extensive chordal attachments to the brim of the ventricular septal defect. Rastelli type B defects are rare and involve the insertion of the left-sided choral structures to the right of the ventricular septum. In Rastelli type C defects, the superior bridging leaflet is *free floating* over the ventricular septum with no specific choral attachments.

Complete AV canal defects are frequently associated with other conotruncal anomalies, including tetralogy of Fallot (most common), double-outlet right ventricle, and transposition of the great arteries. Other congenital heart defects are also common, including PDA, left superior vena cava, and left ventricular outflow tract obstruction. Complete AV canal is particularly common in infants and children with trisomy 21.

Pathophysiology and Clinical Presentation

The pathophysiology of a partial AV canal resembles that of secundum ASD, unless there is significant AV valve insufficiency. For these patients, repair is generally recommended in early childhood. The pathophysiology of a complete AV canal resembles that of a large VSD, with left-to-right shunting at the atrial and ventricular levels, leading to biventricular volume overload, CHF, and failure to thrive. As AV valve insufficiency worsens, the degree of shunting worsens, imposing an additional volume load on the ventricles. The large (nonrestrictive) left-to-right shunt results in a pulmonary artery pressure that is equal to systemic pressure, and these children, by definition, have pulmonary hypertension. Children with a complete AV canal may also have rapid progression of pulmonary obstructive vascular disease (even more so in children with trisomy 21). Therefore, early repair, typically in the first year of life and often before 6 months, is recommended.

Preoperative Evaluation

Chest x-ray generally denotes cardiomegaly with increased pulmonary vascular markings. The electrocardiogram shows a leftward and superior QRS axis with biatrial enlargement and biventricular hypertrophy. Echocardiography is important to delineate the morphology of the papillary muscles, valve attachments, and presence of left ventricular outflow tract obstruction. Cardiac catheterization is not usually required unless concerns of fixed pulmonary vascular disease are present.

Surgical Intervention and Postoperative Care

Repair of a partial AV canal is described earlier in the section on ASD. The ideal age for repair of a complete AV canal remains somewhat controversial, although, because of the rapidity with which these children develop irreversible pulmonary obstructive vascular disease, repair is generally performed between the ages of 3 and 6 months [33–36]. Repair is performed under cardiopulmonary bypass via a median sternotomy and right atriotomy using either a single-patch or two-patch technique.

The common AV valve is separated into right and left atrioventricular valves and the atrial and ventricular defects are closed (reviewed elsewhere [37–39]). Occasionally, a valve annuloplasty or pericardial patch augmentation may be necessary to achieve valve competence. Postoperative management during the first 24–48 hr

after surgery is targeted toward maintaining a lower atrial filling pressure with liberal use of inotropic support since volume loading may worsen AV valve insufficiency. The incidence of postoperative pulmonary hypertension can be high, often necessitating treatment with sedation, neuromuscular blockade, oxygen, inhaled nitric oxide, and newer agents such as sildenafil or bosentan. Additional complications include low cardiac output syndrome, complete heart block, junctional ectopic tachycardia, residual VSD, and atrioventricular valve insufficiency or stenosis.

Aortopulmonary Window Defects

The separation of the great vessels occurs when two opposing tissue cushions form on the right superior and left inferior portions of the common arterial trunk. Failure of these tissue cushions will result in an aortopulmonary defect, placing this defect in the same spectrum as that of truncus arteriosus [40]. Mori et al. have classified aortopulmonary defects into three types based on their location [41].

Type I defects are the most common and exist just above the AV valves. Type II aortopulmonary window defects are located in the most distal aspect of the ascending aorta, with repair being more complicated. Type III defects involve the majority of the ascending aortic pulmonary union. These children usually develop significant CHF within the first few months of life, as soon as the pulmonary vascular resistance drops. Early repair (usually at the time of diagnosis) is generally recommended. Repair is generally performed via a median sternotomy under cardiopulmonary bypass; the defect is closed with a patch via the *sandwich* technique (Figure 8.5) [42]. Postoperative management is usually straightforward, although the postoperative course can be complicated by pulmonary hypertension.

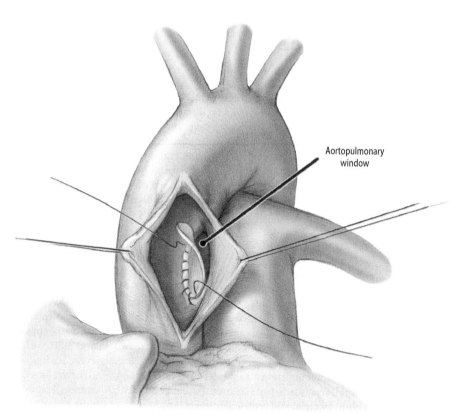

Aortopulmonary window

FIGURE 8.5. Repair of an aortopulmonary window defect (anterior sandwich patch closure). (Courtesy of James D. St. Louis, MD, Medical College of Georgia.)

References

1. Driscoll DJ. Left-to-right shunt lesions. Pediatr Clin North Am 1999;46:355–368.

2. Hillman ND, Mavroudis C, Backer CL. Patent ductus arteriosus. In: Mavroudis C, Backer CL, eds. Pediatric Cardiac Surgery, 3rd ed. Philadelphia: Mosby, 2003:223–233.

3. Gross RE, Hubbard JP. Surgical ligation of a PDA: report of first successful case. JAMA 1939;112:729–730.

4. Gray DT, Fyler DC, Walker AM, et al. Clinical outcomes and costs of transcatheter as compared with surgical closure of PDA. The PDA Closure Comparative Study Group. N Engl J Med 1993;329:517–523.

5. Wheeler DS, Poss WB, Maxwell JM. Surgical ligation of a residually patent arterial duct following failed occlusion using transcatheter coils. Cardiol Young 2003;13:574–575.

6. Galal MO. Advantages and disadvantages of coils for transcatheter closure of patent ductus arteriosus. J Interv Cardiol 2003;16:157–163.

7. Anil SR, Sivakumar K, Philip AK, Francis E, Kumar RK. Clinical course and management strategies for hemolysis after transcatheter closure of patent arterial duct. Catheter Cardiovasc Intervent 2003;59:538–543.

8. Jan SL, Hwang B, Fu YC, Chi CS. Transcatheter closure of a large patent ductus arteriosus in a young child using the Amplatzer duct occluder. Pediatr Cardiol 2005;26:703–706.

9. Wang JK, Hwang JJ, Chiang FT, et al. A strategic approach to transcatheter closure of patent ductus: Gianturco coils for small-to-moderate ductus and Amplatzer duct occluder for large ductus. Int J Cardiol 2006;106:10–15.

10. Masura J, Tittel P, Gavora P, Podnar T. Long-term outcome of transcatheter patent ductus arteriosus closure using Amplatzer duct occluders. Am Heart J 2006;151:755.e7–e755.e10.

11. Shunmacker HB Jr, King H, Waldhausen JA. The persistent left superior vena cava. Surgical implications, with special reference to caval drainage into the left atrium. Ann Surg 1967;165:797–805.

12. Cockerham JT, Martin TC, Gutierrez FR, Hartmann AF Jr, Goldring D, Strauss AW. Spontaneous closure of secundum atrial septal defect in infants and young children. Am J Cardiol 1983;52:1267–1271.

13. Helgason H, Jonsdottir G. Spontaneous closure of atrial septal defects. Pediatr Cardiol 1999;20:195–199.

14. Berger F, Ewert P, Bjornstad PG, et al. Transcatheter closure as standard treatment for most interatrial defects: experience in 200 patients treated with the Amplatzer septal occluder. Cardiol Young 1999;9:468–473.

15. Berger F, Vogel M, Alexi-Meskishvilli V, Lange PE. Comparison of results and complications of surgical and Amplatzer device closure of atrial septal defect. J Thorac Cardiovasc Surg 1999;118:674–680.

16. Thomson JD, Aburawi EH, Watterson KG, Van Doorn C, Gibbs JL. Surgical and transcatheter (Amplatzer) closure of atrial septal defects: a prospective comparison of results and cost. Heart 2002;87:466–469.

17. Durongpisitkul K, Soongswang J, Laohaprasitiporn D, et al. Comparison of atrial septal defect closure using Amplatzer septal occluder with surgery. Pediatr Cardiol 2002;23:36–40.

18. Bialkowski J, Karwot B, Szkutnik M, Banaszak P, Kusa J, Skalski J. Texas Heart Inst J 2004;31:220–223.

19. Mitchell SC, Korones SB, Berendes HW. Congenital heart disease in 56,109 births. Incidence and natural history. Circulation 1971;43:323–332.

20. Mavroudis C, Backer CL, Jacobs JL. Ventricular septal defect. In: Mavroudis C, Backer CL, eds. Pediatric Cardiac Surgery, 3rd ed. Philadelphia: Mosby; 2003:298–220.

21. Soto B, Becker AE, Moulaert AJ, Lie JT, Anderson RH. Classification of ventricular septal defects. Br Heart J 1980;43:332–343.

22. Van Praagh R, Geva AT, Kreutzer J. Ventricular septal defects: how shall we describe, name and classify them? J Am Coll Cardiol 1989;14:1298–1299.

23. Anderson RH, Wilcox BR. The surgical anatomy of ventricular septal defect. J Card Surg 1992;7:17–35.

24. Mace L, Dervanian P, Le Bret E, et al. "Swiss cheese" septal defects: surgical closure using a single patch with intermediate fixings. Ann Thorac Surg 1999;67:1754–1758.

25. Neutze JM, Ishikawa T, Clarkson PM, Calder AI, Barratt-Boyes BG, Kerr AR. Assessment and follow-up of patients with ventricular septal defect and elevated pulmonary vascular resistance. Am J Cardiol 1989;63:327–331.

26. Carminati M, Butera G, Chessa M, Drago M, Negura D, Piazza L. Transcatheter closure of congenital ventricular septal defect with Amplatzer septal occluders. Am J Cardiol 2005;96:52L–58L.

27. Fu YC, Bass J, Amin Z, et al. Transcatheter closure of perimembranous ventricular septal defects using the new Amplatzer membranous VSD occluder: results of the U.S. phase I trial. J Am Coll Cardiol 2006;47:319–325.

28. Walsh MA, Coleman DM, Oslizlok P, Walsh KP. Percutaneous closure of postoperative ventricular septal defects with the Amplatzer device. Cathet Cardiovasc Intervent 2006;67:445–451.

29. Becker AE, Anderson RH. Atrioventricular septal defects: what's in a name? J Thorac Cardiovasc Surg 1982;83:461–469.

30. Wilcox BR, Cook AC, Anderson RH. Abnormal segmental connections. In: Wilcox, BR, Cook AC, Anderson RH, eds. Surgical Anatomy of the Heart, 3rd ed. United Kingdom: Cambridge University Press, 2005:141–157.

31. Penkoske PA, Neches WH, Anderson RH, Zuberbuhler JR. Further observations on the morphology of atrioventricular septal defects. J Thorac Cardiovasc Surg 1985;90:611–622.

32. Rastelli GC. Kirklin JW. Titus JL. Anatomic observations on complete form of persistent common atrioventricular canal with special reference to atrioventricular valves. Mayo Clin Proc 1966;41:296–308.

33. Newfeld EA, Sher M, Paul MH, et al. Pulmonary vascular disease in complete atrioventricular canal defect. Am J Cardiol 1977;39:721–726.

34. Cooney TP, Thurlbeck WM. Pulmonary hypoplasia in Down's syndrome. N Engl J Med 1982;307:1170–1173.

35. Clapp S, Perry BL, Farooki ZQ, et al. Down syndrome, complete atrioventricular canal, and pulmonary vascular obstructive disease. J Thorac Cardiovasc Surg 1990;100:115–121.

36. Yamaki S, Yasui H, Kado H, et al. Pulmonary vascular disease and operative indications in complete atrioventricular canal defect in early infancy. J Thorac Cardiovasc Surg 1993;106:398–405.

37. Pearl JM, Laks H. Intermediate and complete forms of atrioventricular canal. Semin Thorac Cardiovasc Surg 1997;9:8–20.

38. Mavroudis C, Backer CL. The two-patch technique for complete atrioventricular canal. Semin Thorac Cardiovasc Surg 1997;9:35–43.

39. Backer CL, Mavroudis C. Atrioventricular canal defects. In: Mavroudis C, Backer CL, eds. Pediatric Cardiac Surgery, 3rd ed. Philadelphia: Mosby; 2003:321–338.

40. Kutsche LM, Van Mierop LHS. Anatomy and pathogenesis of aortopulmonary septal defects. Am J Cardiol 1987;59:442.

41. Mori K, Ando M, Takao A. Distal type of aortopulmonary window: report of 4 cases. Br Heart J 1978;40:681–689.

42. Ravikumar E, Whight CM, Hawker RE, et al. The surgical management of aortopulmonary window using the anterior sandwich patch closure technique. J Cardiovasc Surg (Torino) 1988;29:629–632.

9

Congenital Heart Disease: Cyanotic Lesions with Decreased Pulmonary Blood Flow

John M. Costello and Peter C. Laussen

Introduction

Patients with cyanotic congenital heart disease and decreased pulmonary blood flow may have a spectrum of abnormalities of the tricuspid valve, right ventricle, pulmonary valve, and pulmonary arteries. Treatment pathways are undertaken with the goals of eliminating cyanosis and optimizing right ventricular function, growth, and development. The impact of each intervention on tricuspid and pulmonary valve integrity, right ventricular systolic and diastolic function, and pulmonary artery anatomy must be carefully considered to achieve optimal outcomes.

Initial Evaluation and Stabilization of the Cyanotic Neonate

In cyanotic neonates, an initial evaluation is undertaken to determine whether the etiology of the cyanosis is cardiac or noncardiac in origin. The algorithm used at Children's Hospital in Boston to triage cyanotic newborns is shown in Figure 9.1. A brief review of the maternal, family, and gestational histories and a directed physical examination may provide clues that favor either cardiac or pulmonary disease. A chest radiograph (CXR), electrocardiogram (ECG), and hyperoxia test should be obtained in all neonates with unexplained cyanosis. The CXR should be inspected for heart size, signs of parenchymal lung disease, increased or decreased pulmonary vascular markings, and sidedness of the aortic arch. For example, a very large heart and decreased pulmonary arterial markings on CXR suggests severe Ebstein's anomaly of the tricuspid valve (Figure 9.2), whereas a normal heart size and decreased pulmonary blood flow suggest tetralogy of Fallot, pulmonary atresia with intact ventricular septum, or tricuspid atresia. Those

with increased pulmonary vascular markings may have truncus arteriosus or total anomalous pulmonary venous return.

During the hyperoxia test (also called an *oxygen challenge test*), an arterial blood gas measurement is obtained from the right radial artery while the neonate is breathing room air, and a second blood gas value is obtained after the patient breathes for 10 min at 100% inspired oxygen. The PaO_2 is often between 25 and 40 mm Hg on room air. In 100% FiO_2, the PaO_2 will usually rise to >80 mm Hg in patients with pulmonary disease (provided that significant pulmonary artery hypertension is not present) but remain unchanged or only increase slightly in most neonates with cyanotic heart disease. The $PaCO_2$ is typically mildly decreased in newborns with cardiac disease and mildly elevated in those with pulmonary disease. Note that the hyperoxia test cannot be used in isolation to exclude critical congenital heart disease, as some neonates with left-sided obstructive lesions may have a PaO_2 >60 mm Hg in any extremity or a PaO_2 >150 mm Hg in the right arm.

If the aforementioned screening tests are suggestive of critical congenital heart disease, an echocardiogram should be obtained in a timely fashion. If pediatric cardiology consultation is readily available, and severe cyanosis (SaO_2 <80%) and metabolic acidosis (pH <7.3) are not present, then the echocardiogram may be obtained prior to initiation of a prostaglandin E_1 (PGE_1) infusion. If the neonate has mild cyanosis (SaO_2 >80%) and the echocardiogram reveals anatomy that does not likely require prompt surgical or transcatheter intervention (e.g., some neonates with tetralogy of Fallot), then observation without PGE_1 is warranted. However, if pediatric cardiology consultation and echocardiography are not readily available, a prolonged transport is anticipated, or the neonate is profoundly cyanotic, then PGE_1 should be administered without delay. If it is unclear from the initial postnatal echocardiogram whether early intervention is needed, then it is preferable to withhold PGE_1 and monitor the neonate's systemic oxygenation as the ductus arteriosus closes. This strategy avoids exposing some neonates to the side effects of PGE_1 and also allows for timely identification of neonates with cyanotic congenital heart diseases who do not have ductal-dependent pulmonary blood flow and can have surgical or transcatheter intervention deferred.

Prostaglandin E_1

Prostaglandin E_1 has been used since the late 1970s to maintain ductal patency in infants with critical congenital heart disease.

D.S. Wheeler et al. (eds.), *Cardiovascular Pediatric Critical Illness and Injury*,
DOI 10.1007/978-1-84800-923-3_9, © Springer-Verlag London Limited 2009

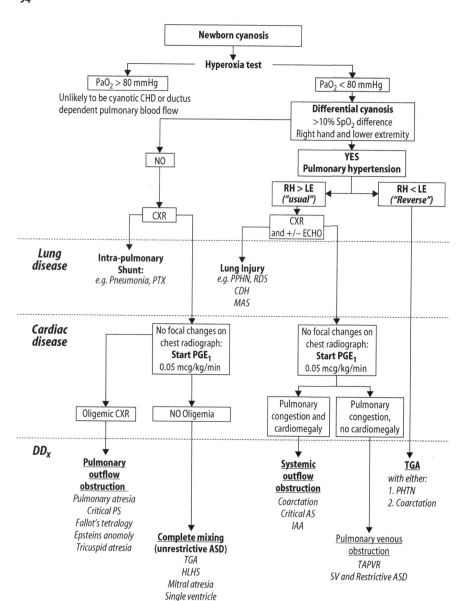

FIGURE 9.1. Algorithm for initial assessment of cyanotic newborns. AS, aortic stenosis; ASD, atrial septal defect; CXR, chest radiograph; CDH, congenital diaphragmatic hernia; CHD, congenital heart disease; ECHO, echocardiogram; HLHS, hypoplastic left heart syndrome; IAA, interrupted aortic arch; LE, lower extremity; MAS, meconium aspiration syndrome; PTX, pneumothorax; PGE_1, prostaglandin E_1; PPHN, primary pulmonary hypertension; PHTN, pulmonary hypertension; PS, pulmonary stenosis; RH, right heart; SV, single ventricle; TAPVR, total anomalous pulmonary venous return; TGA, D-transposition of the great arteries.

Prostaglandin E_1 will maintain systemic blood flow in neonates with severe left ventricular outflow tract obstruction, maintain pulmonary blood flow in those with severe right ventricular outflow tract obstruction, and allow for mixing of systemic and pulmonary blood flow in the setting of parallel anatomic circulation (e.g., D-transposition of the great arteries). Prostaglandin E_1 allows adequate time for interhospital transport, detailed cardiac evaluation, treatment of noncardiac disorders, and semielective scheduling of most cardiac interventions. Neonates who present with shock or severe cyanosis can be given time for recovery of end-organ function before cardiac intervention. Prostaglandin E_1 may be administered through a central or peripheral venous line.

A PGE_1 dose of 0.05–0.1 μg/kg/min is used when the ductus arteriosus is severely constricted or functionally closed and severe cyanosis exists. Lower doses (0.01 μ/kg/min) will safely maintain ductal patency. The most common side effect of PGE_1 is apnea, which occurs in a minority of neonates receiving the drug [1]. The risk of apnea is not an absolute indication for empiric endotracheal intubation and mechanical ventilation. Aminophylline may mini-

mize the occurrence of apnea and need for endotracheal intubation in neonates receiving PGE_1 [2]. Other common side effects are listed in Table 9.1. Uncommonly, the initiation of PGE_1 may cause a significant clinical deterioration. In neonates with congenital absence of the ductus arteriosus (e.g., tetralogy of Fallot with absent pulmonary valve syndrome; some infants with pulmonary atresia, ventricular septal defect, and major aortopulmonary collateral arteries), PGE_1 may lower systemic vascular resistance, decrease pulmonary blood flow, and thus exacerbate cyanosis.

In contrast to neonates with ductal-dependent systemic blood flow, the ductus arteriosus in those with right ventricular outflow tract obstruction is often somewhat restrictive and follows a tortuous course from the aorta to the pulmonary artery. Diastolic runoff from the aorta is thus diminished, and the risk for necrotizing enterocolitis may be diminished. Thus, it is reasonable to introduce enteral feedings in stable neonates with ductal-dependent pulmonary blood flow who are receiving PGE_1, provided that a reasonable diastolic blood pressure (>30 mm Hg) is present.

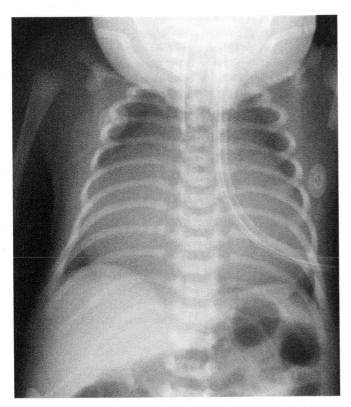

FIGURE 9.2. Chest radiograph of a neonate with severe Ebstein's anomaly.

Preoperative Evaluation

All patients with cyanotic congenital heart disease with decreased pulmonary blood flow require a complete echocardiogram. Detailed anatomic and functional information is obtained for the tricuspid valve and right ventricle. The right ventricular outflow tract is carefully studied, including the infundibulum, pulmonary valve, main pulmonary artery, and the proximal left and right pulmonary arteries. If a ductus arteriosus is present, its size and gradient from the aorta to the pulmonary arteries can be determined. The proximal coronary arteries should be interrogated to ensure that an important coronary vessel does not cross the infundibular region, as this may influence the surgeon's technique for right ventricular outflow tract reconstruction. In selected cases additional diagnostic information may be required. Cardiac magnetic resonance imaging (MRI) in infants and young children usually requires sedation and paralysis but will provide useful anatomic information about extracardiac vessels, including pulmonary artery

TABLE 9.1. Side effects of prostaglandin E₁ infusion.

Respiratory	Respiratory depression,* apnea*
Cardiovascular	Hypotension,* tachycardia,† tissue edema*
Central nervous system	Fever,* seizures†
Endocrine/metabolic	Hypocalcemia,† hypoglycemia,† cortical hyperostosis‡
Gastrointestinal	Diarrhea,† gastric outlet obstruction‡
Hematologic	Inhibition of platelet aggregation†
Dermatologic	Flushing,* harlequin rash*

*Common.
†Rarely of clinical significance.
‡With long-term use.

anatomy and blood supply, as well as the number, size, and location of any major aortopulmonary collateral arteries (MAPCAs). Cardiac catheterization is used selectively to evaluate the branch pulmonary artery anatomy, evaluate the relative contribution of pulmonary blood flow to lung segments from the native pulmonary arteries or MAPCAs, clarify any coronary artery branching abnormalities, or determine the functional significance of coronary artery fistulas arising from the right ventricle. Hemodynamic data are obtained including right ventricular pressure (RVP) and gradients across stenotic valves or vessels. In selected cases, transcatheter interventions are performed during the same catheterization once diagnostic information is complete.

Common Postoperative Concerns

Restrictive Right Ventricular Physiology

The phrase *restrictive right ventricular physiology* is commonly used in the immediate postoperative period in reference to patients who have diastolic dysfunction from a stiff, poorly compliant, and sometimes hypertrophied right ventricle. Restrictive right ventricular physiology is particularly evident following neonatal right ventricular outflow reconstruction, which is required during surgical repair of tetralogy of Fallot, pulmonary atresia, or truncus arteriosus. A right ventriculotomy is required for most of these neonatal repairs and further exacerbates the problem. Additional factors contributing to right ventricular diastolic dysfunction may include myocardial edema following cardiopulmonary bypass, inadequate myocardial protection of the hypertrophied ventricle during aortic cross clamp, myocardial ischemia–reperfusion injury, coronary artery injury, residual outflow tract obstruction, and volume load on the ventricle from a residual ventricular septal defect (VSD) or pulmonary regurgitation. The elevated ventricular end diastolic pressure restricts filling during diastole, causing increased right atrial filling pressure and systemic venous hypertension. Because of the phenomenon of ventricular interdependence, changes in right ventricular diastolic function and septal position will in turn affect left ventricular compliance and function. Stroke volume and preload to the left ventricle are ultimately compromised.

A low cardiac output state with increased right-sided filling pressure (usually >10–15 mm Hg) is a manifestation of neonatal restrictive right ventricular physiology. Tachycardia, hypotension, and a narrow pulse pressure are present. Patients often have cool extremities, oliguria, and a metabolic acidosis. As a result of elevated right atrial pressure, hepatic congestion, ascites, increased chest tube losses, and pleural effusions may develop. Because of the restrictive physiology, a relatively small volume load from a residual VSD or pulmonary regurgitation is poorly tolerated in the early postoperative period.

Treatment includes the maintenance of preload, despite elevation of the right atrial pressure. Inotrope support is often required, typically starting with dopamine at 5–10 μg/kg/min. Milrinone may be added for its lusitropic properties. In advanced cases, low-dose epinephrine (e.g., 0.05–0.1 μg/kg/min) may be beneficial provided that further elevation of the heart rate does not occur. Sedation and paralysis are often necessary for the first 24–48 hours to minimize the stress response and associated myocardial workload.

Although any atrial septal defects are usually closed at the time of surgery in older patients, it is beneficial to leave a small atrial communication following neonatal repair. In the face of diastolic dysfunction and increased right ventricular end diastolic pressure, a right-to-left atrial shunt will maintain preload to the left ventricle and therefore cardiac output. Patients may be desaturated initially following surgery (SaO_2 75%–85%), but, as right ventricular compliance and function improve (usually within 2–3 postoperative days), the amount of shunt decreases and both antegrade pulmonary blood flow and SaO_2 increase.

Mechanical ventilation may influence right ventricular afterload and pulmonary regurgitation. Increased pulmonary vascular resistance caused by hypothermia, acidosis, and either hypo- or hyperinflation of the lung will increase afterload on the right ventricle and pulmonary regurgitation. Intermittent positive pressure ventilation is used with adequate tidal volumes to prevent lung collapse and avoid respiratory acidosis while achieving the lowest possible mean airway pressure. Once right ventricular compliance has improved, as evidenced by a fall in right-sided filling pressures, increased arterial saturation, improved cardiac output with warm extremities, and an established diuresis, sedation or paralysis is discontinued and the patient allowed to slowly wean from mechanical ventilation.

Residual Lesions

Following transcatheter or surgical intervention, important residual anatomic lesions may have a major impact on patient outcome. A combination of factors will lead to the early identification of significant residual lesions, including an appreciation of the "normal" postoperative course, close attention to data obtained by intracardiac monitoring and physical examination, communication with the cardiovascular surgeon, and a high index of suspicion. Residual lesions may exacerbate restrictive right ventricular physiology. Tricuspid valve stenosis or insufficiency, pulmonary valve regurgitation, or right ventricular outflow tract obstruction at any level may be encountered. Residual VSDs or MAPCAs may cause volume overload to the left ventricle and pressure overload to the right ventricle. Compromise of the coronary circulation, either by injury of a coronary vessel during right ventricular outflow tract reconstruction or by decompression of a right ventricle in a patient with right ventricular–dependent coronary circulation (RVDCC) may result in regional or global myocardial dysfunction.

Arrhythmias

Common arrhythmias following right heart surgery include heart block and junctional ectopic tachycardia. It is important to maintain sinus rhythm and the atrial contribution to ventricular filling, particularly in the setting of restrictive right ventricular physiology. Loss of atrioventricular synchrony will further increase right atrial pressure and compromise cardiac output and blood pressure. The use of temporary pacing wires for atrioventricular sequential pacing may be necessary for advanced second degree and third degree heart block. Approximately two thirds of patients with third degree heart block immediately following surgery will recover atrioventricular conduction within 10 days, and those who do not require permanent pacemaker placement. Complete right bundle branch block is typical on the postoperative ECG but usually of little significance in the short term.

Junctional ectopic tachycardia may cause a significant decrease in cardiac output and be difficult to treat. This is a self-limiting, catecholamine-sensitive tachyarrhythmia, usually with an abrupt

onset in the first 12–24 hr following surgery. Treatment includes reducing endogenous sympathetic stimulation by ensuring adequate sedation and analgesia, optimizing mechanical ventilation and volume status, and reducing exogenous catecholamine infusions, if possible. Inducing hypothermia to 34°–35°C may reduce the ectopic rate, thereby enabling the use of temporary atrial pacing at a faster rate to achieve atrioventricular synchrony [3]. If these maneuvers are unsuccessful, procainamide or amiodarone is an appropriate antiarrhythmic drug to achieve junctional rate control.

Tetralogy of Fallot

Anatomy

The primary anatomic features of tetralogy of Fallot are an anterior malalignment VSD, right ventricular outflow tract obstruction, an overriding aorta, and right ventricular hypertrophy (Figure 9.3). Although most commonly a single VSD exists, additional VSDs may be present. Right ventricular outflow tract obstruction may exist in the infundibulum, at the pulmonary valve, and in the main

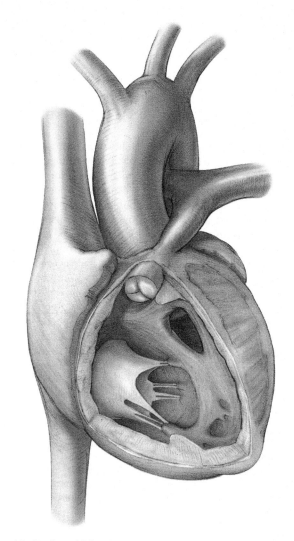

FIGURE 9.3. Tetralogy of Fallot (Courtesy of James D. St. Louis, MD, Medical College of Georgia.)

and branch pulmonary arteries. Patients with tetralogy of Fallot have a spectrum of severity of right ventricular outflow tract obstruction, ranging from minor infundibular and pulmonary valve stenosis (favorable) to pulmonary atresia with inadequate-sized central pulmonary arteries (less favorable). The most problematic anatomy is pulmonary atresia with diminutive or absent central pulmonary arteries and MAPCAs supplying a distal pulmonary vascular bed. There may be multiple stenoses and diminished total cross-sectional area of the pulmonary vascular bed. The aortic arch may be right sided in 25% of cases, which is important if placement of a systemic-to-pulmonary shunt is planned. The proximal coronary artery anatomy must be defined as the left coronary artery arises from the right coronary artery and crosses the right ventricular outflow tract in 5% of cases and may impact on the surgeon's ability to place an infundibular patch [4]. Tetralogy of Fallot is rarely associated with atrioventricular canal defect or absent pulmonary valve syndrome, and these conditions are not discussed further [5,6].

Pathophysiology and Clinical Presentation

The clinical presentation of patients with tetralogy of Fallot is determined to a great extent by the degree of malalignment of the conal septum into the right ventricular outflow tract. The amount of blood that shunts right-to-left through the VSD, and thus the extent of cyanosis, varies with the severity of right ventricular outflow tract obstruction and the systemic vascular resistance. Pulmonary vascular resistance usually falls soon after birth and has minimal influence on intracardiac shunting. Infants with a minimal degree of obstruction to pulmonary blood flow (*pink TETs*) are usually asymptomatic and fairly well oxygenated (SaO_2 >90%) soon after birth. These patients may be discharged from the newborn nursery with close follow up. Occasionally a pink TET will mimic the pathophysiology of an infant with a large VSD and develop congestive heart failure as pulmonary vascular resistance falls. More commonly, progressive right ventricular outflow tract obstruction and worsening cyanosis develop. Neonates with tetralogy of Fallot and more severe right ventricular outflow tract obstruction or pulmonary atresia will develop excessive cyanosis upon closure of the ductus arteriosus. Such patients are stabilized with PGE_1 and are referred for early surgical intervention.

Patients with an unrepaired tetralogy of Fallot are at risk for developing hypercyanotic episodes, which are potentially life-threatening events marked by significant hypoxemia, hyperpnea, and irritability. Dynamic infundibular stenosis and decreased systemic vascular resistance lead to a progressive cycle of decreased pulmonary blood flow, increased right-to-left shunting across the VSD, worsening cyanosis, and, eventually, metabolic acidosis. Although hypercyanotic episodes can occur at any time, the incidence seems to increase after 4–6 months of age. Hypercyanotic episodes can be triggered by any event that provokes significant patient agitation, including placement of intravenous catheters and phlebotomy. Sedation may precipitate a hypercyanotic episode, likely because of a drop in systemic vascular resistance. Treatment is directed toward decreasing patient agitation and heart rate, increasing systemic vascular resistance and pulmonary blood flow, and correcting metabolic acidosis (Table 9.2). Because of the potential morbidity associated with a hypercyanotic episode, many physicians consider their occurrence an indication for urgent surgery.

TABLE 9.2. Treatment options for hypercyanotic episodes, presented in the general sequence that they are administered.

Intervention	Effect on pathophysiology
Knee–chest position	↑ Systemic vascular resistance
Oxygen	↑ Blood oxygen content
Opioids or benzodiazepines	↓ Agitation, ↓ hyperpnea
Ketamine	↓ Agitation, ↑ systemic vascular resistance
Volume	↑ Right ventricular preload (30 cc/kg crystalloid)
β-Blocker	↓ Infundibular spasm, ↓ heart rate
Sodium bicarbonate	↓ Metabolic acidosis
Phenylephrine	↑ Systemic vascular resistance
CPB or ECMO	Rescue therapy when above measures fail

Note: CPB, cardiopulmonary bypass; ECMO, extracorporeal membranous oxygenation.

Preoperative Evaluation

Complete anatomic information is usually obtained by transthoracic echocardiography [4]. If uncertainty persists about the coronary artery anatomy, some surgeons may request a cardiac catheterization, although the coronary anatomy can usually be determined by intraoperative inspection and is not as important if the operation is performed without a ventriculotomy [7]. Details about the pulmonary artery anatomy may be clarified by computed tomography (CT) angiography, MRI or cardiac catheterization. A microdeletion at chromosome 22q11 is present in 15% of patients with tetralogy of Fallot [8].

Surgical or Transcatheter Intervention

Indications for prompt surgical intervention include increasing cyanosis and the occurrence of a hypercyanotic episode [9]. Many centers recommend primary complete repair for asymptomatic patients with tetralogy of Fallot before 6 months of age to alleviate cyanosis, minimize the occurrence of hypercyanotic episodes, prevent progressive infundibular stenosis, and alleviate RVP overload. This strategy avoids the additional surgical procedure and potential morbidity associated with a systemic-to-pulmonary artery shunt (shunt thrombosis, pulmonary artery distortion, overcirculation) [9,10]. However, some centers will selectively place systemic-to-pulmonary shunts in symptomatic neonates and young infants in order to minimize the need for an extensive ventriculotomy and the use of deep hypothermic circulatory arrest [11]. Definitive repair in these patients is then completed at 12–24 months of age.

Complete repair includes VSD closure, resection of muscle bundles in the right ventricular outflow tract, a pulmonary valvotomy or leaflet resection, and, if necessary, patch augmentation of the proximal pulmonary arteries. In many cases, the operation may be accomplished using a transatrial–transpulmonary approach, thus avoiding the short- and long-term sequelae of a right ventriculotomy or transannular patch [7,10]. A small atrial septal defect may be left patent in neonates to allow the right heart to decompress into the left atrium, which serves to maintain left ventricular preload and systemic cardiac output at the expense of mild cyanosis early after surgery.

Postoperative Care and Outcome

The adequacy of tetralogy of Fallot repair may be objectively assessed by a number of modalities, including intraoperative

transesophageal echocardiogram [11], measurement of right ventricular and pulmonary artery pressure, and pulmonary artery
oxygen saturation data [12]. Right ventricular function and compliance are often abnormal because of the combined effects of preexisting right ventricular hypertrophy, myocardial edema from
cardiopulmonary bypass, myocardial ischemia–reperfusion injury,
subpulmonic muscle bundle resection, VSD closure, and (if present)
a ventriculotomy. Significant pulmonary regurgitation or residual
VSDs, right ventricular outflow tract obstruction, or pulmonary
artery stenosis may further exacerbate right heart failure. The
inability of the right heart to provide adequate preload to the left
ventricle, along with adverse effects of ventricular interdependence
and abnormal septal position, may result in left ventricular dysfunction and low cardiac output, particularly in neonates, that
persists for 2–3 days. Loss of sinus rhythm may be poorly tolerated
in the setting of restrictive right ventricular physiology.

Adequate preload is required when right ventricular compliance
is poor, yet volume boluses may contribute to further elevation of
right-sided filling pressures, pleural effusions, and ascites. Inotropic support of the right ventricle is commonly required immediately following surgery. If an atrial communication does not exist
and significant right heart failure exists in the early postoperative
period, the atrial septum may be opened in the cardiac catheterization laboratory. Junctional ectopic tachycardia is the most common
arrhythmia seen early following tetralogy of Fallot repair [9,13].
Ventricular tachycardia is rarely encountered in the early postoperative period. Complete right bundle branch block is commonly
present on the postoperative ECG but is usually of little short-term
significance. Surgical outcomes in the current era are excellent for
uncomplicated tetralogy of Fallot [7,9–11].

Neonates with tetralogy of Fallot who have a systemic-to-
pulmonary artery shunt placed are at risk for developing congestive heart failure, as pulmonary blood flow from the shunt plus the
native flow across the right ventricular outflow tract may be excessive. Acute shunt thrombosis and pulmonary artery distortion are
also complications of this procedure.

Tetralogy of Fallot, Pulmonary Atresia, and Multiple Aortopulmonary Collateral Arteries

Tetralogy of Fallot with pulmonary atresia is a condition notable
for a spectrum of disease severity based on the anatomy of the
pulmonary arteries and MAPCAs. At the best end of the spectrum,
a patient may have tetralogy of Fallot, pulmonary atresia, good-
sized central pulmonary arteries, and no MAPCAs, but this
anatomy is uncommon. Often, the central pulmonary arteries are
diminutive and supplied by one or more duct-like collaterals.
Occasionally the central pulmonary arteries are discontinuous. In
approximately 15%–25% of cases there are no central pulmonary
arteries [14,15]. The MAPCAs are variable in number and usually
arise from the descending aorta, although their origin may be from
the ascending aorta, aortic arch, brachiocephalic vessels, or coronary arteries (Figure 9.4) [14].

A balanced circulation with mild cyanosis, excessive cyanosis,
or congestive heart failure may be evident upon presentation,
depending on the size and number of MAPCAs and the severity of
stenoses within these vessels [15]. By definition, all systemic venous
return must shunt right to left at the atrial or ventricular level in
patients with pulmonary atresia, resulting in complete mixing with
pulmonary venous return in the left heart. Neonates with tetralogy

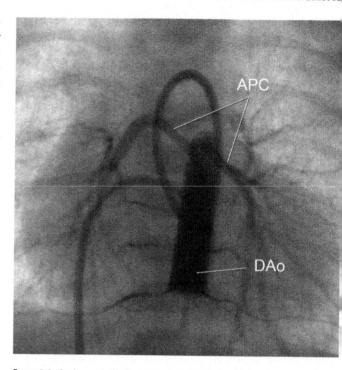

FIGURE 9.4. Angiogram in the descending aorta (DAo) of a patient with tetralogy of Fallot with pulmonary atresia demonstrating two major aortopulmonary collateral arteries (APC).

of Fallot, pulmonary atresia, and multiple MAPCAs are generally
not dependent on PGE$_1$. Although cardiac MRI provides adequate
visualization of central pulmonary arteries and the proximal
course of important MAPCAs, cardiac catheterization is ultimately
required to clarify distal pulmonary artery anatomy and identify
all sources of pulmonary blood flow.

Indications for initial surgical intervention in neonates with
tetralogy of Fallot, pulmonary atresia, and MAPCAs include excessive cyanosis, refractory congestive heart failure, or diminutive
central pulmonary arteries in need of a reliable source of blood flow
to promote growth. In the absence of symptoms, elective surgical
intervention should occur within the first 2–6 months of life to
maximize the growth potential of the central pulmonary arteries.
The ultimate goal of intervention is to optimize the effective cross-
sectional area of the pulmonary arterial vascular bed, eliminate
any MAPCAs that represent dual blood supply in order to minimize
the risk of pulmonary vascular obstructive disease to lung segments, and thus limit right ventricular hypertension following
eventual VSD closure.

Although primary complete repair in early infancy is possible in
selected patients [16], in many cases a staged series of surgical
and transcatheter interventions are required, the timing and
conduct of which must be individualized based on underlying
anatomy and physiology at presentation [14]. If the central
pulmonary arteries are small but confluent, the initial operation
must include the establishment of a reliable source of antegrade
blood flow, which will promote growth of these vessels over time.
Options include placement of a modified Blalock-Taussig shunt,
creation of an aortopulmonary window, or placement of a right
ventricular to pulmonary artery conduit [14,17,18]. The latter
approach may be advantageous in that it provides easy antegrade
transcatheter access to the distal pulmonary arteries for subse-

quent balloon angioplasty. If the central pulmonary arteries are absent, they can be constructed using pericardium or pulmonary allograft [14].

Intervention for each MAPCA is customized depending on its size, the presence or absence of proximal stenosis within the vessel, and a determination as to whether it represents redundant blood supply to individual lung segments. Redundant MAPCAs can be coil occluded in the cardiac catheterization laboratory or ligated at the time of surgery to eliminate left-to-right shunting and prevent the development of pulmonary vascular disease. If an MAPCA represents the sole source of pulmonary blood flow to a lung segment, the proximal end of the MAPCA is removed from its source and incorporated into the native or newly constructed central pulmonary arteries such that blood flow to the lung is supplied from a single source (unifocalization procedure) [14,19].

Once the pulmonary vascular bed has been optimally recruited, intracardiac repair is completed, including VSD closure and (if not previously completed) right ventricular outflow tract reconstruction. The incidence of early postoperative right ventricular failure may be decreased by placement of a fenestrated VSD patch in patients with an inadequate pulmonary vascular bed, which serves to preserve systemic cardiac output at the expense of mild postoperative cyanosis [18]. Although earlier series reported 5-year mortality rates exceeding 50% [15], in contemporary series the midterm mortality ranges from 2% to 16% [14,20].

Pulmonary Valve Stenosis

Anatomy

Pulmonary valve stenosis occurring in isolation is common, representing about 10% of all congenital heart disease. Pulmonary stenosis may be associated with other lesions, including VSD, transposition of the great arteries, Ebstein's anomaly, or atrioventricular canal defect. This section focuses on isolated pulmonary valve stenosis, as the associated lesions are discussed elsewhere. Stenotic pulmonary valves have one to three thickened cusps that often dome in ventricular systole. The pulmonary valve annulus may be hypoplastic, and infundibular hypertrophy may be present. In utero, the stenotic pulmonary valve imposes high afterload on the right ventricle, causing it to hypertrophy. A patent foramen ovale or atrial septal defect is commonly associated with pulmonary valve stenosis.

Pathophysiology and Clinical Presentation

Pulmonary valve stenosis has a wide spectrum of severity and may be classified as mild (0–40 mm Hg gradient across the pulmonary valve or RVP less than half of left ventricular pressure [LVP]), moderate (40–80 mm Hg gradient or RVP greater than half but less than LVP), or severe (>80 mm Hg gradient or RVP equal to or greater than LVP). This classification system assumes that cardiac output is normal and may not be applicable to neonates or the unusual older patient with right ventricular dysfunction. The phrase *critical pulmonary valve stenosis* is commonly used to describe the neonate who is symptomatic with cyanosis and right ventricular failure. A pinhole orifice in the pulmonary valve mandates that nearly all systemic venous return shunts right to left across the atrial septum, where mixing occurs with pulmonary venous return. When compared with infants having severe pulmonary stenosis, those with critical pulmonary stenosis may have smaller tricuspid valves and right ventricles, more tricuspid regurgitation, more right ventricular hypertrophy, and the absence of significant antegrade flow across the right ventricular outflow tract with resultant right to left shunting through an atrial communication (Table 9.3) [21]. Closure of the ductus arteriosus may cause severe cyanosis, which is alleviated by initiating PGE_1. As the transcatheter management for older children with pulmonary valve stenosis is technically straightforward and rarely results in complications requiring intensive care, the remainder of this section focuses on the neonate with critical pulmonary valve stenosis.

Preoperative Evaluation

Echocardiographic evaluation of pulmonary valve stenosis in the neonatal period is focused on the size and function of the tricuspid valve, right ventricle, and pulmonary valve (Figure 9.5). In the presence of a widely patent ductus arteriosus and poor right ventricular function or pulmonary hypertension, color Doppler flow may not be seen across a patent pulmonary valve. Right

TABLE 9.3. Classification and outcomes for balloon dilation for pulmonary valve stenosis.

	Mild PS	Moderate PS	Severe PS	Critical PS
RVP	<40 mm Hg; <50% LVP	40–80 mmHg; 50%–100% LVP	>80 mm Hg; ≥ LVP	>LVP
Cyanosis	None	Rare, mild	Common, mild	≥ Moderate
Ductal-dependent PBF	No	No	No	Yes
Tricuspid valve size	Normal	Normal	Normal	Low–normal range
≥ Mild TR	None	Uncommon	+	++
RVH	None	Mild	Moderate	Moderate–severe
Antegrade RVOT flow	+++	+++	++	Trivial
Probability of successful balloon valvuloplasty*	Not indicated	High	90%	64%–85%

*Success is defined as the lack of need for early surgery [21,25].

Note: LVP, left ventricular pressure; PBF, pulmonary blood flow; PS, pulmonary stenosis; RVH, right ventricular hypertrophy; RVOT, right ventricular outflow tract; RVP, right ventricular pressure; TR, tricuspid regurgitation.

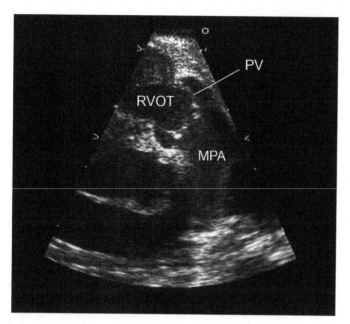

FIGURE 9.5. Two-dimensional echocardiogram demonstrating the thickened doming leaflets in a neonate with pulmonary valve stenosis. MPA, main pulmonary artery; PV, pulmonary valve; RVOT, right ventricular outflow tract.

ventricular pressure is quantified by Doppler interrogation of the tricuspid regurgitation jet. The Doppler gradient across the pulmonary valve may be influenced by right ventricular function and by the main pulmonary artery pressure and thus cannot be interpreted in isolation.

Surgical or Transcatheter Intervention

Neonates with severe or critical pulmonary valve stenosis require prompt referral for balloon valvuloplasty. Surgical valvotomy is now reserved for those neonates who fail transcatheter intervention. During the catheterization, a series of balloons with a final diameter of approximately 120% of the pulmonary valve annulus size are used to dilate the stenotic pulmonary valve [22]. Perforation of the right ventricular outflow tract is a potential complication of this procedure. Prostaglandin E_1 may be discontinued following successful valvuloplasty and the patient returned to the intensive care unit.

Postoperative Care and Outcome

The most common problem encountered following balloon dilation of critical pulmonary valve stenosis in the neonate is persistent cyanosis [23]. In such patients, mild right ventricular hypoplasia and poor right ventricular compliance secondary to right ventricular hypertrophy and elevated end diastolic pressure result in right-to-left shunting at the atrial level. Prostaglandin E_1 may be used to maintain ductal patency for several days, thus providing time for right ventricular compliance to improve [24]. Right ventricular systolic dysfunction, anemia, tricuspid stenosis, or residual pulmonary stenosis may contribute to the cyanosis. Management strategies to support right ventricular function and enhance pulmonary blood flow in the setting of poor right ventricular compliance include maintenance of adequate preload, keeping the hematocrit around 45% to maximize oxygen-carrying capacity,

inotropic support with dopamine if systolic function is compromised, milrinone for its lusitropic properties, avoidance of tachycardia and consideration of short-acting β-blockers to optimize diastolic filling time, and maintenance of low right ventricular afterload by allowing spontaneous ventilation or use of mechanical ventilation with low mean airway pressure. Patience is required while caring for these neonates, and SaO_2 >75% and PaO_2 >35–40 mm Hg are acceptable in the short term. Several trials of observation off PGE_1 may be required.

Surgical intervention is ultimately required in 15%–25% of neonates with critical pulmonary stenosis for either technical failure of the balloon valvuloplasty or persistent cyanosis [22–24]. A systemic-to-pulmonary shunt will provide effective pulmonary blood flow until right ventricle compliance and size improves. If infundibular hypertrophy or residual pulmonary valve stenosis is contributing to the cyanosis, an infundibular patch or pulmonary valvotomy may be required. Mortality for neonates with critical pulmonary stenosis in experienced centers is <5% [22,25].

Pulmonary Atresia with Intact Ventricular Septum

Anatomy

Pulmonary atresia with intact ventricular septum is an uncommon lesion characterized by a membranous or muscular obstruction of the pulmonary valve, associated with hypoplasia of the right ventricle and tricuspid valve. The left and right pulmonary arteries are usually of normal size. Major aortopulmonary collateral arteries are quite uncommon, in contrast to patients with tetralogy of Fallot with pulmonary atresia. Right ventricle to coronary artery fistulas are present in nearly half of cases, particularly in those with advanced tricuspid valve and right ventricular hypoplasia [26–28]. In 9%–34% of patients with pulmonary atresia and intact ventricular septum, stenoses, interruptions, or ostial occlusions are present in one or more coronary vessels. The myocardium supplied by these compromised coronary arteries is thus dependent on flow from the right ventricle through the coronary fistula, a condition known as right ventricular–dependent coronary circulation (RVDCC) [26,28–30]. Ebstein's anomaly of the tricuspid valve is found in 10% of cases [28].

Pathophysiology and Clinical Presentation

All neonates with pulmonary atresia and intact ventricular septum have ductal-dependent pulmonary blood flow, and PGE_1 should be started soon after birth. Complete intracardiac mixing occurs, as all systemic venous return to the right atrium flows through an obligatory atrial communication to the left atrium. The right ventricle is decompressed by tricuspid regurgitation or egress through the coronary fistulas to the aorta. If tricuspid regurgitation is limited, suprasystemic RVP and marked right ventricular hypertrophy are usually present.

In neonates with right ventricular to coronary artery fistulas, right ventricular decompression may compromise myocardial perfusion because of reduced coronary perfusion pressure and runoff or *steal* from the aorta to the right ventricle in diastole [31]. If the coronary anatomy is such that RVDCC is present and the right ventricle is decompressed, myocardial ischemia or infarction may occur [29].

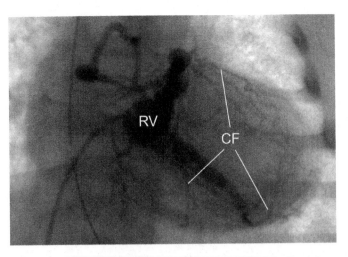

Figure 9.6. Angiographic injection in the right ventricle of a neonate with pulmonary atresia with intact ventricular septum demonstrating multiple fistulous connections to the coronary circulation. RV, right ventricle; CF, coronary fistula.

Preoperative Evaluation

The initial echocardiogram must delineate the size and function of the tricuspid valve and right ventricle and the anatomy of the right ventricular outflow tract. A judgment must be made as to whether the right heart structures are adequate, or have the potential to be adequate in the future, to support a two-ventricle circulation [32]. Right ventricle to coronary artery fistulas may be identified by echocardiogram using color Doppler. Neonates with a tricuspid valve z score of ≤−2.5 are very likely to have RVDCC [27]. The coronary anatomy should be precisely defined by cardiac catheterization (Figure 9.6) [32]. If stenoses, interruptions, or ostial occlusions exist such that a significant amount of myocardium is dependent on flow from the right ventricle through the coronary fistulas, then decompression of the right ventricle is contraindicated.

Surgical or Transcatheter Intervention

Provided that the tricuspid valve and right ventricle are of reasonable size and there is no evidence for RVDCC, the goal is to eventually achieve a two-ventricle repair. Any intervention must enable growth of the tricuspid valve and right ventricle without compromising the coronary circulation. Right ventricular decompression may be accomplished by placement of a right ventricular outflow tract patch to encourage right ventricular growth and allow regression of right ventricular hypertrophy [30,32]. The atrial septal defect is left open to allow for decompression of the right heart and maintenance of systemic cardiac output, and usually a systemic-to-pulmonary shunt is concurrently placed to ensure adequate pulmonary blood flow. The right ventricle may also be decompressed in neonates with membranous pulmonary atresia by transcatheter perforation of the pulmonary valve using a stiff wire or radiofrequency ablation catheter followed by balloon valvuloplasty, which avoids the need for surgical intervention in approximately one third of patients undergoing this procedure (Figure 9.7) [33].

Following neonatal right ventricular decompression, patients are evaluated for interval growth of right-sided heart structures and right ventricular compliance. Provided that cyanosis and systemic venous hypertension do not develop during test occlusions of the

atrial septal defect and systemic-to-pulmonary shunt performed during cardiac catheterization, closure of the atrial communication and takedown or coil occlusion of the shunt are performed to separate the systemic and pulmonary circulations. One-and-one half ventricular repair and Fontan palliation are options for older patients whose right heart has not developed adequately to support the entire circulation [30].

If RVDCC exists, relief of right ventricular outflow obstruction is contraindicated, and the initial operation is a systemic-to-pulmonary artery shunt as the first stage of single-ventricle palliation [34]. Cardiac transplantation may be considered for the unusual infant with severe RVDCC and myocardial dysfunction that precludes single-ventricle palliation [35].

Postoperative Care and Outcome

Following placement of a right ventricular outflow patch in the neonatal period, supportive care as described above for patients with restrictive right ventricular physiology is usually necessary. Care should be taken to avoid excessive systemic vasodilation, particularly in patients with RVDCC, who may benefit from vasopressor support with norepinephrine to maintain aortic root pressure and coronary perfusion. Close ECG monitoring for ST segment changes is required, and, if any signs of myocardial ischemia develop, prompt echocardiography should be obtained to evaluate for wall motion abnormalities. If RVDCC is unrecognized and a right ventricular outflow patch is placed, myocardial ischemia, ventricular dysfunction, and arrhythmias are likely to develop immediately following surgery [29].

Additional concerns related to the systemic-to-pulmonary shunt include the potential for pulmonary overcirculation (high Qp:Qs), poor systemic perfusion, low diastolic blood pressure, and inadequate coronary perfusion in patients with coronary fistulas. In this setting, maneuvers are indicated to increase pulmonary vascular resistance and thus "balance" the circulation, such as use of increased mean airway pressure and the avoidance of supplemental oxygen and respiratory alkalosis. Rarely, a circular shunt may develop following placement of a right ventricular outflow tract patch and systemic to pulmonary shunt (as described in detail later in Ebstein's Anomaly); however, this is uncommon in patients with pulmonary atresia and intact ventricular septum due in part to the elevated end diastolic pressure that serves to limit pulmonary regurgitation. Using appropriate staged interventions in patients with pulmonary atresia and intact ventricular septum, 5-year survival rates as high as 98% may be achieved [30]

Ebstein's Anomaly

Anatomy

In Ebstein's anomaly, the septal and posterior leaflets of the tricuspid valve are displaced to a variable extent into the anatomic right ventricle, and the anterior leaflet, while not inferiorly displaced, may be redundant or *sail-like* and cause obstruction of the right ventricular outflow tract. The tricuspid valve chordae tendinae and papillary muscles may be abnormal, and tricuspid regurgitation may be severe. The functional right atrium may be quite enlarged because of tricuspid regurgitation and the fact that the inlet portion of the right ventricle is *atrialized* by the displaced tricuspid valve leaflets. Atrial septal defects and anatomic pulmonary valve steno-

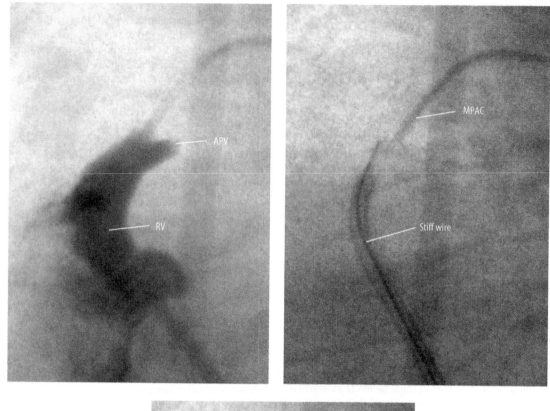

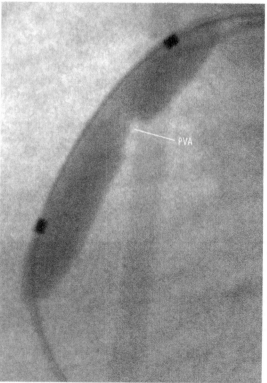

FIGURE 9.7. A series of images obtained during therapeutic cardiac catheterization in a neonate with pulmonary atresia and intact ventricular septum. **(A)** Angiogram in the right ventricle demonstrating no antegrade flow across the pulmonary valve. **(B)** A stiff wire is being advanced across the atretic pulmonary valve, using a catheter in the main pulmonary artery as a target. **(C)** Following perforation of the pulmonary valve, a balloon is advanced across the right ventricular outflow tract and inflated. Note the waist in the balloon that defines the location of the pulmonary valve annulus. APV, atretic pulmonary valve; MPAC, main pulmonary artery catheter; PVA, pulmonary valve annulus; RV, right ventricle.

sis or atresia are associated with Ebstein's anomaly. One or more accessory conduction pathways may exist at the tricuspid valve annulus, creating the necessary substrate for atrioventricular reentrant tachycardia. Pulmonary hypoplasia has been associated with advanced Ebstein's anomaly and thought to contribute to cyanosis and mortality [36]. However, a recent report suggests that, although lung compression may be severe, lung hypoplasia and immaturity are uncommon [37]

Pathophysiology and Clinical Presentation

Many patients with Ebstein's anomaly do not develop symptoms until adolescence or early adulthood, when right-sided congestive heart failure, cyanosis, or arrhythmias develop [38]. A subset of newborns with severe Ebstein's anomaly (i.e., severe tricuspid regurgitation, a large *atrialized* portion of the right ventricle, and severe cardiomegaly) present with hydrops fetalis or severe cyanosis and shock soon after birth [39]. Ebstein's anomaly presenting in the newborn period is one of the most severe forms of congenital heart disease. Often there are limited management options, and the risk for mortality remains high even in the current era. Right-to-left shunting at the atrial level occurs and may be due to pulmonary hypertension, pulmonary valve stenosis or atresia, or right ventricular outflow tract obstruction by the sail-like anterior leaflet of the tricuspid valve. *Functional* or *pseudo* pulmonary atresia exists when severe tricuspid regurgitation results in the inability of the right ventricle to eject blood into the pulmonary artery despite a patent pulmonary valve. Severe tricuspid regurgitation and extreme right atrial enlargement may result in pooling of venous return in the compliant right atrium with limited shunting across the atrial septal defect to the left atrium and left ventricle. The reduced preload to the left ventricle may contribute to underdevelopment of the left side of the heart and a low cardiac output state. Biventricular function may also be diminished by myocardial fibrosis [40,41].

Neonates presenting with significant cyanosis (<80% systemic saturation) should receive PGE₁, and mechanical ventilation with judicious use of positive end-expiratory pressure, as the lungs may be compressed by severe cardiomegaly. If functional atresia of the pulmonary valve may be present, inhaled nitric oxide should be used to decrease pulmonary vascular resistance, which may increase antegrade flow across the right ventricular outflow tract [42]. Despite aggressive supportive care, a subset of neonates with severe Ebstein's anomaly has persistent low cardiac output and profound cyanosis resulting in early mortality [41,42]. We do not currently recommend an "exit-to ECMO" (extracorporeal membrane oxygenation) strategy for these patients.

Preoperative Evaluation

The cardiothoracic ratio on CXR often exceeds 80% in severe cases (see Figure 9.2) [41]. The size of the right atrium, anatomy and function of the tricuspid valve, and the right ventricular outflow tract can all be assessed by echocardiography (Figure 9.8). A trial of nitric oxide during echocardiography may discriminate functional from anatomic pulmonary atresia [42]. Using echocardiographic measurements from the apical four-chamber view, the ratio of the right atrium and atrialized right ventricle to the area of the functional right ventricle, left atrium, and left ventricle of greater than 1 is a strong independent predictor of mortality [38,39,41]. Other predictors of mortality in the neonatal

period include the presence of cyanosis, right ventricular outflow tract obstruction, and left ventricular systolic dysfunction [38,41].

Surgical or Transcatheter Intervention

In some neonates with severe Ebstein's anomaly and cyanosis, medical management with mechanical ventilation, supplemental oxygen, correction of acidosis, and inhaled nitric oxide will allow pulmonary vascular resistance to fall, thereby promoting antegrade flow across the right ventricular outflow tract [41,42]. If this occurs and cyanosis decreases, surgical intervention can be deferred. For symptomatic neonates who fail medical management, there is no single reparative or palliative procedure that has a high success rate. One surgical option is to place a systemic to pulmonary artery shunt, oversew the tricuspid valve annulus, and perform an atrial septectomy as the first stage procedure toward Fontan palliation [43]. Plication of the right atrium is usually necessary to reduce its size and volume and to promote right-to-left shunting across the atrial septum. Although a two-ventricle repair has generally been difficult to achieve in the cyanotic newborn with Ebstein's anomaly, a recent small series described acceptable survival rates with primary complete repair, consisting of a reduction atrioplasty, fenestrated closure of the atrial septum, and complex tricuspid valvuloplasty [44]. Heart transplantation may also be considered, but, despite early listing, it may be difficult to medically manage these patients while waiting for a donor graft to become available.

Older children and adults may develop right-sided heart failure or cyanosis that requires either tricuspid valvuloplasty or tricuspid valve replacement [45,46]. Significant right ventricular volume overload because of severe tricuspid regurgitation may cause septal shift and compromised left ventricular function. In addition to tricuspid valve repair, a bidirectional Glenn operation may reduce the volume load to the right heart [47]. Electrophysiologic study and radiofrequency or surgical ablation may be indicated for patients with supraventricular tachycardia, which is most commonly atrial flutter/fibrillation or accessory pathway-mediated tachycardia [48].

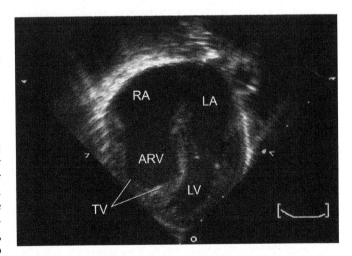

FIGURE 9.8. Two-dimensional echocardiogram demonstrating severe Ebstein's anomaly of the tricuspid valve in a neonate. ARV, atrialized right ventricle; LA, left atrium; LV, left ventricle; RA, right atrium; TV, tricuspid valve.

Postoperative Care and Outcome

Neonates with Ebstein's anomaly who require early surgical intervention are at high risk for mortality because of a persistent, severe low cardiac output state [36,41,42]. Although the lungs may appear small on CXR, excessive mean airway pressures should be avoided, as overdistension of the lungs may increase pulmonary vascular resistance and limit left ventricular preload. In neonates with a systemic-to-pulmonary shunt and residual tricuspid regurgitation without pulmonary atresia, low cardiac output may be partially explained by circular shunting, in which aortic blood flows through the shunt, retrograde through the main pulmonary artery to the right ventricle and tricuspid valve, across the atrial communication, and out the left ventricle and aorta, with resultant inadequate systemic blood flow. If medical therapy is inadequate to reduce the runoff through the systemic to pulmonary shunt in neonates with circular shunting, an emergent reoperation may be required to limit the shunt size, ligate the main pulmonary artery, or reduce tricuspid regurgitation with a valvuloplasty. In those patients with accessory conduction pathways, atrioventricular reentry tachycardia may cause a severe low cardiac output state, and early radiofrequency ablation may be necessary if medical control is unsuccessful.

References

1. Lewis AB, Freed MD, Heymann MA, et al. Side effects of therapy with prostaglandin E₁ in infants with critical congenital heart disease. Circulation 1981;64:893–898.
2. Lim DS, Kulik TJ, Kim DW, et al. Aminophylline for the prevention of apnea during prostaglandin E₁ infusion. Pediatrics 2003;112:e27–e29.
3. Walsh EP, Saul JP, Sholler GF, et al. Evaluation of a staged treatment protocol for rapid automatic junctional tachycardia after operation for congenital heart disease. J Am Coll Cardiol 1997;29:1046–1053.
4. Need LR, Powell AJ, del Nido P, et al. Coronary echocardiography in tetralogy of Fallot: diagnostic accuracy, resource utilization and surgical implications over 13 years. J Am Coll Cardiol 2000;36:1371–1377.
5. Najm HK, Van Arsdell GS, Watzka S, et al. Primary repair is superior to initial palliation in children with atrioventricular septal defect and tetralogy of Fallot. J Thorac Cardiovasc Surg 1998;116:905–913.
6. Hew CC, Daebritz SH, Zurakowski D, et al. Valved homograft replacement of aneurysmal pulmonary arteries for severely symptomatic absent pulmonary valve syndrome. Ann Thorac Surg 2002;73:1778–1785.
7. Karl TR, Sano S, Pornviliwan S, et al. Tetralogy of Fallot: favorable outcome of nonneonatal transatrial, transpulmonary repair. Ann Thorac Surg 1992;54:903–907.
8. Goldmuntz E, Clark BJ, Mitchell LE, et al. Frequency of 22q11 deletions in patients with conotruncal defects. J Am Coll Cardiol 1998;32:492–498.
9. Pigula FA, Khalil PN, Mayer JE, et al. Repair of tetralogy of Fallot in neonates and young infants. Circulation 1999;100:II157–II161.
10. Parry AJ, McElhinney DB, Kung GC, et al. Elective primary repair of acyanotic tetralogy of Fallot in early infancy: overall outcome and impact on the pulmonary valve. J Am Coll Cardiol 2000;36:2279–2283.
11. Fraser CD, Jr., McKenzie ED, Cooley DA. Tetralogy of Fallot: surgical management individualized to the patient. Ann Thorac Surg 2001;71:1556–1561.
12. Lang P, Chipman CW, Siden H, et al. Early assessment of hemodynamic status after repair of tetralogy of Fallot: a comparison of 24 hour (intensive care unit) and 1 year postoperative data in 98 patients. Am J Cardiol 1982;50:795–799.
13. Dodge-Khatami A, Miller OI, Anderson RH, et al. Surgical substrates of postoperative junctional ectopic tachycardia in congenital heart defects. J Thorac Cardiovasc Surg 2002;123:624–630.
14. Duncan BW, Mee RB, Prieto LR, et al. Staged repair of tetralogy of Fallot with pulmonary atresia and major aortopulmonary collateral arteries. J Thorac Cardiovasc Surg 2003;126:694–702.
15. Bull K, Somerville J, Ty E, et al. Presentation and attrition in complex pulmonary atresia. J Am Coll Cardiol 1995;25:491–499.
16. Reddy VM, McElhinney DB, Amin Z, et al. Early and intermediate outcomes after repair of pulmonary atresia with ventricular septal defect and major aortopulmonary collateral arteries: experience with 85 patients. Circulation 2000;101:1826–1832.
17. Rodefeld MD, Reddy VM, Thompson LD, et al. Surgical creation of aortopulmonary window in selected patients with pulmonary atresia with poorly developed aortopulmonary collaterals and hypoplastic pulmonary arteries. J Thorac Cardiovasc Surg 2002;123:1147–1154.
18. Marshall AC, Love BA, Lang P, et al. Staged repair of tetralogy of Fallot and diminutive pulmonary arteries with a fenestrated ventricular septal defect patch. J Thorac Cardiovasc Surg 2003;126:1427–1433.
19. Puga FJ, Leoni FE, Julsrud PR, et al. Complete repair of pulmonary atresia, ventricular septal defect, and severe peripheral arborization abnormalities of the central pulmonary arteries. Experience with preliminary unifocalization procedures in 38 patients. J Thorac Cardiovasc Surg 1989;98:1018–1028.
20. Gupta A, Odim J, Levi D, et al. Staged repair of pulmonary atresia with ventricular septal defect and major aortopulmonary collateral arteries: experience with 104 patients. J Thorac Cardiovasc Surg 2003;126:1746–1752.
21. Kovalchin JP, Forbes TJ, Nihill MR, et al. Echocardiographic determinants of clinical course in infants with critical and severe pulmonary valve stenosis. J Am Coll Cardiol 1997;29:1095–1101.
22. Colli AM, Perry SB, Lock JE, et al. Balloon dilation of critical valvar pulmonary stenosis in the first month of life. Cathet Cardiovasc Diagn 1995;34:23–28.
23. Fedderly RT, Lloyd TR, Mendelsohn AM, et al. Determinants of successful balloon valvotomy in infants with critical pulmonary stenosis or membranous pulmonary atresia with intact ventricular septum. J Am Coll Cardiol 1995;25:460–465.
24. Gournay V, Piechaud JF, Delogu A, et al. Balloon valvotomy for critical stenosis or atresia of pulmonary valve in newborns. J Am Coll Cardiol 1995;26:1725–1731.
25. Tabatabaei H, Boutin C, Nykanen DG, et al. Morphologic and hemodynamic consequences after percutaneous balloon valvotomy for neonatal pulmonary stenosis: medium-term follow-up. J Am Coll Cardiol 1996;27:473–478.
26. Hanley FL, Sade RM, Blackstone EH, et al. Outcomes in neonatal pulmonary atresia with intact ventricular septum. A multiinstitutional study. J Thorac Cardiovasc Surg 1993;105:406–423.
27. Satou GM, Perry SB, Gauvreau K, et al. Echocardiographic predictors of coronary artery pathology in pulmonary atresia with intact ventricular septum. Am J Cardiol 2000;85:1319–1324.
28. Daubeney PE, Delany DJ, Anderson RH, et al. Pulmonary atresia with intact ventricular septum: range of morphology in a population-based study. J Am Coll Cardiol 2002;39:1670–1679.
29. Giglia TM, Mandell VS, Connor AR, et al. Diagnosis and management of right ventricle-dependent coronary circulation in pulmonary atresia with intact ventricular septum. Circulation 1992;86:1516–1528.
30. Jahangiri M, Zurakowski D, Bichell D, et al. Improved results with selective management in pulmonary atresia with intact ventricular septum. J Thorac Cardiovasc Surg 1999;118:1046–1055.
31. Gentles TL, Colan SD, Giglia TM, et al. Right ventricular decompression and left ventricular function in pulmonary atresia with intact ventricular septum. The influence of less extensive coronary anomalies. Circulation 1993;88:II183–II188.
32. Giglia TM, Jenkins KJ, Matitiau A, et al. Influence of right heart size on outcome in pulmonary atresia with intact ventricular septum. Circulation 1993;88:2248–2256.

33. Humpl T, Soderberg B, McCrindle BW, et al. Percutaneous balloon valvotomy in pulmonary atresia with intact ventricular septum: impact on patient care. Circulation 2003;108:826–832.

34. Powell AJ, Mayer JE, Lang P, et al. Outcome in infants with pulmonary atresia, intact ventricular septum, and right ventricle-dependent coronary circulation. Am J Cardiol 2000;86:1272–1274.

35. Rychik J, Levy H, Gaynor JW, et al. Outcome after operations for pulmonary atresia with intact ventricular septum. J Thorac Cardiovasc Surg 1998;116:924–931.

36. Lang D, Oberhoffer R, Cook A, et al. Pathologic spectrum of malformations of the tricuspid valve in prenatal and neonatal life. J Am Coll Cardiol 1991;17:1161–1167.

37. Tanaka T, Yamaki S, Ohno T, et al. The histology of the lung in neonates with tricuspid valve disease and gross cardiomegaly due to severe regurgitation. Pediatr Cardiol 1998;19:133–138.

38. Celermajer DS, Bull C, Till JA, et al. Ebstein's anomaly: presentation and outcome from fetus to adult. J Am Coll Cardiol 1994;23:170–176.

39. Celermajer DS, Cullen S, Sullivan ID, et al. Outcome in neonates with Ebstein's anomaly. J Am Coll Cardiol 1992;19:1041–1046.

40. Celermajer DS, Dodd SM, Greenwald SE, et al. Morbid anatomy in neonates with Ebstein's anomaly of the tricuspid valve: pathophysiologic and clinical implications. J Am Coll Cardiol 1992;19:1049–1053.

41. Yetman AT, Freedom RM, McCrindle BW. Outcome in cyanotic neonates with Ebstein's anomaly. Am J Cardiol 1998;81:749–754.

42. Atz AM, Munoz RA, Adatia I, et al. Diagnostic and therapeutic uses of inhaled nitric oxide in neonatal Ebstein's anomaly. Am J Cardiol 2003;91:906–908.

43. Starnes VA, Pitlick PT, Bernstein D, et al. Ebstein's anomaly appearing in the neonate. A new surgical approach. J Thorac Cardiovasc Surg 1991;101:1082–1087.

44. Knott-Craig CJ, Overholt ED, Ward KE, et al. Repair of Ebstein's anomaly in the symptomatic neonate: an evolution of technique with 7-year follow-up. Ann Thorac Surg 2002;73:1786–1792.

45. Chen JM, Mosca RS, Altmann K, et al. Early and medium-term results for repair of Ebstein anomaly. J Thorac Cardiovasc Surg 2004;127:990–998.

46. Kiziltan HT, Theodoro DA, Warnes CA, et al. Late results of bioprosthetic tricuspid valve replacement in Ebstein's anomaly. Ann Thorac Surg 1998;66:1539–1545.

47. Marianeschi SM, McElhinney DB, Reddy VM, et al. Alternative approach to the repair of Ebstein's malformation: intracardiac repair with ventricular unloading. Ann Thorac Surg 1998;66:1546–1550.

48. Khositseth A, Danielson GK, Dearani JA, et al. Supraventricular tachyarrhythmias in Ebstein anomaly: management and outcome. J Thorac Cardiovasc Surg 2004;128:826–833.

10
Congenital Heart Disease: Left Ventricular Outflow Tract Obstruction

John R. Charpie, Dennis C. Crowley, and Joseph N. Graziano

Valvar Aortic Stenosis

Anatomy

Isolated valvar aortic stenosis (AS) is a common cardiac lesion, accounting for 3%–6% of all congenital heart disease [1]. This defect comprises a spectrum of aortic valve pathologies ranging from a bicuspid valve, which often has minimal hemodynamic significance, to less common abnormalities including fusion of all three leaflets (*unicuspid* valve) or myxomatous, thickened, dysplastic valve leaflets. Aortic annular hypoplasia can occur, and may be more frequently associated with additional left-sided obstructive defects such as mitral valve disease, coarctation of the aorta, and hypoplastic left heart syndrome. Aortic valve abnormalities occur approximately four times more often in males than females, and associated cardiac anomalies are present in nearly 20% of patients, including patent ductus arteriosus (PDA), coarctation of the aorta, and ventricular septal defects (VSD). Although familial cases have been described, there is no known genetic predisposition to valvar AS.

Pathophysiology and Clinical Presentation

Valvar AS is a progressive disease that results in obstruction to egress of blood from the heart, producing a pressure gradient from the left ventricle to the ascending aorta. There is an obligatory increase in left ventricular pressure in order to maintain adequate systemic blood flow. Chronic pressure overload on the left ventricle will stimulate myocardial hypertrophy, leading to altered diastolic properties of the ventricle and eventual elevation of the end diastolic and left atrial pressures. Left ventricular systolic function and cardiac output are generally well maintained. Another consequence of significant left ventricular hypertrophy may be subendocardial ischemia, which is usually manifest only during times of increased myocardial oxygen demand, as with exercise. Subendocardial ischemia may be a stimulus for ventricular tachyarrhyth-

mias that can arise in this setting. Endocardial fibroelastosis, a condition occasionally observed in infants with severe AS and chronic subendocardial ischemia, may impair both systolic and diastolic myocardial performance.

The majority of children with valvar AS are asymptomatic with normal growth and development. The diagnosis is often made by detection of a murmur on routine physical examination. Symptoms, if present, are dependent on the severity of the lesion and the age of the patient. Older children may experience exercise intolerance and easy fatigability. Chest pain and syncope are much less common but are generally considered more ominous signs related to more severe stenosis. Most significant is the small but finite risk of sudden death in patients with moderate or severe AS. In contrast to older children, infants and toddlers may exhibit tachypnea, tachycardia, poor feeding, and delayed growth because of congestive heart failure. Infants with ductal-dependent AS may present in frank cardiogenic shock after closure of the ductus arteriosus.

In many patients, classic cardiac examination findings confirm the diagnosis of valvar AS. Vital signs are usually normal, except for a decreased arterial pulse pressure with severe stenosis. Patients with significant hypertrophy may have a prominent left ventricular impulse, and most patients will have a suprasternal notch thrill, even with mild stenosis. Auscultation often reveals a systolic ejection click heard at the left lower sternal border or apex. However, in severe AS, restricted mobility of the valve leaflets may preclude an audible ejection click. With progression of AS, left ventricular ejection may be prolonged, causing abnormally delayed closure of the aortic valve after pulmonic closure, resulting in paradoxical splitting of the second heart sound.

Valvar AS presents with a systolic ejection murmur that begins immediately following the ejection click and is often best heard at the right upper sternal border with radiation to the carotid vessels. The severity of the stenosis can be estimated by the intensity of the murmur. Murmurs of grade 2 or less are very rarely heard with severe obstruction, whereas a grade 4 murmur (with a thrill) is often associated with gradients of >50 mm Hg [2]. It is important to note that this clinical correlation between intensity and severity assumes a normal cardiac output. Neonates and infants with severe AS and diminished ventricular function often have very soft murmurs because of the markedly diminished cardiac output. An early diastolic murmur of aortic insufficiency may be heard in some patients. Additionally, a fourth heart sound, representing

D.S. Wheeler et al. (eds.), *Cardiovascular Pediatric Critical Illness and Injury*,
DOI 10.1007/978-1-84800-923-3_10, © Springer-Verlag London Limited 2009

decreased ventricular compliance, may be heard in occasional patients with severe AS.

Preoperative Evaluation

The electrocardiogram (ECG) may be quite variable in patients with AS. Children and adults may demonstrate left ventricular hypertrophy on ECG, although the degree does not correlate to the severity of AS [3]. Left ventricular hypertrophy and inverted T waves in the lateral precordial leads (strain pattern) may be the most reliable index of severe AS. In contrast to the older child, infants with severe AS often exhibit right ventricular hypertrophy on ECG. The chest radiograph is generally normal in most patients with AS. Patients with severe AS, particularly infants, may exhibit cardiomegaly and increased pulmonary vascular markings consistent with congestive heart failure.

Two-dimensional echocardiography allows visualization of aortic valve morphology and demonstration of impaired valve leaflet mobility. The echocardiogram also permits assessment of the rest of the left ventricular outflow tract, the degree of left ventricular hypertrophy, and quantification of left ventricular function. Doppler interrogation across the aortic valve estimates the peak instantaneous pressure gradient from left ventricle to ascending aorta, using the simplified Bernoulli equation [gradient = $4 \times$ (velocity)^2]. The Doppler-derived mean gradient across the aortic valve has been shown to correlate reasonably well with the peak systolic gradient measured at cardiac catheterization [4]. Cardiac catheterization remains the gold standard for determination of the degree of AS. However, because of advances in echocardiography, catheterization is rarely required for determination of valve gradients in isolated valvar AS, and it is generally reserved for patients with associated lesions (with multiple levels of obstruction) and for catheter-based intervention.

Surgical or Transcatheter Intervention

Neonates and infants with severe AS and symptoms of congestive heart failure require intervention, regardless of the estimated gradient, because diminished ventricular function and systemic blood flow may underestimate the true gradient across the aortic valve. Furthermore, these neonates often require initiation of prostaglandin E$_1$ (PGE$_1$) at 0.01–0.03 µg/kg/min to maintain ductal patency and augment systemic blood flow while awaiting surgical or catheter-based palliation. Patients who present in cardiogenic shock from ductal closure generally require higher doses of PGE$_1$ at 0.05–0.1 µg/kg/min to reopen the ductus arteriosus. Additional supportive measures, such as mechanical ventilation and inotropic support, are often beneficial to treat severe congestive heart failure in infancy.

Beyond infancy, treatment guidelines are individualized based on patient and physician preference. Generally, patients with trivial AS (gradient <25 mm Hg) do not require intervention or activity restrictions, although follow up is recommended for possible progression. Mild AS (gradient of 25–49 mm Hg) also generally does not require treatment in the absence of symptoms. Although recreational activities are not usually restricted, some clinicians would discourage participation in competitive athletics because of the possibility that the AS gradient might be worse with strenuous exercise. Most physicians would recommend intervention for patients with moderate AS (gradient of 50–75 mm Hg), particularly in the presence of ECG changes or symptomatology (at rest or with exercise). Severe AS (gradient >75 mm Hg), even in the absence of symptoms, requires intervention because of the significant risk of arrhythmias and sudden death.

Balloon aortic valvuloplasty (BAV) was first introduced as a therapeutic option for valvar AS in the mid-1980s [5,6]. In many congenital heart centers, BAV has now become the procedure of choice replacing open surgical valvotomy. Although BAV may be associated with severe arrhythmias, vascular complications, stroke, and even death (particularly in patients with severe AS), registry data show that BAV compares favorably with surgical valvotomy [7]. Furthermore, as catheter technology continues to advance with the introduction of lower profile balloons, the incidence of vascular complications, even in neonates, is improving. The hemodynamic result achieved by BAV appears to be no different from surgery [8,9], with a similar reduction in valve gradient. However, aortic insufficiency remains a potential complication of the procedure, with some series describing at least moderate insufficiency following BAV in 10% of patients [10]. Furthermore, despite adequate reduction in the AS gradient following successful valvuloplasty, progression of the disease is highly likely, and thus BAV is generally considered a palliative and not a curative procedure.

Open surgical valvotomy consists of a commissurotomy of the valve leaflets performed on cardiopulmonary bypass. This surgical approach has been shown to be effective at relieving the valve gradient in nearly all patients [11], although AS may still progress with time. Similar to BAV, valvotomy also may be associated with progressive aortic insufficiency.

For patients in whom BAV has failed to adequately relieve the gradient, or for patients with significant residual aortic insufficiency, replacement of the aortic valve may be the only option. Traditionally, aortic valve replacement has consisted of placing a mechanical prosthesis in the aortic valve position. These mechanical valves have been shown to have excellent long-term durability. However, they carry a significant risk of thromboembolic complications, necessitating life-long anticoagulation (generally with warfarin) and the attendant bleeding risks. Furthermore, mechanical valves are not manufactured in small sizes and have no potential for growth, making them a less desirable option for young children. Tissue valves (bioprostheses) provide an additional replacement option that generally does not requiring anticoagulation. However, bioprosthetic valves have no or limited growth potential, and their long-term durability is also limited, often necessitating replacement within a decade.

More recently, aortic valve replacement using the native pulmonary valve in the aortic position (autograft) with homograft replacement of the pulmonary valve (Ross procedure) has been advocated as a viable surgical option for aortic valve disease in children [12]. This procedure enjoys the dual benefits of avoiding the need for anticoagulation and allowing for native growth of the autograft. In addition, the options for aortic valve replacement in infants and young children are relatively limited. Although impressive early surgical results have been reported in young children and adolescents [13], results in infants and long-term evaluation of autograft growth and function remain to be seen.

Postoperative Care and Outcome

The postoperative course for patients following either surgical aortic valvuloplasty or valve replacement is generally uneventful, and patients are often extubated within 24 hours. Rarely, patients can return from the operating room in low cardiac output. It is important to reevaluate these patients for significant residual aortic stenosis and/or new aortic insufficiency and exclude any additional levels of left ventricular outflow obstruction that may not have been recognized preoperatively, such as aortic coarctation or significant subaortic stenosis. In the absence of significant residual or unrecognized heart disease, patients may benefit from low-dose inotropic support with β-adrenergic agonists. In addition, with significant left ventricular hypertrophy, cardiac output may be preload dependent and responsive to intravascular volume repletion. Postoperative hypertension is frequently observed, and these patients may benefit from β-adrenergic antagonists that slow the heart rate (allowing time for adequate ventricular filling) and simultaneously decrease afterload on the ventricle. Afterload reduction may also be an important adjunctive therapy if there is any residual or new aortic insufficiency. For patients with mechanical valves in the aortic position, heparin infusion may be delayed for 36–48 hours because of bleeding risk. Anticoagulation with warfarin is generally started when the patient begins enteral feedings.

Coarctation of the Aorta

Anatomy

Coarctation of the aorta (CoA) is a common congenital heart defect that may be isolated, but it is frequently associated with bicuspid aortic valve (80%), as well as a variety of other lesions such as VSD and multiple left heart abnormalities. In isolated CoA, the obstruction is usually fairly discrete and is located just opposite the ductus arteriosus (juxtaductal). There is usually some degree of transverse arch or isthmus hypoplasia that may be significant. Rarely, CoA is located in the abdominal aorta near the renal arteries.

Pathophysiology and Clinical Presentation

The pathophysiology of CoA depends on age and severity. In the infant with severe CoA, there is an abrupt increase in left heart afterload following ductal closure, leading to left ventricular failure. If the narrowing is less severe or if ductal closure is incomplete, there is a gradual increase in afterload with compensatory left ventricular hypertrophy, and activation of the renin–angiotensin system leading to upper body hypertension.

Clinical presentation is variable. Symptoms in infancy often include poor feeding, tachypnea, and other signs of congestive heart failure. Neonates with severe CoA may present in shock at the time of ductal closure in the first few weeks of life. Older children are often completely asymptomatic. Symptoms of left heart disease such as dyspnea on exertion, fatigue, chest pain, and decreased blood flow to the legs (claudication) are anticipated but rarely seen in the late-presenting patient.

Classic CoA in the older patient has the examinations findings of upper extremity hypertension with decreased femoral pulses and brachiofemoral pulse delay. There is a normal to mildly increased left ventricular impulse. S1 and S2 are normal. A systolic ejection murmur is heard over the left upper sternal border and left upper back, and if collaterals are present the murmur may be continuous. An apical click is frequently present because of a bicuspid aortic valve, but an AS murmur is unusual. In the infant with severe congestive heart failure or shock, pulses will be globally decreased, and a gallop rhythm is often present. There is frequently absence of a murmur or blood pressure gradient because of severely diminished cardiac output. With abdominal CoA there are decreased femoral pulses, no click or murmur over the precordium, and a bruit heard over the abdomen or lower back.

Preoperative Evaluation

The diagnosis of CoA is usually made clinically, but the echocardiogram is often confirmatory. In the infant with congestive heart failure or shock, the echocardiogram permits an immediate diagnosis, localizes the obstruction, rules out associated lesions, assesses ductal patency, and evaluates ventricular function. In the asymptomatic or older patient the echocardiogram can localize the area of narrowing and assess left ventricular hypertrophy and function. Although occasionally helpful, Doppler gradient measurements tend to overestimate the severity of CoA and therefore are less reliable than cuff pressures for approximation of direct catheterization measurement [14]. Chest x-ray may be helpful for localizing the coarcted area. Plain film reveals the aortic knob, CoA waist, and dilated descending aorta forming the "3" sign. Rib notching from increased intercostal artery collateral flow may be seen in late childhood and adolescence. When the area of CoA cannot be localized by echocardiogram or chest x-ray, magnetic resonance imaging and/or computerized tomography scan are useful modalities for defining the anatomy. Cardiac catheterization is rarely necessary unless there are associated lesions whose severity cannot be assessed by echocardiogram or unless catheter intervention is anticipated. The electrocardiogram may show left ventricular hypertrophy with significant CoA but is generally nonspecific. It may be useful in deciding on an intervention for the borderline patient.

Surgical or Transcatheter Intervention

In the infant with severe congestive heart failure or shock, tracheal intubation and mechanical ventilation, treatment with PGE$_1$, fluid resuscitation, pH correction, and inotropic and pressor agents is indicated. Surgical intervention may be delayed to allow for end-organ recovery if renal and/or hepatic failure occurs [15]. Although urgent surgery would seem to be indicated if ductal patency cannot immediately be established, significant clinical improvement may still be observed with mechanical ventilation and inotropic treatment alone. In the less severely ill infant or child with preserved left ventricular function but early symptoms of congestive heart failure, one can temporize with digoxin and diuretics until elective surgical intervention. Surgical correction usually involves resection of the coarcted segment with direct or extended end-to-end reanastomosis (with arch mobilization), depending on the degree of arch hypoplasia (Figure 10 .1).

Intervention is indicated in the older asymptomatic patient if the blood pressure cuff gradient is greater than 30 mm Hg or if upper body hypertension or significant left ventricular hypertrophy is present. Patients with gradients less than 30 mm Hg can be followed without intervention, but most develop hypertension in early or late adolescence. In native CoA, surgical intervention is usually recommended, although balloon dilation is employed by several centers with good results [16]. In recurrent CoA after initial surgical repair, catheter-directed intervention with balloon angioplasty has been successful [17]. In the older adolescent patient with recurrence or mild CoA with hypertension, intravascular stent placement has been advocated [16].

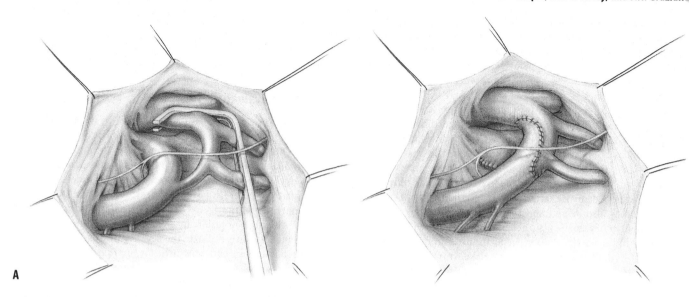

FIGURE 10.1. Repair of coarctation of the aorta (resection of the coarctation with end-to-end anastomosis). **(A)** Exposure through a left thoracotomy. **(B)** The ductus arteriosus is ligated and divided, the coarctation segment is resected, and the two ends of the aorta are re-anastomosed. (Courtesy of James D. St. Louis, MD, Medical College of Georgia.)

Postoperative Care and Outcome

Postoperative care focuses on controlling hypertension, which is mainly observed in older patients but can be seen at any age. The rapid onset and short half-life of esmolol make it ideal for the control of the catecholamine surges that occur in these patients. Adequate pain control and sedation also are necessary, especially if a lateral thoracotomy was performed. In the past, gastrointestinal problems such as mesenteric arteritis were occasionally seen in the older patients. This seems to be a rare complication now. Pretreatment with β-blockers for a short term before surgery has been shown to be effective at blunting postoperative hypertension. In infants who present in shock, postponement of enteral feeding for 5–7 days following surgical repair may help reduce the rare incidence of necrotizing enterocolitis.

Interrupted Aortic Arch

Anatomy

Interrupted aortic arch (IAA) is a rare but serious congenital heart lesion that is frequently associated with VSD (and posterior deviation of the ventricular septum), subaortic narrowing, and PDA [18].

It also can be seen in concert with more complex lesions such as truncus arteriosus, complete atrioventricular septal defect, single ventricle, or aortopulmonary window. A high proportion of patients with IAA also have a genetic defect known as CATCH 22, with half having a chromosome 22q11 deletion and a smaller fraction having the DiGeorge syndrome phenotype [19].

Interrupted aortic arch is generally divided into three subtypes based on the anatomic level of interruption (Figure 10.2). Type A IAA occurs distal to the left subclavian artery (in the region of a classic thoracic coarctation); type B interruption is between the left carotid artery and left subclavian artery, and type C is between the right and left carotid arteries. The diameter of the ascending aorta is usually correlated to the number of vessels that are located proximal to the interrupted segment. Thus, the smallest ascending aorta is often seen in type C IAA with an anomalous right subclavian artery where the right carotid artery is the only vessel arising from the ascending aorta.

Pathophysiology and Clinical Presentation

The pathophysiology of IAA is similar to severe CoA with an acute increase in biventricular afterload and absent systemic blood flow to the trunk and lower extremities occurring with ductal closure

FIGURE 10.2. Anatomic subtypes of interrupted aortic arch. **(A)** Interruption distal to the left subclavian artery. **(B)** Interruption between the left subclavian and left carotid arteries. **(C)** Interruption between the left carotid and innominate arteries. (Courtesy of James D. St. Louis, MD, Medical College of Georgia.)

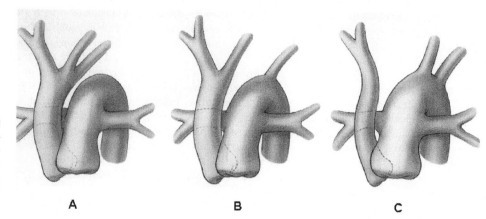

in the first week of life. With a PDA, systemic blood flow is preserved, with the right ventricle supplying the lower body.

Unless detected by routine in utero ultrasound, or if a murmur is appreciated early after birth prompting further work up (including echocardiogram), the most common presentation is cardiogenic shock with severely diminished cardiac output and metabolic acidosis. If ductal patency is present, the physical findings in an infant with IAA may be subtle and are similar to those of a newborn with hypoplastic left heart syndrome or CoA. Usually, however, there is a murmur from subaortic stenosis and occasionally differential cyanosis with lower oxygen saturations in the legs than in the arms. This finding is often obscured by the large intracardiac left-to-right shunt through the VSD, which raises pulmonary artery and hence lower extremity saturations. Following ductal closure, the lack of any perfusion to the lower body leads to severe acidosis, ischemic organ injury, and death unless treatment is initiated immediately.

Preoperative Evaluation

As with CoA, the echocardiogram is a useful diagnostic test for the asymptomatic patient and following resuscitation of the infant presenting in shock. The findings of a VSD with posterior deviation of the outlet ventricular septum and a small ascending aorta strongly support the diagnosis. Precise localization of the area of interruption is usually straightforward, and the size of the PDA can be verified. Electrocardiography is not diagnostic and may appear normal. Chest x-ray has variable findings, but cardiac enlargement and increased pulmonary vascular markings are most common. Cardiac catheterization is generally not indicated because the arch may not be seen well with this study. Magnetic resonance imaging or CT scan may be quite helpful in further delineating the anatomy if the arch is not well visualized by ultrasound.

Surgical Intervention

Immediate treatment with PGE$_1$ is warranted as soon as the diagnosis of IAA is suspected because of the dire consequences to the patient if ductal closure occurs. For this reason, PGE$_1$ should be considered as part of the treatment algorithm for suspected septic shock in the first month of life before evaluation with echocardiogram. Once the diagnosis of IAA is entertained, DiGeorge syndrome precautions should be instituted, including the use of irradiated blood products, when necessary, and careful monitoring of serum calcium levels while chromosome studies are pending.

Definitive treatment for IAA is surgical with a few potential options to consider. One initial option is aortic arch repair and pulmonary artery banding, although there remains a risk of progressive worsening subaortic stenosis using this palliative technique. A second surgical option, particularly with aortic annular hypoplasia, is a combined Norwood-Rastelli operation using the pulmonary valve as the neoaortic valve. Finally, advances in neonatal cardiopulmonary bypass and myocardial preservation techniques make primary aortic arch repair with VSD closure the most common and attractive alternative [20,21].

Postoperative Care and Outcome

The early postoperative care of the patient with IAA is supportive and the use of inotropic agents nearly universal. Because of the complex nature of the underlying anatomic substrate, early echo-

cardiographic evaluation might be considered to look for possible residual lesions such as VSDs and subaortic stenosis, which might impact on morbidity and have long-term consequences. One additional consideration is the possibility of left main bronchial compression following IAA repair, which may complicate weaning from mechanical ventilation. Again, until CATCH 22 has been ruled out, irradiated blood precautions and calcium monitoring must be reinstituted postoperatively.

Supravalvar Aortic Stenosis

Anatomy

Supravalvar aortic stenosis (SVAS) is a rare congenital heart lesion. It presents as a sporadic type, a familial autosomal dominant type, or in association with a genetic defect (Williams syndrome) caused by a microdeletion in the elastin gene at 7q11.23 [19,22]. The fixed area of narrowing is usually at the sinotubular junction just above the sinuses of Valsalva. Frequently there is tethering of the aortic valve leaflets causing interference of flow to the coronary arteries or coronary ostial stenoses. In the familial type, and with Williams syndrome, multiple vessels may have stenoses, especially the peripheral pulmonary arteries, neck vessels, and renal arteries.

Pathophysiology and Clinical Presentation

The overall pathophysiology is one of left ventricular pressure overload. Additionally, because the coronary arteries are below the obstruction, there can be chronic coronary artery hypertension and the development of accelerated coronary arteriosclerosis. The natural history of the disorder is usually progressive, with worsening left ventricular hypertrophy and coronary changes in the first few years of life [23].

Supravalvar aortic stenosis usually presents with the discovery of a murmur. Symptoms are rare in infancy unless coronary obstruction is present, potentially causing anginal pain. Angina in infancy, leading to fussiness around the stress of eating, may be misdiagnosed as colic. Other symptoms with SVAS are similar to those of other forms of left ventricular outflow tract obstruction, and symptoms progress during childhood. These may include dyspnea on exertion, presyncope or syncope with exertion, congestive heart failure, or even sudden death, especially if coronary involvement is present.

Classically SVAS has the findings of a systolic ejection murmur over the right second and third intercostal spaces with radiation especially to the right carotid area. S1 and S2 are normal, and clicks are rare. An increased left ventricular impulse and suprasternal notch thrill are often present. There also is frequently an increased blood pressure in the right arm, even without other vessel narrowing, because of the Coanda effect [24], which is caused by the SVAS jet directed into the first branch off the ascending aorta. One has to be cognizant of the possibility of multiple vessel stenoses, which may make for quite variable pulses and even generalized hypertension if the renal arteries are involved. Abnormal "Elfin" facies and degrees of mental retardation are recognizable in the patients with Williams syndrome.

Preoperative Evaluation

The ECG may show left ventricular hypertrophy depending on the degree of stenosis with varying degrees of right ventricular hypertrophy if peripheral pulmonary artery stenosis is present. ST-T wave changes are ominous, especially if left ventricular hypertrophy is not present, suggesting coronary involvement. Chest x-ray is usually normal, and cardiac enlargement is a late finding in severe cases. Echocardiography is an important tool to examine the degree of left ventricular hypertrophy and ventricular function and can outline the SVAS anatomy. It is also useful in the evaluation of the degree of right heart involvement and peripheral pulmonary artery stenosis [25].

Cardiac catheterization is usually indicated to measure right and left heart pressures, especially if peripheral pulmonary artery stenosis is suspected. Angiography of the pulmonary arteries, ascending aorta and neck vessels, and descending aorta in the area of the renal arteries should be performed because of the risk of multivessel disease. Stenting of the pulmonary arteries may be of benefit before correction of the left-sided lesion. The ability to predict less than systemic right ventricular pressure at the time of relief of the left-sided obstruction probably reduces the risks of surgical interventions. Magnetic resonance imaging and/or CT assessment of anatomy, combined with echocardiography/Doppler studies of the peripheral and renal vessels, may be used instead of catheterization if significant right heart and coronary lesions are not suspected.

Surgical or Transcatheter Intervention

Medical management is usually reserved for patients thought to be inoperable. Surgical intervention of isolated SVAS is indicated for gradients of greater than 25–30 mm Hg or if left ventricular hypertrophy is present by ECG/echocardiography. Stenting of stenotic pulmonary and peripheral vessels has been advocated [16], but stenting or balloon intervention of SVAS is rarely indicated because of the proximity of the aortic valve and coronary arteries. These modalities, however, might be considered in the rare case of membranous stenosis.

Postoperative Care and Outcome

In isolated SVAS the postoperative care is usually straightforward and supportive. If multivessel involvement is present, especially unrelieved peripheral pulmonary artery stenosis with systemic or suprasystemic right ventricular pressure, or uncorrected carotid artery stenoses, maintenance of a generous systemic arterial pressure is probably beneficial.

Subvalvar Aortic Stenosis

Anatomy

Subvalvar aortic stenosis (SAS) encompasses a variety of lesions that produce fixed, or occasionally dynamic, anatomic obstruction to egress of blood across the left ventricular outflow tract (LVOT). The etiology of SAS is incompletely understood and probably multifactorial. Associated cardiac malformations occur in approximately 50% of patients with SAS [26–29], including bicuspid aortic valve, VSD, CoA, mitral valve abnormalities, atrioventricular septal defect, and IAA, suggesting that genetic factors are involved.

A variety of classification schemes for SAS have been proposed based on morphologic, histologic, or anatomic features. From a management perspective, SAS can be divided into discrete, tunnel, and dynamic forms. The discrete form accounts for 70%–80% of SAS and consists of a thin, discrete, fibrous ridge alone or associated with a muscular base circumferentially attached to the LVOT below the aortic valve. In contrast, the tunnel form consists of a diffuse, long segment, fibromuscular narrowing of the LVOT. Subaortic stenosis can also be caused by deviation or malalignment of structures in the LVOT in association with a VSD or by atrioventricular valve tissue in the subaortic area [30,31]. Another form of SAS is dynamic LVOT obstruction, usually as a result of hypertrophy of the interventricular septum. Dynamic SAS may be difficult to distinguish from hypertrophic cardiomyopathy with asymmetric septal involvement, but the latter condition may have a familial inheritance pattern and is often more rapidly progressive and generalizable.

Pathophysiology and Clinical Presentation

Progression of SAS occurs, but the rate is variable and the factors influencing it are unknown. Only the gradient at diagnosis is predictive of the rate of progression of LVOT obstruction [31]. Significant LVOT obstruction ultimately results in concentric left ventricular hypertrophy, which leads to a vicious cycle of further obstruction and localized fibromuscular growth, in addition to decreased left ventricular compliance and left heart failure.

Aortic regurgitation occurs in more than 50% of patients with SAS [32,33], and in some cases it may progress despite surgical intervention [31–34]. The etiology of aortic regurgitation is multifactorial, and in some patients extensions of fibrous tissue onto the valve may result in aortic valve thickening and leaflet distortion. In addition, damage to the valve may result from repetitive trauma and vibrations by the turbulent subaortic systolic jet of blood. A bicuspid aortic valve may also contribute to aortic regurgitation.

Symptoms from SAS, even with severe stenosis, are rare in infancy and uncommon in early childhood. In addition, symptoms of associated congenital heart defects often mask symptoms of SAS. In most cases, SAS is detected either in the course of follow-up care for associated congenital heart defects or during evaluation of a heart murmur. Symptoms, when present, include dyspnea on exertion, effort syncope and presyncope, angina, orthopnea, congestive heart failure, and sudden cardiac death. Most of these symptoms occur in children and young adults with moderate to severe LVOT obstruction and a peak systolic ejection gradient at cardiac catheterization greater than 50 mm Hg.

Somatic growth of the child with SAS is usually normal. Peripheral pulses are symmetric. A palpable carotid thrill and left parasternal thrill are present in approximately one third of patients with mild SAS and in one half of patients with moderate to severe SAS. An increased left ventricular apical impulse is present in most patients with SAS. The first heart sound is normal; the second heart sound can be narrowly split or single (because of prolonged left ventricular systole). Paradoxical splitting of the second heart sound suggests left ventricular dysfunction associated with severe SAS. An ejection click is notably absent (differentiating SAS from valvar AS). A systolic ejection murmur in the second and third left intercostal spaces with radiation to the suprasternal notch is typically present in isolated SAS. A high-pitched early diastolic murmur of aortic regurgitation in the same auscultatory area is present in 30%–50% of patients.

Preoperative Evaluation

Echocardiography provides anatomic definition and localization of SAS, including the extent of LVOT narrowing, degree of left ventricular hypertrophy, and indices of left ventricular systolic and diastolic performance. The peak instantaneous and mean gradient across the LVOT estimated by continuous wave Doppler provide measures of the severity of LVOT obstruction and help guide cardiac intervention. Secondary effects, such as aortic and mitral regurgitation, or poststenotic dilatation of the aorta, may also be assessed by echocardiography. Associated congenital heart defects also may be evaluated. Chest x-ray usually shows mild cardiomegaly and occasionally a dilated ascending aorta. On ECG, a variable degree of left ventricular hypertrophy is often noted, although occasionally ECG findings may be normal. A prominent Q wave in the left precordial leads may be present (indicating septal hypertrophy), and a left ventricular strain pattern is visible in approximately 25% of patients, indicating severe obstruction.

Cardiac catheterization may be indicated in SAS to assess the anatomy and severity of LVOT obstruction, especially if associated with other congenital heart defects. Careful pullback pressure measurements from the left ventricle to the aorta usually delineate the pressure gradient and exact site of obstruction. Left ventriculography can help to define the type of SAS and reveal aortic valve stenosis. An aortogram is useful to assess the degree of aortic regurgitation if present.

Surgical or Transcatheter Interventions

Controversy exists regarding the optimal management and timing of surgery for patients with SAS [31]. Because SAS may be progressive, it often requires intervention to relieve LVOT obstruction sometime during the clinical course of the disease. However, the high rate of postoperative recurrence [35] and the persistence or progression of aortic regurgitation after surgery [31,33,34] may influence the decision to operate. In most centers, a peak systolic ejection gradient >30 mm Hg and presence of mild or more significant aortic regurgitation indicate intervention. Early surgical intervention is usually indicated in tunnel-type and rapidly progressive fibromuscular ridge lesions.

Percutaneous balloon dilation of discrete SAS has been reported [36] and can result in LVOT pressure gradient reduction. However, relief of LVOT obstruction is usually temporary, and thus balloon dilation is only a palliative procedure and generally not recommended. Surgery of choice for discrete SAS is complete resection with or without myomectomy through an aortotomy. Patients with significant aortic regurgitation may also require aortic valvuloplasty or replacement. For tunnel-type or more complex SAS (particularly in the neonate), a modified aortoventriculoplasty (modified Konno procedure) alone or in combination with an aortic valve allograft or pulmonary valve autograft (Ross-Konno procedure) may be required to completely relieve LVOT obstruction.

Postoperative Care and Outcome

The postoperative care of patients with simple SAS is usually uneventful, and early extubation is often performed. An occasional patient may have significant left ventricular hypertrophy and/or residual SAS, and hence it is imperative to maintain adequate preload and avoid β-adrenergic agents if possible. The incidence of early postoperative hypertension (responsive to β-adrenergic antagonists) is probably less than in patients with valvar AS or aortic coarctation. In rare instances, excision of the subaortic membrane may injure the mitral or aortic valves, leading to mitral or aortic insufficiency. With more complex LVOT obstruction

(usually requiring a Ross-Konno procedure), there is a potential for creation of a VSD and a residual left-to-right shunt that may be poorly tolerated in the early postoperative period. Left bundle branch block or even complete heart block can occur secondary to surgical resection in the LVOT or during closure of an associated VSD.

References

1. Hoffman JEI, Christianson R. Congenital heart disease in a cohort of 19,502 births with long-term follow-up. Am J Cardiol 1978;42: 641–647.
2. Braunwald E, Goldblatt A, Aygen MM, et al. Congenital aortic stenosis. I: clinical and hemodynamic findings in 100 patients. Circulation 1963;27:426–462.
3. Wagner HR, Weidman WH, Ellison RC, Miettinen OS. Indirect assessment of severity in aortic stenosis. Circulation 1977;56 (Suppl 1): I-21–I-23.
4. Bengur AR, Snider AR, Serwer GA, Peters J, Rosenthal R. Usefulness of the Doppler mean gradient in evaluation of children with aortic valve stenosis and comparison to gradient at catheterization. Am J Cardiol 1989;64:756–761.
5. Lababidi Z. Aortic balloon valvuloplasty. Am Heart J 1983;106: 751–752.
6. Sanchez GR, Mehta AV, Ewing LL, Brickley SE, Anderson TM, Black IF. Successful percutaneous balloon valvuloplasty of the aortic valve in an infant. Pediatr Cardiol 1985;6:103–106.
7. Rocchini AP, Beekman RH, Ben Shachar G, Benson L, Schwartz D, Kan JS. Balloon aortic valvuloplasty: results of the valvuloplasty and angioplasty congenital anomalies registry. Am J Cardiol 1990;65:784–789.
8. Zeevi B, Keane JF, Castaneda AR, Perry SB, Lock JE. Neonatal critical valvar aortic stenosis: a comparison of surgical and balloon dilation therapy. Circulation 1989;80:831–839.
9. Mosca RS, Iannettoni MD, Schwartz SM, et al. Critical aortic stenosis in the neonate: a comparison of balloon valvuloplasty and transventricular dilation. J Thorac Cardiovasc Surg 1995;109:147–154.
10. Fellows KE, Radtke W, Keane J, Lock JE. Acute complications of catheter therapy for congenital heart disease. Am J Cardiol 1987;60: 679–683.
11. Keane JF, Driscoll DJ, Gersony WM, et al. Second Natural History Study of congenital heart defects: results of treatment of patients with aortic valvar stenosis. Circulation 1993;87(Suppl):I-16–I-27.
12. Gerosa G, McKay R, Ross DN. Replacement of the aortic valve or root with a pulmonary autograft in children. Ann Thorac Surg 1991;51: 424–429.
13. Ohye RG, Gomez CA, Ohye BJ, Goldberg CS, Bove EL. The Ross/Konno procedure in neonates and infants: intermediate-term survival and autograft function. Ann Thorac Surg 2001;72:823–830.
14. Kaine SF, Smith EO, Mott AR, Mullins CE, Geva T. Quantitative echocardiographic analysis of the aortic arch predicts outcome of balloon angioplasty of native coarctation of the aorta. Circulation 1996;94: 1056–1062.
15. Quaegebeur JM, Jonas RA, Weinberg A, Blackstone EH, Kirklin JW, and the Congenital Heart Surgeons Society. Outcomes in seriously ill neonates with coarctation of the aorta: a multiinstitutional study. J Thorac Cardiovasc Surg 1994;108:841–854.
16. Allen HD, Beekman RH, Garson A, et al. Pediatric Therapeutic Cardiac Catheterization. A Statement for Healthcare Professionals from the Council on Cardiovascular Disease in the Young. Am Heart Assoc Circ 1998;97:609–625.
17. Kan JS, White RI, Mitchell SE, Farmlett EJ, Donhado JS, Gardner TJ. Treatment of restenosis of coarctation by percutaneous transluminal angioplasty. Circulation 1983;68:1087–1094.
18. Chin AJ, Jacobs ML. Morphology of the ventricular septal defect in two types of interrupted aortic arch. J Am Soc of Echocardiogr 1996; 9:199–201.

19. Payne RM, Johnson MC, Grant JW, Strauss AW. Toward a molecular understanding of congenital heart disease. Circulation 1995;91:494–504.

20. Kosteka M, Walther T, Geerdts I, et al. Primary repair for aortic arch obstruction with ventricular septal defect. Ann Thorac Surg 2004;58:1989–1993.

21. Haas F, Goldberg CS, Ohye RG, Mosca RS, Bove EL. Primary repair of aortic arch obstruction with ventricular septal defect in preterm low birth weight infants. Eur J Cardiothorac Surg 2000;17:643–647.

22. Morris CA, Mervis CB. Williams syndrome and related disorders. Annu Rev Genomics Hum Genet 2000;1:461–484.

23. Wren C, Oslizlok P, Bull C. Natural history of supravalvular aortic stenosis and pulmonary artery stenosis. J Am Coll Cardiol 1990;15:1625–1630.

24. French JW, Guntheroth WG. An explanation of asymmetric upper extremity blood pressures in supravalvular aortic stenosis: the Coanda effect. Circulation 1970;42:31–36.

25. Tani LY, Minich LL, Pagotto LT, Shaddy RE. Usefulness of Doppler echocardiography to determine the timing of surgery for supravalvar aortic stenosis. Am J Cardiol 2000;86:114–116.

26. Wright GB, Keane JF, Nadas AS, Bernhard WF, Castaneda AR. Fixed subaortic stenosis in the young: medical and surgical course in 83 patients. Am J Cardiol 1983;52:830–835.

27. Newfeld EA, Muster AJ, Paul MH, Idriss FS, Riker WL. Discrete subvalvular aortic stenosis in childhood. Am J Cardiol 1976;38:53–61.

28. Choi JY, Sullivan ID. Fixed subaortic stenosis: anatomical spectrum and nature of progression. Br Heart J 1991;65:280–286.

29. Baltaxe HA, Moller JH, Amplatz K. Membranous subaortic stenosis and its associated malformations. Radiology 1970;95:287–291.

30. Gewillig M, Daenen W, Dumoulin M, Van der Hauwaert L. Rheologic genesis of discrete subvalvular aortic stenosis: a Doppler echocardiographic study. J Am Coll Cardiol 1992;19:818–824.

31. Rohlicek CV, Font del Pino S, Hosking M, Miro J, Cote J-M, Finley J. Natural history and surgical outcomes for isolated discrete subaortic stenosis in children. Heart 1999;82:708–713.

32. Kitchiner D, Jackson M, Malaiya N, Walsh K, Peart I, Arnold R. The incidence and prognosis of left ventricular outflow tract obstruction in Liverpool 1960–1991. Br Heart J 1994;71:588–595.

33. Coleman DM, Smallhorn JF, McCrindle BW, Williams WG, Freedom RM. Post-operative follow-up of fibromuscular subaortic stenosis. J Am Coll Cardiol 1994;24:1558–1564.

34. Brauner R, Laks H, Drinkwater DC, Shvarts O, Eghbali K, Galindo A. Benefits of early surgical repair in fixed subaortic stenosis. J Am Coll Cardiol 1997;30:1835–1842.

35. Stewart JR, Merrill WH, Hammon Jr. JW, Graham TP, Bender HW. Reappraisal of localized resection for subvalvar aortic stenosis. Ann Thorac Surg 1990;50:197–202.

36. Suarez de Lezo J, Pan M, Sancho M, et al. Percutaneous transluminal balloon dilatation for discrete subaortic stenosis. Am J Cardiol 1986;58:619–621.

11

Congenital Heart Disease: Cyanotic Lesions with Increased Pulmonary Blood Flow

Peter B. Manning and James D. St. Louis

Introduction

Cyanosis is a common presenting feature of many congenital cardiac malformations. Although it is common to initially assume that the underlying physiologic cause for the cyanosis is diminished pulmonary blood flow, as in infants with tetralogy of Fallot or critical pulmonic stenosis, a number of anomalies that present with cyanosis are actually associated with normal or increased pulmonary blood flow, a fact that seems quite counterintuitive to many. Cyanosis associated with congenital heart anomalies occurs when some amount of deoxygenated blood returning from the systemic venous system is pumped back out to the aorta, referred to as a *right-to-left shunt*. It is critical to understand the anatomy, physiology, and interactions of the systemic and pulmonary circuits in congenital cardiac lesions to adequately understand their associated signs and symptoms, including cyanosis. *Effective pulmonary blood flow* is defined as the volume of deoxygenated blood pumped to the lungs. In many anomalies oxygenated blood may also be pumped to the lungs, termed *ineffective pulmonary blood flow*, with the resultant total pulmonary blood flow greater than normal, yet a lower than normal effective pulmonary blood flow. This explains how one can see increased *total* pulmonary blood flow in a child with cyanosis (decreased *effective* pulmonary blood flow).

From a more practical standpoint, cyanotic lesions with increased pulmonary blood flow fall into two distinct physiologic groups: complete mixing lesions and transposition of the great arteries. In complete mixing lesions, part of the anatomic defect results in the complete or near-complete mixing of the systemic and pulmonary venous returns prior to blood reaching the systemic arterial system. In many such cases there is little or no restriction to pulmonary blood flow and because of the lower resistance in the pulmonary circuit, pulmonary blood flow is increased. Cyanosis is present because it would take a volume of pulmonary blood flow over four times systemic (assuming normal systemic cardiac output) to raise the oxygen saturation greater than 90% when there is complete mixing of the venous returns. Clinically, the degree of cyanosis depends in large part on the pulmonary vascular resistance, which in the first hours of life is high, resulting in less pulmonary blood flow and more pronounced cyanosis. As pulmonary vascular resistance falls in the first days of life, infants with complete mixing lesions will have milder cyanosis, yet may ultimately develop signs and symptoms of congestive heart failure if pulmonary blood flow increases to excessive degrees. The prime examples of complete mixing lesions are truncus arteriosus, total anomalous pulmonary venous connection (TAPVC), and any single-ventricle anomaly that is associated with limited or no restriction to pulmonary blood flow.

In transposition physiology, the anatomic arrangement of the major cardiac segments is such that, instead of the systemic and pulmonary circuits being connected in series, they are in parallel. Thus, systemic venous return is primarily ejected back to the aorta, and pulmonary venous return is primarily ejected back to the lungs. Completely separated parallel circuits would be incompatible with life, resulting in progressively severe cyanosis and tissue hypoxia. All cases of survivable transposition physiology must be associated with one or multiple levels of communication between the pulmonary and systemic circuits, typically atrial, ventricular septal, and/or ductal level shunts. Because of the lower resistance in the pulmonary circuit, there will be more flow in the pulmonary circuit, but, because of inefficient mixing between the parallel circuits, cyanosis results. D-transposition of the great arteries is the most commonly seen anomaly demonstrating this physiologic picture, but it may also be seen in other anomalies, including some forms of double-outlet right ventricle (DORV).

Clinically apparent cyanosis typically requires systemic oxygen saturation as low as 80%–85%, depending on the hemoglobin level [1]. In cyanotic cardiac defects associated with increased pulmonary blood flow, the degree of cyanosis is most profound in cases of transposition physiology and may be quite mild with complete mixing lesions. Respiratory distress is rarely associated with the cyanosis in the newborn, helping to distinguish cardiac from pulmonary causes of cyanosis. A variety of other signs and symptoms may be seen depending on the specific anomaly and the age of the child.

D.S. Wheeler et al. (eds.), *Cardiovascular Pediatric Critical Illness and Injury*,
DOI 10.1007/978-1-84800-923-3_11, © Springer-Verlag London Limited 2009

Transposition of the Great Arteries

Anatomy

In D-transposition (D-TGA) of the great arteries, the atrial and ventricular anatomy and relationships are normal, but the aorta and pulmonary arteries arise from the wrong ventricle, leading to the systemic and pulmonary circuits functioning in parallel rather than in series. D-TGA is classified as a conotruncal anomaly because of its embryologic origin as a malformation of the conotruncus. During cardiac development, the infundibulum, or conus arteriosus, is the junction of the cardiac tube between the future ventricle and outflow vessels. During early septation of the heart there is an infundibulum beneath both great vessels. Normal alignment of the great vessels with their respective ventricles occurs because of complete involution of the subaortic conus, drawing the aorta posteriorly onto the left ventricle and resulting in fibrous continuity (lack of any muscular infundibulum) between the aortic and mitral annuli. In D-TGA, the subpulmonary conus involutes with persistence of the subaortic conus, resulting in the pulmonary artery aligning with the left ventricle, fibrous continuity between the pulmonary and mitral valves, and a complete, muscular subaortic conus between aorta and right ventricle [2]. In approximately 25% of cases, a ventricular septal defect is seen. The coronary arteries arise in a *typical* fashion from the aorta in 60%–70% of cases, with the right coronary centrally exiting from the right-posterior-facing sinus of Valsalva and the left main, giving rise to the left anterior descending artery and circumflex coronaries, arising from the left-posterior-facing sinus. Variations in coronary artery origin and branching pattern become important issues in the surgical reconstruction of D-TGA via the arterial switch operation [3]. Although not described here, L-transposition of the great vessels is synonymous with anatomically corrected transposition, wherein the aortic valve is anterior and to the left of the pulmonary valve and is connected to the left-sided morphologic right ventricle.

Pathophysiology, Clinical Presentation, and Preoperative Evaluation and Stabilization

As stated in the introduction, complete separation of the pulmonary and systemic circuits in parallel is not compatible with life. Mixing to allow oxygenated blood to pass from the left side of the heart to the right is essential to maintain adequate tissue oxygen delivery. Most neonates with D-TGA are found to be cyanotic in the first hours of life but are generally only mildly tachypneic (*quiet tachypnea*) unless the cyanosis is so severe that it results in acidosis. A murmur is not usually heard, although the second heart sound (S2) is usually loud and single (unless a ventricular septal defect is present). Infants with a significant sized ventricular septal defect will typically have adequate bidirectional mixing to maintain adequate oxygen saturations with no further stabilization required. Although the best mixing will typically occur at the atrial level, a normal patent foramen ovale is usually inadequate for maintaining adequate oxygen exchange in the newborn with D-TGA and intact ventricular septum. Initial stabilization by initiating PGE₁ infusion allows increased pulmonary blood flow via aortic-to-pulmonary ductal blood flow, which results in increased left atrial return and increased left-to-right flow at the atrial septal level. Because ductal flow itself is predominantly aortic to pulmonary, ductal patency alone is not sufficient to stabilize the infant

with D-TGA and intact ventricular septum [4]. In the rare case with a severely restrictive interatrial communication, emergent balloon atrial septostomy may be life saving. Unless operative repair is planned within the first days of life, most centers prefer to perform balloon atrial septostomy in all newborns with D-TGA unless there is a naturally large atrial septal communication. This may allow discontinuation of prostaglandin infusion and will prevent development of left atrial hypertension, which could complicate later management if operative correction is delayed.

The electrocardiogram (ECG) is usually nondiagnostic (the QRS axis is rightward and right ventricular forces are prominent, which is also typical for most newborn infants without D-TGA). Chest radiograph demonstrates the classic *egg-on-a-string* appearance (the mediastinal shadow is narrowed because of the anteroposterior relationship of the aorta and pulmonary artery), often with increased pulmonary vascular markings. Echocardiography is diagnostic, and cardiac catheterization is rarely necessary (with the exception of performing atrial septostomy, see later). Important anatomic features that should be defined during initial stabilization include presence of any septal defects, coronary artery anatomy, relative orientation of the great arteries relative to each other, the presence of outflow tract obstruction on either side of the heart, particularly the left, and presence or absence of a coarctation.

Surgical Intervention

Anatomic surgical reconstruction of D-TGA via the arterial switch operation [5] has become the standard of care since the mid to late 1980s. In most cases the operation is performed in the first week or two of life, before the left ventricle can become *deconditioned* pumping to the low-resistance pulmonary circuit [6]. The arterial switch operation includes closure of any septal defects (atrial and/or ventricular), patent ductus arteriosus division (to allow translocation of the great arteries), independent coronary artery transfer, and division, translocation, and reanastomosis of the aorta and pulmonary arteries at a level a few millimeters above the semilunar valves. Techniques to safely transfer coronary arteries of virtually all variations have been described to avoid kinking or stretching, essentially making any coronary artery anatomy *switchable*. In current practice the operation is performed with moderate hypothermic cardiopulmonary bypass support. Circulatory arrest is rarely, if ever, indicated for this procedure.

Postoperative Care and Outcome

In the majority of patients the postoperative period is uncomplicated. Although concern about coronary arterial insufficiency should be maintained after their translocation, important coronary flow disturbances more often lead to intractable ventricular dysrhythmias or low cardiac output before the patient leaves the operating room [7]. Many recommend limiting volume infusions to smaller aliquots than typical for a postoperative patient because of the possibility that sudden distension of the right ventricular outflow tract may result in stretching of the coronary arteries. As with most newborns undergoing major cardiac reconstruction, a sag in myocardial performance peaking 6–12 hr postoperatively may be clinically evident [8]. The risk of problems related to increased pulmonary vascular reactivity is similar to that seen with any neonate. This risk may actually be increased in patients who have had a period of left atrial hypertension preoperatively, such as a child with a ventricular septal defect and a restrictive atrial septal communication. Currently operative survival for the arterial switch for simple D-TGA exceeds 95% [9]. The most common late postoperative complication observed is proximal pulmonary artery stenosis. In contrast to the Mustard and Senning operations, which had previously been employed for this anomaly, the incidence of late ventricular failure and arrhythmias is virtually nonexistent [10–12].

Truncus Arteriosus

Anatomy

Truncus arteriosus represents postnatal persistence of the early embryologic state of a common arterial trunk arising from the ventricles. There is a large ventricular septal defect in the superior position just beneath the large, single, semilunar truncal valve. The valve is anatomically abnormal with anywhere from two to five or six leaflets, although it typically functions well. The single artery exiting the heart separates into pulmonary arteries and aorta a short distance above the valve, following patterns which have lead to a number of classification schemes [13,14].

Collett and Edwards classified truncus arteriosus based on the origin of the pulmonary artery from the truncal artery (Figure 11.1) [13]. Type I consists of an arterial trunk that originates from the common semilunar valve with its immediate bifurcation into a pulmonary artery and ascending aorta. The type II defect refers to a separate origin of the left and right pulmonary arteries from the posterior wall of the truncal artery. Type III describes a similar anatomy as type II but with the right and left pulmonary arteries originating farther apart. In type IV, often referred to as *pseudotruncus*, there is absence of the main pulmonary artery, with the

lungs receiving its blood supply via pulmonary collaterals. Most would agree this entity should not be described as a truncal defect but rather as a form of pulmonary atresia with ventricular septal defect.

Van Praagh and Van Praagh published a different classification system based on the presence or absence of a common conotruncal septum (see Figure 11.1) [14]. In type A1, the truncal septum is partially developed so that a pulmonary artery and aorta coexist. In type A2, there is complete absence of the truncal septum, with the main pulmonary arteries originating from the truncal arteries separately. Type A3 is characterized by the absence of one pulmonary artery from the truncal artery. Type A4 describes any type of truncus arteriosus associated with an interrupted aortic arch. The arch anomaly is usually a type B interruption with the descending aorta receiving its blood supply from a large ductus arteriosus and the pulmonary arteries originating from the truncal artery.

Pathophysiology, Clinical Presentation, Preoperative Evaluation, and Stabilization

At the level of the ventricular septal defect and the common trunk there is virtually complete mixing of the systemic and pulmonary blood resulting in nearly identical oxygen saturation in the aorta and pulmonary arteries. At birth cyanosis may be more pronounced because of the normally elevated pulmonary resistance seen at this time, but, as the resistance falls, oxygen saturations rise, and these infants will develop signs and symptoms of congestive heart failure [15]. As the pulmonary resistance drops, the peripheral pulses are often bounding with a widened pulse pressure.

Newborns with truncus arteriosus rarely need specific cardiac intervention for stabilization unless associated with interrupted aortic arch. Anatomy is well defined echocardiographically. Size

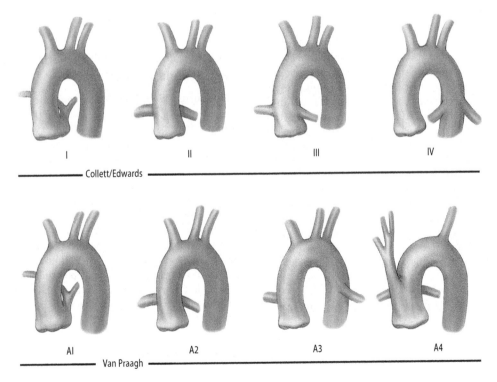

FIGURE 11.1. Two classification schemes for truncus arteriosus. (see text for explanation).

and position of the ventricular septal defect, truncal valve function, and branching of the truncal vessels must be detailed. In most cases a mild-to-moderate flow gradient through the truncal valve is seen that is almost always related to the high volume of flow through the valve rather than to anatomic stenosis. Important truncal regurgitation is far more problematic and represents one of the major identified risk factors for predicting poor outcome. The association of chromosome 22q11 deletion, commonly referred to as DiGeorge syndrome, is reported in 40% of children with truncus arteriosus [16]. All patients with truncus arteriosus should have close monitoring for hypocalcemia and should receive only irradiated blood products to prevent the possibility of graft versus host disease until the microdeletion can be confirmed or ruled out by fluorescence in situ hybridization analysis of the chromosomes.

Surgical Intervention

Currently complete surgical reconstruction is carried out during the initial newborn hospitalization in most cases [17]. Closure of the ventricular septal defect baffles left ventricular flow to the common truncal valve. The pulmonary arteries are separated from the truncal root, and right ventricle to pulmonary artery continuity is established using a valved conduit of homograft or xenograft origin. Later reoperation for replacement of the right ventricle to pulmonary artery conduit will be necessary in all patients as they grow.

Postoperative Care and Outcome

Postoperatively these patients will typically display more pronounced right ventricular dysfunction compared with the newborn undergoing arterial switch operation for D-TGA. Leaving a patent foramen ovale to allow a right-to-left pop-off in the face of right ventricular dysfunction allows better left ventricular function by avoiding right ventricular dilation and allowing better left-sided filling at the expense of mild to moderate cyanosis, which usually begins to resolve within 4 or 5 days following operation. In patients with 22q11 microdeletion, calcium instability is typically more pronounced in the early postoperative period and can result in important hemodynamic instability. In a series from Boston Children's Hospital [18], Hanley et al. identified four risk factors for mortality in patients with truncus arteriosus: coronary artery anomalies, aortic interruption, important truncal valve insufficiency, and age greater than 100 days at the time of operation. Coronary anomalies that influence surgical repair are exceedingly rare. With improvements in surgical techniques the impact of aortic interruption and truncal insufficiency has improved, although the latter is still recognized as a major risk factor [19]. Increased risk in older infants relates to the higher incidence of severe congestive heart failure and the risk of important pulmonary hypertensive changes that may develop rapidly in the first months of life with this anomaly.

Total Anomalous Pulmonary Venous Connection

Anatomy

The development of the pulmonary venous system is more complex than that of other cardiac segments. This system develops from two different components: the pulmonary venous plexus, which devel-

ops into the intraparenchymal pulmonary veins, originates as part of the foregut venous plexus, which drains via the cardinal venous system to the future atrial portion of the heart. The common pulmonary vein begins as an outgrowth of the left atrium and later joins with the pulmonary venous plexus. As the communication between the pulmonary venous plexus and the common pulmonary vein becomes established, the connection of the plexus to the cardinal venous system (future vena cavae and coronary sinus) involutes. Failure of this stage results in persistent drainage of the pulmonary veins to the right atrium and absence of connection to the left atrium.

The classification system for this defect has undergone several revisions, but the system set forth by Darling and associates has been widely accepted by the congenital community [20]. This classification system is based on the origin of the anomalously draining vein. In type I, the anomalous connection is at the supracardiac level, in which the confluence of pulmonary veins drains via a vertical vein to the left side of the innominate vein, then via the superior vena cava to the right atrium. In type II, the connection is directly to the heart, in which the confluence of pulmonary veins drains via the coronary sinus to the right atrium. Type III anomalous veins originate from below the diaphragm, in which the confluence of pulmonary veins drains via a vertical vein that passes through the diaphragm, usually connecting to the portal system with the blood then passing through the hepatic parenchyma before reaching the inferior vena cava and ultimately the right atrium. Finally, type IV consists of a combination of two or more of the other types. Physiologic characterization is based on whether the passage of pulmonary venous blood is either obstructed or unobstructed on its course to the right atrium. Obstructed TAPVC is most commonly associated with infracardiac anatomy but can be seen with other variations. Obstructed TAPVC is associated with severe cyanosis, decreased pulmonary blood flow, and pulmonary venous congestion and represents one of the few neonatal cardiac surgical emergencies as there is no effective means to medically stabilize such an infant.

Pathophysiology, Clinical Presentation, and Preoperative Evaluation and Stabilization

Unobstructed TAPVC results in complete mixing of the systemic and pulmonary venous blood in the right atrium, and therefore cyanosis depends on the relative volumes of blood from each source that is contributed. An atrial septal defect must be present to allow blood flow to enter the left side of the heart to support systemic circulation. In the neonate, cyanosis is usually more pronounced and becomes milder as pulmonary resistance drops and pulmonary blood flow increases. Typical symptoms of congestive heart failure frequently develop in the first weeks or months of life in the untreated infant [21].

Echocardiography can typically define the anatomy of unobstructed TAPVC completely, including the course of pulmonary venous drainage, the absence of obstruction, and the completely right-to-left flow at the atrial septal level. Early management before surgical repair centers on management of congestive heart failure symptoms.

Surgical Intervention

As stated previously, repair of obstructed TAPVC is a surgical emergency as only cardiopulmonary bypass support (either in the operating room or via extracorporeal membrane oxygenation [21]) can establish effective oxygenation in such an infant. In the infant with unobstructed TAPVC, surgical correction is often performed in the first weeks of life, although some centers prefer delaying operation for a month or more if the child is stable. Repair entails direct anastomosis of the confluence of the pulmonary veins to the adjacent left atrium, closure of a vertical vein that connected the pulmonary veins to the systemic vena caval circulation, and closure of the atrial septal communication. Deep hypothermic circulatory arrest of low flow is often used to facilitate exposure during creation of pulmonary vein to left atrial anastomosis.

Postoperative Care and Outcome

Because the left-sided cardiac structures are often slightly small in this anomaly, these infants may be more sensitive to large volume infusions postoperatively with sharp elevations of left atrial pressure seen with relatively small volume boluses. Persistent pulmonary hypertension or accentuated pulmonary vascular reactivity is commonly seen and is often the major cause of morbidity and mortality in this anomaly, particularly in the infant with obstructed TAPVC. Hospital survival for infants with TAPVC without associated cardiac anomalies is currently greater than 90%, including patients who present with obstructed physiology [22,23]. The most feared late complication is the development of restenosis of the pulmonary veins that is seen in 5%–10% of cases, more commonly those who presented with obstruction originally. Although this problem may represent stenosis of the anastomosis that may be addressed well via reoperation, more commonly it represents a diffuse fibrosis of the branch pulmonary veins. In cases of diffuse stenosis, recurrence after reoperation is common, leading to death or referral for heart–lung transplantation, although the more recent application of a *sutureless* technique of repair for pulmonary vein stenosis seems to result in a higher rate of success than older techniques [24].

Single-Ventricle Anomalies with Unobstructed Pulmonary Blood Flow

A variety of single-ventricle anomalies are observed in which pulmonary blood flow is unobstructed. As with other examples of complete mixing lesions, the systemic and pulmonary blood freely mixes before delivery to the systemic arteries, resulting in a level of cyanosis dependent on the relative volumes of pulmonary and systemic blood flow, or Qp:Qs ratio. Symptoms depend on the remaining details of the cardiac anatomy, such as the presence or absence of obstruction to systemic arterial outflow. Hypoplastic left heart syndrome is an example of a single-ventricle anomaly with unobstructed pulmonary blood flow and severe systemic blood flow restriction with the systemic circulation dependent on ductal patency. Tricuspid atresia with normally related great vessels and a large ventricular septal defect is an example of a single-ventricle anomaly with little or no restriction to flow to either pulmonary or systemic circuit.

All infants with single-ventricle cardiac anomalies will typically follow a multistaged reconstruction strategy toward the ultimate creation of a Fontan circulation: the single ventricle committed to the systemic circuit, channeling of the systemic venous return directly to the pulmonary arteries without an interposed ventricle, and near-complete separation of pulmonary and systemic circulations resulting in near-normal oxygen saturations. The basic requirements for successfully attaining a Fontan circulation are a well-functioning ventricle that ejects unobstructed to the systemic circulation and nonstenotic, low-resistance pulmonary arteries. The planning for achieving this goal must begin on the first day of life. The medical and surgical measures that must be taken to accomplish these goals vary with the individual patient's anatomy. Surgical reconstruction is typically performed in three stages, with the first being the most variable depending on individual anomaly. The newborn intervention must create unobstructed communication between the single ventricle and the aorta and a regulated source of pulmonary blood flow. The latter part is critical to prevent both ventricular volume overload and pulmonary hypertensive changes and to ensure an oxygen level compatible with normal growth and development. Depending on the individual anatomy, this may be accomplished via pulmonary artery banding or a systemic-to-pulmonary artery shunt. The second stage in most infants involves creation of a superior cavopulmonary connection (bidirectional Glenn shunt) as the new source of pulmonary blood flow, typically between 4 and 6 months of age. The completion Fontan operation, routing inferior vena caval blood to the pulmonary arteries, is performed between 2 and 4 years of age. Outcomes for children born with single-ventricle anomalies have improved dramatically over the past two decades, with survival of greater than 70% for most children with the most complex lesions such as hypoplastic left heart syndrome to over 90% with more favorable lesions such as tricuspid atresia [25,26].

References

1. Grifka RG. Cyanotic congenital heart disease with increased pulmonary blood flow. Pediatr Clin North Am 1999;46:405–425.
2. Pasquini L, Sanders SP, Parness IA, et al. Conal anatomy in 119 patients with d-loop transposition of the great arteries and ventricular septal defect: an echocardiographic and pathologic study. J Am Coll Cardiol 1993;21:1712–1721.
3. Pasquali SK, Hasselblad V, Li JS, et al. Coronary artery pattern and outcome of arterial switch operation for transposition of the great arteries: a meta-analysis. Circulation 2002;106:2575–2580.
4. Baylen BG, Grzeszczak M, Gleason ME, et al. Role of balloon atrial septostomy before early arterial switch repair of transposition of the great arteries. J Am Coll Cardiol 1992;19:1025–1031.
5. Karl TR, Cochrane A, Brizzard CPR. Arterial switch operation. Surgical solution to complex problems. Tex Heart Inst J 1997;24:322–333.
6. Duncan BW, Poirier NC, Mee RB, et al. Selective timing for the arterial switch operation. Ann Thorac Surg 2004;77:1691–1696.
7. Legendre A, Losay J, Touchot-Kone A, et al. Coronary events after arterial switch operation for transposition of the great arteries. Circulation 2003;108(Suppl 1):II-186–II-1190.
8. Wernovsky G, Wypij D, Jonas RA, et al. Postoperative course and hemodynamic profile after the arterial switch operation in neonates and infants. A comparison of low-flow cardiopulmonary bypass and circulatory arrest. Circulation 1995;92:2226–2235.
9. Dibardino DJ, Allison AE, Vaughn WK, et al. Current expectations for newborns undergoing the arterial switch operation. Ann Surg 2004;239:588–596.
10. Williams WG, McCrindle BW, Ashburn DA, et al. Outcomes of 829 neonates with complete transposition of the great arteries 12–17 years after repair. Eur J Cardiothorac Surg 2003;24:1–9.
11. Colan SD, Boutin C, Castaneda AR, et al. Status of the left ventricle after arterial switch operation for transposition of the great arteries. Hemodynamic and echocardiographic evaluation. J Thorac Cardiovasc Surg 1995;109:311–321.

12. Rhodes LA, Wernovsky G, Keane JF, et al. Arrhythmias and intracardiac conduction after the arterial switch operation. J Thorac Cardiovasc Surg 1995;109:303–310.

13. Collett RW, Edwards JE. Persistent truncus arteriosus: a classification according to anatomic types. Surg Clin North Am 1949;29:1245.

14. Van Praagh R, Van Praagh S. The anatomy of common aorticopulmonary trunk (truncus arteriosus communis) and its embryologic implications: a study of 57 necropsy cases. Am J Cardiol 1965;16:406–425.

15. Calder L, Van Praagh R, Van Praagh S, et al. Truncus arteriosus communis: clinical, angiocardiographic, and pathologic findings in 100 patients. Am Heart J 1976;92:23.

16. McElhinney DB, Driscoll DA, Emanuel BS, Goldmuntz E. Chromosome 22q11 deletion in patients with truncus arteriosus. Pediatr Cardiol 2003;24:569–573.

17. Thompson LD, McElhinney DB, Reddy M, et al. Neonatal repair of truncus arteriosus: continuing improvement in outcomes. Ann Thorac Surg 2001;72:391–395.

18. Hanley FL, Heinemann MK, Jonas RA, et al. Repair of truncus arteriosus in the neonate. J Thorac Cardiovasc Surg 1993;105:1047–1056.

19. Jahangiri M, Zurakowski D, Mayer JE, et al. Repair of the truncal valve and associated interrupted arch in neonates with truncus arteriosus. J Thorac Cardiovasc Surg 2000;119:508–514.

20. Darling RC, Rothney WB, Craig JM. Total pulmonary venous drainage into the right side of the heart: report of 17 autopsied cases not associated wit other major cardiovascular anomalies. Lab Invest 1957;6:44–64.

21. Yee ES, Turley K, Hsieh WR, et al. Infant total anomalous pulmonary venous connection: factors influencing timing of presentation and operative outcome. Circulation 1987;76:III-83.

22. Stewart DL, Mendoza JC, Winston, et al. Use of extracorporeal life support in total anomalous pulmonary venous drainage. J Perinatol 1996;16(3 Pt 1):186–190.

23. Caldarone CA, Najm HK, Kadletz M, et al. Surgical management of total anomalous pulmonary venous drainage: impact of coexisting cardiac anomalies. Ann Thorac Surg 1998;66:1521.

24. Hancock Friesen CL, Zurakowski D, Thiagarajan RR, et al. Total anomalous pulmonary venous connection: an analysis of current management strategies in a single institution. Ann Thorac Surg 2005;79:596–606.

25. Ashburn DA, McCrindle BW, Tchervenkov CI, et al. Outcomes after the Norwood operation in neonates with critical aortic stenosis or aortic valve atresia. J Thorac Cardiovasc Surg 2003;125:1070–1082.

26. Sittiwangkul R, Azakie A, Van Arsdell GS, et al. Outcomes of tricuspid atresia in the Fontan era. Ann Thorac Surg 2004;77:889–894.

12
Single-Ventricle Lesions

Steven M. Schwartz, David P. Nelson, Catherine L. Dent, Ndidi L. Musa, and Derek S. Wheeler

Introduction

The term *single ventricle* or *univentricular heart* applies to a wide variety of anatomic lesions (Table 12.1) and their subsequent postoperative anatomy. Single-ventricle physiology presents unique challenges to the intensive care physician, as these children often respond to common interventions such as supplemental oxygen, mechanical ventilation, and vasoactive infusions differently than children with more conventional circulatory physiology. Infants and children with single-ventricle physiology undergo multiple cardiac operations throughout the course of their lives and may be more adversely affected by intercurrent illnesses than other children with congenital heart disease. As such, these patients are commonly encountered in pediatric critical care medicine and frequently have chronic cardiac problems that often require intensive care. This unique physiology represents the sine qua non of pediatric cardiac intensive care, and it is imperative that pediatric intensivists have a thorough understanding of the nuances of single-ventricle physiology. This chapter addresses the important physiologic issues that arise in the care of infants and children with single-ventricle physiology.

The Neonate with Single-Ventricle Physiology

Although virtually all newborns with single-ventricle physiology have mixing of pulmonary and systemic venous return, the relative amounts of each vary substantially depending on the underlying anatomy. The most important anatomic issue that dictates management is the outflow to and from the systemic ventricle and lungs. The neonate with single-ventricle anatomy may have (1) unobstructed pulmonary blood flow and obstructed systemic blood flow; (2) unobstructed systemic blood flow and obstructed pulmonary blood flow; or (3) bilaterally unobstructed outflow. Additionally, either systemic or pulmonary venous return may also be obstructed in the newborn single-ventricle circulation. Early survival is largely dependent on achieving a balanced circulation without excessive pulmonary blood flow, yet with enough pulmonary blood flow to prevent severe cyanosis.

Systemic Outflow Obstruction

Systemic outflow obstruction is characteristic of hypoplastic left heart syndrome (HLHS) (Figure 12.1) (see later), tricuspid atresia with transposed great arteries [1–4], double-inlet left ventricle (DILV) [1–8], and other less common anatomic variations. Single-ventricle physiology with systemic outflow obstruction also pertains to newborns with critical aortic stenosis, severe coarctation of the aorta, or interrupted aortic arch (discussed in Chapter 10). The important features of this type of anatomy are complete mixing of systemic and pulmonary venous return and ventricular outflow directed primarily to the pulmonary artery. Systemic blood flow (Qs) is provided largely by right-to-left shunting across the patent ductus arteriosus (PDA) and is dependent on the relative pulmonary and systemic vascular resistances. In general, systemic outflow obstruction is poorly tolerated and in the face of single-ventricle anatomy is usually accompanied by signs or symptoms of profound shock.

Hypoplastic left heart syndrome encompasses a continuum of congenital heart lesions producing left-sided obstruction and hypoplasia and generally ranges from severe, with mitral and aortic atresia with a diminutive left ventricle to mitral and/or aortic stenosis with a nonapex-forming left ventricle. Although biventricular repair may be possible for those infants at the more favorable end of the spectrum (i.e., mitral stenosis, aortic stenosis) [9–11], the severe end of the spectrum is universally fatal, with an average life expectancy of around 5 days (untreated) [12]. In contrast to most neonates born with complex congenital heart disease, these children usually are otherwise normal with no abnormalities of other organ systems. Even with a staged surgical approach to palliation (discussed later), HLHS carries a substantial risk of morbidity and mortality, with hospital survival following Norwood stage I palliation as low as 47% [13]. The most optimistic rates of mortality in the current era range from 14% to 25% with a staged surgical approach to palliation [14–20], while the mortality rate in centers that favor heart transplantation is approximately 30%, including those infants who die while waiting for transplant [21,22]. A multicenter review of 323 neonates with HLHS reported an overall

D.S. Wheeler et al. (eds.), *Cardiovascular Pediatric Critical Illness and Injury*,
DOI 10.1007/978-1-84800-923-3_12, © Springer-Verlag London Limited 2009

TABLE 12.1. Anatomic diagnoses commonly associated with single-ventricle physiology in the newborn.

Physiology	Anatomy
Systemic outflow obstruction	Hypoplastic left heart syndrome
	Critical aortic stenosis
	Critical coarctation of the aorta
	Interrupted aortic arch
	Tricuspid atresia with transposition of the great arteries
	Double-inlet left ventricle
	Double-outlet right ventricle (some variations)
Pulmonary outflow obstruction	Tricuspid atresia with normally related great arteries
	Pulmonary atresia with intact ventricular septum
	Tetralogy of Fallot with pulmonary atresia
	Critical pulmonary stenosis
	Severe Ebstein's anomaly of the tricuspid valve
	Double-outlet right ventricle (some variations)

Note: Not all diagnoses listed are anatomically single-ventricle lesions.

30-day mortality rate of 33% for either approach (transplant or staged palliation) [23]. There are many excellent reviews and chapters that discuss the myriad issues pertaining to the evaluation and management of infants with HLHS in great detail—these would be difficult to improve on and to attempt to do so is well beyond the intended scope of the present discussion—the reader is therefore directed to other reviews for additional information [24–34].

Pulmonary Outflow Obstruction

Single-ventricle physiology with pulmonary outflow obstruction is characteristic of lesions such as tricuspid atresia, pulmonary atresia, and severe Ebstein's anomaly of the tricuspid valve. The salient anatomic features are complete mixing of systemic and pulmonary venous return and ventricular outflow predominantly directed out the aorta. Low pulmonary blood flow (Qp) in these patients implies an obligate right-to-left shunt, generally at the atrial level, and results in deoxygenated blood reaching the systemic circulation and, hence, cyanosis. The clinical consequences of low Qp are variable and depend on the degree of pulmonary outflow obstruction. Mild obstruction may permit an inordinate amount of the total cardiac output to go to the pulmonary circulation, sometimes at the expense of systemic cardiac output. Treatment is therefore directed at limiting, rather than increasing, Qp. Infants with this type of anatomy may be only minimally cyanotic and can have signs and symptoms of congestive heart failure. At the other end of the spectrum are those infants with severe pulmonary outflow obstruction or even atresia. These patients are profoundly cyanotic unless an alternate source of Qp is quickly established.

Obstructed Venous Return

Unobstructed pulmonary or systemic venous return in infants with single-ventricle anatomy frequently depends upon an unrestrictive interatrial communication. When one of the atrioventricular (AV) valves is severely stenotic or atretic, as occurs in HLHS, tricuspid atresia, or pulmonary atresia with intact ventricular septum, a large atrial septal defect is mandatory for decompression of the atrium with the inadequate AV valve. Obstruction of the systemic venous atrium causes increased central venous pressures and third spacing of fluid, eventually limiting systemic cardiac output and

producing signs and symptoms of shock. Although a patent foramen ovale allows for some right-to-left shunting of blood across the atrial septum, it may be inadequate to permit unobstructed flow of all systemic venous return.

Obstruction of the pulmonary venous return causes elevated pulmonary venous pressures and pulmonary hypertension. This phenomenon may be helpful in the immediate neonatal period, as it can limit Qp and enhance systemic flow, thereby increasing systemic oxygen delivery (DO_2), even if at the expense of arterial oxygen saturation (SaO_2). Nevertheless, the atrial septum must be opened at the time of the first palliative operation to avoid the long-term consequences of elevated pulmonary vascular resistance. A severely restrictive or intact atrial septum with pulmonary venous hypertension usually requires emergent creation of an atrial level shunt because of profound cyanosis. These procedures carry a high risk of morbidity and may imply a worse prognosis for further palliative surgery [35–38].

Postoperative Anatomy

The goal to any palliative surgery is to establish (1) unobstructed pulmonary and systemic venous return, (2) unobstructed systemic outflow, and (3) a regulated source of pulmonary blood flow. Typically, this is accomplished via a stage I Norwood type procedure (Figures 12.2 and 12.3), modified systemic-to-pulmonary artery (Blalock-Taussig) shunt, or pulmonary artery band (the latter two

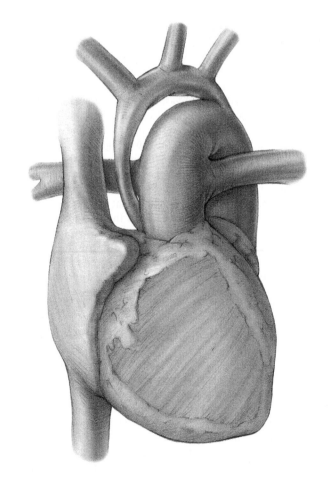

FIGURE 12.1. Hypoplastic left heart syndrome. (Courtesy of James D. St. Louis, MD, Medical College of Georgia.)

palliative procedures are discussed in greater detail in Chapter 7). Although variations on each of these operations exist, they represent the spectrum of postoperative anatomy the intensive care physician is likely to encounter. Because each anatomic arrangement establishes similar physiology, the important differences between them are in the means by which each operation accomplishes its goals.

The Norwood operation requires cardiopulmonary bypass, cardioplegia, and a period of deep hypothermic circulatory arrest, although newer techniques can limit circulatory arrest time [39–41]. The heart, kidneys, brain, and other organs are exposed to a *planned* period of ischemia followed by reperfusion, which often results in a defined period of myocardial, renal, and perhaps endothelial dysfunction in the postoperative period. A Blalock-Taussig shunt, either alone or as part of a stage I Norwood procedure, often results in low diastolic arterial pressure, which may compromise coronary perfusion. Unlike a Blalock-Taussig shunt, a pulmonary artery band is not associated with diastolic systemic arterial runoff, but some investigators have suggested a pulmonary artery band may increase the risk of subaortic obstruction and ventricular hypertrophy [42], although this assertion has also been disputed [2,4–6,43]. Both shunts and bands carry the risk of unilateral

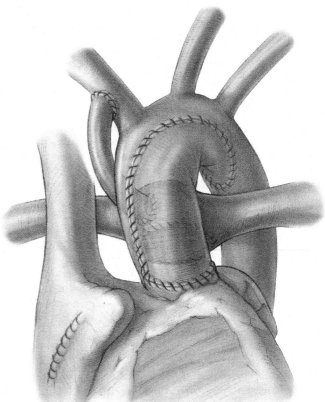

Figure 12.3. The Norwood stage I palliation for hypoplastic left heart syndrome (final appearance). The proximal aorta has been anastomosed to the adjacent pulmonary trunk (usually with a patch of the pulmonary allograft to augment the neoaorta). A modified Blalock-Taussig shunt provides pulmonary blood flow. (Courtesy of James D. St. Louis, MD, Medical College of Georgia.)

pulmonary artery obstruction, and this should be included in the differential of late cyanosis after either of these procedures.

The Sano modification of the stage I Norwood procedure (right ventricle–pulmonary artery conduit in lieu of Blalock-Taussig shunt) is reported to produce favorable results that are comparable to the traditional approach of using the Blalock-Taussig shunt and may simplify postoperative management of these complex patients [44–48]. A multicenter (high-volume centers in the United States), prospective, randomized trial comparing the modified Blalock-Taussig shunt versus right ventricle–pulmonary artery conduit (Single Ventricle Reconstruction Trial) will hopefully provide further answers as to which procedure is associated with better long-term outcome.

A Rational Approach to Single-Ventricle Physiology in the Newborn

Balancing the Circulations (Optimizing Qp : Qs)

Regardless of underlying anatomy, single-ventricle physiology is characterized by (1) the complete mixing of systemic and pulmonary venous return and (2) the partitioning of total cardiac output into Qp and Qs based on the amount of anatomic obstruction and/or vascular resistance to flow in the respective circuits. It is generally assumed that SaO_2 reflects the ratio of Qp to Qs (Qp : Qs) in the

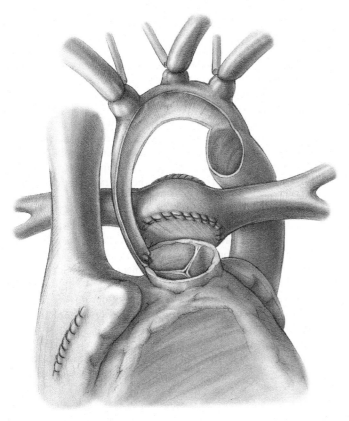

Figure 12.2. The Norwood stage I palliation for hypoplastic left heart syndrome. Arterial cannulation is accomplished through the main pulmonary artery and venous cannulation in the right atrial appendage. The arch vessels are exposed, and snares are placed for occlusion during reconstruction of the neoaortic arch. The arterial cannula is advanced through the ductus arteriosus and the main pulmonary artery is divided, and the distal portion is closed with a polytetrafluoroethylene patch. The main pulmonary trunk is next divided proximal to the bifurcation (in this case under circulatory arrest). The ductus arteriosus is ligated and excised. The aorta is opened proximally and distally in preparation for anastomosis to the adjacent pulmonary trunk. (Courtesy of James D. St. Louis, MD, Medical College of Georgia.)

unoperated, shunted, or banded newborn single-ventricle patient. This assumption is based on manipulation of the Fick principle; Qs and Qp are calculated by the Fick equation:

$$Qs = VO_2/(CaO_2 - CmvO_2)$$
$$Qp = VO_2/(CpvO_2 - CpaO_2)$$

where VO_2 is oxygen consumption, CaO_2 is arterial oxygen content, $CmvO_2$ is mixed venous oxygen content, $CpvO_2$ is pulmonary venous oxygen content, and $CpaO_2$ is pulmonary artery oxygen content. By substituting the equations for oxygen content into the above equations, and because arterial and pulmonary artery saturations are identical in this type of single-ventricle physiology, one can derive a simplified Fick equation for Qp:Qs:

$$Qp:Qs = (SaO_2 - SmvO_2)/(SpvO_2 - SaO_2)$$

where $SmvO_2$ is oxygen saturation of mixed venous blood, SaO_2 is oxygen saturation of arterial blood, and $SpvO_2$ is oxygen saturation of pulmonary venous blood. In the vast proportion of cases, assuming normal function of the respiratory tract, $SpvO_2$ can be assumed to be approximately 95% while breathing room air. If one also assumes that the systemic arterial–venous oxygen saturation difference ($SaO_2 - SmvO_2$) is normal, at approximately 25%, the above equation can be further simplified:

$$Qp:Qs = 25/(95 - SaO_2)$$

This simplified version of the Fick equation allows estimation of Qp:Qs based on SaO_2. Given the ease with which SaO_2 can be obtained in clinical practice, the above equation allows the clinician to estimate DO_2 simply by looking at SaO_2. Thus, one can theoretically assess the effectiveness of any intervention designed to alter Qp:Qs by observing the change in SaO_2. This simplified approach to estimating Qp:Qs is predicated on assumptions regarding $SmvO_2$ and $SpvO_2$. The assumption regarding the systemic arterial–venous oxygen saturation difference is only accurate if DO_2 is normal. In shock, which often occurs in neonates with ductal-dependent Qs or in the face of myocardial dysfunction following surgery, $SmvO_2$ will be low and therefore $SaO_2 - SmvO_2$ will be substantially higher than 25%. When the decrease in $SmvO_2$ is offset by an increase in the amount of well-saturated blood returning from the lungs (increased Qp:Qs), SaO_2 will remain unchanged [49–52]. Many centers have begun to routinely monitor $SmvO_2$ following Norwood palliation for HLHS using a sample from the superior vena cava as representative of mixed venous blood (in single-ventricle anatomy, there is no site of true systemic mixed venous blood).

Although $SpvO_2$ is likely to be normal in the absence of clinical or x-ray evidence of pulmonary parenchymal disease, there are conditions under which this assumption is also false. Taeed and colleagues placed catheters in the left lower pulmonary vein at the time of the Norwood operation in infants with HLHS, and found that unexpected pulmonary venous desaturation occurred commonly, particularly with FiO_2 <0.3 [51]. Failure to account for decreased $SpvO_2$ results in a falsely low calculation of Qp:Qs, as even small errors in estimation of $SpvO_2$ can result in gross inaccuracy in calculated Qp:Qs [53]. The important clinical implication of this principle is that maneuvers that decrease $SpvO_2$ rather than Qp:Qs result in lower SaO_2 and reduced DO_2 because there is no increase in Qs.

The importance of accurately estimating Qp:Qs can be seen when one considers the relationship between Qp:Qs, DO_2, and total cardiac output [54]. Using mathematical modeling and keeping $SpvO_2$ constant at 96%, Barnea et al. generated a series of curves showing DO_2 as a function of Qp:Qs [53]. Because the total cardiac output pumped by the single ventricle is Qp + Qs, an increase in Qp is accompanied by a decrease in Qs and vice versa unless the total cardiac output also increases. The maximum DO_2 occurs between a Qp:Qs of approximately 0.5 and 1 and depends on the total cardiac output. The slope of each isobar for a given cardiac output is steepest on either side of the maximum DO_2, suggesting small changes in Qp:Qs can be associated with large changes in DO_2. The results of this study also suggest that DO_2 can be improved to a far greater degree by increasing total cardiac output than by altering Qp:Qs. One limitation to this type of model for DO_2 is the use of SaO_2 and Qs as interchangeable components of DO_2. Although newborns tolerate cyanosis well, the oxyhemoglobin dissociation curve dictates that once SaO_2 becomes critically low, further decreases can no longer be compensated for by increases in Qs [55]. Nevertheless, when cardiac output is maximized, optimization of Qp:Qs is still very important for improvement of marginal DO_2.

The most commonly used method of balancing Qp:Qs at the bedside is through the differential manipulation of pulmonary and systemic vascular resistances with the use of oxygen, CO_2, and acid–base status [56] (Table 12.2). Subatmospheric oxygen (FiO_2 0.17–0.19) or induction of respiratory acidosis can effectively raise pulmonary vascular resistance, decrease systemic vascular resistance, and thus decrease Qp:Qs in infants with unrestricted Qp. Subatmospheric oxygen should be used with caution, because it can be associated with pulmonary venous desaturation and thus have a less beneficial effect on DO_2, particularly in the postoperative patient [51]. Conversely, the use of inhaled CO_2 (rather than subatmospheric oxygen) may be associated with increased cerebral and/or systemic DO_2 [57–59]. Pulmonary vascular resistance can also be increased independently of systemic vascular resistance with the judicious use of positive end-expiratory pressure (PEEP) [56].

When lung compliance is normal, PEEP increases pulmonary vascular resistance by compressing the interalveolar pulmonary arterioles. To accomplish this, the level of PEEP must result in an end-expiratory lung volume greater than functional residual capacity (FRC). This is because the nadir of pulmonary vascular resistance occurs at FRC rather than at zero PEEP. The initial application of PEEP above zero applies radial traction forces to the pulmonary vasculature and aids vascular recruitment. Further increases in PEEP above FRC compress the vessels. Increased PEEP may also prevent pulmonary venous desaturation by optimizing lung gas exchange and therefore decreasing Qp:Qs while simultaneously maximizing $SpvO_2$.

However, it is less clear that manipulation of pulmonary vascular resistance is useful in altering Qp:Qs in infants with low

TABLE 12.2. Effects of respiratory maneuvers on pulmonary and systemic vascular resistances.

Treatment	PVR	SVR	Qp:Qs
Increase FiO_2	Decrease	Increase	Increase
Increase CO_2	Increase	Decrease	Decrease
Increase pH	Decrease	Increase	Increase
PEEP	Increase	No effect	Decrease

Note: PVR, pulmonary vascular resistance; Qp:Qs, ratio of pulmonary to systemic blood flow; SVR, systemic vascular resistance, FiO_2, fraction of inspired oxygen; PEEP, positive end-expiratory pressure.

pulmonary vascular resistance and anatomically restricted pulmonary blood flow. One study has demonstrated no significant changes in Qp:Qs with subatmospheric oxygen following Norwood palliation [51]. It is likely that Qp becomes limited by the size of the systemic-to-pulmonary artery shunt or pulmonary artery band, and further decreases in downstream resistance are of minimal consequence [60,61]. More recent data suggest that management of total cardiac output (i.e., Qp + Qs, see later) and systemic vascular resistance may be more effective [52]. Sodium nitroprusside, phenoxybenzamine, inamrinone, and milrinone have been used as systemic afterload-reducing agents and to block the α-adrenergic receptor mediated vasoconstriction that occurs with drugs such as epinephrine. Phenoxybenzamine lowers systemic vascular resistance, decreases Qp:Qs, and improves DO_2 after the Norwood operation, even though it is associated with a decrease in systemic blood pressure [52]. β-Adrenergic stimulation of the myocardium in conjunction with systemic vasodilation can further increase total cardiac output (Qp + Qs) without associated vasoconstriction. Other vasodilating agents can potentially be used to accomplish the same goal, although they involve different receptor mechanisms and cellular pathways.

It should be mentioned that not all neonates with single-ventricle physiology demonstrate pulmonary overcirculation. Elevated pulmonary vascular resistance can easily persist in the newborn with single-ventricle physiology and cause severe cyanosis. When Qp is very low ($PaO_2 < 30$ torr), it can effectively increase pulmonary dead space and impair minute ventilation. The occurrence of respiratory acidosis in this setting is of grave concern because this will further increase pulmonary vascular resistance, limiting the ability to hyperventilate or alkalinize the patient. Management of high pulmonary vascular resistance in this population is much the same as in any other population. Alveolar recruitment strategies of ventilation are appropriate when there is atelectasis or pulmonary disease, but otherwise airway pressures should be kept to a minimum. High-frequency ventilation may be effective in inducing hyperventilation at low mean airway pressure [62]. Use of supplemental inspired oxygen, hyperventilation, and alkalosis (i.e., through the administration of sodium bicarbonate) may all be effective. Inhaled nitric oxide and prostaglandin E infusion have been used in these patients to selectively lower pulmonary vascular resistance as well. Raising systemic blood pressure by vasoconstriction may increase Qp and will usually increase SaO_2, but at the expense of some systemic perfusion.

Cardiac Output (Optimizing Qp + Qs)

Low *total* cardiac output (Qp + Qs) in single-ventricle physiology causes both low Qs and low SaO_2 and is thus of critical importance to rapidly diagnose and treat. In the absence of $SmvO_2$ monitoring, low SaO_2 with clinical signs of low cardiac output or shock (e.g., anuria, poor capillary refill, high ventricular filling pressure, or metabolic acidosis out of proportion to the degree of cyanosis) suggests poor cardiac function. Single-ventricle physiology places the newborn at an increased risk of ventricular dysfunction [63,64]. For example, the single ventricle is volume loaded in that it must supply both Qp and Qs (by comparison, in an anatomically normal heart, the left ventricle needs only to supply Qs). Low Qs, particularly with low diastolic blood pressure (as commonly observed in a newborn with a large patent ductus arteriosus or following the modified Blalock-Taussig shunt) or a high end diastolic ventricular pressure (as commonly observed with a volume-loaded heart or ventricular

dysfunction that normally occurs after cardiopulmonary bypass) can cause coronary perfusion pressure to become critically low—this further compromises systolic ventricular function—and further raise end diastolic pressure and lower systemic arterial pressure. If not rapidly corrected, this type of situation can result in profound hemodynamic decompensation.

Inotropic support that increases Qs may also increase SaO_2 simply by increasing $SmvO_2$. The use of particular inotropic agents may also be associated with a change in Qp:Qs in addition to increases in total cardiac output. Riordan et al. [56] studied the effects of epinephrine, dobutamine, and dopamine in an animal model of single-ventricle physiology and found that dobutamine (5 and 15 μg/kg/min) increases Qp:Qs, epinephrine (0.05 and 0.1 μg/kg/min) decreases Qp:Qs, and dopamine (5 and 15 μg/kg/min) has minimal effects on Qp:Qs. In this study, the use of low-dose epinephrine (0.05 μg/kg/min) was associated with the greatest increase in pulmonary vascular resistance/systemic vascular resistance ratio, largely because of a *decrease* in systemic vascular resistance. This probably reflects the predominance of vascular β-receptor stimulation at this dose compared with α-adrenergic activation at a higher dose and illustrates the importance of using vasodilating drugs as an accompaniment to inotropic agents with prominent vasoconstrictor properties. Finally, maintenance of oxygen-carrying capacity by keeping hemoglobin in the range of 13 to 15 mg/dL can have a positive influence on DO_2. Increased hemoglobin concentration increases $SmvO_2$ and SaO_2 and decreases Qp:Qs in single-ventricle physiology [65,66].

A Rational Approach to Single-Ventricle Physiology in the Older Infant and Child

The Bidirectional Cavopulmonary Anastomosis

Second and third stage palliation for single-ventricle lesions result in pulmonary blood flow that is dependent on nonpulsatile venous return. The second stage of single-ventricle palliation is the creation of a bidirectional cavopulmonary anastomosis (BCPA) in which the superior vena cava is connected directly to the pulmonary artery and other sources of Qp are either eliminated or severely restricted. Anatomic variations include the bidirectional Glenn (Figure 12.4) and the hemi-Fontan. These procedures differ in that the hemi-Fontan includes the attachment of the proximal stump of the superior vena cava to the underside of the pulmonary artery, but this connection is then patched to avoid flow of deoxygenated blood into the right atrium from the pulmonary artery. The BCPA has been remarkable for its relatively low level of associated morbidity and mortality, with numerous reviews suggesting an overall mortality rate of 3%–5% [67–69].

The real hemodynamic advantage of the BCPA compared with shunted or banded single-ventricle physiology is in the reduction of the volume load on the ventricle. This occurs because the right-to-left shunt is eliminated and all Qp is effective pulmonary flow. The ventricle now only pumps Qs, not Qp + Qs [70]. Some of the Qs (the portion distributed to the upper body) passes through the lungs before reaching the ventricle again, and thus all blood reaching the lungs is deoxygenated. The advantageous consequences of this volume reduction go beyond simply lowering the amount of blood the ventricle needs to pump to maintain adequate systemic cardiac output. There is an acute increase in wall thickness and decrease in cavity dimension that has been associated with

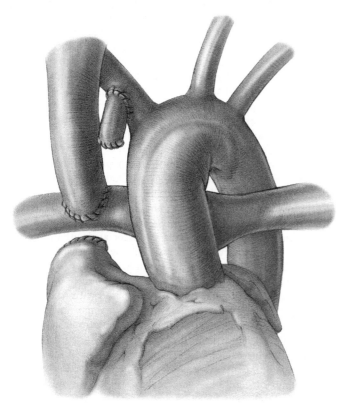

FIGURE 12.4. Completion of the bidirectional cavopulmonary (Glenn) anastomosis—the second stage palliation for hypoplastic left heart syndrome. (Courtesy of James D. St. Louis, MD, Medical College of Georgia.)

improved tricuspid valve function [71]. Preload and afterload are both decreased, although there is not a measurable increase in ventricular contractile state [72]. Coronary blood flow decreases, probably in response to the lower metabolic demand of the myocardium, but coronary flow changes from predominantly systolic to both systolic and diastolic [73].

Because Qp is supplied by upper body systemic venous return, one consequence of conversion to a BCPA is an acute rise in superior vena cava pressure. Selection of patients with low pulmonary vascular resistance as candidates for the BCPA minimizes the risk of clinical complications arising from elevated superior vena cava pressure, but superior vena cava syndrome can occur nonetheless. Failure to maintain low superior vena cava pressure following the BCPA can also lead to problems maintaining an adequate SaO_2. Small venovenous collateral vessels (such as a persistent left superior vena cava or vein of Marshall) may enlarge in size following a BCPA and allow a *pop-off* for desaturated blood in the superior vena cava to bypass the lungs and thus contribute to arterial desaturation [74]. When the anastomosis is performed as part of a hemi-Fontan rather than a bidirectional Glenn, a right-to-left shunt may occur if there is a persistent communication between the superior vena cava and right atrium.

To minimize superior vena cava pressure, it is desirable to minimize the use of positive pressure, including PEEP, following surgery [75–78]. However, setting the ventilator to maintain the PEEP at zero may result in atelectasis and an increase in pulmonary vascular resistance. As in the neonate with single-ventricle physiology (see earlier), favorable hemodynamics are most likely maintained by using ventilator settings that allow the end expiratory lung

volume to approximate FRC, because pulmonary vascular resistance is lowest at FRC. In the patient with healthy lungs, minimal mean airway pressure and early tracheal extubation are often beneficial, because negative pressure ventilation is associated with increased Qp in this type of circulation. When lung disease such as pneumonia or acute respiratory distress syndrome occurs in the patient with a cavopulmonary anastomosis, higher airway pressures may actually promote Qp and minimize pulmonary artery pressure if the higher airway pressure helps maintain FRC.

A unique aspect of the physiology of the BCPA (Glenn shunt) is that pulmonary blood flow is largely dependent on the resistance of two highly but differentially regulated vascular beds [79]. Both the cerebral and pulmonary vasculature have opposite responses to changes in carbon dioxide, acid–base status, and oxygen. This can make treatment of elevated pulmonary resistance or low arterial saturation particularly challenging. Hyperventilation and alkalosis, for example, may have limited utility in this setting. Although they are effective pulmonary vasodilators, hyperventilation and alkalosis cause cerebral vasoconstriction [80,81]. Because Qp is dependent on venous return via the superior vena cava (largely made up of cerebral blood flow), maneuvers that limit cerebral blood flow may decrease pulmonary flow and exacerbate hypoxemia [82]. Other frequently used techniques for decreasing pulmonary resistance such as deep sedation/anesthesia may also reduce cerebral blood flow and therefore fail to increase Qp even if they successfully reduce resistance. Inhaled nitric oxide, which acts selectively on the pulmonary vasculature, has been reported to be effective in reducing the transpulmonary pressure gradient for patients after the BCPA and may therefore be the best treatment for high pulmonary resistance and hypoxemia [83]. For the patient with normal pulmonary vascular resistance, mild hypoventilation will generally result in improved cerebral blood flow and increased pulmonary blood flow [84]. Patients with a cavopulmonary anastomosis will also benefit from return to spontaneous ventilation as soon as their clinical state allows.

When a significant left-to-right shunt persists following BCPA because of additional sources of Qp or aortopulmonary collateral blood vessels, persistent pleural effusions, high central venous pressures and low cardiac output may result [85–87]. It is also important to recognize that there are changes in ventricular geometry that occur with these operations because of reduction in left-to-right shunt, particularly with the bidirectional Glenn. When systemic outflow is dependent on flow through a ventricular septal defect or bulboventricular foramen, acute decreases in ventricular dimension may precipitate effective subaortic stenosis. The appearance of an ejection murmur in a patient with susceptible anatomy following BCPA should prompt a complete assessment for this phenomenon.

Total Cavopulmonary Anastomosis

The Fontan operation (Figure 12.5) has several commonly used anatomic variants, all designed to achieve optimum fluid dynamics and minimize the risk of long-term complications. Although one may still encounter older individuals with direct right atrial to pulmonary artery connections, the most common current approaches to the Fontan operation are the creation of either an intracardiac lateral tunnel or an extracardiac conduit. The lateral tunnel involves placement of a semicircular tube, usually Gore-Tex (WL Gore & Associates, Flagstaff, AZ), along the lateral wall of the

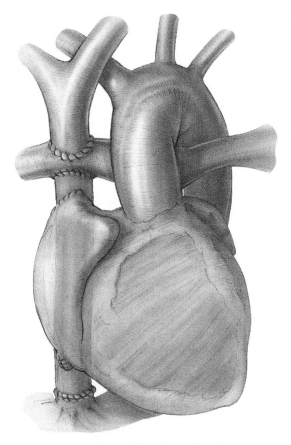

FIGURE 12.5. The Fontan procedure (in this case, an intracardiac lateral tunnel Fontan)—the third and final stage palliation for hypoplastic left heart syndrome. (Courtesy of James D. St. Louis, MD, Medical College of Georgia.)

Fontan physiology is a hybrid of bidirectional Glenn and normal cardiovascular physiology. Like the bidirectional Glenn, Qp is dependent on systemic venous pressure, and all Qp is effective [70]. If the Fontan baffle is fenestrated, there may still be a right-to-left shunt causing some mild systemic arterial desaturation, but the systemic and pulmonary circulations are largely separated, as with a normal heart. Important issues for the intensive care physician arise when there is elevated pulmonary artery pressure. This can occur in the setting of elevated pulmonary vascular resistance, mechanical pulmonary artery obstruction, or elevated pressures in the pulmonary venous atrium because of myocardial dysfunction.

Numerous studies have demonstrated an association between elevated pulmonary artery pressure (>10–15 mm Hg) and poor outcome in Fontan patients [91–93], largely because of third space losses of fluid that occur with elevated central venous pressures. As these fluid losses progress, patients develop pleural effusions, ascites, and generalized edema. In the face of a full abdomen, heavy chest wall, and smaller effective pleural cavities, it often becomes necessary to increase ventilator pressures to maintain adequate FRC and tidal volume. Increased intrathoracic pressure, particularly in the absence of parenchymal lung disease, effectively raises pulmonary resistance and necessitates even higher venous pressures to maintain cardiac output, creating a vicious circle. Furthermore, as central venous and intraabdominal pressure rise, renal perfusion pressure decreases, especially in the face of low cardiac output and borderline hypotension. In general, Fontan fenestration can lower the risk of some of these complications by providing a source of Qs that is not dependent on passing through the pulmonary circulation [94,95]. Fenestration can also decrease pulmonary artery pressure enough to reduce third space losses of fluid.

When an individual with Fontan physiology is in a low cardiac output state, it is essential to determine and treat the underlying cause. It is common for postoperative Fontan patients to need large amounts of volume in the first day after surgery. Persistently low central venous and left atrial pressures strongly suggest the need for volume. Pulmonary artery obstruction should be considered as the cause of low output when left atrial pressure is low and central venous pressure is high. If central venous pressure is not monitored, large third space fluid losses with a low or normal left atrial pressure should raise the suspicion of this diagnosis. Even in the presence of a fenestrated Fontan, the capability of the fenestration to preserve cardiac output in the face of anatomic or physiologic obstruction to pulmonary blood flow is significantly limited compared with the situation after the BCPA. Therefore, limited pulmonary flow can result in low cardiac output and, when a fenestration is present, significant cyanosis. Cyanosis can also result from intrapulmonary arteriovenous malformations or ventilation–perfusion mismatch related to low cardiac output [96,97].

If high pulmonary resistance is responsible for the elevation of central venous pressure, institution of the standard therapies of supplemental oxygen, hyperventilation, and alkalosis is indicated. As with the bidirectional Glenn patient, the use of high positive pressures to achieve these ends may be counterproductive. Negative pressure ventilation can augment stroke volume and cardiac output, and high-frequency jet ventilation may lower PaCO₂ at low mean airway pressures [62,98,99]. Intravenous vasodilators such as prostacyclin or prostaglandin E should be used with caution because of the risk of systemic vasodilation with limited cardiac output. Inhaled nitric oxide has been reported to be effective in lowering the transpulmonary pressure gradient [100].

right atrium from the inferior vena cava to the superior vena cava. Patients with a prior bidirectional Glenn then need to have the proximal portion of the superior vena cava reconnected to the pulmonary artery, whereas those who have had a prior hemi-Fontan need only to have the patch between the pulmonary artery and right atrium taken down. The extracardiac conduit uses a complete circular tube of Gore-Tex or pericardium to connect the inferior vena cava to the pulmonary artery. The conduit is placed along the outer surface of the right atrium and thus creates a connection incapable of dilating over time, unlike the classic Fontan, or even potentially the lateral tunnel. Either variation on the Fontan can be fenestrated by leaving a hole of known size in the baffle. In the case of the extracardiac Fontan, fenestration requires connection of the conduit to the atrial wall.

The different approaches to the Fontan connection may have implications for postoperative physiology, although no consensus on which technique is preferable has yet been reached. The arguments in favor of the lateral tunnel are that it is less thrombogenic, can be done at a younger age, and retains the possibility for growth without the likelihood of severe dilation. Those who favor the extracardiac approach argue that it preserves kinetic energy better, that it can be performed without cardioplegia, thereby reducing the incidence of postoperative myocardial dysfunction, and that it is less arrhythmogenic because there is no atrial suture line [88–90]. In the absence of a conclusive study, the differences between Fontan techniques remain largely theoretical.

Low cardiac output with high left atrial and central venous pressures indicates myocardial dysfunction in the patient with Fontan physiology. Myocardial dysfunction can occur from ischemia-reperfusion injury if aortic cross-clamping and cardioplegia are used to create the Fontan baffle. It may also be related to poor preoperative myocardial function. The only effective long-term therapy for low cardiac output with ventricular dysfunction following a Fontan operation is to improve cardiac output and reduce left atrial pressure. The use of inotropic agents that do not increase ventricular afterload, such as phosphodiesterase inhibitors, dobutamine, and low-dose epinephrine ($\leq 0.05\,\mu g/kg/min$) may be helpful. If systemic blood pressure will tolerate it, aggressive afterload reduction with vasodilating agents may also lower left atrial pressure significantly. If there is good reason to believe the insult to ventricular function is reversible, mechanical circulatory support can also be effective therapy. Because persistent aortopulmonary collateral vessels can be associated with hemodynamics similar to those of ventricular dysfunction, aggressive assessment and embolization of these vessels may be useful in this situation [101–103].

References

1. Jacobs ML, Rychik J, Murphy JD, Nicolson SC, Steven JM, Norwood WI. Results of Norwood's operation for lesions other than hypoplastic left heart syndrome. J Thorac Cardiovasc Surg 1995;110:1555–1562.
2. Jensen RA Jr, Williams RG, Laks H, Drinkwater D, Kaplan S. Usefulness of banding of the pulmonary trunk with single ventricle physiology at risk for subaortic obstruction. Am J Cardiol 1996;77:1089–1093.
3. Daebritz SH, Nollert GD, Zurakowski D, et al. Results of Norwood stage I operation: comparison of hypoplastic left heart syndrome with other malformations. J Thorac Cardiovasc Surg 2000;119:358–367.
4. Lan YT, Chang RK, Laks H. Outcome of patients with double-inlet left ventricle or tricuspid atresia with transposed great arteries. J Am Coll Cardiol 2004;43:113–119.
5. Cerillo AG, Murzi B, Giusti S, Crucean A, Redaelli S, Vanini V. Pulmonary artery banding and ventricular septal defect enlargement in patients with univentricular atrioventricular connection and the aorta originating from an incomplete ventricle. Eur J Cardiothorac Surg 2002;22:192–199.
6. Lan YT, Chang RK, Drant S, et al. Outcome of staged surgical approach to neonates with single left ventricle and moderate size bulboventricular foramen. Am J Cardiol 2002;89:959–963.
7. Clarke AJ, Kasahara S, Andrews DR, et al. Mid-term results for double-inlet left ventricle and similar morphologies: timing of Damus-Kaye-Stansel. Ann Thorac Surg 2004;78:650–657.
8. Earing MG, Cetta F, Driscoll DJ, et al. Long-term results of the Fontan operation for double-inlet left ventricle. Am J Cardiol 2005;96:291–298.
9. Minich LL, Tani LY, Hawkins JA, et al. Possibility of postnatal left ventricular growth in selected infants with non-apex-forming left ventricles. Am Heart J 1997;133:570–574.
10. Blaufox AD, Lai WW, Lopex L, et al. Survival in neonatal biventricular repair or left-sided cardiac obstructive lesions associated with hypoplastic left ventricle. Am J Cardiol 1998;82:1138–1140.
11. Tchervenkov CI, Tahta SA, Justras LC, et al. Biventricular repair in neonates with hypoplastic left heart complex. Ann Thorac Surg 1998;66:1350–1357.
12. Roberts WC, Perry LW, Chandra RS, et al. Aortic valve atresia: a new classification based on necropsy study of 73 cases. Am J Cardiol 1976;37:753–756.
13. Iannettoni MD, Bove EL, Mosca RS, et al. Improving results with first-stage palliation for hypoplastic left heart syndrome. J Thorac Cardiovasc Surg 1994;107:934–940.
14. Gutgesell HP, Massaro TA. Management of hypoplastic left heart syndrome in a consortium of university hospitals. Am J Cardiol 1995;76:809–811.
15. Bove EL, Lloyd TR. Staged reconstruction for hypoplastic left heart syndrome. Contemporary results. Ann Surg 1996;224:387–935.
16. Bando K, Turrentine MW, Sun K, et al. Surgical management of hypoplastic left heart syndrome. Ann Thorac Surg 1996;62:70–77.
17. Tweddell JS, Hoffman GM, Musatto KA, et al. Improved survival of patients undergoing palliation of hypoplastic left heart syndrome: lessons learned from 115 consecutive patients. Circulation 2002;106:I82–I89.
18. Chang RK, Chen AY, Klitzner TS. Clinical management of infants with hypoplastic left heart syndrome in the United States, 1988–1997. Pediatrics 2002;110:292–298.
19. Stasik CN, Goldberg CS, Bove EL, Devaney EJ, Ohye RG. Current outcomes and risk factors for the Norwood procedure. J Thorac Cardiovasc Surg 2006;131:412–417.
20. Mitchell ME, Ittenback RF, Gaynor JW, et al. Intermediate outcomes after the Fontan procedure in the current era. J Thorac Cardiovasc Surg 2006;131:172–180.
21. Johnston JK, Chinnock RE, Zuppan CW, et al. Limitations to survival for infants with hypoplastic left heart syndrome before and after transplant: the Loma Linda experience. J Transplant Coord 1997;7:180–186.
22. Chrisant MR, Naftel DC, Drummond-Webb J, et al. Fate of infants with hypoplastic left heart syndrome for cardiac transplantation: a multi-center study. J Heart Lung Transplant 2005;24:575–582.
23. Jacobs ML, Blackstone EH, Bailey LL. Intermediate survival in neonates with aortic atresia: a multi-institutional study. The Congenital Heart Surgeons Society. J Thorac Cardiovasc Surg 1998;116:417–431.
24. Bailey LL, Gundry SR. Hypoplastic left heart syndrome. Pediatr Clin North Am 1990;37:137–150.
25. Hennein HA, Bove EL, eds. Hypoplastic Left Heart Syndrome. Armonk, NY: Futura; 2002.
26. Goldberg CS, Gomez CA. Hypoplastic left heart syndrome: new developments and current controversies. Semin Neonatol 2003;8:461–468.
27. Pearl JM, Nelson DP, Schwartz SM, et al. First-stage palliation for hypoplastic left heart syndrome in the twenty-first century. Ann Thorac Surg 2002;73:331–340.
28. Rychik J, Wernovsky G. Hypoplastic Left Heart Syndrome. Norwell, MA: Kluwer Academic; 2003.
29. Bove EL, Ohye RG, Devaney EJ. Hypoplastic left heart syndrome: conventional surgical management. Semin Thorac Cardiovasc Surg Pediatr Card Surg Annu 2004;7:3–10.
30. Walker SG, Stuth EA. Single-ventricle physiology: perioperative implications. Semin Pediatr Surg 2004;13:188–202.
31. Quintessenza JA, Morell VO, Jacobs JP. Achieving a balance in the current approach to the surgical treatment of hypoplastic left heart syndrome. Cardiol Young 2004;14:127–130.
32. Anderson RH, Pozzi M, Hutchinson S. Hypoplastic Left Heart Syndrome. London, UK: Springer-Verlag; 2005.
33. Theilen U, Shekerdemian L. The intensive care of infants with hypoplastic left heart syndrome. Arch Dis Child Fetal Neonatal Ed 2005;90:F97–F102.
34. Sedmera D, Cook AC, Shirali G, McQuinn TC. Current issues and perspectives in hypoplasia of the left heart. Cardiol Young 2005;15:56–72.
35. Atz AM, Feinstein JA, Jonas RA, et al. Preoperative management of pulmonary venous hypertension in hypoplastic left heart syndrome with restrictive atrial septal defect. Am J Cardiol 1999;83:1224–1228.
36. Rychik J, Rome JJ, Collins MH, et al. The hypoplastic left heart syndrome with intact atrial septum: atrial morphology, pulmonary vascular histopathology and outcome. J Am Coll Cardiol 1999;34:554–560.
37. Vlahos AP, Lock JE, McElhinney DB, van der Velde ME. Hypoplastic left heart syndrome with intact or highly restrictive atrial septum:

outcome after neonatal transcatheter atrial septostomy. Circulation 2004;109:2326–2330.

38. Photiadis J, Urban AE, Sinzohahamvya N, et al. Restrictive left atrial outflow adversely affects outcome after the modified Norwood procedure. Eur J Cardiothorac Surg 2005;27:962–967.

39. Imoto Y, Kado H, Shiokawa Y, et al. Norwood procedure without circulatory arrest. Ann Thorac Surg 1999;68:559–561.

40. Pigula FA, Siewers RD, Nemoto EM. Regional perfusion of the brain during neonatal aortic arch reconstruction. J Thorac Cardiovasc Surg 1999;117:1023–104.

41. Photiadis J, Asfour B, Sinzobahamvya, et al. Improved hemodynamics and outcome after modified Norwood operation on the beating heart. Ann Thorac Surg 2006;81:976–981.

42. Freedom RM, Sondheimer H, Sische R, et al. Development of "subaortic stenosis" after pulmonary arterial banding for common ventricle. Am J Cardiol 1977;39:78–83.

43. Webber SA, LeBlanc JG, Keeton BR, et al. Pulmonary artery banding is not contraindicated in double inlet left ventricle with transposition and aortic arch obstruction. Eur J Cardiothorac Surg 1995;9: 515–520.

44. Mair R, Tulzer G, Sames E, et al. Right ventricular to pulmonary artery conduit instead of modified Blalock-Taussig shunt improves postoperative hemodynamics in newborns after the Norwood operation. J Thorac Cardiovasc Surg 2003;126:1378–1384.

45. Bradley SM, Simsic JM, McQuinn TC, et al. Hemodynamic status after the Norwood procedure: a comparison of right ventricle-to-pulmonary artery connection versus modified Blalock-Taussig shunt. Ann Thorac Surg 2004;78:933–941.

46. Sano S, Ishino K, Kawada M, Honjo. Right ventricle-pulmonary artery shunt in first-stage palliation of hypoplastic left heart syndrome. Semin Thorac Cardiovasc Surg Pediatr Card Surg Annu 2004; 7:22–31.

47. Azakie A, Martinez D, Sapru A, et al. Impact of right ventricle to pulmonary artery conduit on outcome of the modified Norwood procedure. Ann Thorac Surg 2004;77:1727–1733.

48. Tabbutt S, Dominquez TE, Ravishankar C, et al. Outcomes after the stage I reconstruction comparing the right ventricular to pulmonary artery conduit with the modified Blalock Taussig shunt. Ann Thorac Surg 2005;80:1582–1591.

49. Hoffman GM, Ghanayem NS, Kampine JM, et al. Venous saturation and the anaerobic threshold in neonates after the Norwood procedure for hypoplastic left heart syndrome. Ann Thorac Surg 2000;70:1515–1521.

50. Riordan CJ, Locher JP Jr, Santamore WP, et al. Monitoring systemic venous oxygen saturations in the hypoplastic left heart syndrome. Ann Thorac Surg 1997;63:835–837.

51. Taeed R, Schwartz SM, Pearl JM, et al. Unrecognized pulmonary venous desaturation early after Norwood palliation confounds Qp : Qs assessment and compromises oxygen delivery. Circulation 2001; 103:2699–2704.

52. Tweddell JS, Hoffman GM, Fedderly RT, et al. Phenoxybenzamine improves systemic oxygen delivery after the Norwood procedure. Ann Thorac Surg 1999;67:161–168.

53. Barnea O, Santamore WP, Rossi A, et al: Estimation of oxygen delivery in newborns with a univentricular circulation. Circulation 1998;98: 1407–1413.

54. Barnea O, Austin EH, Richman B, et al: Balancing the circulation: theoretic optimization of pulmonary/systemic flow ratio in hypoplastic left heart syndrome. J Am Coll Cardiol 1994;24:1376–1381.

55. Francis DP, Willson K, Thorne SA, et al: Oxygenation in patients with a functionally univentricular circulation and complete mixing of blood: are saturation and flow interchangeable? Circulation 1999;100: 2198–2203.

56. Riordan CJ, Randsbeck F, Storey JH, et al. Effects of oxygen, positive end-expiratory pressure, and carbon dioxide on oxygen delivery in an animal model of the univentricular heart. J Thorac Cardiovasc Surg 1996;112:644–654.

57. Ramamoorthy C, Tabbutt S, Kurth CD, et al. Effects of inspired hypoxic and hypercapnic gas mixtures on cerebral oxygen saturation in neonates with univentricular heart defects. Anesthesiology 2002;96:283–288.

58. Tabbutt S, Ramamoorthy C, Montenegro LM, et al. Impact of inspired gas mixtures on preoperative infants with hypoplastic left heart syndrome during controlled ventilation. Circulation 2001;104: I159–I164.

59. Bradley SM, Simsic JM, Atz AM. Hemodynamic effects of inspired carbon dioxide after the Norwood procedure. Ann Thorac Surg 2001;72:2088–2094.

60. Nakano T, Kado H, Shiokawa Y, et al. The low resistance strategy for the perioperative management of the Norwood procedure. Ann Thorac Surg 2004;77:908–912.

61. Bradley SM, Atz AM, Simsic JM. Redefining the impact of oxygen and hyperventilation after the Norwood procedure. J Thorac Cardiovasc Surg 2004;127:473–480.

62. Meliones JN, Bove EL, Dekeon MK, et al. High-frequency jet ventilation improves cardiac function after the Fontan procedure. Circulation 1991;84:III364–III368.

63. Donnelly JP, Raffel DM, Shulkin BL, et al. Resting coronary flow and coronary flow reserve in human infants after repair or palliation of congenital heart defects as measured by positron emission tomography. J Thorac Cardiovasc Surg 1998;115:103–110.

64. Williams RV, Ritter S, Tani LY, et al. Quantitative assessment of ventricular function in children with single ventricles using the Doppler myocardial performance index. Am J Cardiol 2000;86: 1106–1110.

65. Lister G, Hellenbrand WE, Kleinman CS, et al. Physiologic effects of increasing hemoglobin concentration in left-to-right shunting in infants with ventricular septal defects. N Engl J Med 1982;306: 502–506.

66. Beekman RH, Tuuri DT. Acute hemodynamic effects of increasing hemoglobin concentration in children with a right to left ventricular shunt and relative anemia. J Am Coll Cardiol 1985;5:357–362.

67. Forbess JM, Cook N, Serraf A, et al. An institutional experience with second- and third-stage palliative procedures for hypoplastic left heart syndrome: the impact of the bidirectional cavopulmonary shunt. J Am Coll Cardiol 1997;29:665–670.

68. Lamberti JJ, Mainwaring RD, Spicer RL, et al. Factors influencing perioperative morbidity during palliation of the univentricular heart. Ann Thorac Surg 1995;60:S550–S553.

69. Reddy VM, McElhinney DB, Moore P, et al. Outcomes after bidirectional cavopulmonary shunt in infants less than 6 months old. J Am Coll Cardiol 1997;29:1365–1370.

70. Santamore WP, Barnea O, Riordan CJ, et al. Theoretical optimization of pulmonary-to-systemic flow ratio after a bidirectional cavopulmonary anastomosis. Am J Physiol 1998;274:H694–H700.

71. Rychik J, Jacobs ML, Norwood WI Jr. Acute changes in left ventricular geometry after volume reduction operation. Ann Thorac Surg 1995;60:1267–1274.

72. Donofrio MT, Jacobs ML, Spray TL, et al. Acute changes in preload, afterload, and systolic function after superior cavopulmonary connection. Ann Thorac Surg 1998;65:503–508.

73. Fogel MA, Rychik J, Vetter J, et al. Effect of volume unloading surgery on coronary flow dynamics in patients with aortic atresia. J Thorac Cardiovasc Surg 1997;113:718–777.

74. Filippini LH, Ovaert C, Nykanen DG, et al. Reopening of persistent left superior caval vein after bidirectional cavopulmonary connections. Heart 1998;79:509–512.

75. Alvarado O, Sreeram N, McKay R, et al. Cavopulmonary connection in repair of atrioventricular septal defect with small right ventricle. Ann Thorac Surg 1993;55:729–736.

76. Kim YH, Walker PG, Fontaine AA, et al. Hemodynamics of the Fontan connection: an in-vitro study. J Biomech Eng 1995;117:423–428.

77. Redington AN, Penny D, Shinebourne EA. Pulmonary blood flow after total cavopulmonary shunt. Br Heart J 1991;65:213–217.

78. Sievers HH, Gerdes A, Kunze J, et al. Superior hydrodynamics of a modified cavopulmonary connection for the Norwood operation. Ann Thorac Surg 1998;65:1741–1745.

79. Fogel MA, Durning S, Wernovsky G, Pollock AN, Gaynor JW, Nicolson S. Brain versus lung: hierarchy of feedback loops in single-ventricle patients with superior cavopulmonary connection. Circulation 2004;110:II147–II152.

80. Simsic JM, Bradley SM, Muvihill DM. Sodium nitroprusside infusion after bidirectional superior cavopulmonary connection: preserved cerebral blood flow velocity and systemic oxygenation. J Thorac Cardiovasc Surg 2003;126:186–190.

81. Kawaguchi M, Ohsumi H, Ohnishi Y, Nakajima T, Kuro M. Cerebral vascular reactivity to carbon dioxide before and after cardiopulmonary bypass in children with congenital heart disease. J Thorac Cardiovasc Surg 1993;106:823–827.

82. Bradley SM, Simsic JM, Mulvihill DM. Hyperventilation impairs oxygenation after bidirectional superior cavopulmonary connection. Circulation 1998;98:II372–II377.

83. Gamillscheg A, Zobel G, Urlesberger B, et al. Inhaled nitric oxide in patients with critical pulmonary perfusion after Fontan-type procedures and bidirectional Glenn anastomosis. J Thorac Cardiovasc Surg 1997;113:435–442.

84. Bradley SM, Simsic JM, Mulvihill DM. Hypoventilation improves oxygenation after bidirectional superior cavopulmonary connection. J Thorac Cardiovasc Surg 2003;v126:1033–1039.

85. Frommelt MA, Frommelt PC, Berger S, et al. Does an additional source of pulmonary blood flow alter outcome after a bidirectional cavopulmonary shunt? Circulation 1995;92:II240–II244.

86. Triedman JK, Bridges ND, Mayer JE Jr, Lock JE. Prevalence and risk factors for aortopulmonary collateral vessels after Fontan and bidirectional Glenn procedures. J Am Coll Cardiol 1993;22:207–215.

87. Ichikawa H, Yagihara T, Kishimoto H, et al. Extent of aortopulmonary collateral blood flow as a risk factor for Fontan operations. Ann Thorac Surg 1995;59:433–437.

88. McElhinney DB, Petrossian E, Reddy VM, et al. Extracardiac conduit Fontan procedure without cardiopulmonary bypass. Ann Thorac Surg 1998;66:1826–1828.

89. Uemura H, Yagihara T, Yamashita K, et al. Establishment of total cavopulmonary connection without use of cardiopulmonary bypass. Eur J Cardiothorac Surg 1998;13:504–508.

90. Azakie A, McCrindle BW, Van Arsdell G, et al. Extracardiac conduit versus lateral tunnel cavopulmonary connections at a single institution: impact on outcomes. J Thorac Cardiovasc Surg 2001;122:1219–1228.

91. Celermajer DS, Bull C, Till JA, et al. Ebstein's anomaly: presentation and outcome from fetus to adult. J Am Coll Cardiol 1994;23:170–176.

92. Gentles TL, Mayer JE, Jr., Gauvreau K, et al. Fontan operation in five hundred consecutive patients: factors influencing early and late outcome. J Thorac Cardiovasc Surg 1997;114:376–391.

93. Kaulitz R, Luhmer I, Bergmann F, Rodeck B, Hausdorf G. Sequelae after modified Fontan operation: postoperative haemodynamic data and organ function. Heart 1997;78:154–159.

94. Bridges ND, Mayer JE, Jr., Lock JE, et al. Effect of baffle fenestration on outcome of the modified Fontan operation. Circulation 1992;86:1762–1769.

95. Bridges ND, Lock JE, Castaneda AR. Baffle fenestration with subsequent transcatheter closure. Modification of the Fontan operation for patients at increased risk. Circulation 1990;82:1681–1689.

96. Buheitel G, Hofbeck M, Tenbrink U, Leipold G, vd Emde J, Singer H. Possible sources of right-to-left shunting in patients following a total cavopulmonary connection. Cardiol Young 1998;8:358–363.

97. Premsekar R, Monro JL, Salmon AP. Diagnosis, management, and pathophysiology of post-Fontan hypoxaemia secondary to Glenn shunt related pulmonary arteriovenous malformation. Heart 1999;82:528–530.

98. Shekerdemian LS, Bush A, Shore DF, Lincoln C, Redington AN. Cardiopulmonary interactions after Fontan operations: augmentation of cardiac output using negative pressure ventilation. Circulation 1997;96:3934–3942.

99. Shekerdemian LS, Shore DF, Lincoln C, Bush A, Redington AN. Negative-pressure ventilation improves cardiac output after right heart surgery. Circulation 1996;94:II49–II55.

100. Goldman AP, Delius RE, Deanfield JE, et al. Pharmacological control of pulmonary blood flow with inhaled nitric oxide after the fenestrated Fontan operation. Circulation 1996;94:II44–II48.

101. Kanter KR, Vincent RN. Management of aortopulmonary collateral arteries in Fontan patients: occlusion improves clinical outcome. Semin Thorac Cardiovasc Surg Pediatr Card Surg Annu 2002;5:48–54.

102. Kanter KR, Vincent RN, Raviele AA. Importance of acquired systemic-to-pulmonary collaterals in the Fontan operation. Ann Thorac Surg 1999;68:969–975.

103. Spicer RL, Uzark KC, Moore JW, Mainwaring RD, Lamberti JJ. Aortopulmonary collateral vessels and prolonged pleural effusions after modified Fontan procedures. Am Heart J 1996;131:1164–1168.

13
Vascular Rings and Associated Malformations

Carl L. Backer, Constantine Mavroudis, and Lauren D. Holinger

Historical Perspective and Surgical Milestones

The phrase *vascular ring* was introduced to the medical literature by Dr. Robert E. Gross. Gross was Chief of Surgery at Boston Children's Hospital and in 1945 reported the first successful division of a double aortic arch in a 1-year-old infant [1]. In that surgical report, Gross recalled the findings of an autopsy that he had performed 14 years earlier in 1931. The description of that infant is classic for patients with vascular rings causing tracheoesophageal compression.

In 1931, I performed an autopsy on a five-month-old baby who had had wheezing respirations since birth and had recently developed difficulty in swallowing. At this examination a ring of blood vessels was found encircling the intrathoracic portion of the esophagus and trachea in such a way that the esophagus was indented from behind, whereas the trachea was compressed on its anterior surface. The pathological findings at once suggested that a division of some part of the so-called "vascular ring" during life would probably have relieved the pressure on the constricted esophagus and trachea.

The phrase, *vascular ring* has now come to encompass a constellation of entities marked by a congenital compression of the trachea, the esophagus, or both. Vascular rings can be either complete rings or partial rings. The classification scheme that we have used at Children's Memorial Hospital is the one endorsed by the International Congenital Heart Surgery Nomenclature and Database Committee (Table 13.1) [2]. The two true anatomically complete vascular rings are the double aortic arch and the right aortic arch with left ligamentum. The *partial* rings that are included in this classification scheme are innominate artery compression syndrome and the pulmonary artery sling. Both partial and complete vascular rings present with similar symptoms, are evaluated by similar diagnostic techniques, and have similar surgical interventions, thus, it is logical to group them together under the heading *vascular rings*.

The operation performed by Gross that successfully treated a patient with a double aortic arch was followed by several other historical milestones in the field of vascular ring surgery. In 1948, Gross and Neuhauser were the first to suspend the innominate artery to the posterior sternum to treat innominate artery compression syndrome [3]. In 1953, Willis J. Potts and colleagues from Children's Memorial Hospital in Chicago performed the first successful repair of a pulmonary artery sling in a 5-month-old child with wheezing, dyspnea, and episodes of cyanosis [4]. The first successful use of pericardium to patch open the stenotic trachea of a child with complete tracheal rings was reported by Farouk Idriss and colleagues from Children's Memorial Hospital in 1984 [5]. These historical milestones are reviewed in Table 13.2.

Most children with vascular rings present with symptoms in the first few months of life and often require surgery within the first year of life. Because of the tracheal compression many of these patients have critical airway issues requiring specialized intensive care unit management. Fortunately, the great majority of these patients after surgical intervention will have essentially complete recovery of their airway and resolution of their respiratory symptoms. The first successful operation for a vascular ring was performed at our institution by Dr. Willis J. Potts when he divided a double aortic arch in 1947 [6]. Since that time we have operated on nearly 350 patients with different types of vascular rings. With the strong support from our Division of Otolaryngology, we have developed a comprehensive program here at Children's Memorial Hospital to treat these patients. This experience forms the basis for this chapter.

Embryology/Pathology

An understanding of the embryology of vascular ring development and the resultant pathology helps one understand the clinical presentation and surgical alternatives. The two classic studies of the embryonic development of vascular rings were reported by Congdon [7] and Edwards [8]. Congdon studied the human aortic arch system. Edwards proposed the model of the double aortic arch system and bilateral ductus arteriosus. Stewart, Kincaid, and Edwards published the classic *An Atlas of Vascular Rings and Related Malformations of the Aortic Arch System*, which summarized the pathologic, embryologic, and roentgenographic studies of these lesions [9].

D.S. Wheeler et al. (eds.), *Cardiovascular Pediatric Critical Illness and Injury*,
DOI 10.1007/978-1-84800-923-3_13, © Springer-Verlag London Limited 2009

TABLE 13.1. Classification scheme used at Children's Memorial Hospital.

Complete vascular rings
   Double aortic arch
   Right aortic arch with left ligamentum arteriosum
Partial vascular rings
   Innominate artery compression syndrome
   Pulmonary artery sling

TABLE 13.2. Historical milestones in treatment.

Year	Procedure	Surgeon
1945	Division of double aortic arch	Robert Gross
1948	Innominate artery suspension	Robert Gross
1953	Pulmonary artery sling repair	Willis J. Potts
1982	Pericardial tracheoplasty	Farouk Idriss

The possible embryonic aortic arch development patterns are shown in Figure 13.1. All humans start with six pairs of aortic arches connected to the primitive ventral and dorsal aorta. The development of a vascular ring results from preservation or deletion of specific segments of the rudimentary aortic arch complex that is different from normal. In most humans the first, second, and fifth aortic arches regress. The third aortic arches become the carotid arteries. A branch from the ventral bud of the sixth aortic arch meets the lung bud to form the pulmonary artery. On the right side the dorsal contribution to the sixth arch usually disappears. On the left side it persists as the ductus arteriosus. The subclavian arteries develop from the seventh intersegmental arteries arising from the dorsal aorta. Normally the right fourth arch involutes at 36 days to leave the usual aortic arch configuration. The apex of the aortic arch in this (normal situation) is to the left of the trachea. Whether a patient has a right aortic arch or a left aortic arch is defined by the relationship of the apex of the aortic arch to the trachea.

Double Aortic Arch

If both the right and left fourth arches persist, a double aortic arch is formed. The arches pass on both sides of the trachea and esophagus and join the descending aorta, producing a true complete vascular ring (Figure 13.2). The right arch is the posterior arch and gives rise to the right carotid and subclavian arteries. The left carotid and subclavian arteries arise from the usually smaller left anterior arch. In our surgical series, 75% of these patients had a dominant right sided arch. In 20% the left arch was dominant, and in 5% the arches were equal in size [10].

Right Aortic Arch with Left Ligamentum

If the left fourth arch involutes, a right aortic arch system is created (Figure 13.3). Depending on the site of interruption of the left arch and the branching pattern of the left subclavian artery, different configurations of right aortic arch are possible. The two most

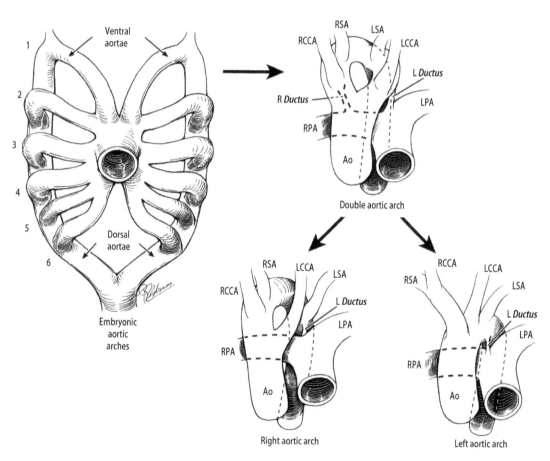

FIGURE 13.1. The embryonic aortic arches. In the embryonic aortic arch system the ventral and dorsal aorta (AO) are connected by six primitive aortic arches. The first, second, and fifth arches involute to form Edwards' classic double aortic arch. If the right fourth arch involutes, a normal left arch is formed. If the left fourth arch involutes, a right arch is formed. LCCA, RCCA, left, right common carotid artery; L, left; LPA, RPA, left, right pulmonary artery; R, right; LSA, RSA, left, right subclavian artery.

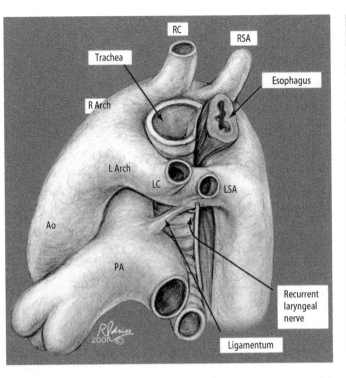

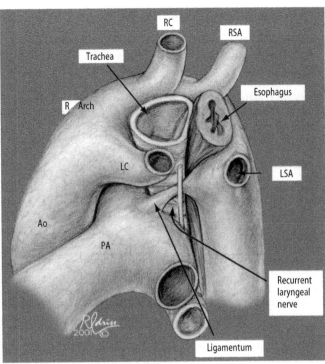

FIGURE 13.2. Double aortic arch, right arch dominant. The left carotid artery (LC) and left subclavian artery (LSA) originate separately from the left aortic arch (L Arch). Note tracheal and esophageal compression within the ring. Ao, aorta; PA, pulmonary artery; R Arch, right aortic arch; RC, right carotid artery; FSA, right subclavian artery.

FIGURE 13.3. Right aortic arch (R arch) with retroesophageal left subclavian artery (LSA) and left ligamentum arteriosum. The ring is formed by the right arch, pulmonary artery (PA), and ligamentum. Ao, aorta; LC, left carotid artery; RC, right carotid artery; RSA, right subclavian artery.

common variations are retroesophageal left subclavian artery (65%) and mirror-image branching (35%) [11]. It is the ligamentum arteriosum that completes the vascular ring in these patients. When the left subclavian artery has a retroesophageal origin from the descending thoracic aorta, the ligamentum typically extends from the descending aorta to the pulmonary artery, creating a vascular ring. If there is mirror-image branching of the left subclavian artery from a left innominate artery, typically the ligamentum originates from the innominate artery and a complete vascular ring is not formed. In an interesting embryologic association, one-third of patients with tetralogy of Fallot and truncus arteriosus have a right aortic arch. However, most commonly these patients have mirror-image branching and do not have a complete vascular ring.

Pulmonary Artery Sling

Pulmonary artery sling occurs when the developing left lung captures its arterial supply from derivates of the right sixth arch (not the normal left sixth arch) through capillaries caudad (rather than cephalad) to the developing tracheobronchial tree [12]. The left pulmonary artery originates from the right pulmonary artery instead of the main pulmonary artery. The left pulmonary artery courses around the right main bronchus and between the trachea and esophagus, forming a sling that compresses the distal trachea and right main bronchus (Figure 13.4). There is a strong association embryologically with complete cartilage tracheal rings causing congenital tracheal stenosis, the so-called ring-sling complex [13].

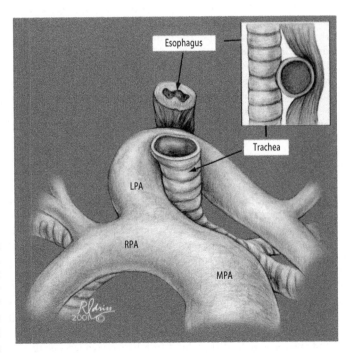

FIGURE 13.4. Pulmonary artery sling. The left pulmonary artery (LPA) originates from the right pulmonary artery (RPA) and courses between the esophagus and trachea to reach the left lung. **Inset:** Lateral view shows anterior compression of the esophagus.

Innominate Artery Compression

Innominate artery compression of the anterior trachea occurs when the innominate artery has a more distal take-off from the aorta than usual. Why the innominate artery in some patients causes severe compression of the anterior trachea and in others does not remains a question. It may be that some patients are more prone to tracheomalacia from the innominate artery compression than others.

Aberrant Right Subclavian Artery

In some patients with a left aortic arch the right subclavian artery originates from the descending thoracic aorta. In these patients the right subclavian artery traverses the mediastinum posterior to the esophagus. This produces a posterior indentation of the esophagus but does not form a complete vascular ring. This is the most common vascular anomaly of the aortic arch system and occurs in 0.5% of all humans. Because this is so common it has been blamed in the past for vague swallowing symptoms. It has hence earned the label *dysphagia lusoria* [14] or *difficulty in swallowing due to a trick of nature*. In actuality the aberrant right subclavian artery is nearly always a red herring and not the true etiology of the child's symptoms. At Children's Memorial Hospital we have not operated on a child with this diagnosis since 1973.

Rare Vascular Rings

There are other rare vascular rings that can be caused by various unusual deletions or failure of involution of portions of the embryonic aortic arch system. One of these is a left aortic arch, right descending aorta, and right ligamentum arteriosum. Another is a ductus arteriosus traveling from the right pulmonary artery to the descending aorta with an aberrant right subclavian artery (ductus arteriosus sling). Another is right aortic arch, right ligamentum, and absent left pulmonary artery. Robotin and colleagues reported three groups of unusual tracheoesophageal compression syndromes in a series of over 500 patients with vascular rings [15]. Patients with the *circumflex aorta* have a right aortic arch, left-sided descending aorta, and ligamentum arteriosum. They also described an unusual group of patients who had airway compression after the ascending aorta was moved during an arterial switch operation.

Presentation and Clinical Evaluation

An understanding of the embryology of these lesions and their anatomy leads to a better appreciation of their clinical presentation and the algorithm underlying a systematic clinical diagnostic evaluation. Most patients with vascular rings present with either symptoms of airway compression or swallowing issues when they progress from formula to solid food. The most common respiratory symptoms are stridor (noisy breathing), a *seal bark* cough, wheezing, respiratory distress, apnea, and recurrent respiratory tract infections. Dysphagia is usually for solid foods such as bread and meat and typically occurs in patients over 1 year of age. Neonates and infants may hold their head in a hyperextended position to splint the trachea and lessen the anatomic effect of the obstruction to improve their breathing. Patients with innominate artery compression syndrome may have apneic or cyanotic episodes precipi-

TABLE 13.3. Potential diagnostic imaging modalities.

Chest x-ray
Barium swallow
Bronchoscopy
Computed tomography with contrast
Magnetic resonance imaging
Echocardiography
Cardiac catheterization

tated when they swallow food. The food presses on the soft posterior trachea within the restrictive confines of the vascular compression formed by the anterior compression on the innominate artery on the trachea.

The diagnosis of a vascular ring requires a high index of suspicion because of the relative infrequency of this diagnosis compared with other conditions that may cause respiratory issues in children. These include asthma, gastroesophageal reflux, and upper respiratory tract infections. The diagnosis of a vascular ring should progress in a stepwise fashion. Once the diagnosis has been made, further studies are not necessarily required if the surgeon has enough information to proceed with operative intervention. The diagnosis of a vascular ring starts with a plain chest radiograph. The other potential imaging modalities to be selected from are listed in Table 13.3. The chest x-ray should be evaluated for the location of the aortic arch in relationship to the trachea and tracheal compression sites (Figure 13.5). The chest-x-ray will also rule out other causes of respiratory distress, such as aspiration of a foreign body, pneumonia, and pneumothorax. Historically, the next recommended study for suspected vascular ring patients was a barium esophagram. The impressions produced in the barium-filled esophagus by the anomalous aortic arch or its branches are

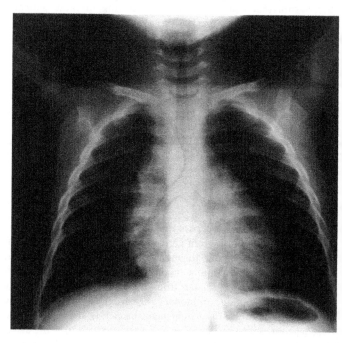

FIGURE 13.5. Chest roentgenogram of a 10-month-old boy with stridor. This film is significant for absence of left aortic knob. The tracheal air column has been highlighted to show the prominent right-sided compression of the trachea by a right aortic arch. The left side of the trachea is relatively straight.

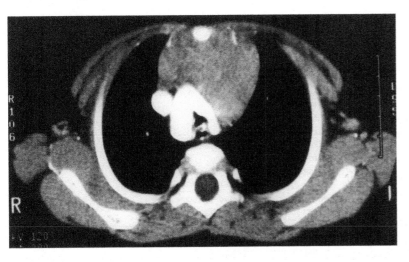

FIGURE 13.6. Computed tomographic scan with contrast of the mediastinum of an 11-month-old boy with severe stridor from a double aortic arch. Both the dominant right and smaller left arches are patent and enhanced by contrast.

characteristic for each of the lesions. However, determining the precise specific type of vascular ring with a chest radiograph and an esophagram alone is not always possible. With the evolution of computed tomographic (CT) imaging and the speed with which images can be obtained, the CT scan is now our diagnostic procedure of choice for patients with a suspected vascular ring [16]. A CT scan gives a precise anatomic diagnosis and demonstrates the degree and location of tracheal compression (Figure 13.6). The ultrafast CT scans are now obtainable in less than 20 sec of imaging time. A CT scan with contrast can be used for even the smallest neonate. The use of three-dimensional reconstruction gives a superb *road map* for the surgeon.

Although the barium esophagram may indeed strongly suggest the diagnosis of a vascular ring, it does not give the precise anatomic detail provided by the CT scan. In addition, an equivocal barium swallow is often of little use. The CT scan truly surpasses the barium swallow in its ability to transmit an incredible amount of information in a short period of time. The diagnostic sign that is most specific for a vascular ring is the *four-artery sign* [17]. This sign is seen on CT sections obtained cephalic to the aortic arch and consists of the two dorsal subclavian arteries and the two ventral carotid arteries evenly spaced about the trachea (Figure 13.7). The four-artery sign is present when the two dorsal subclavian arteries arise directly from the aortic arch and not from the brachial cephalic artery. This will occur with both the double aortic arch in

the patients with a right aortic arch with aberrant left subclavian artery. In patients with innominate artery compression syndrome the CT scan will show the anterior compression of the trachea by the innominate artery. In patients with a pulmonary artery sling the CT scan will demonstrate the left pulmonary artery originating from the right pulmonary artery encircling the trachea and coursing to the hilum of the left lung anterior to the esophagus and the aorta. In addition the trachea can be evaluated for tracheal stenosis caused by complete tracheal rings.

At some institutions magnetic resonance imaging (MRI) is more frequently used for the diagnosis of a vascular ring than a CT scan with contrast [18]. The disadvantages of MRI scans are that they require the patients to remain still for an extended period of time. This is not always possible for a small infant with respiratory distress. This may require more sedation than clinicians are comfortable with administering to a patient with respiratory issues. In our experience evaluating many outside films, frequently the MRIs are not of sufficient quality to be useful for preparing a surgical intervention. The advantages of MRI are that there is no requirement for intravenous contrast material and there is no ionizing radiation.

In a recent review of our patients with vascular rings, we found a high incidence of associated cardiac and airway abnormalities. Because of this we recommend routine echocardiography and bronchoscopy for all patients diagnosed with a vascular ring [16].

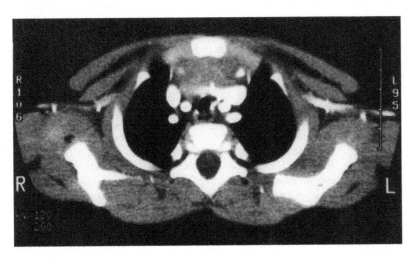

FIGURE 13.7. Computed tomographic scan with contrast of the same child shown in Figure 13.6. Note the four brachiocephalic vessels grouped symmetrically around the trachea.

The echocardiogram is performed to rule out associated congenital intracardiac anomalies, which were found in 12% of our patients. Bronchoscopic evaluation is used to assess the degree of tracheobronchomalacia and help to provide a prognosis for the family. In addition, in some patients unsuspected aspirated material has been discovered, such as chicken bones and pieces of plastic. Our routine currently is to obtain the intraoperative bronchoscopy at the time of the surgical approach to the vascular ring so that the patient does not require two general anesthetics. Some vascular ring abnormalities are of course discovered at the time of bronchoscopy for airway issues.

Cardiac catheterization was formerly used to diagnose vascular rings. Because of the noninvasive nature of the CT scan and MRI imaging and their precise anatomic diagnoses they have completely supplanted cardiac catheterization. The only patients for whom we now use cardiac catheterization are those with associated congenital cardiac anomalies that require catheterization.

Echocardiography can detect aortic arch anomalies but because of the limited windows it has not become a dominant diagnostic tool. The main problem with echocardiography is that the vascular ring segment without a lumen cannot be displayed. Hence, although the echocardiogram can occasionally pick up or suggest a vascular ring based on aortic arch branching, we do not use this for the definitive diagnosis of the anatomy of a vascular ring. The one area where we have found echocardiography to be very useful, however, is the evaluation of a patient known to have complete tracheal rings and tracheal stenosis for an associated pulmonary artery sling. Many of these patients are in the intensive care unit on a ventilator, and it is difficult to move them because of the precarious nature of their endotracheal tube. In this patient subpopulation, transthoracic echocardiography with color Doppler imaging can be used to diagnose a pulmonary artery sling and allow the surgeon to prepare the operative approach appropriately.

Surgical and Intensive Care Unit Management

An operation to repair a vascular ring is indicated for all patients diagnosed with a vascular ring that has symptoms. Early and appropriate surgical intervention is important to avoid serious complications that may arise from attempted medical management of a vascular ring. Some of these patients, particularly those with innominate artery compression syndrome, may have significant apneic or hypoxic episodes. Patients with a double aortic arch or right aortic arch with left ligamentum can develop respiratory syncytial virus infection or other pneumonias requiring tracheal intubation and prolonged hospitalization. Improper management of these patients with prolonged tracheal intubation and nasogastric feeding tubes can lead to an occasional catastrophic erosion of the aortic arch into the trachea or the esophagus [19,20]. Late complications of an unrepaired vascular ring include aortic dissection and aneurysm formation [21]. The surgical approaches to vascular rings are summarized in Table 13.4.

Double Aortic Arch

In nearly all instances, a double aortic arch can be approached through a left thoracotomy. The exception to this is the patient with a dominant left arch and a left-sided descending aorta. In these patients (who are quite rare), the safer approach is through a right thoracotomy to divide the smaller anterior right arch. The left tho-

TABLE 13.4. Surgical approaches to vascular rings.

Double aortic arch
- Left thoracotomy
- Division of smaller of two aortic arches between vascular clamps
- Preservation of blood flow to carotid and radial arteries
- Ligation and division of ligamentum arteriosum
- Pleura left open

Right aortic arch/left ligamentum
- Left thoracotomy
- Division and oversewing of ligamentum arteriosum
- Possible resection of Kommerell's diverticulum with transfer of left subclavian to left carotid artery
- Leave pleura open

Innominate artery compression syndrome
- Right anterolateral thoracotomy
- Resect right lobe of thymus
- Suspend innominate artery and ascending aorta to posterior sternum
- Intraoperative bronchoscopy

Pulmonary artery sling
- Median sternotomy/extracorporeal circulation
- Division and oversewing of origin of left pulmonary artery from right pulmonary artery
- Implantation of left pulmonary artery into main pulmonary artery anterior to the trachea
- Surgical attention to complete tracheal rings if present

racotomy is performed with a muscle-sparing technique, sparing both the serratus and latissimus muscles. The thorax is entered through the fourth intercostal space. The lung is retracted anteriorly. The mediastinal pleura is opened. Careful dissection of the posterior mediastinum is performed to define the anatomy of the vascular ring. In particular, structures that are identified are the left subclavian artery, the ligamentum arteriosum, and the descending thoracic aorta. Most frequently the left or anterior arch is the smaller of the two arches and is often atretic where it inserts into the descending thoracic aorta.

The vascular ring is released by dividing the smaller of the two arches most frequently at the posterior insertion site into the descending thoracic aorta (Figure 13.8). The arches are divided between vascular clamps after establishing preservation of flow to the carotid and subclavian arteries. In the patient with balanced aortic arches care must be taken to ensure preservation of blood flow to the lower half of the body. The arches are divided between vascular clamps carefully oversewing the two stumps with fine running polypropylene suture. In patients with a dominant right aortic arch the left ligamentum is always doubly ligated and divided to prevent the ligamentum from contributing to a vascular ring. If the left aortic arch is dominant, the ligamentum may be left in place as it will not contribute to vascular compression. Adhesive bands around the esophagus and trachea are lysed. The recurrent laryngeal nerve and phrenic nerve are identified and protected throughout the case. The mediastinal pleura is left open. This is an important technical point. Many of the patients that I have had to reoperate on had their pleura closed at the time of the original operation elsewhere. This later lead to scar tissue that caused recurrent tracheal or esophageal compression. In the majority of patients, the chest is closed without the use of a chest tube. The thorax is evacuated of air with a small suction catheter passed through the incision and pulled out as the incision is being closed. Most patients are extubated in the operating room. The patients spend an hour or two in the recovery room and are then transferred to the regular ward or the pediatric intensive care unit (PICU). The mean hospital

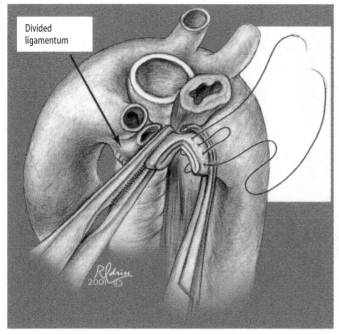
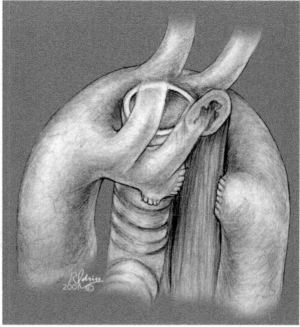

Divided ligamentum

A

B

FIGURE 13.8. Double aortic arch division. **(A)** Left arch partially divided between vascular clamps. Note the ligamentum has already been divided and oversewn. **(B)** Left arch divided, both stumps oversewn with fine Prolene suture. Note the esophagus and trachea are no longer compressed.

stay for an isolated double aortic arch repair is now 2 days. Because of the tracheobronchomalacia that was created by the vascular compression, many patients require up to a year for the barky cough to completely disappear.

The postoperative management of these patients can in some instances be rather tricky. Because of the preoperative tracheobronchomalacia from the tracheal compression when they are extubated, they show initial signs of respiratory distress with tachypnea and retractions. They frequently require treatment with humidified oxygen and often small doses of sedation to calm them and to prevent a vicious cycle of pain, increased respiratory rate, worsened tracheomalacia, followed by increased difficulty of work of breathing and more tachypnea. This cycle can be broken by the careful use of intravenous sedation with fentanyl, morphine, lorazepam, or midazolam. Often there is a sense that the patient may require reintubation. This impulse should be resisted as much as possible as the great majority of these patients will improve significantly in the first several hours following the procedure and often by the next morning will appear to have almost no respiratory issues whatsoever. The subgroup of patients like this requires monitoring in the PICU postoperatively.

Other modalities in the postoperative intensive care unit should the patient have respiratory issues are the use of helium–oxygen (heliox) [22] and a high-flow nasal cannula (Vapotherm) [23]. Heliox works by allowing passage of less dense air through a narrow trachea, easing the child's work of breathing. Vapotherm provides positive pressure and humidity, which is very important to keep the patient's airway from drying out with a high flow of gas. Other modalities that we have used in the postoperative period are inhaled corticosteroids, albuterol treatments, and intravenous corticosteroids. In our experience, if the patient can remain extubated for the first 4 to 6 hr postoperatively, they will almost always maintain that

extubated status and go on to steady improvement in their airway. In a few rare circumstances we have had to provide these infants with prolonged intubation and, in even rarer circumstances, tracheostomy.

Right Aortic Arch with Left Ligamentum

The surgical management of patients with right aortic arch with left ligamentum is similar to that of the double aortic arch patients. The approach is nearly always through a left thoracotomy with a muscle-sparing approach. The lung is retrached anteriorly and the pleura is opened. The ligamentum arteriosum is identified, along with the left subclavian artery and the descending thoracic aorta. The ligamentum can be either doubly ligated and divided or doubly clamped and divided with the two stumps oversewn (Figure 13.9). Adhesive bands are lysed, and attention is paid to preserving the recurrent laryngeal nerve and phrenic nerves. The pleura is left open. Closure and postoperative management are similar to those for the double aortic arch patients, but the postoperative course in general is more benign.

There is an interesting subpopulation of patients with a right aortic arch and left ligamentum who have aneurysmal dilatation of the base of the left subclavian artery where it originates from the descending thoracic aorta. This aneurysm is called a Kommerell's diverticulum and it is embryologically a remnant of the left fourth aortic arch (Figure 13.10). This diverticulum may enlarge to a size where it can independently compress the esophagus or trachea. Our experience with having to perform a reoperation on patients with a Kommerell's diverticulum that was left in place during the initial ligamentum division has led us to recommend primary resection of the Kommerell's diverticulum and transfer of the left subclavian artery to the left carotid artery (Figure 13.11) [24]. We have now

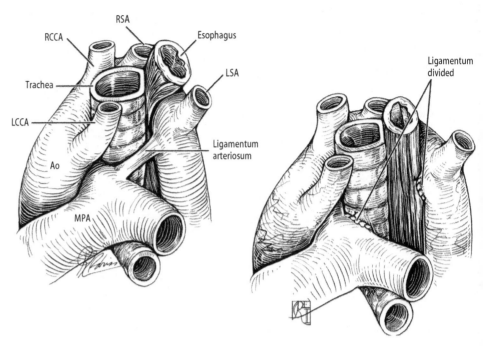

Figure 13.9. Right aortic arch—division and over-sewing of ligamentum arteriosum. Ao, Aorta; LCCA, RCCA, left, right common carotid artery; LSA, RSA, left, right subclavian artery; MPA, main pulmonary artery.

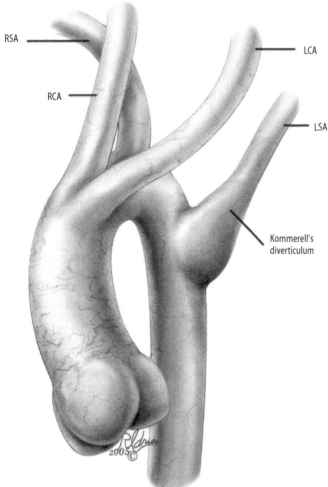

Figure 13.10. The origin of the left subclavian artery (LSA) in some patients with a right aortic arch is an aneurysmal embryologic remnant of the left fourth arch. This is called a Kommerell's diverticulum. RCA, right carotid artery; RSA, right subclavian artery; LCA, left carotid artery.

performed this as a secondary procedure (reoperation) in 10 patients and as a primary operation in 7 patients.

Another unusual group of patients have a right aortic arch, a left ligamentum, and a left-sided descending aorta, the *circumflex aorta*. Because the aorta crosses posteriorly behind the trachea, the tracheal compression may not be significantly relieved by division of the ligamentum. In a very small group of patients, an aortic uncrossing procedure may be required. We have performed this in one patient at Children's Memorial Hospital. Robotin et al. reported 3 patients out of 468 vascular ring patients having this procedure in France [15]. This operation is performed through a median sternotomy with the use of cardiopulmonary bypass and circulatory arrest. The aorta is divided and then brought anterior to the trachea, where an anastomosis is performed to recreate a normal left aortic arch.

Innominate Artery Compression Syndrome

Innominate artery compression syndrome was originally treated by Gross through a left anterolateral thoracotomy with suspension of the innominate artery to the posterior aspect of the sternum. That technique is still used at Boston Children's Hospital [25]. At our institution we have preferred a small right inframammary anterolateral thoracotomy. The innominate artery is secured with pledget-supported sutures to the posterior periosteum of the sternum. Typically three separate mattress sutures are used. One is on the anterior surface of the ascending aorta, the second is at the junction between the innominate artery and the aorta, and the third is on the innominate artery itself. Intraoperative bronchoscopy is performed to confirm the suspension, providing relief of the tracheal compression. The right radial pulse is monitored with pulse oximetry or an arterial line to confirm that there is no compression of the subclavian or innominate artery. An alternative technique has been described using a median sternotomy incision with division and transfer of the innominate artery to a site more to the right and anterior to the native site [26]. We have not utilized this technique, as it sacrifices the active suspending mechanism provided by pulling the innominate artery anteriorly, leaving the adhesions between the trachea and innominate artery intact.

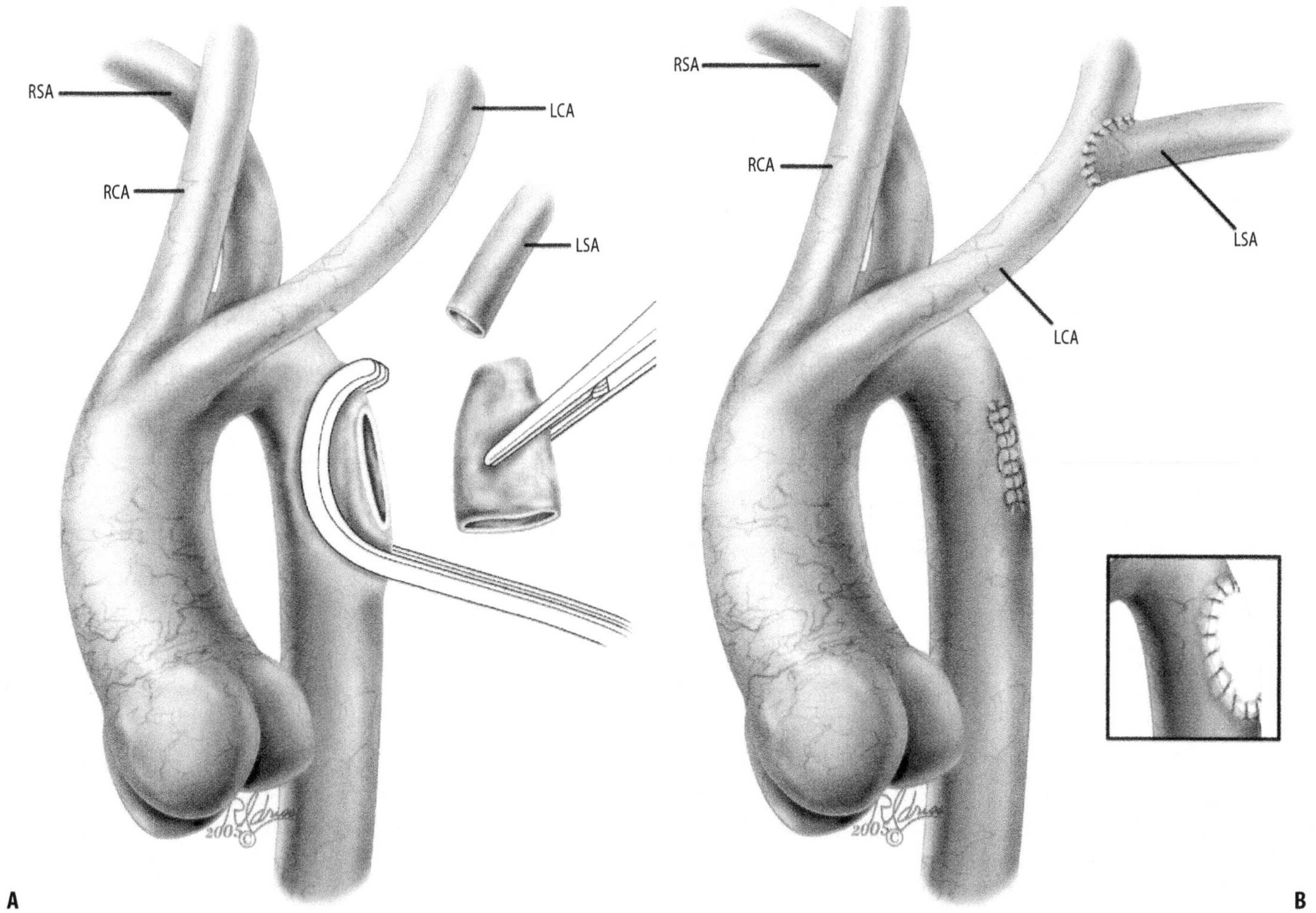

FIGURE 13.11. (A) Resection of a Kommerell's diverticulum through a left thoracotomy. There is a vascular clamp partially occluding the descending thoracic aorta at the origin of the Kommerell's diverticulum. The clamp on the left subclavian artery is not illustrated. The Kommerell's diverticulum has been completely resected. (B) The completed repair. The orifice at which the Kommerell's diverticulum was resected is usually closed primarily. The orifice can also be patched with polytetrafluoroethylene if necessary (as shown in the **inset**). The left subclavian artery has been implanted into the side of the left common carotid artery with fine running polypropylene sutures. LCA, left carotid artery; RCA, right carotid artery; LSA, left subclavian artery; RSA, right subclavian artery.

Pulmonary Artery Sling

The first pulmonary artery sling repair was performed at our institution by Willis Potts in 1953 [4]. Potts operated on a patient who did not have a precise preoperative diagnosis. His approach was through a right thoracotomy. He made the diagnosis intraoperatively and doubly clamped and then divided the left pulmonary artery. He translocated the left pulmonary artery anterior to the trachea and reimplanted it into the main pulmonary artery. The child survived the operation and had relief of his tracheal compression. However, on long-term follow-up, he was found to have an occluded left pulmonary artery [27].

The next group of patients operated on for this diagnosis at our hospital were approached through a left thoracotomy. Again, the pulmonary artery was transected and reimplanted into the main pulmonary at a site approximating its normal origin. This approach continued to be associated with a high incidence of left pulmonary artery stenosis. Since 1985, all patients with pulmonary artery sling have been approached at our institution through a median sternotomy [28]. Cardiopulmonary bypass is used to support the respiratory function of the lungs while the operation is being performed.

The right pulmonary artery is mobilized and the origin of the left pulmonary artery from the right pulmonary artery divided between vascular clamps. The left pulmonary artery is then identified in the left posterior pericardium and is pulled up from posterior to the trachea into the pericardium anterior to the trachea. A site is selected for implantation of the left pulmonary artery into the main pulmonary artery that approximates the normal anatomy. This anastomosis is performed with interrupted suture technique to prevent late vascular anastomosis stenosis (Figure 13.12). With this technique (median sternotomy, cardiopulmonary bypass), all patients have had a patent left pulmonary artery. Mean flow to the left lung assessed by postoperative nuclear medicine perfusion scan has been 32%.

An alternative technique to division and reimplantation is to translocate the left pulmonary artery anterior to the trachea by dividing the trachea [29]. Many of these patients have associated tracheal stenosis and will require attention to their trachea. In particular, when a tracheal resection is performed, the trachea can be transected and the left pulmonary artery can be translocated anterior to the trachea. The difficulty with this technique is that, because of the severe rightward take-off of the left pulmonary

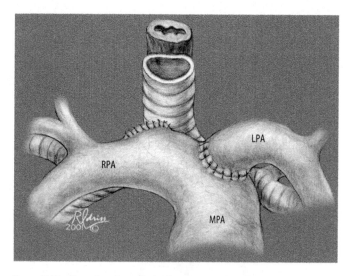

FIGURE 13.12. Illustration of a repaired pulmonary artery sling. The left pulmonary artery (LPA) has been implanted into the main pulmonary artery (MPA) anterior to the trachea. The origin of the LPA from the right pulmonary artery (RPA) has been oversewn with interrupted Prolene suture.

artery from the right pulmonary artery, even when the pulmonary artery is translocated anteriorly it still may be compressed and kinked because of its take-off so far to the right. van Son and colleagues compared the two techniques and thought that the translocation technique had a significantly higher incidence of left pulmonary artery stenosis [30].

If the patient with pulmonary artery sling does not have associated tracheal stenosis, the patient can usually be extubated within the first 24 to 48 hr following the procedure. The time to extubation in our experience is usually related to the age of the patient, with newborns needing somewhat longer to be extubated than older patients. The oldest patient in our series to undergo pulmonary artery sling repair was 10 years old.

For patients with tracheal stenosis associated with a pulmonary artery sling, an operation to repair the tracheal stenosis is indicated. We have utilized tracheal resection, pericardial tracheoplasty, tracheal autograft repair, and slide tracheoplasty for these patients [31]. Tracheal resection is our procedure of choice if the length of the tracheal stenosis is less than one third of the total tracheal length. For patients with a longer stenosis (long segment congenital tracheal stenosis), we prefer the slide tracheoplasty or tracheal autograft. These patients typically require postoperative ventilation for several days and in some cases longer. The tracheal tube acts as a stent to hold the trachea open in the initial phases of the healing process. The issue of tracheal stenosis has been addressed previously in this textbook.

Outcomes

Our experience at the Children's Memorial Hospital from 1947 through 2005 with vascular ring surgery has been excellent. There has been no operative mortality from repair of an isolated double aortic arch since 1952. One patient out of 121 has required a reoperation for persistent symptoms arising from scar tissue near the divided posterior arch. There have been 105 patients with a diagnosis of a right aortic arch with left ligamentum; all have had

division of the left ligamentum. Seven patients have had simultaneous resection of a Kommerell's diverticulum and transfer of the left subclavian artery to the left carotid artery. All anastomoses are patent. There has been no operative mortality in this group since 1959.

We have had excellent results with innominate artery suspension, now having operated on 85 patients with no operative mortality and only two patients requiring reoperation for resuspension. All patients have had cessation of their episodes of apnea.

A total of 36 patients with pulmonary sling have been operated on at Children's Memorial Hospital, 28 with cardiopulmonary bypass. Tracheal stenosis requiring surgical intervention was present in 21 of those 36 patients (58%). The only mortality after pulmonary artery sling repair has been in those patients with associated long segment tracheal stenosis (3 deaths out of 36 patients = 8% mortality).

Conclusion

The diagnosis of vascular ring in infancy requires a high index of suspicion. These babies present with noisy breathing and varying degrees of respiratory distress. A CT scan with contrast is the single best diagnostic study to confirm the diagnosis and delineate the anatomy in preparation for an operation.

Double aortic arch and right aortic arch with left ligamentum are approached through a left thoracotomy. The innominate artery compression syndrome is treated by right or left anterolateral thoracotomy with suspension of the innominate artery to the posterior aspect of the sternum. Pulmonary artery sling is repaired through a median sternotomy with the use of cardiopulmonary bypass by reimplanting the pulmonary artery into the main pulmonary artery anterior to the aorta. These patients have a high incidence of associated tracheal stenosis, which can be addressed at the time of pulmonary artery sling repair.

Overall the outcomes of these children are quite good, and the long-term prognosis is excellent. Their airways will require attention from dedicated ear, nose, and throat and intensive care unit services in many instances during the first several days following the operative repair. Optimal outcomes depend on close collaboration between the divisions of cardiovascular–thoracic surgery; ear, nose, and throat; and the intensive care unit.

References

1. Gross RE: Surgical relief for tracheal obstruction from a vascular ring. N Engl J Med 1945;235:586–590.
2. Backer CL, Mavroudis C: Congenital Heart Surgery Nomenclature and Database Project: vascular rings, tracheal stenosis, pectus excavatum. Ann Thorac Surg 2000;69(Suppl):S308–S318.
3. Gross RE: Neuhauser EBD: Compression of the trachea by an anomalous innominate artery: an operation for its relief. Am J Dis Child 1948;75:370–374.
4. Potts WJ, Holinger PH, Rosenblum AH: Anomalous left pulmonary artery causing obstruction to right main bronchus: report of a case. JAMA 1954;155:1409–1411.
5. Idriss FS, DeLeon WY, Ilbawi MN, et al.: Tracheoplasty with pericardial patch for extensive tracheal stenosis in infants and children. J Thorac Cardiovasc Surg 1984;88:527–536.
6. Potts WJ, Gibson S, Rothwell R: Double aortic arch: report of two cases. Arch Surg 1948;57:227.

7. Congdon ED: Transformation of the aortic arch system during the development of the human embryo. Contrib Embryol 1922; 14:47.

8. Edwards JE: Anomalies of the derivatives of the aortic arch system. Med Clin North Am 1948;32:925.

9. Stewart JR. Kincaid OW, Edwards JE: An Atlas of Vascular Rings and Related Malformations of the Aortic Arch System. Springfield, IL: Charles C Thomas; 1964.

10. Backer CL, Ilbawi MN, Idriss FS, DeLeon SY. Vascular anomalies causing tracheoesophageal compression. Review of experience in children. J Thorac Cardiovasc Surg 1989;97:725–731.

11. Felson B, Palayew MJ. The two types of right aortic arch. Radiology 1963;81:745–759.

12. Sade RM, Rosenthal A, Fellows K, Castaneda AR. Pulmonary artery sling. J Thorac Cardiovasc Surg 1975;69:333–346.

13. Berdon WE, Baker DH, Wung JT, Chrispin A, Kozlowski K, deSilva M, Bales P, Alford B. Complete cartilage-ring tracheal stenosis associated with anomalous left pulmonary artery: the right-sling complex. Radiology 1984;152:57–64.

14. Beabout JW, Stewart JR, Kincaid OW. Aberrant right subclavian artery: dispute of commonly accepted concepts. Am J Roentgen 1964;92: 855–864.

15. Robotin MC, Bruniaux J, Serraf A, et al. Unusual forms of tracheobronchial compression in infants with congenital heart disease. J Thorac Cardiovasc Surg 1996;112:415–423.

16. Backer CL, Mavroudis C, Rigsby CK, Holinger LD. Trends in vascular ring surgery. J Thorac Cardiovasc Surg 2005;139:1339–1347.

17. Lowe GM, Donaldson JS, Backer CL: Vascular rings: 10-year review of imaging. RadioGraphics 1991;11:637–646.

18. Azarow KS, Pearl RH, Hoffman MA, et al.: Vascular ring: does magnetic resonance imaging replace angiography? Ann Thorac Surg 1992; 53:882–885.

19. Othersen HB Jr, Khalil B, Zellner J, Sade R, Handy J, Tagge EP, Smith CD. Aortoesophageal fistula and double aortic arch: two important points in management. J Pediatr Surg 1996;31: 594–595.

20. Heck HA Jr, Moore HV, Lutin WA, Leatherbury L, Truemper EJ, Steinhart CM, Pearson-Shaver AL. Esophageal-aortic erosion associated with double aortic arch and tracheomalacia. Experience with 2 infants. Texas Heart Inst J 1993;20:126–129.

21. Midulla PS, Dapunt OE, Sadeghi AM, Quintana CS, Griepp RB. Aortic dissection involving a double aortic arch with a right descending aorta. Ann Thorac Surg 1994;58:874–875.

22. Martinon-Torres F, Rodriguez-Nunez A, Martinon-Sanchez JM. Heliox therapy in infants with acute bronchiolitis. Pediatrics 2002;109:68–73.

23. Waugh JB, Granger WM. An evaluation of 2 new devices for nasal high-flow gas therapy. Respir Care 2004;49:902–906.

24. Backer CL, Hillman N, Mavroudis C, Holinger LD. Resection of Kommerell's diverticulum and left subclavian artery transfer for recurrent symptoms after vascular ring division. Eur J Cardiothorac Surg 2002;22:64–69.

25. Adler SC, Isaacson G, Balsara RK. Innominate artery compression of the trachea: diagnosis and treatment by anterior suspension. A 25-year experience. Ann Otol Rhinol Laryngeal 1995;104:924–927.

26. Hawkins JA, Bailey WW, Clark SM. Innominate artery compression of the trachea. Treatment by reimplantation of the innominate artery. J Thorac Cardiovasc Surg 1992;103:678–682.

27. Campbell CD, Wernly JA, Koltip PC, Vitullo D, Replogle RL. Aberrant left pulmonary artery (pulmonary artery sling): successful repair and 24 year follow-up report. Am J Cardiol 1980;45:316–320.

28. Backer CL, Mavroudis C, Dunham ME, Holinger LD. Pulmonary artery sling: results with median sternotomy, cardiopulmonary bypass, and reimplantation. Ann Thorac Surg 1999;67:1738–1745.

29. Jonas RA, Spevak PJ, McGill T, Castaneda AR. Pulmonary artery sling: primary repair by tracheal resection in infancy. J Thorac Cardiovasc Surg 1989;97:548–550.

30. van Son JA, Hambsch J, Haas GS, Schneider P, Mohr FW. Pulmonary artery sling: reimplantation versus antertracheal translocation. Ann Thorac Surg 1999;68:989–994.

31. Backer CL, Mavroudis C, Gerber ME, Holinger LD. Tracheal surgery in children: an 18-year review of four techniques. Eur J Cardiothorac Surg 2001;19:777–784.

14
Cardiopulmonary Bypass

Kelly M. McLean, John P. Lombardi, and Jeffrey M. Pearl

Historical Perspective

Before the advent and widespread availability of cardiopulmonary bypass (CPB), repair of congenital heart disease was limited primarily to palliative procedures such as shunts and pulmonary artery bands, or to brief intracardiac repairs with associated high mortality and morbidity rates. Fortunately, the development of CPB and subsequent advances has allowed the field of intracardiac repair to grow and develop over the past 50 years. John Gibbon first conceived of the idea in the 1930s, motivated by the death of a patient from a massive pulmonary embolus [1]. Heparin had already been discovered [2]. Dr. Gibbon and his wife, Mary, built the first CPB prototype from household items. The collaboration between the Gibbons and Thomas Watson Jr. of IBM [3] resulted in the first real prototype bypass machine. In 1953, Cecelia Bavolek became famous after undergoing the first successful heart repair with CPB. Unfortunately, subsequent attempts by Gibbon and others were unsuccessful [4]. The use of CPB fell out of favor in preference for vena caval occlusion with hypothermia and direct visualization. However, the inherent time limitations and risks of this technique precluded repair of more complex lesions [5–7].

To extend the safe period of cardiopulmonary support, cross-circulation utilizing an adult, usually the parent, was attempted. Not only did cross-circulation both lengthen available support time and improve visualization of defects, it also decreased the reaction to bypass in comparison with the earlier attempts at heart–lung machines [8–10]. Approximately 45 successful repairs were performed with this technique. Although no mortalities were reported, the technique put a healthy adult at risk [11]. Concurrently, research efforts focused on developing an adequate way to circulate and oxygenate blood outside of the body. By 1955, Kirklin et al. reported a successful series of repairs utilizing extracorporeal circulation [12]. Improved understanding and continued experience led to the introduction of the concepts of hypothermia [13], circulatory arrest [14], hemodilution [15], and myocardial oxygen demand.

The oxygenator, which facilitates the oxygenation of blood and the removal of carbon dioxide, is the key component of CPB. The first oxygenator capable of perfusing the entire body was a rotating screen. Blood was spread in a thin film over a screen that was rotated in a cylinder of oxygen. Agitation of the blood from the texture of the screen combined with the rotation increased oxygen exchange 800% over previous oxygenators [16,17]. Secondary to inefficient gas exchange, previous oxygenators could only provide adequate perfusion for a single organ and not the entire body [18]. Since then, three main types of oxygenators have been employed in CPB: film, bubble, and membrane [19]. Film oxygenators, of which the rotating screen is an example, were limited by their inefficiency of gas exchange with hemodilution, excessive prime volumes of up to five units of blood, and difficulty cleaning and sterilizing, although the rotating disk oxygenator, developed by Kay and Cross, was in clinical use for nearly 20 years.

The advent of the bubble oxygenator by DeWall and Lillehei in 1955 was a breakthrough because it required a smaller priming volume and was easy to clean and sterilize. Gases diffused through the large surface area of bubbles passing through the blood, allowing effective exchange of oxygen and carbon dioxide. Addition of a chamber in which the bubbles could settle out of the blood and incorporation of in-line filters reduced, but did not completely eliminate, gaseous emboli [20]. Because the design was efficient, inexpensive, and able to be mass produced, bubble oxygenators persisted as the oxygenator of choice until the development of the membrane oxygenator. The design was not without its limitations, however. The stress from the stream of bubbles and the direct contact of blood with gas traumatized the blood, creating microemboli and hemolysis [21,22].

The membrane oxygenator developed in parallel with the bubble oxygenator. In a membrane oxygenator, oxygen and carbon dioxide are exchanged through a microporous, gas-permeable membrane without actually contacting the blood. Avoiding introduction of bubbles directly into the blood significantly reduces the cause of bubble and microparticulate emboli and minimizes the trauma to the blood. The original membrane oxygenators were not without their drawbacks, however. Initially, membrane oxygenators required higher prime volumes, had a greater leak rate, and were

D.S. Wheeler et al. (eds.), *Cardiovascular Pediatric Critical Illness and Injury*,
DOI 10.1007/978-1-84800-923-3_14, © Springer-Verlag London Limited 2009

more expensive than the bubble oxygenators. Membrane oxygenators were saved for longer operations and extracorporeal membrane oxygenation (ECMO) [23]. In the 1980s, development of hollow polycarbonate siloxane fibers and improvements in manufacturing techniques neutralized the disadvantages of membrane oxygenators. Up to 7 m² of surface area could be generated with the hollow fibers [24]. Soon they replaced bubble oxygenators in CPB. Further material development of microporous membranes and other advances such as incorporation of heat exchangers continued to increase the flexibility and efficiency of membrane oxygenators [19].

Although advances in oxygenator development have had the most significant impact on CPB, other aspects of the CPB circuit have not been immune from evolution. In the early 1960s it was discovered that contact between the blood and artificial surface of the CPB circuit created microemboli. The material of the CPB circuit adsorbs protein onto its surface, altering both the balance and the structure of clotting factors in the blood [25,26]. In addition, clumps of platelets adhere to this protein monolayer, forming aggregates in the blood [27]. Incorporation of filters into the circuit reduced some but not all of the particles. Various materials for the CPB circuit have been investigated in order to alter its thrombogenicity. For example, heparin [28,29], phospholipids [30], and poly-2-methoxyethylacrylate [31] have been bonded onto CPB circuits or the plasticizer removed from the tubing [32] in hopes of decreasing the inflammatory response and consumptive coagulopathy triggered by CPB. In addition, advances such as integration of components, vacuum-assisted drainage, smaller cannulas and tubing, and remote pump heads, which miniaturize circuits, decrease the surface area over which blood and foreign material interact, thus decreasing the inflammatory response. Simultaneously, miniaturization decreases the circuit prime volume, further pushing the limit of the size of children who can be operated on without blood transfusion [32,33].

Components of the Cardiopulmonary Bypass Circuit

The CPB circuit consists of both hardware and disposable units. The hardware consists of several mechanical pumps positioned on a base with wheels. The pumps are interfaced with a computerized control panel that manages various monitors and safety devices associated with the pump. The disposables that make up the extracorporeal circuit are the venous reservoir, oxygenator, hemoconcentrator, cardioplegia delivery system, and arterial line filter.

Pumps: Roller Versus Centrifugal

The two main types of pumps used for CPB are the roller pump and the centrifugal pump. With the roller pump, polyvinylchloride (PVC) tubing is inserted into a raceway. The pump has two rollers that press the PVC tubing against a backing plate. As the rollers rotate, blood is propelled forward. Adjusting the rate of rotation changes the flow rate accordingly. With the roller pump, the degree to which the roller squeezes against the backing plate, also referred to as the *occlusion of the pump*, must be properly set. Over-occluding the roller pump damages the cellular components of the blood. Under-occlusion results in lower actual flow than measured.

Changes in afterload do not affect the roller pump. The roller pump, therefore, gives a constant output, regardless of changes in the patient's systemic vascular resistance. Historically, the roller pump provides continuous, nonpulsatile flow. New generations of roller pumps, however, can provide pulsatile flow.

The centrifugal pump uses a different mechanism for propelling the blood. Spinning impellors or cones draw blood into the pump inlet, located in the center of the pump. The centrifugal force placed on the blood by the spinning action of the cones/impellors propels the blood through an outlet located on the outer circumference of the pump. Centrifugal pumps can be set to a pulsatile mode, which some institutions believe to be more beneficial to the patient. The centrifugal pump is both preload and afterload dependent. At a given rate of rotation, pump output can fluctuate, depending on the systemic vascular resistance of the patient. Previously, research comparing pulsatile to nonpulsatile flow has not shown the superiority of one type over the other. More recently, however, pulsatile flow has demonstrated improved coronary artery flow [34], renal perfusion [35] and function [36], and pulmonary function, as well as lower interleukin-8, endothelin-1, and catecholamine levels [36,37].

Cannulas

To initiate bypass, large-bore catheters are placed in the heart. Venous cannulas, designed for insertion into the right side of the heart, come in three designs: two stage, right angle, and lighthouse tip. The appropriate cannula type is selected based on the type of surgical repair and the cardiac anatomy of the patient. A single venous cannula is placed in the right side of the heart when the repair is limited to the left heart and no septal defects are present or if complete isolation of venous return to the heart is needed for visualization. For cases involving repair to the right side of the heart or in the presence of atrioventricular septal defects, both vena cavae are cannulated directly. The presence of a left superior vena cava requires a third cannulation. A cannula inserted in the ascending aorta returns blood to the patient.

"Venting" the Heart During Bypass

Distension of the left ventricle is extremely detrimental to the myocardium and must be avoided. An additional catheter, a left ventricular vent, may be inserted in the left heart via the superior right pulmonary vein or left atrial appendage in order to remove volume accumulating during CPB. Sources of blood that empty directly into the heart chambers include coronary vessels (arterial luminal, thebesian veins, and arteriosinusoidal vessels), collateral vessels from the pericardial circulation, and aortopulmonary collaterals. The volume in the left ventricle is actively removed via roller pump. The heart is also de-aired via the left ventricle vent. After the intracardiac repair is complete, the surgeon fills the heart with irrigation. Any air in the heart is evacuated via the left ventricle vent before removal of the aortic cross clamp. An additional "vent" may be placed in the ascending aorta by attaching tubing from the cardioplegia cannula to the low-pressure venous line. The vent aids clearance of air before cross-clamp removal, as well as allowing any residual air ejected by the heart to be removed before and after termination of CPB. Because this passive vent siphons off aortic flow, an increased pump flow rate may be required to compensate.

The Venous Reservoir

At the initiation of CPB, the venous line is opened. Blood returning to the right side of the heart is drained out of the patient into the venous reservoir. Simultaneously, the pump is turned on to provide arterial flow to the patient. The reservoir allows the perfusionist to monitor venous drainage while CPB is ongoing and provides a margin of safety during CPB. Adequate venous drainage keeps the operative field free from blood and the patient well perfused. The two main types of venous reservoir are open and closed. In an open system, the reservoir, also referred to as a *hard-shell* reservoir because it is made of polycarbonate, is vented to the atmosphere. The hard-shell reservoir has an integral filter coated with anti-foam A that prevents any large gaseous or particulate emboli in the venous line from entering the CPB circuit. If the reservoir empties completely, however, air may be introduced into the CPB circuit. The closed system, also called a *soft-shell reservoir*, on the other hand, consists of a soft bag that safeguards the system. If venous drainage is compromised, the bag collapses, preventing room air from entering the circuit. Because the blood is not continuously exposed to an integral filter or air, as in the open reservoir, the closed system is less traumatic to the blood than the open system [38].

Cardiopulmonary bypass utilizes three types of venous drainage: gravity, kinetic assist, and vacuum-assisted venous return (VAVR). The size of the cannula placed in the heart, the tubing size of the venous line, and the height difference between the patient and the venous reservoir all determine the effectiveness of gravity drainage. In essence, blood is siphoned from the patient. Gravity drainage is the most widely accepted mechanism for venous drainage. With the advent of minimally invasive surgery and microcircuitry, other methods have been developed to overcome the limitations of gravity drainage. In kinetic assist, a centrifugal pump placed in the venous line actively draws volume out of the patient. Similarly, in VAVR, a regulated vacuum applied to the venous reservoir suctions volume away from the patient. Addition of these advancements to gravity venous return enables the cannula and tubing size to be decreased while still providing adequate venous drainage. Vacuum-assisted venous return may, however, pass more gaseous microemboli to the patient than gravity drainage alone [39–42].

Cardiotomy Suction

Cardiotomy suction allows conservation of blood during CPB. Via an additional roller pump, blood and irrigation are removed from the operative field and returned to the venous reservoir, becoming part of the patient's circulating blood volume. Cardiotomy suction may begin once both arterial and venous cannulas are placed, the patient is fully heparinized, and the coagulation status of the patient is confirmed by an activated clotting time greater than 480 sec. Pump suction must be discontinued once protamine is administered.

The Oxygenator with Integral Heat Exchanger

The oxygenator provides the gas exchange in the CPB circuit. The practice of CPB did not become routine until inexpensive, disposable oxygenators were designed. Currently, the hollow fiber membrane oxygenator is used for CPB. Desaturated blood from the venous reservoir is actively pumped over the outside of the hollow fibers within the oxygenator housing while an oxygen/air mixture flows through the interior lumen of the hollow fibers, with gas exchange occurring across the fiber. Adjusting the rate of sweep gas across the oxygenator normalizes the pCO_2, whereas adjusting the FiO_2 alters the pO_2.

The efficiency of an oxygenator, compared with the native lung, is limited by two factors. The first is the diffusion distance. In the native lung, red blood cells pass through the pulmonary capillary one cell at a time, where the membrane thickness is only 0.5 μm. With the oxygenator, however, the membrane thickness is 150 μm. Surface area is the other limiting factor. The oxygenator typically has a surface area less than 10% that of the native lung. Modern engineering has incorporated designs that overcome these limitations. Increasing the length the blood travels across the gas exchange surface (250,000 μm for the oxygenator vs. only 200 μm for the native lung) increases the effective surface area. In addition, the surface of the hollow fiber is irregular promoting mixing of the desaturated blood that improves oxygenation. Furthermore, ventilating the oxygenator with 1.00 FiO_2 increases the gradient across the membrane [43].

In the early days of CPB, the heat exchanger was a separate component of the circuit. Today, the oxygenators contain an integral heat exchanger, a metal coil that contacts the blood as it enters the oxygenator. Water passing through the coil alters the core temperature of the patient accordingly. For longer procedures, the patient is actively cooled to decrease metabolic requirements. The heat exchanger allows the patient temperature to be controlled during CPB.

Hemofiltration and Ultrafiltration

A hemofilter concentrates diluted blood during CPB. Originally utilized when patients with compromised renal function were placed on CPB, the hemofilter consists of a semipermeable membrane filter that removes plasma water and low-molecular-weight solutes from the cellular components and plasma proteins in the blood. This process is more simplistic than hemodialysis in that a dialysate solution is not required. Instead, the hydrostatic pressure gradient across the filter membrane is the driving force. The membrane pore size determines what soluble plasma molecules will be removed. The pore size is usually 10–35 Å, allowing molecules up to 20,000 Daltons to be filtered [44].

Cardioplegia Delivery

The cardioplegia delivery system is the portion of the circuit that infuses cardioplegic solution into the aortic root, the coronary sinus, or directly into the coronary ostia. The system consists of a roller pump, heat exchanger, and tubing. For blood cardioplegia, arterial blood is drawn off the main CPB circuit and mixed with the high-potassium cardioplegic solution. When mixed 4:1 with the blood, a concentration of 20–25 mEq/L of potassium (high-K solution) or 8–12 mEq/L (low-K solution) is delivered to the myocardium. The blood passes through a heat exchanger, cooling it to 2°–4°C for cold doses. The solution arrests the heart in diastole. The system pressure is closely monitored to avoid exposing the coronary circulation to excessive pressure.

When administering antegrade cardioplegia, the cardioplegia cannula is placed in the ascending aorta, between the aortic cannula and the base of the heart. With the aorta cross-clamped, this cannula infuses cardioplegia into the coronary arteries in a forward direction. The aortic valve must be competent in order to give antegrade cardioplegia. Retrograde and ostial perfusions are alternatives to antegrade cannulation. In retrograde cardioplegia, the coronary sinus is cannulated with a balloon tip catheter, and perfusate is delivered to the coronary arteries in a retrograde fashion. For ostial cardioplegia, another specialized cannula is used in which the surgeon holds the tip of in the coronary ostia while cardioplegia is administered.

Tubing

All of the components of the circuit described above are connected together with tubing. Tubing within the extracorporeal circuit needs to meet several specifications. Cardiopulmonary bypass tubing needs to be transparent, flexible, and kink resistant. In addition, it must re expand after compression, resist cracks and rupture, have a low spallation rate, tolerate heat sterilization, and be compatible with blood. Medical grade PVC tubing has all of these characteristics [45]. Polyvinylchloride tubing has been modified with heparin coating, but research has failed to show that adding heparin coating is truly more biocompatible. More recently, new types of surface-modified additive tubing have been developed. This new process attempts to mimic the endothelial cell surface by using two copolymers on the inner lumen of the tubing, with alternating hydrophilic and hydrophobic groups. Research has shown that these new types of coatings better preserve platelet levels [46] and, when used in combination with methylprednisolone, significantly decrease inflammatory mediators after CPB [47].

Prime Constituents

The entire extracorporeal circuit is primed using a pH-balanced electrolyte solution. Before prime solution is added, the circuit is flushed with CO_2 to displace the air within the circuit. This makes the circuit easier to de-air, because CO_2 is more soluble than room air. Once the circuit is primed and de-aired, heparin, mannitol, and bicarbonate are added. Other additives may include corticosteroids, antibiotics, and albumin. At our institution, we keep our hematocrit greater than 25 during CPB which, for patients less than 10 kg, requires the addition of blood to the prime. The blood is *normalized* by washing with plasmalyte A and adding bicarbonate. The blood gas of the prime is adjusted to the normal values for arterial blood, with the exception of the ionized calcium, which is left below normal. Whole blood is added for patients under 10 kg and for reoperative patients under 40 kg although the advantage is controversial [48]. The circuit may be primed with either fresh packed red blood cells (PRBCs) or old PRBCs that contain storage media. Although the initial potassium and lactate levels are higher and the glucose level and pH are lower when priming with old blood, the differences can resolve after circulation of the priming solution for 20 min [49]. Although another study found that, upon initiation of CPB, lactate levels increased in the old-blood group, outcomes were not affected [50]. To avoid graft-versus-host disease, at our institution all PRBCs for immunocompromised patients and patients younger than 6 months are irradiated and leukocyte depleted.

Safety Features

Many safety features are integrated into the extracorporeal circuit. With open venous reservoirs, a level detector is placed on the reservoir. This electronic sensor is interfaced with the arterial pump to give visual and acoustic alarms and can be set to automatically shut the pump off if the level in the reservoir drops below the sensor, preventing room air from entering the circuit in the event that venous drainage is compromised. Another safety device, the bubble detector, is an ultrasonic sensor that is clamped around the extracorporeal tubing either between the oxygenator and arterial line filter or distal to the arterial line filter. When bubbles with a diameter greater than or equal to 300 µm (Stockert S III System COBE Cardiovascular, Inc.) are detected, the pump automatically shuts off. Several filters used within the extracorporeal circuit reduce the gaseous and particulate microemboli passed to the patient. During the priming process, a pre-bypass filter removes any debris that may be present from the manufacturing process as well as reduces contamination from the endotoxins found in priming solutions [51]. Because of its small pore size (0.2 µm), this filter is removed from the circuit before the addition of blood. An arterial line filter with a pore size of 32 µm is placed distal to the oxygenator, the last point at which emboli can be removed from the perfusate.

Conduct of Cardiopulmonary Bypass

Phases of Cardiopulmonary Bypass: Initiation, Cross-Clamping, and Termination

Cardiopulmonary bypass is initiated by opening the venous line and simultaneously dialing the arterial pump to the appropriate flow rate. A cardiac index of 2.5–3.0 L/min/m^2 is the target flow rate at normothermia. Once the target pump flow rate is achieved, the patient's ventilator is turned off. Desaturated blood returning to the right side of the heart is diverted to the venous reservoir. This point, when the heart is ejecting very little volume, is known as *partial bypass*. If necessary, a left ventricle vent is inserted, and the heart is allowed to fill in order to avoid entrainment of room air. The cardioplegia cannula is inserted into the ascending aorta, between the aortic cannula and the base of the heart. During this time, the patient is cooled to the prescribed temperature. A cross-clamp is applied between the aortic cannula and cardioplegia cannula. Cold cardioplegia mixed 4:1 with blood is infused into the aortic root, filling the coronaries and arresting the heart. The initial dose of cardioplegia is 30 mL/kg, with a maximum dose of 1,000 mL. The snares on the venous cannula are tightened. This point, when all of the patient's blood is diverted to the CPB circuit and the heart is no longer beating, is termed *full bypass*. The surgeon is now able to begin an intracardiac repair.

During full bypass, cardioplegia is administered every 20 min to provide myocardial protection. Hypothermia is also held constant. As the repair is completed, the cardioplegia is warmed to 30°–37°C, and the systemic temperature is increased. The heart is de-aired via the active and passive vents. Warm cardioplegia is given for 1 min, and then the crystalloid portion is removed and the heart is perfused with warm blood. Electrical activity should return during this time. The cross-clamp is removed, and the patient is fully rewarmed. Calcium is normalized, the left ventricle vent is removed, and the patient's ventilator is restarted. The patient is now ready to be separated from CPB. This is known as *termination of bypass*. The venous line is gradually occluded while arterial pump flow is decreased, allowing the heart to fill and take over the work of pumping blood throughout the body. Arterial pressure, left atrial pressure, and central venous pressure are monitored to assess the hemodynamics of the patient. Once the hemodynamics are optimized, the arterial pump is turned completely off, the patient is *off bypass*, and the cannulas may be removed.

Coagulation

By definition, CPB fulfills all major criteria for a procoagulant state: exposure of blood to foreign surfaces, potential stagnation of flow, and activation of the clotting cascade. Elevated levels of thrombin-antithrombin (TAT) [52], plasmin, antiplasmin, α_2-antiplasmin-plasmin, prothrombin fragment F1.2, and kallikrein and decreased prekallikrein and kallikrein inhibitor levels have been associated with CPB, indicating activation of the fibrinolytic, coagulation, and kallikrein pathways [53]. Contact of blood with the foreign surface of the CPB circuit deposits fibrinogen and fibrin onto the circuit, to which thrombin and platelets adhere. This collection of thrombin transforms prothrombin to thrombin, perpetuating the cascade. Although heparin may prevent thrombus formation, because of a conformational change in thrombin, it cannot inhibit thrombin bound to the circuit [54]. Increased secretion of tissue plasminogen activator (tPA), generation of plasmin, and degradation of fibrin indicate activation of the fibrinolytic pathway as well. This milieu sets up the potential for a consumptive coagulopathy associated with both clotting and bleeding [55].

Multiple factors, including hemodilution, transfusion, cyanosis, and an immature coagulation system [56], combine to place the neonate and infant at greater risk of bleeding. Cyanotic children have higher levels of TAT and tPA antigen [52], as well as increased tissue factor expression on endothelial surfaces [57] promoting a procoagulant state with a potential consumptive coagulopathy [58]. Hemodilution lowers platelet counts [59], whereas platelet contractile force [60] is increased after CPB. Platelet dysfunction, which results from CPB and from the generation of thrombin, a source of activation and degranulation of platelets [61], may be another cause of bleeding after cardiac surgery.

Anticoagulation for Bypass

Heparin, the common method of anticoagulation during CPB, is a cofactor for antithrombin III, an inhibitor of thrombin. Heparin may also anticoagulate by stimulating release of tissue factor pathway inhibitor, which inhibits tissue factor. Classically, heparin dosage is determined by measurement of the activated clotting time (ACT). This, however, may not truly reflect the level of heparin in the blood or the state of the coagulation system [62]. It has been suggested that heparin dosing based on heparin concentration rather than ACT results in less blood product usage and postoperative bleeding [63]. In general, heparin is administered at a dose of 300–400 units/kg, and a minimum ACT of 480 sec is required to initiate CPB. Heparin resistance can occur, and, if unrecognized, can result in low-grade activation of coagulation with consumption of platelets and procoagulants, resulting in both microemboli as well as postoperative bleeding.

Patients with prior heparin exposure can also develop heparin-induced thrombocytopenia (HIT) secondary to antiplatelet antibodies. On occasion, alternate modalities of anticoagulation are required for bypass in patients with contraindications to heparin. Two approaches have been used to anticoagulate patients with HIT. The first is to use direct thrombin inhibitors such as bivalrudin [64,65], lepirudin, or argatroban [66,67]. Hypersensitivity reactions

have been reported with lepirudin [68], and antibodies developed against lepirudin may cross-react with bivalrudin [69]. The other alternative is to inhibit platelet aggregation with agents such as tirofiban or epoprostenol, which then allows unfractionated heparin to be used for anticoagulation during bypass [70]. Warfarin therapy should be avoided until platelet levels return to normal, as earlier administration has been associated with limb gangrene and skin necrosis [71]. Danaparoid, which consists of heparin, dermatan, and chondroitin sulfates, has been successfully used to treat HIT but is not available in the United States [72,73].

Following termination of CPB, heparin is reversed with protamine sulfate. Derived from fish sperm, protamine, which is strongly cationic, binds to anionic heparin, forming an inactive compound. Heparin–protamine interactions occur in proportion to the weight rather than the activity of heparin. One milligram of protamine neutralizes 1 mg of heparin. Protamine dosing is generally based on the total amount of heparin given at 1–1.5 mg protamine for every 1 mg (100 units) of heparin. A heparin dose–response curve can also be utilized. Heparin bound to protein, or stored in fat, is not neutralized by protamine; thus, as it is released, a heparin rebound phenomenon may occur, necessitating additional small doses of protamine. Additionally, saved pump blood that is administered postoperatively contains heparin that can reanticoagulate the patient.

Reactions to protamine can occur, being more common in adults than in children. Diabetics who have received porcine-based insulin and men who have undergone vasectomy are at increased risk of protamine reactions. Protamine reactions are of three general types: systemic hypotension, pulmonary hypertension, and anaphylaxis [74]. Excess protamine may exacerbate bleeding tendencies by interfering with platelet function [63,75].

Antifibrinolytic Agents

Aprotinin is a serine protease inhibitor that inhibits plasmin and, at higher doses, kallikrein. Plasmin inhibition results in a significant antifibrinolytic effect yet does not increase thrombosis. Inhibition of kallikrein, which is produced from prekallikrein during activation of factor XII by the bypass circuit and surgical trauma, reduces activation of complement and decreases bradykinin release [76]. Initially, aprotinin was administered as either low dose or high dose. Early experience suggested an increased risk of thrombosis with aprotinin. Soon, however, it was recognized that this was secondary to inadequate heparin anticoagulation related to interference of aprotinin with ACT measurement using the standard Celite methods. Conversion to the Kaolin method allowed proper determination of ACT and, hence, heparin dosing. One of the benefits of aprotinin is its ability to preserve platelet function, even in patients treated with aspirin preoperatively. The favorable effects on platelets can be achieved with either the low-dose or high-dose protocol [77–79]. This effect on platelets has been hypothesized to be from inhibition of plasmin by aprotinin [80].

Significant data support the benefits of aprotinin. Mössinger and colleagues [81] found that high-dose aprotinin reduced both postoperative blood loss, as measured by chest tube drainage, and postoperative blood product usage in patients with a variety of cardiac anomalies. Both prothrombin fragments F1.2 and D-dimer levels were lower in the group receiving aprotinin, indicating reduced fibrinolysis. Times to extubation and to discharge from the intensive care unit were also shorter in the aprotinin group [81]. Dietrich and colleagues [82] had similar results. Comparison of three groups—high-dose aprotinin, low-dose aprotinin, or no aprotinin—demonstrated a dose-dependent reduction in markers of fibrin activation. Only high-dose aprotinin impacted blood loss after surgery [82]. Other groups have not demonstrated any difference in blood loss or blood product usage when aprotinin, either high or low dose, has been administered [76,77].

At our institution, we utilize a high-dose protocol that consists of an intravenous load of $1,715,000\,KIU/m^2$ and a pump prime load of a similar amount. A maximum combined loading dose is 4 million KIU for patients greater than $10\,kg$ and 2 million KIU for patients less than $10\,kg$. A continuous infusion of $400,000\,KIU/m^2/hr$ is infused during the operation and is usually stopped when the patient leaves the operating room. Aprotinin is a bovine protein that can induce hypersensitivity reactions, including hypotension, bronchial reactivity and spasm, and cardiac arrest. Although initial exposure is rather benign, repeated exposure carries risk. Beierlein and colleagues [83], in a literature review of all patients receiving aprotinin, found 124 reported cases of hypersensitivity reactions of which over 50% were life-threatening and 9% were fatal. Eighty percent of these patients had had previous exposure, the majority within 3 months [83]. Although rare, reactions can occur with first-time exposures. Administering a test dose before initiation of bypass is a standard of care, although it does not identify all hypersensitivity reactions. A test dose of $10,000\,KIU$ ($1\,mL$) is given. Presensitization may occur without prior intravenous administration by the use of synthetic cryoprecipitate glues, such as tisseal, which contain aprotinin.

Antihistamines may attenuate the hypersensitivity reaction [84]. In patients with previous exposure, absence of IgG in serum [83] or negative skin test has a high negative predictive value for hypersensitivity reaction [85], but positive correlation with either IgG or IgE levels is poor with only very high levels of IgG correlating with reaction [86]. In contrast, Jaquiss and colleagues reported equal occurrence of hypersensitivity reactions to aprotinin in spite of previous and number of times of exposure, 1% to 2.9% in pediatric cardiac patients.

Alternate anti-fibrinolytic agents used include episolon-aminocaproic acid (EACA), or Amicar®. The main anti-fibrinolytic property of Amicar is inhibition of plasminogen activator substances and an antiplasmin effect. Amicar is given as a bolus of $100\,mg/kg$ to the patient and a second dose in the bypass circuit. An infusion of $10\,mg/kg/hr$ is continued during the operation and can be continued for as long as 24 hours postoperatively. Although able to decrease perioperative bleeding, Amicar lacks the antiinflammatory properties of aprotinin.

In an effort to further decrease potential microemboli as well as consumption of clotting factors and platelets to decrease postoperative bleeding, heparin based coating of the CPB circuit has been introduced. Studies have shown lower fibrinopeptide A [87], tPA, tPA antigen, prothrombin activator peptide [88,89] and TAT levels [52], indicating both decreased coagulation and fibrinolysis. Heparin bonded circuits, along with improving pulmonary function, also decreased complement activation in pediatric patients resulting in improved coagulation after surgery as evidenced by lower prothrombin time [90].

Blood Gas Management During Cardiopulmonary Bypass: Alpha-Stat Versus pH-Stat

At our institution, we utilize both alpha-stat and pH-stat blood gas management: alpha-stat when the patient temperature is above 26°C and switching to pH-stat when cooling below 26°C. The main difference between the two strategies is the management of pCO_2. As the patient is cooled, CO_2 becomes more soluble because weak acids reassociate, which creates an alkalosis by reducing the H^+ concentration. With alpha-stat, blood samples are warmed to 37°C and management is based on these results, regardless of actual patient temperature. With pH-stat, blood gas results are corrected to the actual temperature of the patient. To maintain normal values for pH and pCO_2, the CO_2 must be increased relative to alpha-stat management.

Debate exists as to the best way to manage acid–base status while on bypass. In alpha-stat, as the patient cools the blood becomes more alkalotic. As a result, alpha-stat preserves intracellular pH, enzyme activity [91], cerebral autoregulation, and appropriate flow-metabolism coupling [92,93]. On the other hand, organ cooling is neither efficient nor homogenous [94]. With pH-stat management, pH and pCO_2 are maintained at 7.4 and $40\,mmHg$ at the patient's actual temperature. Hypercapnia vasodilates cerebral and coronary arteries, increasing blood flow to the organs. In addition, pH-stat shifts the oxygen–hemoglobin dissociation curve to the right, releasing more oxygen to the tissues [95]. As a result, organs receive both more oxygen and a more even distribution of oxygen/blood flow. Both warming and cooling are faster and more homogeneous [96]. Disadvantages are that pH-stat may place a greater acid load on the cell because normal buffering capabilities are impaired at hypothermic temperatures. Greater cerebral vessel dilatation is thought to increase the risk of cerebral microemboli and enhance reperfusion injury during rewarming [92].

At moderate hypothermia or warmer, little difference in effect is appreciated [97]. For deep hypothermia with circulatory arrest (DHCA), however, many centers use a combined approach to acid–base management. pH-stat is used for cooling when the vasodilator principles can be used to advantage by oxygen loading the tissues particularly when combined with hyperoxia before arrest. Postoperative acid–base status is improved in infants managed with a combination of hyperoxia and pH-stat [98].

More recent studies have demonstrated a definite advantage of pH-stat management over alpha-stat, while disproving the previously held beliefs that pH-stat increases microemboli and acid load. Infants treated with pH-stat over alpha-stat had decreased troponin T levels, decreased intensive care unit stay, and decreased time of ventilation [95]. Duebener et al. [94] demonstrated improved tissue oxygenation, decreased whole body lactate levels, and faster return of tissue oxygenation to baseline with pH-stat. Leukocyte adherence was not different between the two groups, although steroids were used in the pump prime [94,99]. Other studies have shown decreased rate of brain O_2 depletion [100], faster return of cerebral adenosine triphosphate and phosphocreatinine [101], and improved survival and neurologic outcome in piglets [102,103] and infants [104].

Myocardial Protection

Basic strategies for adult and pediatric myocardial protection are similar—reduce metabolic demand and provide an energy source and oxygen. Traditionally, CPB has accomplished these goals by arresting and cooling the heart, delivering oxygen either intermittently or continuously, maintaining acid–base balance, providing a metabolic substrate, and modifying reperfusion. Current innovative fields of research in myocardial protection include pre-ischemic conditioning, membrane channel openers, antiinflammatory agents, direct inhibitors of specific injury pathways, and gene therapy.

Sonnenblick et al. identified four determinants of myocardial oxygen consumption: intramyocardial tension, heart rate, basal metabolism, and energy associated with shortening against a load [105]. The combination of asystole, decompression, and hypothermia lowers myocardial oxygen demand by 97% [106,107]. The extent of ischemia determines the severity of reperfusion injury. Although ischemia itself may induce damage such as necrosis and cell death, greater injury occurs upon reperfusion. Minimize ischemia, and reperfusion injury will be minimized as well [108].

High-dose potassium cardioplegia arrests the heart in diastole by preventing myocyte repolarization. Because intramyocardial tension is reduced in diastole, traditionally this is considered a lower energy consuming state. Membrane ion channels, however, still require active transport to maintain depolarization. According to Cohen et al., however, arrest in hyperpolarization, the myocyte's normal resting state, may actually consume less energy [109]. Re-administration of cold, low-potassium cardioplegia every 20 min maintains myocardial protection by continuing to cool the heart, oxygenating and nourishing it, and washing out metabolites.

Systemic–pulmonary collateral vessels often complicate cyanotic congenital heart anomalies. Collateral blood flow threatens myocardial protection by washing out the cardioplegia solution, rewarming the heart, returning electromechanical activity, and distending the myocardium [110], which all increase myocardial oxygen demand. Decompressing the myocardium alone lowers oxygen demand by 30%–40% [111,112]. Blood from collaterals, in addition to coronary sinus return and leakage around the vena cavae cannulas, may also obscure the operating field. Placement of a left atrial or ventricular vent and snaring the vena cavae keeps the heart decompressed and the field clear [113,114].

Hemodilution

The additional volume of the CPB circuit requires priming with fluid to displace air in the circuit and maintain sufficient circulatory volume, particularly at initiation and termination of bypass. Originally, whole blood was used to prime the circuit, requiring as little as 2 units and as many as 5 or 6 units for one patient. As the increased frequency of cardiac surgery strained blood banks and the risks of blood transfusion became known, a shift to crystalloid-based primes occurred, hemodiluting patients' blood [115]. Although in adults this dilution may be negligible because the prime volume is only 25%–30% of the patient's total blood volume, in neonates the prime may be 200%–300% of the patient's total blood volume [114]. At our institution, the smallest circuit requires a prime of 600 mL. Most patients below 12 kg receive blood in their prime. Miniaturization of CPB circuits has reduced prime volumes, allowing asanguinous prime for infants as low as 5 kg, although some institutions are challenging even these limits. In a study of children of Jehovah's Witness, a 3.5-kg child with tetralogy of Fallot was successfully repaired without blood transfusion. The lowest hemoglobin on CPB was 7.3 g/dL [116]. In addition, Hubler and colleagues recently reported operating on a 2.2-kg neonate without blood transfusion while maintaining hemoglobin greater than 8 g/mL [117]. Techniques to minimize prime volumes included ultra-filtration throughout surgery, incorporation of a remote pump head, decreased tubing size to 5/32 inch, use of colloid in the prime and postoperatively, administration of furosemide postoperatively,

and transfusion of residual circuit blood after bypass. Ando and colleagues reported a series of limited or no blood exposure utilizing miniaturized circuits with low prime volumes. The lowest recorded hematocrit on bypass was 15.2% ± 2.4%, [118]. Although perfusion may appear adequate at low hematocrits, especially when hypothermic, evidence suggests detrimental neurologic effects of low hematocrits on bypass.

Lowering the hematocrit of blood decreases its viscosity and perfusion pressure, which then decreases the resistance of flow through smaller vessels where flow is usually lowest and viscosity highest [119]. In theory, this increases microperfusion, thus improving tissue perfusion [120], counteracting the effects of hypothermia [121]. At hypothermia microcirculatory flow is impeded at a hematocrit of 40% [122]. Increased passive venous return has been demonstrated in both dogs [123] and humans [124] with hemodilution. At normothermia hemodiluted kidneys (hematocrit of 21%) have demonstrated increased urine output and creatinine clearance versus nondiluted kidneys (hematocrit of 33%), supporting the theory that hemodilution may improve end-organ function with normal temperatures [125].

The apparent benefits of hemodilution, however, may not be so straightforward. Potential improvements in microvascular distribution must be balanced against decreased oxygen delivery at comparable flow rates and lower perfusion pressures. Although oxygen delivery to tissues can be maintained with a hematocrit as low as 10% [126], multiple studies demonstrate that higher hematocrits are necessary to maintain adequate end-organ oxygenation, particularly during cooling and warming. With cooling before DHCA, lower cerebral phosphocreatinine and increased cerebral intracellular acidosis were seen in piglets with a hematocrit of 10% compared with 20% and 30%. In addition, postoperative recovery of neurologic function was slower [127]. During warming after DHCA, microcirculation, as evidenced by lower functional capillary diameter, is also impaired at a hematocrit of 10%. At a hematocrit of 30%, microcirculation was not impaired [128]. Sakamoto and colleagues did show that with fixed perfusion blood flow cerebral blood flow did increase at a lower hematocrit [129]. In this study, however, microcirculation was not investigated, nor did the increased flow adequately compensate for the increased cerebral metabolic rates in the low hematocrit group. As a result, the increased blood flow may instead increase reperfusion injury, embolic phenomena, or edema [129].

The ideal hematocrit may be as high as 30%. In a prospective, randomized trial, Jonas and colleagues compared the psychomotor development at 1 year of age of children who had undergone hypothermic CPB as infants [130]. Those children whose hematocrit on bypass was less than 22% had lower psychomotor development scores that those whose hematocrit was maintained at greater than 27% [130]. In addition, the minimal tolerated hematocrit may vary with cardiac lesion. In a study comparing the repair of tetralogy of Fallot with ventricular septal defects, patients with tetralogy of Fallot repair became hemodynamically unstable and had impaired oxygen delivery at a 40% dilution, whereas the ventricular septal defect repairs were able to tolerate a dilution of 50% [131].

Hemodilution also dilutes clotting factors and plasma proteins. Neonatal livers are underdeveloped, particularly with a deficiency of vitamin K-based clotting factors. Hemodilution exacerbates this deficiency, as well as impairs liver function, thus increasing the risk of bleeding [132]. In a neonatal piglet model, liver perfusion was decreased in a low hematocrit (15%) versus high hematocrit (25%) group at all temperatures. Liver metabolism was also lower, with the lower hematocrit indicating decreased liver function [133].

For older, larger patients hemodilution can be used to advantage by deliberately lowering the hematocrit to 30% by removing pre-bypass blood. This sequestered blood has a full complement of clotting factors, functional platelets, and none of the inflammatory proteins activated by bypass. The blood is then transfused after CPB is completed. Few recent studies exist to evaluate this technique [134,135].

The Inflammatory Response to Cardiopulmonary Bypass

Multiple aspects of CPB initiate the inflammatory response. Initially, blood, particularly under high shear stress, contacting the artificial surface of the bypass circuit activates the alternative pathway of the complement system [136,137], triggering inflammatory proteins and activating leukocytes. Reversal of heparin with protamine at the termination of bypass forms heparin–protamine complexes that further activate the complement cascade via the classic pathway [138]. In many patients a baseline inflammatory response secondary to preoperative and surgical stress may also exist [139,140].

The early inflammatory proteins released during CPB, interleukin 1-β (IL-1β)) and tumor necrosis factor-α (TNF-α)) [141], synergistically [142] stimulate vasodilatation, increase vascular permeability [143], and propagate the immune response by production of the proinflammatory cytokines IL-6 and IL-8 [144]. Initially, TNF-α and IL-1β depress myocardial function by impeding calcium handling [145,146] and desensitizing β-adrenergic receptors [147]. Myocardial depression is sustained via the nitric oxide–inducible nitric oxide synthase pathway, which may contribute to myocardial stunning [148]. Additionally, both stimulate necrosis and apoptosis [149]. Interleukin-8 also attracts leukocytes and T lymphocytes [150], augmenting endothelial and myocardial cell death and potentially contributing to lung injury. Interleukin-6, on the other hand, has both pro- and antiinflammatory properties, stimulating the liver to produce acute phase proteins such as C-reactive protein and stimulating the production of IL-10 and IL-1β receptor antagonist (IL-1ra), both anti-inflammatory molecules [151]. Cytokine levels increase with increased bypass duration [152].

The cytokine profile has been correlated with both organ-specific injury and overall outcome. In sepsis, an increased IL-6 to IL-10 ratio is related to worse postoperative outcome [153]. In cardiac surgery, an increased level of TNF-α is related to worse postoperative heart, lung, liver, kidney, and ileum histologic tissue damage, whereas elevated IL-10 levels prevented damage [154,155]. Hövels-Gürich and colleagues also correlated elevated levels of IL-6 and IL-8 with increased myocardial damage postoperatively [156]. Postoperative arrhythmias have also been related to levels of IL-6 and histamine [157]. Additionally, a higher degree of complement activation and higher leukocyte elastase levels correlate with the development of multisystem organ failure postoperatively [158].

Children with congenital heart defects may enter surgery with already elevated levels of cytokines. Particularly, IL-6 and the ratio between IL-6 and IL-10 are chronically elevated in children with heart failure and/or hypoxemia. In addition, postoperatively levels remain higher longer than in other patients [159]. Although neonates tend to have an exaggerated stress response to cardiac surgery

with elevated levels of epinephrine, norepinephrine, and cortiso [160], they may still suffer a relative adrenal insufficiency [161] from a dissociation of the hypothalamic–pituitary–adrenal axis [162] Adrenal insufficiency has been correlated with increased inotropi requirement. Shore and colleagues demonstrated that postoperative steroid administration decreased inotrope dependence in neo nates after cardiac surgery [163].

Although minimized, CPB creates an ischemia–reperfusion injury in the heart characterized by intracellular build up o calcium that triggers an inflammatory response. The immature myocardium, with a lack of metabolic reserve and altered calcium handling, is particularly susceptible to injury [164,165]. Recent evidence implicates calpain and calpastatin, an endogenous inhibitor of calpain, as mediators of ischemia–reperfusion injuries [166,167] Calpains are a family of calcium-dependent cysteine proteases that degrade cytoskeletal proteins, contractile proteins such as troponin I, and regulatory proteins such as inhibitor of κ B (IκB). During reperfusion the intracellular concentration of sodium ions increases potentially as a result of a deactivated Na^+/K^+-ATPase pump [168,169], a reversed Na^+/Ca^{2+} exchange pump [170], and an accelerated Na^+/H^+ exchange pump [171,172]. Sodium ions are transported extracellularly in exchange for calcium ions, increasing the intracellular concentration of calcium. This intracellular accumulation of calcium activates calpain that degrades IκB, leaving nuclear factor κ B (NF-κB) free to translocate to the nucleus and initiate transcription of inflammatory proteins.

Pulmonary hypertension, particularly after the chronic hypoxia of cyanotic heart disease, is common after CPB [173]. Activated neutrophils accumulate in the lung [159,174], and markers of neutrophil activation such as myeloperoxidase activity are elevated [175]. Increased endothelin-1, a pulmonary vasoconstrictor [140,176], combined with decreased endothelial nitric oxide synthase (eNOS) activity [174,177], contributes to this phenomenon. Activation of calpain may also drive this complication, as inhibition of calpain decreases postoperative pulmonary hypertension, reduces endothelin-1 levels, and maintains eNOS activity [178]. Postoperative pulmonary hypertension is initially treated with inhaled nitric oxide. If the condition persists, patients can be transitioned to an oral phosphodiesterase-5 inhibitor such as sildenafil [179].

Multiple ways of inhibiting the immune response or mitigating the damage from it have been explored. Miniaturization of circuits reduces inflammation by both limiting contact between blood and artificial surfaces and reducing the need for blood transfusion. In piglets, Karamlou and colleagues demonstrated lower TNF-α and improved postoperative cardiopulmonary function in the group with a miniaturized circuit and no blood transfusion [180]. Whether the reduction in inflammation resulted from decreased blood–artificial surface contact or lack of blood transfusion is difficult to discern [180].

Heparin-coated circuits decrease the activation of complement and recruitment of neutrophils [181]. Controversy exists as to whether coating the circuit with heparin actually makes a difference when systemic heparinization is used [182]. The results have varied with type of coating/circuit used [181,183]. In a study by de Vroege and colleagues, patients placed on bypass with Bioline heparin-coated circuit were more hemodynamically stable intraoperatively and postoperatively than those with nonheparin-coated circuits [184]. Bradykinin, complement activation, and elastase, an indicator of neutrophil activity, were lower in the heparin-coated group even when patients also received aprotinin and dexamethasone [184]. Another study, by the same group, demonstrated improved pulmonary function as measured by PaO_2/FiO_2 ratio and pulmonary vascular resistance [185]. Tayama and colleagues demonstrated lower IL-6 and IL-8 levels, in addition to lower complement and elastase levels, in patients having a heparin-bonded circuit over a nonheparin-bonded circuit [186]. Neither study, however, demonstrated that the suppression of inflammation improved time to extubation, intensive care unit stay, or time to discharge. Palatianos and colleagues, on the other hand, did demonstrate a decrease in intensive care unit stay in patients treated with a heparin-coated circuit [187]. They also found lower TNF-α levels. Interestingly, they did not show a difference between the group treated with an entire circuit bonded with heparin and the group in which only the oxygenator and filter were treated [187].

Aldea and colleagues demonstrated decreased neutrophil elastase with the Duraflo II heparin-bonded circuit [188]. Removing cardiotomy suction further reduced neutrophil activation [188]. Cardiotomy suction is a significant source of red cell hemolysis and a potential source of cytokine and leukocyte activation [189] secondary to air–blood intermixing. A new technology—Smart System—reduces air–blood intermixing by turning on only in the presence of blood [190]. Although Smart technology does reduce hemolysis, it may not contribute significantly to reducing the inflammatory response [191]. Further studies are necessary to evaluate this technology. Intraoperative blood salvage devices themselves may reduce inflammatory mediators [192]. The minimal extracorporeal circulation system (MECC system), which combines all of the above features—reduced tubing length, full heparin bonding, and removal of cardiotomy suction—had lower postoperative complications and perioperative blood loss [193] as well as lower intraoperative levels of TNF-α, IL-6, and neutrophil elastase [194] compared with conventional circuits.

Aprotinin, a serine-protease inhibitor introduced initially for decreasing blood loss especially in patients on aspirin, may also decrease the inflammatory response to bypass. Aprotinin inhibits endothelial cell expression of intercellular adhesion molecule-1 (ICAM-1) and vascular cell adhesion molecule-1 (VCAM-1), potent adhesion molecules for extravasation of neutrophils [195], and shedding of L-selectin from neutrophils, a marker of neutrophil activation [196]. It has been suggested that, by inhibiting adhesion, aprotinin may decrease neutrophil-mediated injury [197,198].

Glucocorticoids, a potent inhibitors of the inflammatory response, given either preoperatively or in the bypass prime, decrease the immune response and resulting tissue injury initiated by CPB. Schroeder and colleagues showed lower levels of the proinflammatory proteins RANTES, MCP-1, IL-6, and ICAM-1 and increased serum concentration of the proinflammatory cytokine IL-10 in infants undergoing CPB who received glucocorticoids both in the pump prime and before surgery [199]. This may translate to improved postoperative function. In a neonatal piglet model, glucocorticoids decreased myocardial troponin degradation, apoptosis, and inflammatory mediatory expression [200,201]. Traditionally, methylprednisolone (30 mg/kg) is given in the pump prime in most centers. The addition of a preoperative dose of 10–30 mg/kg of solumedrol given 4–6 hr pre-bypass has been advocated by some and is used routinely in our center for all neonates. Bourbon and colleagues examined the effects of lower doses (5 and 10 mg/kg) given as one dose just before bypass [202]. Tumor necrosis factor-α, IL-6, and free-radical levels were lower in the 10 mg/kg group, indicating that lower steroid doses may be as effective as higher doses [202].

Moderate hypothermia, which has traditionally been employed in cardiac surgery to decrease metabolic demands, may also decrease the inflammatory response by increasing IL-10 production via the signal transducer and activator of transcription (STAT)-3/suppressor of cytokine signaling (SOCS)-3 pathway. In a porcine model, Qing and colleagues demonstrated increased IL-10 production with resultant lower TNF-α levels and diminished hepatic necrosis with cooling to 28°C on CPB compared with normothermia (37°C) and deep hypothermia (20°C) [154,203]. Studies in adults do not support these findings. Ohata and colleagues found an attenuated inflammatory response accompanied by improved postoperative lung function in adults when placed on normothermic (34°C) bypass compared with moderate hypothermia (28°C) [204].

Although preventing proinflammatory cytokine release altogether might be ideal, only modest attenuation of the inflammatory response has been achieved with the available modalities. This fact has prompted work on ways to eliminate circulating cytokines once they are released. Ultrafiltration throughout bypass and rewarming removes low-molecular-weight proteins [205], including inflammatory mediators [206], and complement [207], improving postoperative blood loss, complement activation, hemodynamics, inflammatory protein levels, and time to extubation [208]. Modified ultrafiltration, now a common practice in pediatric cardiac surgery, removes additional excess fluid and inflammatory proteins after CPB [206].

Blood Flow Strategies: Circulatory Arrest and Regional Perfusion

Certain types of cardiac repair, mainly of the aortic arch, require either very low flow rates during CPB or complete circulatory arrest (no flow). Deep hypothermia is utilized for these cases to decrease the metabolic requirements of the patient. Recently, new techniques have been developed that provide neuroprotection during periods of circulatory arrest. Antegrade cerebral perfusion, or regional perfusion, is achieved by cannulating the innominate artery and snaring the head vessels. The brain is perfused at a rate of 30 mL/kg/min. During regional perfusion, flow is distributed to both the right subclavian and common carotid arteries. Back bleeding of the descending thoracic aorta during regional perfusion demonstrates that there is some degree of flow to the systemic circulation [209].

Ultrafiltration: Conventional, Modified, and Zero Balance

At any time during bypass, but most commonly during rewarming, the fluid in the CPB circuit can be hemoconcentrated through ultrafiltration (UF) in order to restore proper fluid balance before weaning from bypass. Neonates, particularly, are prone to third space excess fluid during CPB secondary to capillary leak from inflammatory mediators, hemodilution from the bypass prime, and decreased colloid oncotic pressure from hemodilution [210,211]. Passage of blood past a semipermeable membrane across a hydrostatic pressure gradient removes low-molecular-weight proteins [205], including inflammatory mediators [206], complement [207], and excess fluid. As a result of UF, blood loss, complement activation, hemodynamics, inflammatory protein levels, and time to extubation are improved postoperatively [208]. Conventional UF, however, does not impact weight gain or myocardial edema compared with no filtration [212].

In addition, neonates and infants do not tolerate removal of large amounts of fluid from the bypass circuit. As a result, a second type of UF, zero-balance ultrafiltration (Z-BUF), has been developed. Commonly, Z-BUF initiates soon after the start of bypass and runs throughout bypass. To maintain circuit volume, a balanced salt crystalloid solution replaces the volume of filtrate removed. Studies evaluating Z-BUF are scarce. In adult patients, C3a and IL-6 briefly increased postoperatively with Z-BUF compared with no filtration, returning to similar levels by 12 hr after surgery [213]. In pediatric patients, combining Z-BUF during rewarming with post-bypass UF compared with post-bypass UF alone has decreased postoperative blood loss, decreased time to extubation, and decreased levels of TNF-α, IL-10, myeloperoxidase, and C3a [214].

In 1991, Naik and colleagues introduced a third permeation of UF—modified ultrafiltered (MUF) [215]. For MUF, the circuit contents are ultrafiltrated immediately after bypass, returning all the blood in the circuit to the patient while removing dilutional fluid without compromising hemodynamics. Blood is removed from the patient via the aortic cannula, passed through a hemoconcentrator, and returned to the patient via the venous line. During the second stage of MUF, fluid is removed and ultrafiltered, and only the concentrated blood is reinfused, resulting in a net decrease in patient blood volume–the "dry-out" phase. Once the patient shows signs of hypovolemia, that is, hypotension, the aortic cannula is removed and the very concentrated blood reinfused into the patient. At this point, protamine is given to reverse heparinization. Hematocrits can increase as high as 10 points.

With MUF, immediate improvements are seen in pulmonary vascular resistance, systemic resistance, and blood pressure [215,216]. Patients receiving MUF have better postoperative cardiac function and decreased inotropic requirements compared with patient who are not ultrafiltered [217]. Echocardiograms after MUF show decreased ventricular wall thickness [213]. Fontan patients demonstrated decreased pericardial and pleural effusions [218]. Modified ultrafiltration has been associated with improved pulmonary compliance and decreased airway pressures, probably as a result of decreased lung water [219]. Infants who underwent low-flow CPB with deep hypothermia had faster return of cerebral oxygen consumption [96], potentially a result of decreased cerebral edema. Postoperative hematocrits are increased while chest tube drainage and blood product usage are decreased in patients receiving MUF compared with patients not receiving filtration [220], all potentially resulting from hemoconcentration.

Modified ultrafiltration is helpful not for only its ability to remove fluid but also for its ability to remove inflammatory myocardial depressants. In neonatal piglets, Daggett and colleagues compared UF, MUF and no filtration [212]. In the MUF group, total body weight gain was less, myocardial wet/dry ratio was less, mean arterial pressure increased, and left ventricular preload recruitable stroke work increased over both the UF and no-filtration groups. In addition, infusion of small amounts of MUF ultrafiltrate into hearts depressed cardiac function, demonstrating the presence of deleterious cytokines in the effluent [212]. Wang and colleagues found that total body water removed by ultrafiltration was greater with MUF than with UF [206]. Because of the greater volume of fluid removed, more TNF-α and IL-6 were removed. The efficacy, however, of removal between the two groups was the same [206]. When the volume of fluid removed was held constant between patients receiving MUF and UF, Thompson and colleagues did not find a difference in hemodynamics, ventricular function, or blood product usage [221].

Ultrafiltration or Z-BUF combined with MUF may interact synergistically, pulling on the strengths of each technique. Particularly for patients with pulmonary hypertension, the addition of MUF to UF has decreased blood product usage, chest tube output, time to extubation, intensive care unit stay [222], endothelin-1 levels, and pulmonary hypertensive crises [223], although these results were not reproduced by Pearl and colleagues [224].

References

1. Gibbon JH Jr. Artificial maintenance of circulation during experimental occlusion of the pulmonary artery. Arch Surg 1937;34:1105–1137.
2. McLean J. The thromboplastic action of cephalin. Am J Physiol 1916;41:250–257.
3. Gibbon JH Jr. The maintenance of life during experimental occlusion of the pulmonary artery followed by survival. Surg Gynecol Obstet 1939;69:602.
4. Gibbon JH Jr. The application of a mechanical heart and lung apparatus to cardiac surgery. Minn Med 1954;37:171–180.
5. Lewis FJ, Taufic M. Closure of atrial septal defects with the aid of hypothermia; experimental accomplishments and the report of one successful case. Surgery 1953;33:52–59.
6. Lewis FJ, Varco RL, Taufic M. Repair of atrial septal defects in man under direct vision with the aid of hypothermia. Surgery 1954;36:538–556.
7. Lewis FJ. Hypothermia in cardiac and general surgery. Minn Med 1955;38:77–81.
8. Warden HE, Cohen M, Read RC, Lillehei CW. Controlled cross circulation for open intracardiac surgery. J Thorac Surg 1954;28:331.
9. Lillehei CW. Controlled cross circulation for direct vision intracardiac surgery correction of ventricular septal defects, atrioventricularis communis, and tetralogy of Fallot. Postgrad Med 1955;17:388–396.
10. Lillehei CW, Cohen M, Warden HE, Varco RL. The direct vision intracardiac correction of congenital anomalies by controlled cross circulation; results in 32 patients with ventricular septal defects, tetralogy of Fallot, and atrioventricular communis defects. Surgery 1955;38:11.
11. Lillehei CW, Varco RL, Cohen M, Warden HE, Patton C, Moller JH. The first open heart repairs of ventricular septal defect, atrioventricular communis, and tetralogy of Fallot using extracorporeal circulation by cross circulation: a 30-year follow-up. Ann Thorac Surg 1986;41:4–21.
12. Kirklin JW, Dushane JW, Patrick RT, et al. Intracardiac surgery with the aid of a mechanical pump-oxygenator system (Gibbon type): report of eight cases. Mayo Clin Proc 1955;30:201–206.
13. Sealy WC, Brown IW Jr, Young WG Jr. A report on the use of both extracorporeal circulation and hypothermia for open heart surgery. Ann Surg 1958;147:603–613.
14. Sealy WC, Young WG Jr, Brown IW Jr, Smith WW, Lesage AM. Profound hypothermia combined with extracorporeal circulation for open heart surgery. Surgery 1960;48:432.
15. Zudhi N, McCollough B, Carey J, Greer A. Double-helical reservoir heart–lung machine. Arch Surg 1961;82:320–325.
16. Stokes TL, Flick JB Jr. An improved vertical cylinder oxygenator. Proc Soc Exp Biol Med 1950;73:528.
17. Dennis C, Spreng DS Jr, Nelson GE, et al. Development of a pump-oxygenator to replace the heart and lungs; an apparatus applicable to human patients, and application to one case. Ann Surg 1951;134:709–721.
18. Edmunds LH. The evolution of cardiopulmonary bypass: lessons to be learned. Perfusion 2002;17:243–251.
19. Iwahashi H, Yuri K, Nosé Y. Development of the oxygenator: past, present, and future. J Artif Organs 2004;7:111–120.

20. Dewall RA, Gott VL, Lillehei CW, et al. A simple, expendable, artificial oxygenator for open heart surgery. Surg Clin North Am 1956;103:1025–1034.

21. Kessler J, Patterson RH Jr. The production of microemboli by various oxygenators. Ann Thorac Surg 1970;9:221–228.

22. Solis RT, Kennedy PS, Beall ACJ, Noon GP, CeBakey ME. Cardiopulmonary bypass, microembolization and platelet aggregation. Circulation 1975;52:103.

23. Haworth WS. The development of the modern oxygenator. Ann Thorac Surg 2003;76:S2216–S2219.

24. Leonard RJ. The transition from the bubble oxygenator to the microporous membrane oxygenator. Perfusion 2003;18:179–183.

25. Baier RE, Dutton RC. Initial events in interactions of blood with a foreign surface. J Biomater Res 1969;3:191–206.

26. Lillehei CW. Historical development of cardiopulmonary bypass in Minnesota. In: Gravlee GP, Davis RF, Kurusz M, Utley JR, eds. Cardiopulmonary Bypass: Principles and Practice, 2nd ed. Philadelphia: Lippincott, Williams, & Wilkins, 2000:3–21.

27. Zucker MB, Vroman L. Platelet adhesion induced by fibrinogen adsorbed onto glass. Proc Soc Exp Biol Med 1969;131:318–320.

28. Gu YJ, van Oeveren W, Akkerman C, Boonstra PW, Huyzen RJ, Wildevuur CR. Heparin-coated circuits reduce the inflammatory response to cardiopulmonary bypass. Ann Thorac Surg 1993;55:917–922.

29. Olsson C, Siegbahn A, Henze A, et al. Heparin-coated cardiopulmonary bypass circuits reduce circulating complement factors and interleukin-6 in paediatric heart surgery. Scand Cardiovasc J 2000;34:33–40.

30. De Somer F, Francois K, van Oeveren W, et al. Phosphorylcholine coating of extracorporeal circuits provides natural protection against blood activation by the material surface. Eur J Cardiothorac Surg 2000;18:602–606.

31. Saito N, Motoyama S, Sawamoto J. Effects of new polymer-coated extracorporeal circuits on biocompatibility during cardiopulmonary bypass. Artif Organs 2000;24:547–554.

32. Gourlay T. Biomaterial development for cardiopulmonary bypass. Perfusion 2001;16:381–390.

33. von Segesser LK, Tozzi P, Mallbiabrrena I, Jegger D, Horisberger J, Corno A. Miniaturization in cardiopulmonary bypass. Perfusion 2003;18:219–224.

34. Son HS, Sun K, Fang YH, et al. The effects of pulsatile versus nonpulsatile extracorporeal circulation on the pattern of coronary artery blood flow during cardiac arrest. Int J Artif Organs 2005;28:609–616.

35. Kim HK, Son HS, Fang YH, Park SY, Hwang CM, Sun K. The effects of pulsatile flow upon renal tissue perfusion during cardiopulmonary bypass: a comparative study of pulsatile and nonpulsatile flow. ASAIO J 2005;51:30–36.

36. Sezai A, Shiono M, Nakata K, et al. Effects of pulsatile CPB in interleukin-8 and endothelin-1 levels. Artif Organs 2005;29:708–713.

37. Ündar A. Benefits of pulsatile flow during and after cardiopulmonary bypass procedures. Artif Organs 2005;29:688–689.

38. Schonberger JP, Everts PA, Hoffmann JJ. Systemic blood activation with open and closed venous reservoirs. Ann Thorac Surg 1995;59:1549–1555.

39. Rider SP, Simon LV, Rice BJ, Poulton CC. Assisted venous drainage, venous air, and gaseous microemboli transmission into the arterial line: an in vitro study. Extra Corpor Technol 1998;30:160–165.

40. Willcox TW, Mitchell SJ, Gorman DF. Venous air in the bypass circuit: a source of arterial line emboli exacerbated by vacuum-assisted drainage. Ann Thorac Surg 1999;68:1285–1289.

41. LaPietra A, Grossi EA, Pua BB, et al. Assisted venous drainage presents the risk of undetected air microembolism. J Thorac Cardiovasc Surg 2000;120:856–862.

42. Jones TJ, Deal DD, Vernon JC, Blackburn N, Stump DA. Does vacuum-assisted venous drainage increase gaseous microemboli during cardiopulmonary bypass? Ann Thorac Surg 2002;74:2132–2137.

43. High KM, Bashein G, Kurusz M. Principles of oxygenator function: gas exchange, heat transfer, and operation. In: Gravlee GP, Davis RF, Kurusz M, Utley JR, eds. Cardiopulmonary Bypass: Principles and Practice, 2nd ed. Philadelphia: Lippincott, Williams, & Wilkins, 2000:49–68.

44. Moore RA, Laub GW. Hemofiltration, dialysis, and blood salvage techniques during cardiopulmonary bypass. In: Gravlee GP, Davis RF, Kurusz M, Utley JR, eds. Cardiopulmonary Bypass: Principles and Practice, 2nd ed. Philadelphia: Lippincott, Williams, & Wilkins, 2000:105–130.

45. Hessel EA II, Hill AG. Circuitry and cannulation technique. In: Gravlee GP, Davis RF, Kurusz M, Utley JR, eds. Cardiopulmonary Bypass: Principles and Practice, 2nd ed. Philadelphia: Lippincott, Williams, & Wilkins, 2000:69–97.

46. Defraigne JO, Pincemail J, Dekoster G, et al. SMA circuits reduce platelet consumption and platelet factor release during cardiac surgery. Ann Thorac Surg 2000;70:2075–2081.

47. Rubens FD, Nathan H, Labow R, et al. Effects of methylprednisolone and a biocompatible copolymer circuit on blood activation during cardiopulmonary bypass. Ann Thorac Surg 2005;79:655–665.

48. Mou SS, Giroir BP, Molitor-Kirsch EA, et al. Fresh whole blood versus reconstituted blood for pump priming in heart surgery in infants. N Engl J Med 2004;351:1635–1644.

49. Keidan I, Amir G, Mandel M, Mishali D. The metabolic effects of fresh versus old stored blood in the priming of cardiopulmonary bypass solution for pediatric patients. J Thorac Cardiovasc Surg 2004;127:949–952.

50. Schroeder TH, Hansen M. Effects of fresh versus old stored blood in the priming solution on whole blood lactate levels during paediatric cardiac surgery. Perfusion 2005;20:17–19.

51. Merkle F, Bottcher W, Hetzer R. Prebypass filtration of cardiopulmonary bypass circuits: an outdated technique? Perfusion 2003;18(Suppl 1):81–88.

52. Jensen E, Andréasson S, Bengtsson A, et al. Changes in hemostasis during pediatric heart surgery: impact of a biocompatible heparin-coated perfusion system. Ann Thorac Surg 2004;77:962–967.

53. Saatvedt K, Lindberg H, Michelsen S, Pedersen T, Geiran OR. Activation of the fibrinolytic, coagulation and plasma kallikrein-kinin systems during and after open heart surgery in children. Scand J Clin Lab Invest 1995;55:359–367.

54. Weitz JI, Hudoba M, Massel D, Maraganore J, Hirsh J. Clot-bound thrombin is protected from inhibition by heparin-antithrombin III but is susceptible to inactivation by antithrombin III–independent inhibitors. J Clin Invest 1990;86:385–391.

55. Laffey JG, Boylan JF, Cheng DCH. The systemic inflammatory response to cardiac surgery, implications for the anesthesiologist. Anesthesiology 2002;97:215–252.

56. Andrew M. The relevance of developmental hemostasis to hemorrhagic disorders of newborns. Semin Perinatol 1997;21:70–85.

57. Jaggers JJ, Neal MC, Smith PK, Ungerleider RM, Lawson JH. Infant cardiopulmonary bypass: a procoagulant state. Ann Thorac Surg 1999;68:513–520.

58. Levin E, Wu J, Devine DV, et al. Hemostatic parameters and platelet activation marker expression in cyanotic and acyanotic pediatric patients undergoing cardiac surgery in the presence of tranexamic acid. Thromb Haemost 2000;83:54–59.

59. Kestin AS, Valeri CR, Khuri SF, et al. The platelet function defect of cardiopulmonary bypass. Blood 1993;82:107–117.

60. Greilich PE, Brouse CF, Beckham J, Jessen ME, Martin EJ, Carr ME. Reductions in platelet contractile force correlate with duration of cardiopulmonary bypass and blood loss in patients undergoing cardiac surgery. Thromb Res 2002;105:523–529.

61. Esmon CT. Role of coagulation inhibitors in inflammation. Thromb Haemost 2001;86:51–56.

62. Despotis GJ, Summerfield AL, Joist JH, et al. Comparison of activated coagulation time and whole blood heparin measurements with

laboratory plasma anti-Xa heparin concentration in patients having cardiac operations. J Thorac Cardiovasc Surg 1994;108:1076–1082.

63. Despotis GJ, Levine V, Alsoufiev A, Joist H, Goodnough LT, Pasque M. Recurrent thrombosis of biventricular-support devices associated with accelerated intravascular coagulation and increased heparin requirements. J Thorac Cardiovasc Surg 1996;112:538–540.

64. Bott JN, Reddy K, Krick S. Bivalirudin use in off-pump myocardial revascularization in patients with heparin-induced thrombocytopenia. Ann Thorac Surg 2003;76:275.

65. Dyke CM, Koster A, Veale JJ, Maier GW, McNiff T, Levy JH. Preemptive use of bivalirudin for urgent on-pump coronary artery bypass grafting in patients with potential heparin-induced thrombocytopenia. Ann Thorac Surg 2005;80:299–303.

66. Furukawa K, Ohteki H, Hirahara K, Narita Y, Koga S. The use of argatroban as an anticoagulant for cardiopulmonary bypass in cardiac operations. J Thorac Cardiovasc Surg 2001;122:1255–1256.

67. Edwards JT, Hamby JK, Worrall NK. Successful use of argatroban as a heparin substitute during cardiopulmonary bypass: heparin-induced thrombocytopenia in a high-risk cardiac surgical patient. Ann Thorac Surg 2003;75:1622–1624.

68. Greinacher A, Lubenow MD, Eichler P. Anaphylactic and anaphylactoid reactions associated with lepirudin in patients with heparin-induced thrombocytopenia. Circulation 2003;108:2062–2065.

69. Eichler P, Lubenow N, Strobel U, Greinacher A. Antibodies against lepirudin are polyspecific and recognize epitopes on bivalrudin. Blood 2004;103:613–616.

70. Warkentin TE, Greinacher A. Heparin-induced thrombocytopenia and cardiac surgery. Ann Thorac Surg 2003;76:638–648.

71. Bartholomew JR. Transition to an oral anticoagulant in patients with heparin-induced thrombocytopenia. Chest 2005;127:27–34.

72. Ibbotson T, Perry CM. Danaparoid: a review of its use in thromboembolic and coagulation disorders. Drugs 2002;62:2283–2314.

73. Hassell K. The management of patients with heparin-induced thrombocytopenia who require anticoagulant therapy. Chest 2005;127:1–8.

74. Ammar T, Fisher CF. The effects of heparinase 1 and protamine on platelet reactivity. Anesthesiology 1997;86:1382–1386.

75. Shigeta O, Kojima H, Hiramatsu Y, et al. Low-dose protamine based on heparin-protamine titration method reduces platelet dysfunction after cardiopulmonary bypass. J Thorac Cardiovasc Surg 1999;118:354–360.

76. Davies MJ, Allen A, Kort H, et al. Prospective, randomized, double-blind study of high-dose aprotinin in pediatric cardiac operations. Ann Thorac Surg 1997;63:497–503.

77. Boldt J, Knothe C, Zickmann B, Wege N, Dapper F, Hempelmann G. Aprotinin in pediatric cardiac operations: platelet function, blood loss, and use of homologous blood. Ann Thorac Surg 1993;55:1460–1466.

78. Orchard MA, Goodchild CS, Prentice CRM, et al. Aprotinin reduces cardiopulmonary bypass-induced blood loss and inhibits fibrinolysis without influencing platelets. Br J Haematol 1993;85:533–541.

79. Wahba A, Black G, Koksch M, et al. Aprotinin has no effect on platelet activation and adhesion during cardiopulmonary bypass. Thromb Haemost 1996;75:844–848.

80. Huang H, Ding W, Su Z, Zhang W. Mechanism of the preserving of aprotinin on platelet function and its use in cardiac surgery. J Thorac Cardiovasc Surg 1993;106:11–18.

81. Mössinger H, Dietrich W, Braun SL, Jochum M, Meisner H, Richter JA. High-dose aprotinin reduces activation of hemostasis, allogeneic blood requirement, and duration of postoperative ventilation in pediatric cardiac surgery. Ann Thorac Surg 2003;75:430–437.

82. Dietrich W, Mossinger H, Spannagl M, et al. Hemostatic activation during cardiopulmonary bypass with different aprotinin dosages in pediatric patients having cardiac operations. J Thorac Cardiovasc Surg 1993;105:712–720.

83. Beierlein W, Scheule AM, Dietrich W, Ziemer G. Forty years of clinical aprotinin use: a review of 124 hypersensitivity reactions. Ann Thorac Surg 2005;79:741–748.

84. Dietrich W, Spath P, Ebell A, Richter JA. Prevalence of anaphylacti reactions to aprotinin: analysis of two hundred forty-eight reexpo sures to aprotinin in heart operations. J Thorac Cardiovasc Sur 1997;113:194–201.

85. Jaquiss RDB, Ghanayem NS, Zacharisen MC, Mussatto KA, Twedde JS, Litwin SB. Safety of aprotinin use and re-use in pediatric cardic thoracic surgery. Circulation 2002;106:I90–I94.

86. Dietrich W, Späth P, Zühlsdorf M, et al. Anaphylactic reactions t aprotinin reexposure in cardiac surgery. Anesthesiology 2001;9 64–71.

87. Moen O, Fosse E, Braten J, et al. Differences in blood activation relate to roller/centrifugal pumps and heparin-coated/uncoated surfaces i a cardiopulmonary bypass model circuit. Perfusion 1996;11:113–123

88. Spiess BD, Vocelka C, Cochran RP, Soltow L, Chandler WL. Heparin coated bypass circuits (Carmeda) suppress the release of tissue plas minogen activator during normothermic coronary artery bypass graf surgery. J Cardiothorac Vasc Anesth 1998;12:299–304.

89. Johnell M, Elgue G, Larsson R, Larsson A, Thelin S, Siegbahn A. Coag ulation, fibrinolysis, and cell activation in patients and shed medias tinal blood during coronary artery bypass grafting with a new heparin-coated surface. J Thorac Cardiovasc Surg 2002;124:321 332.

90. Grossi EA, Kallenbach K, Chau S, et al. Impact of heparin bonding o pediatric cardiopulmonary bypass: a prospective randomized study Ann Thorac Surg 2000;70:191–196.

91. White FN. A comparative physiological approach to hypothermia J Thorac Cardiovasc Surg 1981;82:821–831.

92. Henriksen L. Brain luxury perfusion during cardiopulmonary bypas in humans. A study of the cerebral blood flow response to changes i CO_2, O_2, and blood pressure. J Cereb Blood Flow Metab 1986;6:366– 378.

93. Murkin JM, Farrar JK, Tweed WA, McKenzie FN, Guiraudon G. Cere bral autoregulation and flow/metabolism coupling during cardiopul monary bypass: the influence of $PaCO_2$. Anesth Analg 1987;66 825–832.

94. Duebener LF, Hagino I, Sakamoto T, et al. Effects of pH managemen during deep hypothermic bypass on cerebral microcirculation: alpha stat versus pH-stat. Circulation 2002;106:I103–I108.

95. Nagy ZL, Collins M, Sharpe T, et al. Effect of two different bypass techniques on the serum troponin-T levels in newborns and children does pH-stat provide better protection? Circulation 2003;108:577– 582.

96. Skaryak LA, Kirshbom PM, DiBernardo LR, et al. Modified ultrafiltra tion improves cerebral metabolic recovery after circulatory arrest J Thorac Cardiovasc Surg 1995;109:744–751.

97. Murkin JM, Martzke JS, Buchan AM, Bentley C, Wong CJ. A random ized study of the influence of perfusion technique and pH manage ment strategy in 316 patients undergoing coronary artery bypass surgery. II. Neurologic and cognitive outcomes. J Thorac Cardiovasc Surg 1995;110:349–362.

98. Pearl JM, Thomas DW, Grist G, Duffy JY, Manning PM. Hyperoxia for management of acid–base status during deep hypothermia with cir culatory arrest. Ann Thorac Surg 2000;70:751–755.

99. Nollert G, Nagashima M, Bucerius J, et al. Oxygenation strategy and neurologic damage after deep hypothermic circulatory arrest. II. Hypoxic versus free radical injury. J Thorac Cardiovasc Surg 1999;117:1172– 1179.

100. Kurth CD, O'Rourke MM, O'Hara IB, Uher B. Brain cooling efficiency with pH-stat and alpha-stat cardiopulmonary bypass in newborn pigs. Circulation 1997;96:II358–II363.

101. Hiramatsu T, Miura T, Forbess JM, et al. pH strategies and cerebral energetics before and after circulatory arrest. J Thorac Cardiovasc Surg 1995;109:948–957.

102. Priestley MA, Golden JA, O'Hara IB, McCann J, Kurth CD. Compari son of neurologic outcome after deep hypothermic circulatory arrest with alpha-stat and pH-stat cardiopulmonary bypass in newborn pigs. J Thorac Cardiovasc Surg 2001;121:336–343.

103. Pokela M, Dahlbacka S, Biancari F, et al. pH-stat versus alpha-stat perfusion strategy during experimental hypothermic circulatory arrest: a microdialysis study. Ann Thorac Surg 2003;76:1215–1226.

104. du Plessis AJ, Jonas RA, Wypij D, et al. Perioperative effects of alpha-stat versus pH-stat strategies for deep hypothermic cardiopulmonary bypass in infants. J Thorac Cardiovasc Surg 1997;114:991–1000.

105. Sonnenblick EH, Ross JJ, Braunwald E. Oxygen consumption of the heart: newer concepts of its multifactorial determination. Am J Cardiol 1968;22:328–336.

106. Rosenkrantz ER, Vinten-Johansen J, Buckberg GD, Okamoto F, Edwards H, Bugyi H. Benefits of normothermic induction of blood cardioplegia in energy-depleted hearts, with maintenance of arrest by multidose cold blood cardioplegic infusions. J Thorac Cardiovasc Surg 1982;84:667–677.

107. Vinten-Johansen J, Ronson RS, Thourani VH, Wechsler AS. Surgical myocardial protection. In: Gravlee GP, Davis RF, Kurusz M, Utley JR, eds. Cardiopulmonary Bypass: Principles and Practice, 2nd ed. Philadelphia: Lippincott, Williams, & Wilkins, 2000:214–264.

108. Opie LH. Reperfusion injury and its pharmacologic modification. Circulation 1989;80:1049–1062.

109. Cohen NM, Wise RM, Wechsler AS, Damiano RJ Jr. Elective cardiac arrest with a hyperpolarizing adenosine triphosphate–sensitive potassium channel opener. A novel form of myocardial protection? J Thorac Cardiovasc Surg 1993;106:317–328.

110. Hetzer R, Warnecke H, Wittrock H, Engel HJ, Borst HG. Extracoronary collateral myocardial blood flow during cardioplegic arrest. Thorac Cardiovasc Surg 1980;28:191–196.

111. Mills SA, Hansen K, Vinten-Johansen J, Howe HR, Geisinger KR, Cordell AR. Enhanced functional recovery with venting during cardioplegic arrest in chronically damaged hearts. Ann Thorac Surg 1985;40:566–573.

112. Allen BS, Okamoto F, Buckberg GD, Bugyi H, Leaf J. Studies of controlled reperfusion after ischemia. XIII. Reperfusion conditions: critical importance of total ventricular decompression during regional reperfusion. J Thorac Cardiovasc Surg 1986;92:605–612.

113. Kern FH, Ungerleider RM, Reves JG, et al. Effect of altering pump flow rate on cerebral blood flow and metabolism in infants and children. Ann Thorac Surg 1993;56:1366–1372.

114. Jaggers JJ, Ungerleider RM. Cardiopulmonary bypass in infants and children. Semin Thorac Cardiovasc Surg Pediatr Card Surg Annu 2000;3:82–109.

115. Cooper JRJ, Giesecke NM. Hemodilution and priming solutions. In: Gravlee GP, Davis RF, Kurusz M, Utley JR, eds. Cardiopulmonary Bypass: Principles and Practice, 2nd ed. Philadelphia: Lippincott, Williams, & Wilkins, 186–196.

116. Alexi-Meskishvili V, Stiller B, Koster A, et al. Correction of congenital heart defects in Jehovah's Witness children. Thorac Cardiovasc Surg 2004;52:141–146.

117. Hubler M, Boettcher W, Koster A, et al. Transfusion-free cardiac surgery with cardiopulmonary bypass in a 2.2-kg neonate. J Card Surg 2005;20:180–182.

118. Ando M, Takahashi Y, Suzuki N. Open heart surgery for small children without homologous blood transfusion by using remote pump head system. Ann Thorac Surg 2004;78:1717–1722.

119. Gordon RJ, Ravin M, Rawitscher RE, Daicoff GR. Changes in arterial pressure, viscosity and resistance during cardiopulmonary bypass. J Thorac Cardiovasc Surg 1975;69:552–561.

120. Messmer K. Hemodilution. Surg Clin North Am 1975;55:659–678.

121. Rand PW, Lacombe E, Hunt HE, Austin WH. Viscosity of normal human blood under normothermic and hypothermic conditions. J Appl Physiol 1964;19:117–122.

122. Utley JR, Wachtel C, Cain RB, Spaw EA, Collins JC, Stephens DB. Effects of hypothermia, hemodilution, and pump oxygenation on organ water content, blood flow and oxygen delivery, and renal function. Ann Thorac Surg 1981;31:121–133.

123. Guyton AC, Richardson TQ. Effect of hematocrit on venous return. Circ Res 1961;9:157–163.

124. Cooley DA, Beall AC, Grondin P. Open-heart operations with disposable oxygenators, 5 percent dextrose prime, and normothermia. Surgery 1962;52:713–719.

125. Dittrich S, Schuth A, Aurich H, vonLoeper J, Grosse-Siestrup C, Lange PE. Haemodilution improves organ function during normothermic cardiopulmonary bypass: investigations in isolated perfused pig kidneys. Perfusion 2000;15:225–229.

126. Cain SM. Oxygen delivery and uptake in dogs during anemic and hypoxic hypoxia. J Appl Physiol 1997;42:228–234.

127. Shin'oka T, Shum-Tim D, Jonas RA, et al. Higher hematocrit improves cerebral outcome after deep hypothermic circulatory arrest. J Thorac Cardiovasc Surg 1996;112:1610–1620.

128. Duebener LF, Sakamoto T, Hatsuoka SI, et al. Effects of hematocrit on cerebral microcirculation and tissue oxygenation during deep hypothermic bypass. Circulation 2005;104:I260–I264.

129. Sakamoto T, Nollert GDA, Zurakowski D, et al. Hemodilution elevates cerebral blood flow and oxygen metabolism during cardiopulmonary bypass in piglets. Ann Thorac Surg 2004;77:1656–1663.

130. Jonas RA, Wypij D, Roth SJ, et al. The influence of hemodilution on outcome after hypothermic cardiopulmonary bypass: results of a randomized trial in infants. J Thorac Cardiovasc Surg 2003;126:1765–1774.

131. Kawamura M, Minamikawa O, Yokochi H, Maki S, Yasuda T, Mizukawa Y. Safe limit of hemodilution in cardiopulmonary bypass—comparative analysis between cyanotic and acyanotic congenital heart disease. Jpn J Surg 1980;10:206–211.

132. Kern FH, Morana NJ, Sears JJ, Hickey PR. Coagulation defects in neonates during cardiopulmonary bypass. Ann Thorac Surg 1992;54:541–546.

133. Nollert G, Sperling J, Sakamoto T, Jaeger BR, Jonas RA. Higher hematocrit improves liver blood flow and metabolism during cardiopulmonary bypass in piglets. Thorac Cardiovasc Surg 2001;49:226–230.

134. Gillon J, Desmond M, Thomas MJ. Acute normovolaemic haemodilution. Transfus Med 1999;9:259–264.

135. Cross MH. Autotransfusion in cardiac surgery. Perfusion 2001;16:391–400.

136. Chenoweth DE, Cooper SW, Hugli TE, Stewart RW, Blackstone EH, Kirklin JW. Complement activation during cardiopulmonary bypass: evidence for generation of C3a and C5a anaphylatoxins. N Engl J Med 1981;304:497–503.

137. Kirklin JK, Westaby S, Blackstone EH, Kirklin JW, Chenoweth DE, Pacifico AD. Complement and the damaging effects of cardiopulmonary bypass. J Thorac Cardiovasc Surg 1983;86:845–857.

138. Kirklin JK, Chenoweth DE, Naftel DC, et al. Effects of protamine administration after cardiopulmonary bypass on complement, blood elements, and the hemodynamic state. Ann Thorac Surg 1986;41:193–199.

139. Asimakopoulos G. Mechanisms of the systemic inflammatory response. Perfusion 1999;14:269–277.

140. Tárnok A, Hambsch J, Emmrich F, et al. Complement activation, cytokines, and adhesion molecules in children undergoing cardiac surgery with or without cardiopulmonary bypass. Pediatr Cardiol 1999;20:113–125.

141. Hattler BG, Zeevi A, Oddis CV, Finkel MS. Cytokine induction during cardiac surgery: analysis of TNF-alpha expression pre- and postcardiopulmonary bypass. J Card Surg 1995;10:418–422.

142. Kumar A, Thota V, Dee L, Olson J, Uretz E, Parrillo JE. Tumor necrosis factor alpha and interleukin 1-beta are responsible for in vitro myocardial cell depression induced by human septic shock serum. J Exp Med 1996;183:949–958.

143. Royall JA, Berkow RL, Beckman JS, Cunningham MK, Matalon S, Freeman BA. Tumor necrosis factor and interleukin 1-alpha increase vascular endothelial permeability. Am J Physiol 1989;257:L399–L410.

144. Meldrum DR. Tumor necrosis factor in the heart. Am J Physiol 1998;274:R577–R595.

145. Krown KA, Yasui K, Brooker MJ, et al. Tumor necrosis factor alpha receptor expression in rat cardiac myocytes: tumor necrosis factor

alpha inhibition of L-type Ca^{2+} current and Ca^{2+} transients. FEBS Lett 1995;376:24–30.

146. Oral H, Dorn GH, Mann DL. Sphingosine mediates the immediate negative inotropic effects of tumor necrosis factor-alpha in the adult mammalian cardiac myocyte. J Biol Chem 1997;8:4836–4842.

147. Gulick T, Chung MK, Pieper SJ, Lange LG, Schreiner GF. Interleukin-1 and tumor necrosis factor inhibit cardiac myocyte beta-adrenergic responsiveness. Proc Natl Acad Sci USA1989;86:6753–6757.

148. Finkel MS, Oddis CV, Jacob TD, Watkins SC, Hattler BG, Simmons RL. Negative inotropic effects of cytokines on the heart mediated by nitric oxide. Science 1992;257:387–389.

149. Larrick JW, Wright SC. Cytotoxic mechanism of tumor necrosis factor-alpha. FASEB J 1990;4:3215–3223.

150. Finn A, Naik S, Klein N, Levinsky RJ, Strobel S, Elliot M. Interleukin-8 release and neutrophil degranulation after pediatric cardiopulmonary bypass. J Thorac Cardiovasc Surg 1993;105:234–241.

151. Heinrich PC, Behrmann I, Haan S, Hermanns HM, Müller-Newen G, Schaper F. Principles of interleukin-6 type cytokine signalling and its regulation. Biochem J 2003;374:1–20.

152. Steinberg JB, Kapelanski DP, Olson JD, Weiler JM. Cytokine and complement levels in patients undergoing cardiopulmonary bypass. J Thorac Cardiovasc Surg 1993;106:1008–1016.

153. Taniguchi T, Koido Y, Aiboshi J, Yamashita T, Suzaki S, Kurokawa A. Change in the ratio of interleukin-6 to interleukin-10 predicts a poor outcome in patients with systemic inflammatory response syndrome. Crit Care Med 1999;27:1262–1264.

154. Qing M, Vazquez-Jimenez JF, Klosterhalfen B, et al. Influence of temperature during cardiopulmonary bypass on leukocyte activation, cytokine balance, and post-operative organ damage. Shock 2001;15: 372–377.

155. Vazquez-Jimenez JF, Qing M, Hermanns B, et al. Moderate hypothermia during cardiopulmonary bypass reduces myocardial cell damage and myocardial cell death related to cardiac surgery. J Am Coll Cardiol 2001;38:1216–1223.

156. Hövels-Gürich HH, Vazquez-Jimenez JF, Silvestri A, et al. Production of proinflammatory cytokines and myocardial dysfunction after arterial switch operation in neonates with transposition of the great arteries. J Thorac Cardiovasc Surg 2002;124:811–820.

157. Seghaye MC. The clinical implications of the systemic inflammatory reaction related to cardiac operations in children. Cardiol Young 2003;13:228–239.

158. Seghaye MC, Duchateau J, Grabitz RG, et al. Complement activation during cardiopulmonary bypass in infants and children. Relation to post-operative multiple organ system failure. J Thorac Cardiovasc Surg 1993;106:978–987.

159. Hövels-Gürich HH, Schumacher K, Vazquez-Jimenez JF, et al. Cytokine balance in infants undergoing cardiac operation. Ann Thorac Surg 2002;73:601–608.

160. Anand KJ, Hansen DD, Hickey PR. Hormonal-metabolic stress responses in neonates undergoing cardiac surgery. Anesthesiology 1990;73:661–670.

161. Sasidharan P. Role of corticosteroids in neonatal blood pressure homeostasis. Clin Perinatol 1998;25:723–740.

162. Roth-Isigkeit AK, Schmucker P. Postoperative dissociation of blood levels of cortisol and adrenocorticotropin after coronary artery bypass grafting surgery. Steroids 1997;62:695–699.

163. Shore S, Nelson DP, Pearl JM, et al. Usefulness of corticosteroid therapy in decreasing epinephrine requirements in critically ill infants with congenital heart disease. Am J Cardiol 2001;88:591–594.

164. Julia P, Kofsky E, Buckberg GD, Young HH, Bugyi HI. Studies of myocardial protection in the immature heart: IV. Models of ischemic and hypoxic/ischemic injury in the immature puppy heart. J Thorac Cardiovasc Surg 1991;101:14–22.

165. Kofsky ER, Julia PL, Buckberg GD, Young H, Tixier D. Studies of myocardial protection in the immature heart. V. Safety of prolonged aortic clamping with hypocalcemic glutamate/aspartate blood cardioplegia. J Thorac Cardiovasc Surg 1991;101:33–43.

166. Chen M, Won DJ, Krajewski S, Gottlieb RA. Calpain and mitochondria in ischemia/reperfusion injury. J Biol Chem 2002;277:29181–29186.

167. Enns D, Karmazyn M, Mair J, Lercher A, Kountchev J, Belcastro A. Calpain, calpastatin activities and ratios during myocardial ischemia–reperfusion. Mol Cell Biochem 2002;241:29–35.

168. Nawada R, Murakami T, Iwase T, et al. Inhibition of sarcolemmal Na^+,K^+-ATPase activity reduces the infarct size-limiting effect of preconditioning in rabbit hearts. Circulation 1997;96:599–604.

169. Inserte J, Garcia-Dorado D, Hernando V, Soler-Soler J. Calpain-mediated impairment of Na^+/K^+-ATPase activity during early reperfusion contributes to cell death after myocardial ischemia. Circ Res 2005;97:465–473.

170. Schafer C, Ladilov Y, Inserte J, et al. Role of the reverse mode of the Na^+/Ca^{2+} exchanger in reoxygenation-induced cardiomyocyte injury. Cardiovasc Res 2001;51:241–250.

171. Tani M, Neely JR. Role of intracellular Na^+ in Ca^{2+} overload and depressed recovery of ventricular function of reperfused ischemic rat hearts. Possible involvement of H^+-Na^+ and Na^+-Ca^{2+} exchange. Circ Res 1989;65:1045–1056.

172. Vandeberg JI, Metcalfe JC, Grace AA. Mechanisms of pHi recovery after global ischemia in the reperfused heart. Circ Res 1993;72:993–1003.

173. Franke A, Lante W, Fackeldey V, et al. Proinflammatory and antiinflammatory cytokines after cardiac operation: different cellular sources at different times. Ann Thorac Surg 2002;74:363–370.

174. Pearl JM, Nelson DP, Wellmann SA, et al. Acute hypoxia and reoxygenation impairs exhaled nitric oxide release and pulmonary mechanics. J Thorac Cardiovasc Surg 2000;119:931–938.

175. Serraf A, Robotin M, Bonnet N, et al. Alteration of the neonatal pulmonary physiology after total cardiopulmonary bypass. J Thorac Cardiovasc Surg 1997;114:1061–1069.

176. Levy JH, Tanaka KA. Inflammatory response to cardiopulmonary bypass. Ann Thorac Surg 2003;75:S715–S720.

177. Nelin LD, Thomas CJ, Dawson CA. Effect of hypoxia on nitric oxide production in neonatal pig lung. Am J Physiol 1996;271: H8–H14.

178. Duffy JY, Schwartz SM, Lyons JM, et al. Calpain inhibition decreases endothelin-1 levels and pulmonary hypertension after cardiopulmonary bypass with deep hypothermic circulatory arrest. Crit Care Med 2005;33:623–628.

179. Lyons JM, Duffy JY, Wagner CJ, Pearl JM. Sildenafil citrate alleviates pulmonary hypertension after hypoxia and reoxygenation with cardiopulmonary bypass. J Am Coll Surg 2004;199:607–614.

180. Karamlou T, Schultz JM, Silliman C, et al. Using a miniaturized circuit and an asanguineous prime to reduce neutrophil-mediated organ dysfunction following infant cardiopulmonary bypass. Ann Thorac Surg 2005;80:6–13.

181. Moen O, Hogasen K, Fosse E, et al. Attenuation of changes in leukocyte surface markers and complement activation with heparin-coated cardiopulmonary bypass. Ann Thorac Surg 1997;63:105–111.

182. Ovrum E, Brosstad F, Am Holen E, Tangen G, Abdelnoor M. Effects on coagulation and fibrinolysis with reduced versus full systemic heparinization and heparin-coated cardiopulmonary bypass. Circulation 1995;92:2579–2584.

183. Ovrum E, Mollnes TE, Fosse E, et al. Complement and granulocyte activation in two different types of heparinized extracorporeal circuits. J Thorac Cardiovasc Surg 1995;110:1623–1632.

184. de Vroege R, Huybregts R, van Oeveren W, et al. The impact of heparin-coated circuits on hemodynamics during and after cardiopulmonary bypass. Artif Organs 2005;29:490–497.

185. de Vroege R, van Oeveren W, van Klarenbosch J, et al. The impact of heparin-coated cardiopulmonary bypass circuits on pulmonary function and the release of inflammatory mediators. Anesth Analg 2004;98:1586–1594.

186. Tayama E, Hayashida N, Akasu K, et al. Biocompatibility of heparin-coated extracorporeal bypass circuits: new heparin bonded bioline system. Artif Organs 2000;24:618–623.

187. Palatianos GM, Foroulis CN, Vassili MI, et al. A prospective, double-blinded study on the efficacy of the bioline surface-heparinized extracorporeal perfusion circuit. Ann Thorac Surg 2003;76:129–135.

188. Aldea GS, Soltow LO, Chandler WL, et al. Limitation of thrombin generation, platelet activation, and inflammation by elimination of cardiotomy suction in patients undergoing coronary artery bypass grafting treated with heparin-bonded circuits. J Thorac Cardiovasc Surg 2002;123:742–755.

189. Mueller XM, Tevaearai HT, Horisberger J, Augstburger M, Boone Y, von Segesser LK. Smart suction device for less blood trauma: a comparison with Cell Saver. Eur J Cardiothorac Surg 2001;19:507–511.

190. Tevaearai HT, Mueller XM, Horisberger J, et al. In situ control of cardiotomy suction reduces blood trauma. ASAIO J 2005;44:M380–M383.

191. Svenmarker S, Engstrom KG. The inflammatory response to recycled pericardial suction blood and the influence of cell-saving. Scand Cardiovasc J 2003;37:158–164.

192. Amand T, Pincemail J, Blaffart F, Larbuisson R, Limet R, Defraigne JO. Levels of inflammatory markers in the blood processed by autotransfusion devices during cardiac surgery associated with cardiopulmonary bypass circuit. Perfusion 2002;17:117–123.

193. Wiesenack C, Liebold A, Philipp A, et al. Four years' experience with a miniaturized extracorporeal circulation system and its influence on clinical outcome. Artif Organs 2004;28:1082–1088.

194. Fromes Y, Gaillard D, Ponzio O, et al. Reduction of the inflammatory response following coronary bypass grafting with total minimal extracorporeal circulation. Eur J Cardiothorac Surg 2002;22:527–533.

195. Asimakopoulos G, Lidington EA, Mason J, Haskard DO, Taylor KM, Landis RC. Effects of aprotinin on endothelial cell activation. J Thorac Cardiovasc Surg 2001;122:123–128.

196. Asimakopoulos G, Taylor KM, Haskard DO, Landis RC. Inhibition of neutrophil L-selectin shedding: a potential anti-inflammatory effect of aprotinin. Perfusion 2000;15:495–499.

197. Seghaye MC, Duchateau J, Grabitz RG, et al. Influence of low-dose aprotinin on the inflammatory reaction due to cardiopulmonary bypass in children. Ann Thorac Surg 1996;61:1205–1211.

198. Wippermann CF, Schmid FX, Eberle B, et al. Reduced inotropic support after aprotinin therapy during pediatric cardiac operations. Ann Thorac Surg 1999;67:173–176.

199. Schroeder VA, Pearl JM, Schwartz SM, Shanley TP, Manning PB, Nelson DP. Combined steroid treatment for congenital heart surgery improves oxygen delivery and reduces postbypass inflammatory mediator expression. Circulation 2003;107:2823–2828.

200. Pearl JM, Nelson DP, Schwartz SM, et al. Glucocorticoids reduce ischemia–reperfusion-induced myocardial apoptosis in immature hearts. Ann Thorac Surg 2002;74:830–837.

201. Schwartz SM, Duffy JY, Pearl JM, Goins S, Wagner CJ, Nelson DP. Glucocorticoids preserve calpastatin and troponin I during cardiopulmonary bypass in immature pigs. Pediatr Res 2003;54:91–97.

202. Bourbon A, Vionnet M, Leprince P, et al. The effect of methylprednisolone treatment on the cardiopulmonary bypass-induced systemic inflammatory response. Eur J Cardiothorac Surg 2004;26:932–938.

203. Qing M, Nimmesgern A, Heinrich PC, et al. Intrahepatic synthesis of tumor necrosis factor-alpha related to cardiac surgery is inhibited by interleukin-10 via the janus kinase (Jak)/signal transducers and activator of transcription (STAT) pathway. Crit Care Med 2003;31:2769–2775.

204. Ohata T, Sawa Y, Kadoba K, Masai T, Ichikawa H, Matsuda H. Effect of cardiopulmonary bypass under tepid temperature on inflammatory reactions. Ann Thorac Surg 1997;64:124–128.

205. FitzGerald DJ, Cecere G. Hemofiltration and inflammatory mediators. Perfusion 2002;17:23–28.

206. Wang MJ, Chiu IS, Hsu CM, et al. Efficacy of ultrafiltration in removing inflammatory mediators during pediatric cardiac operations. Ann Thorac Surg 1996;61:651–656.

207. Andreasson S, Gothberg S, Berggren H, Bengtsson A, Eriksson E, Risberg B. Hemofiltration modifies complement activation after extracorporeal circulation in infants. Ann Thorac Surg 1993;56:1515–1517.

208. Journois D, Pouard P, Greeley WJ, Mauriat P, Vouche P, Safran D. Hemofiltration during cardiopulmonary bypass in pediatric cardiac surgery. Effects on hemostasis, cytokines, and complement components. Anesthesiology 1994;81:1181–1189.

209. Pigula FA, Gandhi SK, Siewers RD, Davis PJ, Webber SA, Nemoto EM. Regional low-flow perfusion provides somatic circulatory support during neonatal aortic arch surgery. Ann Thorac Surg 2001;72:401–406.

210. Maehara T, Novak I, Wyse RK, Elliot MJ. Perioperative monitoring of total body water by bio-electrical impedance in children undergoing open heart surgery. Eur J Cardiothorac Surg 1991;5:258–264.

211. Shin'oka T, Shum-Tim D, Laussen PC, et al. Effects of oncotic pressure and hematocrit on outcome after hypothermic circulatory arrest. Ann Thorac Surg 1998;65:155–164.

212. Daggett CW, Lodge AJ, Scarborough JE, Chai PJ, Jaggers J, Ungerleider RM. Modified ultrafiltration versus conventional ultrafiltration: a randomized prospective study in neonatal piglets. J Thorac Cardiovasc Surg 1998;115:336–341.

213. Tallman RD, Dumond M, Brown D. Inflammatory mediator removal by zero-balance ultrafiltration during cardiopulmonary bypass. Perfusion 2002;17:111–115.

214. Journois D, Israel-Biet D, Pouard P, et al. High-volume, zero-balanced hemofiltration to reduce delayed inflammatory response to cardiopulmonary bypass in children. Anesthesiology 1996;85:965–976.

215. Naik SK, Knight A, Elliot MJ. A successful modification of ultrafiltration for cardiopulmonary bypass in children. Perfusion 1991;6:41–50.

216. Elliot MJ. Ultrafiltration and modified ultrafiltration in pediatric open heat operations. Ann Thorac Surg 1993;56:1518–1522.

217. Davies MJ, Nguyen K, Gaynor JW, Elliot MJ. Modified ultrafiltration improves left ventricular systolic function in infants after cardiopulmonary bypass. J Thorac Cardiovasc Surg 1998;115:361–369.

218. Koutlas TC, Gaynor JW, Nicolson SC, Steven JM, Wernovsky G, Spray TL. Modified ultrafiltration reduces postoperative morbidity after cavopulmonary connection. Ann Thorac Surg 1997;64:37–42.

219. Meliones JN, Gaynor JW, Wilson BG. Modified ultrafiltration reduces airway pressures and improves lung compliance after congenital heart surgery. J Am Coll Cardiol 1995;25:S271A.

220. Draaisma AM, Hazekamp MG, Frank M, Anes N, Schoof PH, Huysmans HA. Modified ultrafiltration after cardiopulmonary bypass in pediatric cardiac surgery. Ann Thorac Surg 1997;64:521–525.

221. Thompson LD, McElhinney DB, Findlay P, et al. A prospective randomized study comparing volume-standardized modified and conventional ultrafiltration in pediatric cardiac surgery. J Thorac Cardiovasc Surg 2001;122:220–228.

222. Bando K, Turrentine MW, Vijay P, et al. Effect of modified ultrafiltration in high-risk patients undergoing operations for congenital heart disease. Ann Thorac Surg 1998;66:821–827.

223. Bando K, Vijay P, Turrentine MW, et al. Dilutional and modified ultrafiltration reduces pulmonary hypertension after operations for congenital heart disease: a prospective randomized study. J Thorac Cardiovasc Surg 1998;115:517–525.

224. Pearl JM, Manning PM, McNamara JL, Saucier MM, Thomas DW. Effect of modified ultrafiltration on plasma thromboxanes B2, leukotriene B4, and endothelin-1 in infants undergoing cardiopulmonary bypass. Ann Thorac Surg 1999;68:1369–1375.

15
Pediatric Myocardial Protection

Jeffrey M. Pearl, Jodie Y. Duffy, and Kelly M. McLean

Introduction

Although the basic principles of myocardial protection are similar for adult and pediatric hearts, major differences exist between the metabolic profiles and preoperative states of adult and pediatric hearts undergoing surgery [1,2]. Although the immature myocardium is attributed with increased tolerance to ischemia, much of the data are from models in which the hearts are not stressed preoperatively or in isolated preparations where deep hypothermia is maintained. In general, irreversible myocardial injury occurs after 20 min of warm, global, nonarrested ischemia in both mature and immature myocardia [3–5]. The impression that neonatal myocardium is "more tolerant of ischemia" than mature myocardium is based partially on studies demonstrating the neonate's overall tolerance to hypoxia and the ability to protect the myocardium by hypothermia alone [1,6,7]. For those involved with the clinical care of neonates undergoing cardiac surgery, however, the neonatal myocardium seems anything but tolerant of ischemic arrest and cardiopulmonary bypass (CPB). In fact, in early studies suggesting greater tolerance to long periods of ischemia, the neonatal heart still demonstrates suboptimal functional recovery, approximately 40% of baseline function [8].

In an elaborate study with crystalloid cardioplegia in infants and children undergoing cardiac surgery, Imura and colleagues demonstrated that children had significantly less reperfusion injury and better clinical outcomes than infants [9]. This difference was related, at least in part, to longer ischemic times in the infants. Although cyanosis did not impact clinical outcome in infants, cyanotic children showed worse reperfusion injury. These findings demonstrate the difficulty in applying generalities to pediatric hearts and the complexities of studying myocardial protection in this nonhomogeneous population.

Although chronic hypoxia may result in a form of ischemic preconditioning that increases the heart's tolerance for subsequent ischemia, acute periods of hypoxia may make hearts more susceptible to injury. In addition, the reintroduction of high oxygen levels to hypoxic tissue results in reoxygenation injury, analogous to reperfusion injury in many ways [6,7,10–14].

A further problem in determining the relative tolerance to ischemia involves defining the age at which the myocardium transitions from immature to mature and when data from animal models can be extrapolated to humans. It is clear that neonatal myocardium expresses fetal genes that may influence its ability to withstand cyanosis, but not necessarily ischemia [15]. As with many therapies in pediatrics, modalities designed for adults are applied to pediatrics without sufficient testing and evaluation. Furthermore, the ability to extrapolate animal studies to human neonates and infants is speculative at best. In this chapter, we attempt to define the unique features of pediatric myocardial protection and explore the scientific bases for modalities employed and under investigation.

Special Features of the Neonatal Myocardium

A significant difference between the immature and mature myocardium is the primary source of adenosine triphosphate (ATP) production. Oxidation of long chain fatty acids provides for the majority, 90%, of ATP production in adult hearts [16]. This reliance on fatty acids makes mature myocardium dependent on aerobic metabolism through the Krebs cycle and therefore highly susceptible to tissue hypoxia. In contrast, glucose is the major source of ATP production in the immature myocardium (Figure 15.1). Furthermore, the immature heart has the ability to oxidize lactate from the blood to pyruvate, in essence utilizing lactate for energy production [17]. Heart muscle exclusively oxidizes lactate to carbon dioxide and water in the presence of oxygen with the direction of lactate dehydrogenase dependent on the ratio of $NADH:NAD^+$. Although the immature heart can utilize fatty acids, ketones, and amino acids when oxygen is present, ATP can still be produced via glycolysis under anaerobic conditions. This feature may explain the ability of neonates and infants to tolerate hypoxia [2]. However, this feature does not necessarily translate into ischemia tolerance

D.S. Wheeler et al. (eds.), *Cardiovascular Pediatric Critical Illness and Injury,*
DOI 10.1007/978-1-84800-923-3_15, © Springer-Verlag London Limited 2009

FIGURE 15.1. Schematic of myocardial energy metabolism demonstrating the major differences between immature and mature myocardium. Acetyl-CoA, acetyl coenzyme A; ADP, adenosine diphosphate; AMP, adenosine 5′-phosphate; ATP, adenosine triphosphate; 5′NT, 5′-nucleotidase.

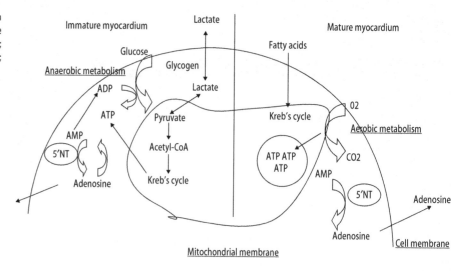

where the lack of glucose delivery and failure to washout accumulated lactate affects myocyte function.

Extrapolating from adult data, the ability to oxidize glucose following ischemia correlates with return of contractile function [18]. Explanations for the superiority of glucose metabolism in the peri-ischemic period include (1) carbohydrates carry more of their own oxygen and, hence, glucose use is more efficient; (2) oxidation of glucose at the pyruvate dehydrogenase step consumes protons generated during ischemia; and (3) glycogen metabolism may be associated with maintenance of sarcoplasmic reticulum function. As immature hearts preferentially utilize glucose, it seems reasonable to expect longer ischemic tolerance than nonglucose-utilizing mature hearts [19].

Additional unique features of the immature myocardium are its dependence on extracellular calcium for contractility because of an underdeveloped sarcoplasmic reticulum and lower sarcoplasmic calcium ATPase activity [20]. Calcium is not only important for contractility, but regulates several pathways involved in ischemia–reperfusion injury. Because of its increased dependence on extra-cellular calcium and reduced ability to handle intracellular calcium, especially when sodium-potassium and sodium-calcium pumps are inhibited, the immature myocardium is particularly sensitive to the calcium fluxes during ischemia–reperfusion. However, great controversy still exists as to the optimal calcium content of cardioplegia and reperfusates [21,22].

A notable difference between adult and pediatric myocardial protection that influences the method, more than the type, of cardioplegia is the inadequate coronary distribution secondary to atherosclerosis often seen in the adult. This is rarely an issue in pediatrics. However, the microvascular distribution and capillary density may play an important role in both the ability to protect the immature heart and in its long-term function, especially where the right ventricle is concerned [23–25].

The preoperative state of the heart may have the largest impact on tolerance of the myocardium to the global ischemia imposed by aortic cross-clamping during surgery. The presence of preoperative cyanosis in many infants and children influences subsequent ability of the heart to tolerate a period of ischemia [26–29]. β-Adrenergic receptor agonists administered preoperatively, as is often required in neonates, may stimulate other processes affecting the heart's ability to tolerate ischemia, as well as result in decreased β-agonist responsiveness postoperatively [30].

As agents have become available to selectively open or block membrane channels and ATP-driven pumps, increased interest into the role of these cell membrane processes in reperfusion injury has occurred. This area of interest has expanded to the neonatal myocardium. The Na^{2+}/H^+ exchanger is active in neonatal hearts and plays an important role in reperfusion injury in the immature heart. Intracellular accumulation of sodium ions increases the activity and exchange of the sodium-calcium pump, thereby increasing detrimental intracellular calcium during ischemia and early reperfusion [31,32].

Oxidant injury at reperfusion is a main mechanism of myocardial injury, and the antioxidant defense system of the myocardium correlates with its ability to withstand oxidant injury. Oxidant stress occurs in pediatric hearts undergoing aortic cross-clamping [33]. It has been hypothesized that immature hearts have reduced levels of endogenous antioxidants, such as catalase and superoxide dismutase. In addition, studies demonstrate that glutathione reductase is markedly decreased in patients with tetralogy of Fallot [34,35].

Although the basic principles of myocardial protection are similar between mature and immature myocardium, the best way to accomplish these goals varies. The basic tenants of myocardial protection have been reduction of metabolic demand and provision of metabolic substrates and oxygen. Traditionally, this has been accomplished by (1) diastolic arrest of the contractile components and cessation of electrical activity, (2) reduction of metabolic activity by hypothermia, (3) intermittent or continuous oxygen delivery, (4) maintaining acid–base balance, (5) metabolic enhancement, and (6) modifying reperfusion. In addition to these basic tenants, additional concepts and modalities are being studied. These include (1) pre-ischemic conditioning, (2) membrane channel openers, (3) antiinflammatory agents, (4) direct inhibitors of specific injury pathways, and (5) gene therapy.

Effects of Cardiopulmonary Bypass on the Myocardium

The role of CPB and its effects on all organs are covered in detail elsewhere. Certainly, the inflammatory response to CPB affects not only the myocardium but other organs as well. However, the conditions of the myocardium before ischemic arrest, that is, the adequacy and composition of perfusate supplied to the heart before placement of the aortic cross-clamp, can have a significant impact on the heart and its response to subsequent ischemia. It has recently been shown that using a pH-stat strategy for management of acid–base status during cooling results in lower troponin T release than does the alpha-stat strategy. Postoperative ventilation and length of intensive care unit stay were longer with an alpha-stat strategy than with a pH-stat strategy [36]. This emphasizes that myocardial injury and function are related to multiple factors, not only ischemic arrest and cardioplegia type.

Reoxygenation of a chronically cyanotic infant, as occurs with the institution of CPB, results in myocardial injury from the reintroduction of oxygen and subsequent formation of oxygen-derived free radicals [6,7,12,14]. Particularly in cyanotic patients, CPB should be instituted with a PO_2 of no greater than 200 mm Hg to prevent oxidant-mediated reoxygenation injury.

Administration of agents in anticipation of cardiac surgery has been advocated to decrease myocardial injury and improve functional recovery. Glucocorticoids are undoubtedly the most widely used. Despite numerous experimental studies showing the benefits of either priming the myocardium for subsequent ischemia or direct pre-ischemic conditioning, few have been studied clinically and even fewer applied in clinical practice.

Glucocorticoids are routinely and somewhat empirically added to the pump prime in many cardiac centers. The presumed mechanisms of glucocorticoids have been to decrease the inflammatory response to cardiopulmonary bypass and thereby limit the deleterious effects of bypass on cardiopulmonary function. Preoperative administration of glucocorticoids has been shown to be even more advantageous than intraoperative dosing alone [37]. In particular, glucocorticoids decrease myocyte intracellular adhesion molecule-1 (ICAM-1) and monocyte chemoattractant protein-1 (MCP-1) expression, apoptosis, and troponin I degradation, resulting in improved myocardial function.

As blood cardioplegia is made from pump blood mixed with a crystalloid component, the composition of the pump blood is likely to affect myocardial protection. The colloid oncotic pressure of the pump blood affects the degree of myocardial edema present following cardioplegic arrest and reperfusion [38]. In addition, the calcium content of the pump blood can influence the calcium content of the blood cardioplegia, which has significant effects on myocardial protection.

Cardiopulmonary bypass increases expression of both E-selectin and ICAM-1 in cardiac and skeletal tissue in children [39]. Neutrophil CD11 integrins are also elevated with CPB, leading to increased neutrophil adhesion and activation [40]. Techniques of leukocyte depletion or neutrophil blocking have been applied to the entire bypass circuit with the same constraints and difficulties encountered as when applying it selectively to cardioplegia.

Delivery Systems

Traditionally, cardioplegia was administered in an antegrade fashion into the aortic root. However, primarily because of inadequate antegrade delivery in the presence of occluded coronaries in adults undergoing bypass grafting, retrograde delivery via the coronary sinus was developed. Retrograde delivery distributes cardioplegia fairly well to the myocardium and provides good protection. Retrograde cardioplegia is also useful during aortic valve or root surgery where repeated antegrade doses cannot be administered, except by direct coronary ostial infusion. Retrograde cardioplegia is also invaluable when effective antegrade delivery is not feasible, as in the case of significant aortic valve incompetence.

Retrograde cardioplegia, however, provides heterogeneous and poor protection of the right ventricle in comparison to the left ventricle. Using magnetic resonance spectroscopy to assess myocardial perfusion in piglets, Oriaku and colleagues demonstrated perfusion deficits in the right ventricular wall and a portion of the left ventricular posterior wall [41]. Intracellular pH was 6.83 and phosphocreatine was 53.5% of baseline following ischemic arrest with retrograde cardioplegia protection alone. Despite this heterogeneous perfusion, ATP levels remained normal, and functional recovery was complete. The incomplete ability of retrograde cardioplegia to protect the right ventricle may be particularly problematic in patients with hypoplastic left heart syndrome where the right ventricle is the systemic pump and antegrade cardioplegia cannot be repeated during the Norwood arch reconstruction. Oriaku and colleagues demonstrated in immature porcine hearts that retrograde cardioplegia distribution, especially to the right ventricle, was heterogeneous and unable to maintain metabolic demands under normothermic conditions [41]. Placement of a purse-string in the ostium of the coronary sinus and insertion of only the very tip of the retrograde catheter have been shown to improve the distribution of cardioplegia to the right ventricle. Ostial occlusion resulted in an increase in the ratio of nutrient flow/total cardioplegic flow from 32.3% to 61.3% in explanted adult hearts [42]. Other studies have demonstrated that retrograde cardioplegia perfuses the microvascular bed similar to antegrade and in some studies reach between 14% and 30% of areas not perfused by antegrade cardioplegia [43].

A typical pediatric myocardial protection strategy includes a 30 mL/kg antegrade dose of *high-potassium* (delivered potassium concentration of 12 mEq/L) cardioplegia given at a perfusion pressure of around 40–60 mm Hg. Subsequent doses of 10–15 mL/kg of *low-potassium* (delivered potassium concentration of 8 mEq/L) cardioplegia are given every 20 min either antegrade or retrograde. Topical cooling is generally employed intermittently as well.

Hypothermia and Cardioplegia

Hypothermia alone has a significant impact on limiting myocardial injury during ischemia. Myocardial oxygen consumption decreases linearly with hypothermia, reaching 1% of baseline at temperatures below 12°C [44]. In fact, hypothermia alone can provide adequate myocardial protection, especially for neonatal hearts [45]. It has been suggested that the main benefit of cardioplegia in neonatal hearts is its ability to maintain adequate cooling of the heart. However, the benefits of hypothermia alone appear to be age dependent, limited to immature myocardium. The additional benefits of cardioplegia increase with age [1]. Although hypothermia alone may provide reasonable myocardial protection, maintaining adequate myocardial hypothermia, less than 12°C, in the clinical setting is difficult and unreliable. In an important study by Ganzel et al., it was demonstrated that at a systemic perfusion temperature of 28°C myocardial temperature increased above 15°C within 10 min and is at 20°C within 20 min of perfusing the heart with a dose of cold cardioplegia at 12°C [46]. Even the addition of cardioplegia at 15°C can result in an increase of 20% in myocardial recovery.

The addition of cardioplegia to hypothermia has become a widely accepted modality to maximize myocardial protection and prolong safe ischemic times needed for complex repairs. Although numerous solutions exist, the basic mechanism and goal of cardioplegia are similar, namely, depolarizing or hyperpolarizing the myocyte membrane and arresting cardiac mechanical activity. Energy consumption even at normothermic temperatures is markedly diminished in the arrested noncontractile heart.

Although it may be difficult to tease out the relative benefits of cardioplegia from hypothermia alone, a period of "protected arrest" following a period of ischemia in stressed hearts is preferable to ischemic insult without a subsequent period of myocardial arrest. In a study of hypoxic piglets undergoing a 20-min period of ischemia, none survived without subsequent therapy. Warm induction cardioplegia with subsequent intermittent cold doses partially reversed the stress injury and resulted in survivors, although function remained depressed [47]. In a recent randomized pediatric trial of three different cardioplegic solutions, no significant differences in clinical outcome, ATP levels, ATP:ADP ratio, or glutamate levels were seen in acyanotic patients. The three strategies employed were (1) cold crystalloid, (2) cold-blood cardioplegia, and (3) cold blood cardioplegia with a terminal warm shot. In cyanotic patients, however, cold-blood cardioplegia with terminal warm reperfusion was superior to cold-crystalloid cardioplegia in terms of improved ATP levels, ATP:ADP ratio, and glutamate levels at the end of ischemia and after reperfusion. Blood cardioplegia alone without warm reperfusion was intermediate between the other two strategies in terms of preservation of these energy metabolites [48].

In a piglet model, Bolling and colleagues demonstrated complete functional recovery using either crystalloid or blood cardioplegia in nonstressed heart [49]. However, in hearts subjected to 60 min of hypoxia before arrest, blood cardioplegia was superior to crystalloid with end systolic elastance of 106% versus 40%; preload recruitable stroke work index of 103% versus 40%; and diastolic stiffness of 153% versus 240%. This study once again emphasizes the discrepancies seen in many laboratory studies of cardioplegia where nonischemic and acyanotic animals were studied or nonblood-perfused isolated preparations were utilized.

As the controversy of blood versus crystalloid cardioplegia continues, attempts have been made to apply more sophisticated basic science to determine the effects of various cardioplegia solutions on the myocardium. Understanding the importance of the apoptotic process, Feng and colleagues demonstrated preservation of antiapoptotic pathways and decreased caspase-3 activation with blood cardioplegia compared with crystalloid cardioplegia [50]. Increased phosphorylation of Bad was seen with blood cardioplegia, which preserved the antiapoptotic protein Bcl-2. Blood cardioplegia results in less release of soluble E-selectin and ICAM-1 than crystalloid cardioplegia [51]. Similar to the deleterious effects of hyperoxic bypass on cyanotic hearts, the oxygen content of the initial cardioplegia may also influence myocardial protection in cyanotic infants.

As mentioned, the benefits of cardioplegia in general, and more specifically the impact of the type and composition of cardioplegia used, are highly dependent on the pre-ischemic state of the myocardium. In general, however, the data support the superiority of blood cardioplegia over crystalloid cardioplegia.

Additives and Compositions of Cardioplegia

Incorporation of Krebs cycle intermediates into cardioplegia ha been advocated as a means to resuscitate the heart rather tha simply protecting it from further ischemic damage. This may b particularly applicable to hearts that are stressed before cardiople gic arrest, such as in ischemic or cyanotic heart disease and i transplantation. Glutamate and aspartate are most commonl applied as a means of metabolic enhancement of the myocardiun Other substances such as pyruvate [19] or fumarate [52] are als used with similar results. In general, amino acid–enriched cardic plegia is limited to warm induction and/or warm terminal reperfu sion and withheld from the intervening cold doses.

It has been suggested that hyperkalemic-based cardioplegia doe not completely depress myocardial oxygen consumption, especiall when adequate hypothermia is not achieved. In fact, the restin membrane potential of a potassium-arrested heart is around - 50 mV compared with a nonarrested heart where the resting mem brane potential is −85 mV. Even in the phase of apparent myocardia quiescence, hearts undergoing hyperkalemic cardioplegia arres and subsequent reperfusion still demonstrate myocyte and micro vascular injury [53]. As a result, recent studies have focused o using either a polarizing cardioplegia based on lidocaine and ade nosine or sodium-potassium channel openers.

Antioxidants added to cardioplegia have been studied experi mentally as a means of decreasing oxidant injury during reperfu sion [54]. However, adequate delivery of these agents clinically i problematic and, despite supportive evidence of potential benefit this modality has not readily been adapted.

Adenosine

The beneficial effects of adenosine in cardioplegia have been knowr for some time. Although the exact mechanisms by which adenosine is beneficial are not clear, and likely multifactorial, recent data suggest that adenosine may be an important mediator of pre-ischemic conditioning. Most of the prior focus on adenosine has been on its effect on the A1 receptor and the subsequent effect on sodium-potassium channels. More recently it has been suggested that adenosine may also exert myocardial protective effects via A2 receptors and subsequent downstream regulation of ERK1/2 [55] and PI$_3$ kinase-dependent pathways [30]. Immature myocardium is less capable of converting AMP to adenosine because of reduced levels of 5′ nucleotidase [56]. Hence, adenosine levels are maintained at a higher level in immature hearts, which may result in ischemic tolerance. This may also account for the diminished effectiveness of adenosine supplementation in immature hearts compared with adults.

Calcium and Magnesium

The calcium content of cardioplegia is a hotly debated and controversial topic. Proponents of hypocalcemic cardioplegia cite evidence of calcium's role in reperfusion injury and evidence that calcium influx in the face of ischemia can result in contracture. Advocates of maintaining calcium levels in cardioplegia provide evidence that completely acalcemic solutions can result in "stone heart" and the important role of extracellular calcium in contractility, especially in neonatal myocardium. This controversy arises, in part, from the models used to test the responses to various levels of calcium in cardioplegia. Hearts in which no preceding ischemic or hypoxic insult is present tend to recover close to normal function with hypocalcemic cardioplegia and normal or supranormal function with normocalcemic cardioplegia [45]. However, it appears that stressed hearts, which is often the case in both adult ischemic heart disease and cyanotic infants and children, have better functional recovery and decreased injury with hypocalcemic, but not acalcemic, cardioplegia.

In a study looking at the effects of cardioplegia calcium concentration on myocardial protection of acutely hypoxic piglet hearts, Kronon and colleagues clearly demonstrate improved results with hypocalcemic solution compared with normocalcemic cardioplegia [57]. Systolic function after CPB, measured as end systolic elastance, is 49% with normocalcemic cardioplegia versus 101% with hypocalcemic cardioplegia. Diastolic stiffness and preload recruitable stroke work index are also superior in the normocalcemic group [57]. Although to emphasize the continued controversy regarding the optimal calcium concentration in cardioplegia, a follow-up study by the same researchers shows incomplete protection and recovery with hypocalcemic cardioplegia unless magnesium is added [47].

Accumulation of intracellular calcium during ischemia and reperfusion results in cellular injury. Although it is clear that limiting intracellular calcium during ischemia and reperfusion is important, the best method to achieve this remains unclear. Calcium channel blockers show benefits, but may be undesirable following reperfusion when calcium influx is needed for contraction. Pediatric hearts, being more dependent on extracellular calcium, are particularly sensitive to calcium channel blockers. Decreasing, but not eliminating, calcium from cardioplegia is probably the simplest way to control calcium content during ischemia and reperfusion. The use of citrate-phosphate-dextrose (CPD) in the crystalloid component of cardioplegia is often not necessary, as the pump blood calcium content is usually low due to CPD in the blood and dilution with crystalloid. As a result, most cardioplegia solutions contain reduced calcium concentrations, obtained by either the use of CPD or simply by diluting the blood with a hypocalcemic cardioplegia solution, such as plegisol. It is preferable to avoid additional CPD, if possible, as there is a potential for calcium chelation that impacts myocardial function after reperfusion.

Magnesium's important role in both myocardial protection and function is becoming increasingly apparent. Magnesium interacts with calcium, has a role in potassium's effect on the heart, and is antiarrhythmic. In a study by Kronon and colleagues, normocalcemic cardioplegia was detrimental to hypoxic neonatal piglet hearts, and magnesium supplementation was able to attenuate the harmful effects of normocalcemic cardioplegia [47]. By competing with calcium for entry sites, magnesium in cardioplegia may limit or negate the effects of calcium during ischemia and reperfusion. Magnesium is a routine component of cardioplegia, in part due to the difficulty with precise control of calcium in blood cardioplegia.

Leukocyte Depletion

Leukocytes are an important mediator of inflammation and in particular of reperfusion injury in ischemic tissues. Leukocyte-depleted reperfusion of ischemic tissues has been shown to reduce injury in many tissue types, including the heart. This strategy can be applied to the CPB circuit as a whole, to the induction dose of cardioplegia, to the terminal reperfusate, or to all doses of cardio-

plegia. However, maintaining an adequate degree of leukocyte depletion with available technology remains the limiting factor. Current leukocyte-depleting filters are limited by their volume and flow. As a result of mostly technical and cost constraints, mechanical leukocyte depletion has not been widely applied or become routine, except in transplant reperfusion.

In a clinical study, Hayashi and colleagues demonstrate reduced oxidant injury, lower CPK-MB, and less inotrope requirement in 25 patients receiving leukocyte-depleted cardioplegia compared with 25 receiving nondepleted blood cardioplegia [58]. A more feasible approach to using leukocyte depletion might be to limit it to the final warm reperfusion dose of cardioplegia [59]. Other modalities aimed at preventing leukocyte injury have included prevention of leukocyte adhesion using monoclonal antibodies to CD18, ICAM-1, or selectins [60–63]. Despite encouraging animal studies, a multicenter clinical study failed to show significant benefit for leukocyte depletion.

Terminal Reperfusion

Terminal reperfusate is the final dose of cardioplegia or blood the heart receives before removal of the aortic cross-clamp. The goal of terminal reperfusion is to warm the heart but maintain arrest, so that metabolic pathways can recover, before the increased demand imposed by contraction. In a study of children, not neonates or infants, Toyoda and colleagues demonstrated improved lactate extraction ratio, lower postreperfusion troponin T, and heart-type fatty acid binding protein in both cyanotic and acyanotic patients receiving terminal warm reperfusion [64]. They concluded that terminal warm reperfusion enhanced myocardial protection by improving aerobic energy metabolism and decreasing myocardial injury. Terminal warm reperfusion reduces myocardial oxidative stress and improves heart recovery after cardioplegic arrest [33].

The impact of the type of cardioplegia and the use of terminal reperfusion may vary depending on the pre-ischemic state of the myocardium. In a clinical study, cold blood cardioplegia with terminal warm reperfusion resulted in improved energy state of the myocardium in cyanotic patients, but was of no additional benefit in acyanotic patients [48].

Utilizing an animal model of acute hypoxia followed by aortic cross-clamping with intermittent cold-blood cardioplegia, Kronon demonstrated a significant decrease in end systolic elastance and preload recruitable stroke work index along with increased diastolic stiffness when no terminal reperfusate was used. In contrast, when warm-blood cardioplegia enriched with the Krebs cycle precursors glutamate and aspartate was used before removal of the aortic cross-clamp, there was complete recovery of end systolic elastance and preload recruitable stroke work index compared with either no reperfusate or warm, nonenriched terminal reperfusate (end systolic elastance of 105% vs. 41% and 50%, respectively; preload recruitable stroke work index of 103% vs. 41% and 52%, respectively). Adenosine triphosphate levels were also preserved with terminal warm enriched reperfusate at 15.5 versus 10.7 and 11.9 µg/g of tissue [47].

Ischemic Preconditioning

Ischemic preconditioning increases the tolerance to later ischemia–reperfusion [65–68]. Preconditioning prevents both necrosis and apoptosis and moderates the degree of myocardial stunning. Two phases have been identified in ischemic preconditioning, an acute phase lasting a few hours and a delayed phase appearing at 24 hr. The acute phase is, in part, based on the release of substances such as adenosine and bradykinin that affect ATP-sensitive potassium channels and mitochondrial permeability transition pores. The delayed phase requires the synthesis of new proteins such as inducible nitric oxide synthase and heat shock proteins. The second phase of ischemic preconditioning is related to opening of mitochondrial potassium-ATP (K-ATP) channels and activation of protein kinase C and p38 MAP kinase.

Ischemic preconditioning clearly reduces infarct size and improves functional recovery in infarct models of regional myocardial ischemia. However, whether this phenomenon is applicable to the more global ischemia associated with hypothermic arrest used for repair of congenital heart disease or is even present in immature myocardium is less clear. Furthermore, the effect of agents used for pre-ischemic conditioning overlaps considerably, with apparent equal benefit, when used either at the time of ischemia or reperfusion [69].

Although the classic modality of inducing pre-ischemic conditioning is a short, controlled period of nonlethal ischemia before the main ischemic–reperfusion event, improved understanding of the underlying mechanisms has permitted more focused modalities [68]. As mentioned, a key component of ischemic preconditioning appears to involve activation of K-ATP channels. Both adenosine (acutely) and nitric oxide (delayed) mediate this effect. Stimulation of these substances by either an antecedent brief ischemic event, the traditional definition of ischemic preconditioning, or pharmacologic manipulation accomplishes similar effects [70–72].

Heat shock proteins have a protective effect on subsequent tolerance of myocardium to ischemia–reperfusion. Induction of heat shock proteins may occur with CPB itself, as well as with cardioplegic arrest. Hearts demonstrating increased levels of heat shock protein 72 have decreased injury following ischemic arrest [73]. Elevated levels of heat shock proteins have been correlated with decreased myocardial injury following cardioplegic arrest and are a possible mechanism of pre-ischemic conditioning. The mechanisms of action underlying heat shock proteins' inhibition of myocardial injury are not fully known.

Manipulation of mitochondrial transition pores has also been identified as a potential mechanism of ischemic preconditioning [74,75]. Volatile anesthetics are known to stimulate pathways involved in ischemic preconditioning. Volatile anesthetics prime the activation of the sarcolemmal and mitochondrial K-ATP channels by stimulating adenosine receptors and subsequent activation of protein kinase C. Inhaled anesthetics also increase formation of nitric oxide and oxygen-derived free radicals [76,77]. Desflurane, which stimulates α- and β-adrenergic receptors, is the preferred inhalational agent for cardiac anesthesia in some centers.

Experimental Myocardial Protection

Not surprisingly, because of its regulation of nitric oxide pathways, sildenafil citrate (Viagra, Pfizer, Groton, CT) has been studied for its possible effects on myocardial ischemia–reperfusion injury and myocardial protection. A recent study using the phosphodiesterase-5 inhibitor sildenafil citrate demonstrated reduced infarct size and improved functional recovery following regional ischemia-reperfusion in rabbits [78]. Our own studies of sildenafil in hypoxia and reoxygenation on CPB demonstrated improved post-reoxygen-

ation left ventricular systolic function compared with untreated animals [79]. Sildenafil has also been shown to prevent endothelial dysfunction induced by ischemia–reperfusion via opening of adenosine-sensitive potassium channels [80].

Administration of L-arginine is also beneficial as a means to augment nitric oxide production. L-arginine can decrease myocardial reperfusion injury and prevent endothelial cell dysfunction [81]. The role of nitric oxide in myocardial protection, however, remains controversial. Supplementation of nitric oxide by providing L-arginine in cardioplegia has had mixed results. It has been suggested that nitric oxide and cGMP may play a role in metabolic adaptation of glucose metabolism to oxygen deprivation [82]. Endothelin-1 is also involved in ischemia–reperfusion injury, and its blockade reduces myocardial dysfunction [83]. Endothelin-1 blockade is associated with decreased leukocyte-mediated injury that may be, in part, due to preservation of nitric oxide activity that is inhibited by endothelin-1.

Traditionally, cardioplegia's greatest effect is hyperkalemia that results in diastolic arrest by affecting the gradient between the potassium-sodium exchange pump [84]. Newer agents that specifically target these pumps are being developed. This modality may provide for a more effective and complete way to achieve diastolic arrest and avoid the potentially harmful effects on the coronary endothelium of hyperkalemic solutions. In a study of adults undergoing coronary bypass grafting, the addition of nicorandil, a hybrid potassium channel opener, to the standard cardioplegic regiment resulted in quicker arrest, better spontaneous recovery, decreased markers of myocardial injury, and lower doses of catecholamines required after surgery [85,86]. Similarly, exogenous K-ATP channel activation by pinacidil pretreatment and cardioplegic enrichment significantly improved the tolerance of neonatal myocardium to cardioplegic arrest in animal studies [50].

Antioxidants such as catalase and superoxide dismutase reduce oxidant injury during reperfusion. However, despite some encouraging clinical studies, this modality has not been incorporated into routine clinical practice. Desferroxamine has been studied for some time as an antioxidant capable of reducing myocardial reperfusion injury. A recent clinical study in adults undergoing coronary artery bypass grafting demonstrated that the anti-oxidant properties can be translated to the clinical setting [87].

In animal studies, poly(adenosine 5′-diphosphate-ribose) synthetase inhibition has been shown to attenuate myocardial ischemia–reperfusion injury by inhibiting oxidative stress and energy depletion [88]. The role of mitochondrial transition pores in myocardial ischemic–reperfusion injury is a relatively new and exciting area of investigation. Reperfusion of the heart following ischemia results in opening of a nonspecific pore in the inner mitochondrial membrane called *mitochondrial transition pore* [75,89,90]. This results in an uncoupling of the mitochondria, making it capable of hydrolyzing rather than synthesizing ATP. The prevention of pore opening correlates with the degree of injury and functional recovery [91]. Inhibition of mitochondrial transition pore opening can be accomplished by cyclosporine A or by decreasing calcium loading and oxidant formation. This is an exciting area of investigation but, as of yet, is not clinically applicable.

Recent evidence has demonstrated an important and perhaps critical role of the calpain–calpastatin system in myocardial ischemia–reperfusion. Calpain is a proteolytic enzyme that is activated by the dissociation of its natural inhibitor calpastatin during reperfusion. Calpain is the only identified substance that is a specific for degrading troponin I. The calcium influx occurring with reperfusion results in calpain activation and subsequent injury. In fact, calpain inhibition has been shown experimentally to reduce myocardial injury, including troponin degradation and apoptosis [92]. Calpastatin, the endogenous inhibitor of the proteolytic enzyme calpain, also regulates L-type calcium channels [93]. Ischemia-reperfusion decreases calpastatin while increasing calpain activity. Glucocorticoids exert a protective effect, at least in part by maintaining myocardial calpastatin levels and attenuating calpain activation [94].

Intracoronary gene therapy utilizing adenoviral vectors can increase myocardial expression of beneficial genes. This modality is being investigated as a means of providing both pre-ischemic conditioning acute protection and resuscitation of myocardium. Experimentally, increased adenoviral vector expression of β-adrenergic receptors with subsequent improved left ventricular function was demonstrated [95–97]. Delivery of either β-adrenergic receptor kinase inhibitor or heat shock protein 70 has been applied to donor heart preservation [96,98]. Gene delivery with CPB, avoiding the need for direct coronary injection, has been successful [99]. Adenoviral gene transfer to the myocardium during cardiopulmonary bypass has been effective in increasing β-adrenergic receptor density in animal models. The implications for this modality are intriguing as a means to not only protect and prevent injury but also provide a means of actually restoring myocardial viability and function. It is likely that gene therapy will have a significant impact on both myocardial protection and resuscitation in the ensuing years.

Myocardial Protection During Transplantation

Several features of myocardial protection are unique to transplantation. In general, longer ischemic times are tolerated compared with hearts arrested in situ because of the ability to keep a donor heart cold during storage and transport. However, unlike in situ hearts, where repeated doses of cardioplegia are administered, typically only a single dose of cardioplegia is given to a donor organ at the time of explantation. Furthermore, cardioplegia solution used for transplant myocardial protection is usually crystalloid based. Because of these unique parameters, donor ischemia times of 6hr or longer are acceptable, especially with pediatric hearts. However, there is still poor long-term graft survival with prolonged ischemic periods.

Two crystalloid solutions are currently used by most transplant centers for donor heart preservation. The electrolyte composition and the presence of other additives are the main differences between the two solutions. Stanford solution, one of the first widely used transplant cardioplegia, was based on data from other crystalloid cardioplegia used for routine myocardial protection. As such, its electrolyte composition was extracellular, similar to plasma but with a potassium concentration around 20 mEq. In contrast, University of Wisconsin (UW) solution, which was initially developed for liver preservation but soon applied to heart transplantation, has an electrolyte composition similar to intracellular fluid, with a potassium concentration of around 120 mEq. A study by Breda and colleagues demonstrated the superiority of intracellular solutions compared with extracellular solution in animal models [100]. Subsequent studies with UW solution confirmed its role as an outstanding transplant cardioplegia [101]. Theoretically, intracellular cardioplegia more completely ceases Na-K pump activity on the membrane because of equal electrolyte concentrations with no gradient across the membrane to drive the shifts of ions and fluid. This has been shown to reduce myocardial edema compared with extracellular solutions that primarily affect potassium pumps. In addition, UW solution contains several additives that act as free-radical scavengers and metabolic substrates, in addition to osmotic agents that decrease edema.

Concern has been raised regarding potential endothelial injury related to the high potassium concentration of UW solution. Cold ischemia in UW solution is associated with acute damage to the coronary endothelium and results in a slightly higher incidence of coronary graft atherosclerosis during midterm follow up. In fact, UW solution experimentally impairs endothelial-dependent coronary relaxation. In addition, UW solution is associated with an increased incidence of coronary disease 2 years after transplant in a clinical study [102].

References

1. Baker EJ, Boerboom LE, Olinger GN. Tolerance of the developing heart to ischemia: impact of hypoxemia from birth. Am J Physiol 1995;268: H1165–H1173.
2. Bull DA, Connors RC, Albanil A, et al. Aprotinin preserves myocardial biochemical function during cold storage through suppression of tumor necrosis factor. J Thorac Cardiovasc Surg 2000;119:242–250.
3. Sellak H, Franzini E, Hakim J, Pasquier C. Reactive oxygen species rapidly increase endothelial ICAM-1 ability to bind neutrophils without detectable upregulation. Blood 1994;83:2669–2677.
4. Reimer KA, Jennings RB, Tatum AH. Pathobiology of acute myocardial ischemia: metabolic, functional and ultrastructural studies. Am J Cardiol 1983;52:72A–81A.
5. Zouki C, Baron C, Fournier A, Filep JG. Endothelin-1 enhances neutrophil adhesion to human coronary artery endothelial cells: role of ET(A) receptors and platelet-activating factor. Br J Pharmacol 1999;127:969–979.
6. Pearl JM, Nelson DP, Wellmann SA, et al. Acute hypoxia and reoxygenation impairs exhaled nitric oxide release and pulmonary mechanics. J Thorac Cardiovasc Surg 2000;119:931–938.
7. Pearl JM, Nelson DP, Wagner CJ, Lombardi JP, Duffy JY. Endothelin receptor blockade reduces ventricular dysfunction and injury after reoxygenation. Ann Thorac Surg 2001;72:565–570.
8. Yano Y, Braimbridge MV, Hearse DJ. Protection of the pediatric myocardium. Differential susceptibility to ischemic injury of the neonatal rat heart. J Thorac Cardiovasc Surg 1987;94:887–896.
9. Imura H, Caputo M, Parry A, Pawade A, Angelini GD, Suleiman MS. Age-dependent and hypoxia-related differences in myocardial protection during pediatric open heart surgery. Circulation 2001;103: 1551–1556.
10. Ihnken K, Morita K, Buckberg GD, et al. Studies of hypoxemic/reoxygenation injury: without aortic clamping. II. Evidence of reoxygenation damage. J Thorac Cardiovasc Surg 1995;110:1171–1181.
11. Ihnken K, Morita K, Buckberg GD, Sherman MP, Young HH. Studies of hypoxemic/reoxygenation injury: without aortic clamping. VI. Counteraction of oxidant damage with exogenous antioxidants: N-(2-mercaptopropionyl)-glycine and catalase. J Thorac Cardiovasc Surg 1995;110:1212–1220.
12. Ihnken K, Morita K, Buckberg GD, Winkelman B, Young HH, Beyersdorf F. Controlling oxygen content during cardiopulmonary bypass to limit reperfusion/reoxygenation injury. Transplant Proc 1995;27:2809–2811.
13. Ihnken K, Morita K, Buckberg GD, et al. Nitric oxide–induced reoxygenation injury in the cyanotic immature heart is prevented by controlling oxygen content during initial reoxygenation. Angiology 1997;48:189–202.
14. Ihnken K, Morita K, Buckberg GD. Delayed cardioplegic reoxygenation reduces reoxygenation injury in cyanotic immature hearts. Ann Thorac Surg 1998;66:177–182.

15. Sharma S, Razeghi P, Shakir A, Keneson BJ 2nd, Clubb F, Taegtmeyer H. Regional heterogeneity in gene expression profiles: a transcript analysis in human and rat heart. Cardiology 2003;100:73–79.

16. Goodwin AT, Amrani M, Gray CC, Chester AH, Yacoub MH. Inhibition of endogenous endothelin during cardioplegia improves low coronary reflow following prolonged hypothermic arrest. Eur J Cardiothorac Surg 1997;11:981–987.

17. Allen BS, Barth MJ, Ilbawi MN. Pediatric myocardial protection: an overview. Semin Thorac Cardiovasc Surg 2001;13:56–72.

18. Depre C, Rider MH. Mechanisms of control of heart glycolysis. Eur J Biochem 1998;258:277–290.

19. Olivencia-Yurvati AH, Blair JL, Baig M, Mallet RT. Pyruvate-enhanced cardioprotection during surgery with cardiopulmonary bypass. J Cardiothorac Vasc Anesth 2003;17:715–720.

20. Gombosova I, Bokink P, Kirchhefer U, et al. Postnatal changes in contractile time parameters, calcium regulatory proteins, and phosphatase. Am J Physiol 1998;274:H2123–2132.

21. Allen BS, Veluz JS, Buckberg G, Aeberhard E, Ignarro LJ. Deep hypothermic circulatory arrest and global reperfusion injury: avoidance by making a pump prime reperfusate—a new concept. J Thorac Cardiovasc Surg 2003;125:625–632.

22. Malhtra SP, Thelitz S, Riemer RK, Reddy VM, Suleman S, Hanley FL. Fetal myocardial protection is markedly improved by reduced cardioplegic calcium content. Ann Thorac Surg 2003;75:1937–1941.

23. Porter GA, Bankston PW. Maturation of myocardial capillaries in the fetal and neonatal rat heart: an ultrastructural study with a morphometric analysis of the vesicle populations. Am J Anat 1987;178:116–125.

24. Porter GA, Bankston PW. Functional maturation of the capillary wall in the fetal and neonatal rat heart, permeability characteristics of developing myocardial capillaries. Am J Anat 1987;180:323–331.

25. Maki T, Gruver EJ, Davidoff AJ, et al. Regulation of calcium channel expression in neonatal myocytes by catecholamines. J Clin Invest 2005;97:656–659.

26. Li HT, Honbo NY, Karlinger JS. Chronic hypoxia increases beta 1-adrenergic receptor mRNA and density but not signaling in neonatal rat cardiac myocytes. Circulation 1996;94:3303–3310.

27. Novotny J, Bourová L, Málková O, Svoboda P, Kolár F. G proteins, β-adrenoceptors and β-adrenergic responsiveness in immature and adult rat ventricular myocardium: influence of neonatal hypo- and hyperthyroidism. J Mol Cell Cardiol 1999;31:761–772.

28. Sun L, Chang J, Kirchhoff SR, Knowlton AA. Activation of HSF and selective increase in heat-shock proteins by acute dexamethasone treatment. Am J Physiol 2000;278:H1091–1097.

29. Rohlicek CV, Viau S, Trieu F, Herbert TE. Effects of neonatal hypoxia in the rat on inotropic stimulation of the adult heart. Cardiovasc Res 2005;65:861–868.

30. Boucher M, Pesant S, Falcao S, et al. Post-ischemic cardioprotection by A2A adenosine receptors: dependent of phosphatidylinositol 3-kinase pathway. J Cardiovasc Pharmacol 2004;43:416–422.

31. Alto LE, Elimban V, Lukas A, Dhalla NS. Modification of heart sarcolemmal Na$^+$/K$^+$-ATPase activity during development of the calcium paradox. Mol Cell Biochem 2000;207:87–94.

32. Baron O, Saiki Y, Rebeyka IM. pH paradox and neonatal heart. J Cardiovasc Surg 2001;42:475–480.

33. Calza G, Lerzo F, Perfumo F, et al. Clinical evaluation of oxidative stress and myocardial reperfusion injury in pediatric cardiac surgery. J Cardiovasc Surg 2002;43:441–447.

34. del Nido PJ, Mickle DA, Wilson GJ. Evidence of myocardial free radical injury during elective repair of tetralogy of Fallot. Circulation 1987;76:174–179.

35. Teoh KH, Mickle DAG, Weisel RD, Tumiati LC, Coles JG, Williams WG. Effect of oxygen tension and cardiovascular operations on the myocardial antioxidant enzyme activities in patients with tetralogy Fallot and aorto-coronary bypass. J Thorac Cardiovasc Surg 1992;104:159–164.

36. Nagy ZL, Collins M, Sharpe T, et al. Effect of two different bypa techniques on the serum troponin-T levels in newborns and childre does pH-stat provide better protection? Circulation 2003;108:577 582.

37. Pearl JM, Nelson DP, Schwartz SM, et al. Glucocorticoids reduce isch emia–reperfusion-induced myocardial apoptosis in immature heart Ann Thorac Surg 2002;74:830–837.

38. Mehlhorn U, Allen SJ, Davis KL, Geissler HJ, Warters RD, Rainer d Vivie E. Increasing the colloid osmotic pressure of cardiopulmonar bypass prime and normothermic blood cardioplegia minimizes myc cardial oedema and prevents cardiac dysfunction. Cardiovasc Sur 1998;6:274–281.

39. Kilbridge PM, Mayer JE, Newburger JW, Hickey PR, Walsh AZ, Neufel EJ. Induction of intercellular adhesion molecule-1 and E-selecti mRNA in heart and skeletal muscle of pediatric patients undergoin cardiopulmonary bypass. J Thorac Cardiovasc Surg 1994;107:1183 1192.

40. Le Deist F, Menasche P, Kucharski C, Bel A, Piwnica A, Bloch G. Hypo thermia during cardiopulmonary bypass delays but does not preven neutrophil–endothelial cell adhesion. A clinical study. Circulatio 1995;92:II354–II358.

41. Oriaku G, Xiang B, Dai G, et al. Effects of retrograde cardioplegia o myocardial perfusion and energy metabolism of immature porcin myocardium. J Thorac Cardiovasc Surg 2000;119:1102–1109.

42. Rudis E, Gates RN, Laks H, et al. Coronary sinus ostial occlusio during retrograde delivery of cardioplegic solution significantl improves cardioplegic distribution and efficacy. J Thorac Cardiovas Surg 1996;111:683.

43. Gates RN, Laks H, Drinkwater DC, et al. Evidence of improved micro vascular perfusion when using antegrade and retrograde cardiople gia. Ann Thorac Surg 1996;62:1388–1391.

44. Niazi SA, Lewis FJ. Effect of carbon dioxide on ventricular fibrillatio and heart block during hypothermia in rats and dogs. Surg Forun 1955;5:106–109.

45. Pearl JM, Laks H, Drinkwater DC, et al. Normocalcemic blood o crystalloid cardioplegia provides better neonatal myocardial protec tion than does low-calcium cardioplegia. J Thorac Cardiovasc Surg 1993;105:201–206.

46. Ganzel BL, Katzmark SL, Mavroudis C. Myocardial preservation in the neonate. Beneficial effects of cardioplegia and systemic hypother mia on piglets undergoing cardiopulmonary bypass and myocardia ischemia. J Thorac Cardiovasc Surg 1988;96:414–422.

47. Kronan MT, Allen BS, Hernan J, et al. Superiority of magnesium cardioplegia in neonatal myocardial protection. Ann Thorac Surg 1999;68:2285–2291.

48. Modi P, Suleiman MS, Reeves B, et al. Myocardial metabolic changes during pediatric cardiac surgery: a randomized study of three cardioplegic techniques. J Thorac Cardiovasc Surg 2004;128:67–75.

49. Bolling K, Kronon M, Allen BS, Wang T, Ramon S, Feinberg H. Myocardial protection in normal and hypoxically stressed neonatal hearts: the superiority of blood versus crystalloid cardioplegia. J Thorac Cardiovasc Surg 1997;113:994–1003.

50. Feng J, Bianchi C, Li J, Sellke FW. Improved profile of bad phosphorylation and caspase 3 activation after blood versus crystalloid cardioplegia. Ann Thorac Surg 2004;77:1384–1389.

51. Kalawski R, Majewski M, Kaszkowiak E, Wysocki H, Siminiak T. Transcardiac release of soluble adhesion molecules during coronary artery bypass grafting: effects of crystalloid and blood cardioplegia. Chest 2003;123:155–160.

52. Pearl JM, Hiramoto J, Laks H, Drinkwater DC, Chang PA. Fumarate-enriched blood cardioplegia results in complete functional recovery of immature myocardium. Ann Thorac Surg 1994;57:1636–1641.

53. Dobson GP, Jones MW. Adenosine and lidocaine: a new concept in nondepolarizing surgical myocardial arrest, protection, and preservation. J Thorac Cardiovasc Surg 2004;127:794–805.

54. Morita K, Ihnken K, Buckberg G, Matheis G, Sherman MP, Young HH. Studies of hypoxemic/reoxygenation injury: with aortic clamping. X.

Exogenous antioxidants to avoid nullification of the cardioprotective effects of blood cardioplegia. J Thorac Cardiovasc Surg 1995;110:1245–1254.

55. Kis A, Baxter GF, Yellon DM. Limitation of myocardial reperfusion injury by AMP579, an adenosine A1/A2A receptor agonist: role of A2A receptor and Erk1/2. Cardiovasc Drugs Ther 2003;17:415–425.

56. Ahmet I, Sawa Y, Nishimura M, Kitakaze M, Matsuda H. Cardioprotective effect of diadenosine tetraphosphate (AP4A) preservation in hypothermic storage and its relation with mitochondrial ATP-sensitive potassium channels. Transplantation 2005;16:16–20.

57. Kronon M, Bolling KS, Allen BS, et al. The relationship between calcium and magnesium in pediatric myocardial protection. J Thorac Cardiovasc Surg 1997;114:1010–1019.

58. Hayashi Y, Sawa Y, Nishimura M, et al. Clinical evaluation of leukocyte-depleted blood cardioplegia for pediatric open heart operation. Ann Thorac Surg 2000;69:1914–1919.

59. Civelek A, Roth M, Lemke P, Klovekorn WP, Bauer EP. Leukocyte-depleted secondary blood cardioplegia attenuates reperfusion injury after myocardial ischemia. J Thorac Cardiovasc Surg 2003;51:249–254.

60. Miura T, Nelson DP, Schermerhorn ML, et al. Blockade of selectin-mediated leukocyte adhesion improves postischemic function in lamb hearts. Ann Thorac Surg 1996;62:1295–1300.

61. Nagashima M, Shinoka T, Nollert G, et al. Effects of a monoclonal antibody to P-selectin on recovery of neonatal lamb hearts after cold cardioplegia ischemia. Circulation 1998;98:II391–II397.

62. Schermerhorn ML, Tofukuji M, Khoury PR, et al. Sialyl Lewis oligosaccharide preserves cardiopulmonary and endothelial function after hypothermia circulatory arrest in lambs. J Thorac Cardiovasc Surg 2000;120:230–237.

63. Sauer HH, Allen SJ, Cox JR, CS JR, Laine GA. Effect of Sialyl Lewis (x) selectin blockade on myocardial protection during cardioplegic arrest and reperfusion. Heart Surg Forum 2001;4:216–222.

64. Toyoda Y, Yamaguchi M, Yoshimura N, Oka S, Okita Y. Cardioprotective effects and the mechanisms of terminal warm blood cardioplegia in pediatric cardiac surgery. J Thorac Cardiovasc Surg 2003;125:1242–1251.

65. Nakamura Y, Takemoto N, Kuroda H, Ohgi S. Mechanisms of ischemic preconditioning effects on Ca^{2+} paradox-induced changes in heart. Surg Today 1999;29:884–889.

66. Olivson A, Berman E, Houminer E, et al. Glucose metabolism, energetics, and function of rat hearts exposed to ischemic preconditioning and oxygenated cardioplegia. J Card Surg 2002;17:214–225.

67. Rajesh KG, Sasaguri S, Suzuki R, Xing Y, Maeda H. Ischemic preconditioning prevents reperfusion heart injury in cardiac hypertrophy by activation of mitochondrial KATP channels. Int J Cardiol 2004;96:41–49.

68. Riksen NP, Smits P, Rongen GA. Ischaemic preconditioning: from molecular characterisation to clinical application–part I. Neth J Med 2004;62:353–363.

69. Budde JM, Morris CD, Velez DA, et al. Reduction of infarct size and preservation of endothelial function by multidose intravenous adenosine during extended reperfusion. J Surg Res 2004;116:104–115.

70. McCully JD, Levitsky S. Alternatives for myocardial protection: adenosine-enhanced ischemic preconditioning. Ann NY Acad Sci 1999;874:295–305.

71. McCully JD, Uematsu M, Levitsky S. Adenosine-enhanced ischemic preconditioning provides myocardial protection equal to that of cold blood cardioplegia. Ann Thorac Surg 1999;67:699–704.

72. Uchiyama, Otani H, Okada T, et al. Integrated pharmacological preconditioning in combination with adenosine, a mitochondrial KATP channel opener and a nitric oxide donor. J Thorac Cardiovasc Surg 2003;126:148–159.

73. Giannessi D, Caselli V, Vitale RL, et al. A possible cardioprotective effect of heat shock proteins during cardiac surgery in pediatric patients. Pharmacol Res 2003;48:519–529.

74. Hausenloy D, Wynne A, Duchen M, Yellon D. Transient mitochondrial permeability transition pore opening mediates preconditioning-induced protection. Circulation 2004;109:1714–1717.

75. Hausenloy DJ, Yellon DM. The mitochondrial permeability transition pore in myocardial preconditioning. Cardiovasc J S Afr 2004; 15:S5.

76. Zaugg CE, Hornstein PS, Zhu P, et al. Endothelin-1-induced release of thromboxane A$_2$ increases the vasoconstrictor effect of the endothelin-1 in postischemic reperfused rat hearts. Circulation 1996;94:742–747.

77. Zaugg M, Luccinetti E, Uecker M, Pasch T, Schaub MC. Anaesthetics and cardiac preconditioning. Part I. signaling and cytoprotective mechanisms. Br J Anaesth 2003;91:551–565.

78. Bremer YA, Salloum F, Ockaili R, Chou E, Moskowitz WB, Kukreja RC. Sildenafil citrate (Viagra) induces cardioprotective effects after ischemia/reperfusion in infant rabbits. Pediatr Res 2005;57:22–27.

79. Lyons JM, Duffy JY, Wagner CJ, Pearl JM. Sildenafil citrate alleviates pulmonary hypertension after hypoxia and reoxygenation with cardiopulmonary bypass. J Am Coll Surg 2004;199:607–614.

80. Gori T, Sicuro S, Dragoni S, Donati G, Forconi S, Parker JD. Sildenafil prevents endothelial dysfunction induced by ischemia and reperfusion via opening of adenosine triphosphate–sensitive potassium channels: a human in vivo study. Circulation 2005;111:742–746.

81. Hayashida N, Tomoeda H, Oda T, et al. Effects of supplemental L-arginine during warm blood cardioplegia. Ann Thorac Cardiovasc Surg 2000;6:27–33.

82. Depre C, Vanoverschelde Jl, Goudemant JF, Mottet I, Hue l. Protection against ischemic injury by nonvasoactive concentrations of nitric oxide synthase in the perfused rabbit heart. Eur J Biochem 1998;258:277–290.

83. Pearl JM, Nelson DP, Wagner CJ, Lombardi JP, Duffy JY. Endothelin receptor blockade reduces ventricular dysfunction and injury after reoxygenation. Ann Thorac Surg 2001;72:570.

84. Fleming W. New strategies for intraoperative myocardial protection. Curr Opin Cardiol 1995;10:577–583.

85. Hayashi Y, Sawa Y, Ohtake S, Nishimura M, Ichkawa H, Matsuda H. Controlled nicorandil administration for myocardial protection during coronary artery bypass grafting under cardiopulmonary bypass. J Cardiovasc Pharmacol 2001;38:21–28.

86. Miura T, Miki T. ATP-sensitive K$^+$ channel openers: old drugs with new clinical benefits for the heart. Curr Vasc Pharmacol 2003;1:251–258.

87. Paraskevaidis IA, Iliodromitis EK, Vlahakos D, et al. Desferroxamine infusion during coronary artery bypass grafting ameliorates lipid peroxidation and protects the myocardium against reperfusion injury: immediate and long-term significance. Eur Heart J 2005;3:263–270.

88. Bloch W, Mehlhorn U. Poly-adenosine diphosphate-ribose polymerase inhibition for myocardial protection: pathophysiologic and physiologic considerations. J Thorac Cardiovasc Surg 2004;128:323–324.

89. Zingarelli B, Cuzzocrea S, Zsengeller Z, Salzman AL, Szabó C. Inhibition of poly(ADP ribose) synthase protects against myocardial ischemia and reperfusion injury. Cardiovasc Res 1997;36:205–212.

90. Yamazaki K, Miwa S, Ueda K, et al. Prevention of myocardial reperfusion injury by poly (ADP-ribose) synthetase inhibitor, 3-aminobenzamide, in cardioplegic solution: in vitro study of isolated rat heart model. Eur J Cardiothorac Surg 2004;26:270–275.

91. Halestrap AP, Clarke SJ, Javadov SA. Mitochondrial permeability transition pore opening during myocardial reperfusion–a target for cardioprotection. Cardiovasc Res 2004;61:372–385.

92. Duffy JY, Schwartz SM, Lyons JM, et al. Calpain inhibition decreases endothelin-1 levels and pulmonary hypertension after cardiopulmonary bypass with deep hypothermic circulatory arrest. Crit Care Med 2005;33:623–628.

93. Hao L-Y, Kameyama A, Kuroki S, et al. Calpastatin domain L is involved in the regulation of L-type Ca^{2+} channels in guinea pig

cardiac myocytes. Biochem Biophys Res Commun 2000;279:756–761.

94. Pearl JM, Nelson DP, Schwartz SM, et al. Glucocorticoids reduce ischemia–reperfusion-induced myocardial apoptosis in immature hearts. Ann Thorac Surg 2002;74:830–837.

95. Tevaearai HT, Eckhart AD, Shotwell KF, Wilson K, Koch WJ. Ventricular dysfunction after cardioplegic arrest is improved after myocardial gene transfer of a beta-adrenergic receptor kinase inhibitor. Circulation 2001;104:2069–2074.

96. Tevaearai HT, Walton GB, Eckhart AD, Keys JR, Koch WJ. Donor heart contractile dysfunction following prolonged ex vivo preservation can be prevented by gene-mediated beta-adrenergic signaling modulation. Eur J Cardiothorac Surg 2002;22:733–737.

97. Jones JM, Wilson KH, Steenbergen C, Koch WJ, Milano CA. Dose dependent effects of cardiac beta$_2$ adrenoceptor gene therapy. J Surg Res 2004;122:113–120.

98. Jayakumar J, Suzuki K, Khan M, et al. Gene therapy for myocardial protection: transfection of donor hearts with heat shock protein 70 gene protects cardiac function against ischemia–reperfusion injury. Circulation 2000;102:III302–III306.

99. Davidson MJ, Jones JM, Emani SM, et al. Cardiac gene delivery with cardiopulmonary bypass. Circulation 2001;104:131–133.

100. Breda M, Drinkwater D, Laks H, et al. Improved neonatal heart preservation with an intracellular cardioplegia and storage solution. J Surg Res 1998;47:212–219.

101. Stein DG, Drinkwater DC, Laks H, et al. Cardiac preservation in patients undergoing transplantation. A clinical trial comparing University of Wisconsin solution and Stanford solution. J Thorac Cardiovasc Surg 1991;102:657–665.

102. Stringham JC, Love RB, Welter D, Canver CC, Mentzer RM. Does University of Wisconsin solution harm the transplanted heart? J Heart Lung Transplant 1991;18:587–596.

16
Postoperative Care of the Pediatric Cardiac Surgical Patient

Catherine L. Dent and Steven M. Schwartz

Introduction

We review the major issues involved in the intensive care of the postoperative pediatric cardiac surgical patient. Although there are many aspects of care common among these patients, the basis of pediatric cardiac intensive care is an understanding of how specific cardiac lesions, operations, and types of cardiovascular physiology influence the postoperative state. A thorough knowledge and understanding of these principles can guide the anticipation and prevention of most postoperative problems.

Preoperative Evaluation

Anatomy

Appropriate postoperative care of pediatric cardiac patients requires a fundamental understanding of a patient's preoperative cardiac anatomy. Preoperative anatomy may guide surgical decision making such as the suitability for complete, two-ventricle *repair* versus single-ventricle *palliation* as well as postoperative concerns such as the likelihood for residual anatomic defects after surgery. The patient with two ventricles undergoing a complete repair will generally emerge from the operating room with a normal circulatory pattern. This allows application of the basic and well-understood principles of cardiovascular hemodynamics in the treatment of low cardiac output, hypotension, or other common postoperative problems. Palliation for single-ventricle lesions is more complex. The palliative nature of surgical intervention for single-ventricle lesions implies an abnormal postoperative hemodynamic burden on the cardiovascular system. The specifics of postoperative care following single-ventricle palliation are discussed later in this chapter.

Preoperative Clinical State

The clinical status of the patient in the preoperative period should be carefully reviewed. This applies not only to the presence of congestive heart failure or cyanosis but also to general pediatric issues such as failure to thrive, feeding difficulties, airway obstruction, and other end-organ abnormalities. Knowledge of current or recent upper respiratory symptoms and febrile illnesses are extremely important, especially during the winter months when respiratory syncytial virus (RSV) and influenza are prevalent. Respiratory infections may significantly complicate postoperative convalescence and prolong mechanical ventilation and overall cardiac intensive care unit (CICU) and hospital stays [1]. The likelihood of anesthetic complications is increased when surgery and anesthesia are performed on a patient with an upper respiratory infection [2–4], and postoperative complications are more likely when cardiac surgery is performed in the presence of concurrent RSV infection [5]. The abnormal pulmonary mechanics associated with RSV infection may be particularly deleterious in patients in whom low pulmonary vascular resistance is crucial (e.g., following a cavopulmonary shunt or Fontan procedure) and in patients prone to right ventricle dysfunction or pulmonary hypertension (e.g., following repair of tetralogy of Fallot). Optimal timing for cardiac surgery after RSV infection remains controversial, although most centers advocate a 6-week waiting period if cardiopulmonary bypass is anticipated.

Preoperative Cardiac Catheterization and Hemodynamics

The results of all preoperative cardiac testing should be reviewed before admission to the CICU. These tests will generally include a chest radiograph, echocardiogram, and electrocardiogram (ECG) and may include computerized tomography (CT), magnetic resonance imaging (MRI), or cardiac catheterization with angiography. These tests will provide insight into the patient's myocardial function, potential for dysrhythmia, and presence of pulmonary congestion.

The advancement in echocardiographic techniques and the increasing use of CT and MRI have decreased the need for diagnostic cardiac catheterization in most patients. However, some patients with congenital cardiac anomalies will require cardiac catheterization before surgery. This is usually done under three circumstances: (1) the anatomic abnormalities are incompletely defined by the

D.S. Wheeler et al. (eds.), *Cardiovascular Pediatric Critical Illness and Injury*,
DOI 10.1007/978-1-84800-923-3_16, © Springer-Verlag London Limited 2009

available noninvasive methods (echocardiography, CT, or MRI); (2) hemodynamic evaluation is required before correction or further palliation; and (3) a therapeutic intervention is necessary.

It is imperative that the physicians caring for the patient be familiar with the anatomic and hemodynamic information obtained by cardiac catheterization. This is especially important for those patients with anatomic or physiologic single ventricles who are undergoing staged palliation with cavopulmonary anastomoses (Glenn shunt, hemi-Fontan, or Fontan procedure). Pre- or postoperative elevations in pulmonary vascular resistance may alter pulmonary blood flow and/or cardiac output in these patients. Resistance values must be interpreted with regard to pulmonary blood flow, because low-flow states may increase resistance measurements without actual vascular changes. Large inequities in blood flow distribution between the right and left lungs or significant aortopulmonary collateral vessels can also make resistance calculations inaccurate or misleading. If vasodilator testing has occurred during the catheterization, specific drug responses may help guide interventions to manipulate pulmonary vascular resistance in the postoperative period. Finally, evidence of pulmonary venous desaturation during the catheterization may assist in managing those patients who are unexpectedly hypoxic after surgery.

It is important to recognize the limitations of invasive hemodynamic data, particularly with regard to diastolic ventricular function. The most common indicator of diastolic function is the ventricular end diastolic pressure. Although a high ventricular end diastolic pressure indicates dysfunction, a normal reading may not accurately predict postoperative performance, particularly in patients with single-ventricle anatomy.

Previous Cardiothoracic Surgery

Outcomes after previous cardiothoracic operations should be noted. In particular, duration of mechanical ventilation, inotropic requirement, and any associated anesthetic complications should be reviewed. Prior unexpected episodes of hemodynamic instability, arrhythmias, or sedation and pain control problems are of particular importance. Ventilator course and previous airway complications should also be noted. This pertains to patients at risk for vocal cord paralysis (such as those with previous aortic arch surgery) and to those who may have prior mechanical vocal cord damage. A history of airway compromise may alter the way that ventilator weaning and extubation are performed.

Intraoperative Course

Procedure/Postoperative Hemodynamics

To provide comprehensive directed management, the intensive care physician must be aware of the intraoperative course. Details regarding the surgical procedure and any complications must be communicated from the surgical team to the intensive care team. It has become routine in most centers to perform pre- and postoperative transesophageal echocardiography (TEE) to evaluate the adequacy of intracardiac surgical repairs. It is imperative that the critical care team be aware of any residual lesions such as intracardiac shunts, valvar stenosis or insufficiency, and outflow obstruction. These lesions can have profound effects on the types of investigations and interventions that the CICU team considers for postoperative problems.

Confirmation of the hemodynamic impact of lesions identifie by TEE may also be sought through invasive hemodynamic mea surements in the operating room. Transvalvar or transpulmonar gradients can be measured directly, and oximetric studies to asses for residual shunts can also be performed. The results of any c these analyses should be conveyed to the CICU team. The surgica team should also communicate the hemodynamic details of th patient's course since weaning from cardiopulmonary bypass. Thi includes heart rate and rhythm, relationships between filling pres sures, blood pressure, and, when applicable, arterial oxygen satura tion and the amount of inotropic support.

Cardiopulmonary Bypass

Repair or palliation of most forms of congenital heart diseas requires use of cardiopulmonary bypass (CPB) for circulatory support. The CPB circuit serves to replace the function of both the heart and lungs during cardiac surgery. Venous drainage result from placement of a single cannula into the right atrium or from bicaval cannulation, depending on the type of surgery and size o the patient. The aortic cannula is placed into the ascending aorta The size of the cannulas and the flow rates on the pump depend or the size of the patient and the degree of hypothermia. Variou reservoirs and filters are built into the circuit to protect the patient from air bubbles, thrombi, or acute changes in volume or hemodynamics.

Because of the need for reduced perfusion flow rates to minimize venous return to the heart during many types of congenital heart surgery, varying degrees of hypothermia are used during CPB Hypothermia preserves organ function by decreasing cellular metabolism and preserving phosphate stores. As temperature is lowered, both basal and functional cellular metabolism is reduced, and the rate of adenosine triphosphate and phosphocreatine consumption is substantially decreased [6]. Three methods of CPB may be used, based on the required surgical conditions, patient size, type of operation, and the potential physiologic impact on the patient:

Moderate hypothermic CPB (25° to 35°C) is the principle method of CPB used for older children and adolescents and for the repair of less demanding cardiac lesions such as atrial or ventricular septal defects. In these patients, the cannulas are less obtrusive and bicaval cannulation allows for adequate drainage of the right atrium.

Deep hypothermic CPB (15° to 20°C) is usually reserved for neonates and infants who require complex cardiac repairs. It allows the surgeon to operate under conditions of low-flow CPB, which improves the operating conditions by providing a near bloodless field and generally allows the use of only a single atrial cannula. This results in better visualization of atrial anatomy and allows for repairs through a right atriotomy.

Deep hypothermic CPB with circulatory arrest (DHCA) allows the surgeon to remove the atrial and if necessary the aortic cannulas and leaves a bloodless and cannula-free operative field. This procedure may be necessary when undertaking extensive aortic reconstructions, because there may not be any practical site in which to place the aortic cannula during this type of surgery. Clinical studies have indicated that the duration of safe circulatory arrest period to be between 45 to 60 min [7,8]. However, mild neurologic deficits may be present in neonates after 30 min of DHCA, and impairment is more common if a ventricular septal defect is present, suggesting that systemic air embolus may also contribute to the long-term deficits. Other organs generally tolerate circulatory arrest fairly well. Because of the neurologic consequences of DHCA, however, many centers have adopted the technique of regional low-flow cerebral perfusion (RLFP) during the aortic arch reconstruction in lieu of DHCA. Regional low-flow cerebral perfusion provides low-flow perfusion to the brain either directly via the innominate artery or through the distal end of an innominate shunt. Regional low-flow cerebral perfusion has been shown to limit the period of cerebral ischemia by limiting decreases in cerebral blood volume and oxygen saturation and has been associated with better neurologic outcome in animals [9].

Support with CPB is geared toward maintaining adequate organ perfusion and systemic oxygen delivery. Flows are based on calculated rates for body surface area and are adjusted based on mixed-venous saturation, acid–base status, and lactic acid levels. Although complications from CPB are relatively rare, it is important for the intensive care physician to be aware of any intraoperative issues with the conduct of bypass and the general risks associated with its use.

Despite advances in perfusion technology, patients undergoing CPB uniformly develop a systemic inflammatory response resulting in tissue injury with transient myocardial dysfunction, which contributes to postoperative morbidity and mortality [10,11]. The use of CPB has been associated with upregulation or activation of numerous inflammatory cytokines, including tumor necrosis factor and interleukins 6, 8, and 10, most likely due to the extensive contact of blood with artificial surfaces and possibly the nonpulsatile nature of CBP flow [10,12]. There is also evidence of a stress response, with increases in many stress-related hormones. The response to CPB is similar to the systemic inflammatory response that occurs in sepsis, with a major difference being the inherent time-limited nature of bypass-related injury. One important consequence of bypass related injury is pulmonary endothelial dysfunction that increases the endothelin/nitric oxide ratio present in the pulmonary vasculature and leads to postoperative pulmonary hypertension [13]. This occurs because the pulmonary endothelium is deprived of its major nutritive source of blood flow during CPB as the lungs are bypassed. Similar aberrations of systemic endothelial function resulting in inappropriate systemic vasoconstriction are thought to occur after DHCA [11].

Other clinical manifestations of systemic inflammation can include capillary leak with third space loss of fluids, alterations in systemic vascular resistance, and transiently diminished renal function [12,14]. The time course of CPB-related injury generally peaks at 12–18 hr following CPB so that it is reasonable to expect some clinical worsening during this time frame, although in practice it is often relatively minor. However, for patients with particular risk factors that might be exacerbated by CPB such as preoperative elevations in pulmonary vascular resistance or poor myocardial function, the initial postoperative period is when these problems are likely to manifest.

Cardioplegia and Myocardial Protection

Most repairs of congenital heart disease require the surgeon to open the heart so as to repair septal defects, construct baffles, or replace or repair valves. Such procedures generally require the use of cardioplegia. The goal of cardioplegia is not only to arrest the heart in a relaxed state, but also to preserve the myocardium during this period of ischemia. Cardioplegic solution contains many additives, and the composition varies from surgeon to surgeon. Many of the additives provide substrate for myocardial energy metabolism, and others are thought to enhance preservation. Cardioplegia is usually administered cold (4° to 8°C) and is often mixed with oxygenated blood. Topical hypothermia (ice slush) may also be used but has been associated with an increase in phrenic nerve injury [15]. Cardioplegia is a high-potassium solution that is usually administered into the aortic root (i.e., antegrade) after cross-clamping the aorta above the coronary arteries. The cardioplegic solution perfuses the coronary circulation and causes the myocardium to arrest in diastole. Repeated doses are given throughout the case to ensure myocardial preservation. Cardioplegic solution can also be administered in a retrograde fashion via the coronary sinus when the coronaries have been removed from the aorta (arterial switch operation) or when there is severe aortic insufficiency, which can cause run-off of the solution into the ventricle.

Despite the effort to maximize myocardial preservation during cardioplegia, its use is associated with an increased likelihood of myocardial dysfunction following surgery. The longer the period of aortic cross-clamp, the more damage the myocardium is likely to sustain. Similar to bypass-related injury, myocardial ischemia–reperfusion injury involves activation of inflammatory mediators within the myocardium and has also been associated with protease activation, degradation of contractile proteins, and myocyte apoptosis [16–18]. Despite the transient nature of postoperative myocardial injury, there may be some element of permanent damage, particularly after very long procedures, multiple episodes of ischemia and reperfusion, or when adequate myocardial protection is difficult such as with aortic insufficiency. Nevertheless, the benefits of repairing residual lesions often tip the risk/benefit ratio in favor of returning to CPB to repair residual lesions identified by postoperative TEE. Strategies to prevent myocardial injury include the use of aprotinin, pre- and intraoperative steroids, and modified ultrafiltration (see below) [19–21].

Modified Ultrafiltration

Cardiopulmonary bypass results in a significant inflammatory response with increased capillary permeability and total body water. In addition, the relatively small blood volume of children relative to the priming volume of the CPB circuit causes significant hemodilution. Hemofiltration is a process that uses convection to remove water and low-molecular-weight substances from plasma under a hydrostatic pressure gradient. This process effectively removes excess body water and several major inflammatory mediators and results in hemoconcentration after termination of CPB. It has been shown to improve hemodynamics, cardiac contractility, and oxygenation and to reduce postoperative blood loss and duration of mechanical ventilation [22,23]. The process currently used is called *modified ultrafiltration* (MUF) and occurs after separation from CPB. The venous cannula is clamped or removed, and the arterial cannula is used to circulate blood from the patient through a hemofilter. The gas exchanger on the main CPB circuit is excluded from the system, and blood is then directed slowly through the hemofilter to a small vent inserted into the right atrium. During MUF, all hemodynamic parameters are carefully monitored, and the hematocrit is measured at regular intervals.

Basic Principles of Postoperative Care

General Principles

The goal of postoperative care in all cases is optimum oxygen delivery and perfusion at an acceptable blood pressure and, in the case of cyanotic patients, saturation. It is essential to realize that blood pressure is not the same as perfusion, although it is often used as a surrogate marker for adequacy of cardiac output. Cardiac output is the product of stroke volume and heart rate, whereas blood pressure is a product of both cardiac output and systemic vascular resistance. Furthermore, increases in systemic vascular resistance represent an increase in afterload on the systemic ventricle and therefore function to diminish cardiac contractility. Thus, blood pressure that is maintained by an increase in systemic resistance at the expense of cardiac contractility and cardiac output may represent decreased tissue oxygen delivery compared with a low resistance/high cardiac output state. Nevertheless, a certain minimum (age-dependent) blood pressure is necessary to maintain adequate organ perfusion.

As soon as practically feasible, the postoperative patient should receive a full examination. This includes the obvious assessment of hemodynamic stability and adequacy of tissue perfusion, as well as the presence of any murmurs, rubs or gallops, air entry into the lung fields, and degree of hepatosplenomegaly. The patient may still be under the systemic effects of general anesthesia, so a full neurologic examination may not be possible. However, the fontanel (if still present) and pupil responses should be checked. A more complete neurologic examination should be completed when appropriate. The sites of in-dwelling catheters, wires, and monitoring devices should be noted and carefully examined for position and function. This includes peripheral and central intravenous lines, arterial catheters, atrial lines, tracheal, nasogastric, mediastinal, and pleural tubes, epicardial pacing wires, and urinary catheters. A chest radiograph is usually obtained upon admission to the CICU and should be checked in a timely fashion noting positions of the various in-dwelling catheters and tubes, heart size, presence of pleural effusions, and pneumothorax.

Hemorrhage and Clotting

The volume of mediastinal drainage should decrease rapidly hour to hour during the first 6 hr, and the nature of the drainage should change from frankly bloody to serosanguinous and ultimately serous during the first 18 to 24 hr. Factors that may promote persistent hemorrhage include preoperative cyanosis with polycythemia, reoperations, and multiple suture lines. In an attempt to avoid excessive fibrinolysis in the immediate postoperative period, some patients are treated with intravenous aprotinin, a systemic antifibrinolytic. Bloody drainage that continues at a volume greater than 10 mL/kg over the first 2 hr or 4 mL/kg thereafter should raise concern, and, if it continues despite blood product and clotting factor replacement, reexploration may be indicated. Conversely, if the mediastinal drainage suddenly ceases and clots are noted within the tube, the possibility of contained intrathoracic hemorrhage and cardiac tamponade should be entertained. An activated clotting time is measured at the completion of bypass. This is a moderately sensitive screening test for deficiencies in the intrinsic and common pathways of the clotting cascade. This tests for potentially all types of clotting factor deficiencies with the exception of factor VII of the extrinsic cascade, but it is practically used to assess

the persistent post-bypass effects of circulating heparin. Normal values vary between 120 and 150 sec. Protamine is used to reverse heparin effects and is given in the operating room in a dose based on the amount of heparin given before and during CBP. For the patient who continues to bleed in the intensive care unit, a second dose of protamine is often given. This dose should be less than the initial dose, because overdoses of protamine can actually promote bleeding. It is also important to realize that the hypothermia associated with CPB inactivates platelets. Like protamine, platelets are usually given at the conclusion of CPB, but it is common for patients to have a normal platelet count with diminished platelet function. It is therefore often helpful to repeat the platelet transfusion in the CICU for the patient with persistent bleeding. If the prothrombin and partial thromboplastin times are elevated in the bleeding patient, treatment with cryoprecipitate or fresh-frozen plasma is indicated. Finally, recombinant factor VIIa has been shown to help terminate postoperative bleeding.

Acid–Base Status

Acid–base status is monitored frequently following cardiac surgery. It gives information about oxygenation, ventilation, and tissue perfusion. Although in most patients the goal is to maintain a normal acid–base status, many patients will tolerate a mild respiratory acidosis during an attempt at early weaning from mechanical ventilation, and those with a bidirectional superior cavopulmonary anastomosis (bidirectional Glenn shunt) may actually benefit from a respiratory acidosis because of the associated increase in cerebral and thus pulmonary blood flow. Alternatively, when elevated pulmonary vascular resistance is a concern, it may be desirable to maintain a mild to moderate respiratory alkalosis because of the beneficial effect this has on the pulmonary vasculature.

The PaO_2 measurement on the blood gas may be particularly helpful in cyanotic patients. Because pulse oximetry may not be as accurate at low oxygen tension, the direct measurement of arterial oxygen levels can help the clinician evaluate the adequacy of pulmonary blood flow. As a general rule, a PaO_2 <28–30 mm Hg is not well tolerated for prolonged periods of time. When pulmonary blood flow reaches a critically low level as reflected by a PaO_2 <30 mm Hg, CO_2 removal is often hampered as well, leading to respiratory acidosis, increase in pulmonary vascular resistance, and metabolic acidosis from impaired oxygen delivery. This is an unstable situation and must be corrected in a timely fashion by medical means to improve pulmonary blood flow, mechanical support, or, when appropriate, reoperation.

In the postoperative patient, a metabolic acidosis should be considered an indication of low cardiac output and inadequate tissue perfusion until proven otherwise. Common causes of low cardiac output immediately following surgery include arrhythmia, tamponade, hypovolemia, anemia, myocardial dysfunction, pulmonary hypertension, and residual lesions. Many of these causes can be ruled out with a thorough knowledge of the preoperative and intraoperative course, including the results of the postoperative TEE, as well as a thorough examination of the patient, ECG, and assessment of information from indwelling hemodynamic monitoring lines.

Recently, investigators have proposed blood lactate levels as a marker of diminished systemic perfusion and as a predictor of outcome after heart surgery. Elevated or rising lactate levels in the early postoperative period indicate inadequate oxygen delivery and suggest an increased risk of morbidity and mortality [24–26]. Furthermore, progressive increases in serum lactate levels may enhance the predictive value of monitoring lactate levels postoperatively [27]. Unfortunately, blood lactate levels may become elevated only with significant circulatory dysfunction, after the anaerobic threshold has been reached, below the point when oxygen consumption becomes dependent on oxygen delivery [28]. In addition, elevated blood lactate might not reflect the current state of well-being but rather relate to prior (pre- or intraoperative) periods of diminished tissue perfusion with end-organ injury and inability to metabolize existing lactate.

Hemodynamic Assessment

Almost all patients who have undergone surgery for congenital heart disease will have arterial and central venous catheters. Those who have had more complex procedures will also have transthoracic intracardiac lines to monitor atrial pressure (right, left, or common) or pulmonary artery pressure. In some cases these lines may be placed so that the tip allows sampling of blood from a particular site such as the superior vena cava, or they may be capable of providing continuous oximetric data. The data gathered from such monitoring lines can be extremely helpful for assessing ventricular function or volume status when determining the cause of postoperative problems such as hypotension, poor perfusion, or low urine output. High left-sided or systemic filling pressures suggest the possibility of systemic ventricular dysfunction, residual left-to-right shunt, or valve dysfunction, depending on the particular anatomy and repair. High left-sided filling pressures will also lead to pulmonary venous hypertension and thereby increase pulmonary artery pressure, which can be problematic after cavopulmonary anastomoses (Glenn shunt or Fontan operation). High right-sided filling pressures are suggestive of right ventricular diastolic dysfunction often seen after repair of lesions associated with significant right ventricular hypertrophy such as tetralogy of Fallot. Other causes of high right-sided filling pressures include severe pulmonary stenosis or insufficiency, tricuspid stenosis (rare), and pulmonary hypertension. It is important to realize that right-sided filling pressures are only indirectly reflective of pulmonary artery pressure. Elevated filling pressures in both atria indicate biventricular dysfunction because of either primary myocardial dysfunction or failure of one ventricle with subsequent influence on the other via septal position and ventricular–ventricular interactions. Elevated filling pressures in both atria also raise the possibility of cardiac tamponade, although tamponade can occur in the absence of elevated filling pressures if there is a localized collection of blood or fluid that impedes cardiac filling.

Careful analysis of waveforms may also provide insight into myocardial performance, the status of the atrioventricular (AV) valves, or cardiac rhythm. The atrial tracing may have canon a-waves, which occur when the atria contract against a closed AV valve. This indicates lack of AV synchrony and can occur with severe first degree AV heart block, second or third degree heart block, junctional rhythms, or atrial flutter. Large a-waves may also occur in the presence of AV valvar stenosis. Exaggerated v-waves can indicate AV valve insufficiency.

Oximetric Assessment

Mixed venous oxygen saturation (SvO_2) and the arterial-venous oxygen saturation difference ($SaO_2 - SvO_2$) are often used to assess cardiac output and oxygen delivery. In patients with intracardiac shunts, superior vena cava saturation is the best estimate of SvO_2 [29], and many investigators have advocated continuous or intermittent monitoring of superior vena cava saturation in postoperative patients [30–33]. Low SvO_2 and $SaO_2 - SvO_2$ are sensitive predictors of low systemic blood flow and inadequate oxygen delivery; an $SaO_2 - SvO_2$ greater than 40 mm Hg suggests significant impairment in cardiac output and inadequate tissue delivery of oxygen (34). Monitoring of superior vena cava saturation is particularly useful after Norwood palliation, because systemic output in these patients depends on both myocardial performance and the balance of systemic and pulmonary blood flow. In patients after Norwood procedure, anaerobic metabolism and metabolic acidosis are more common when the absolute SvO_2 falls below 30% (35).

Measurement of mixed cerebral oxygen saturation (ScO_2) by continuous near-infrared spectroscopy has been used to estimate the balance between cerebral oxygen delivery and consumption. Near-infrared spectroscopy has been applied to both adults and children during CPB and to children during deep hypothermic circulatory arrest to assess adequacy of cerebral oxygen delivery [36,37]. Its use has become more routine in the postoperative setting [38], and recent reports suggest an association between low postoperative ScO_2 and cerebral ischemia [39]. It has also been suggested that ScO_2 values may correlate with SvO_2 to thus provide a noninvasive measure of cardiac output [40], but further confirmatory studies are necessary.

Mechanical Ventilation

Mechanical ventilation is usually fairly straightforward following surgery for congenital heart disease. Most patients have healthy lungs, so the purpose of mechanical ventilation is to ensure airway protection and adequate gas exchange until the heart and lungs have recovered sufficiently to undertake these activities without assistance. Either volume- or pressure-limited ventilation is usually acceptable, and support can be rapidly weaned as the patient resumes wakefulness. Respiratory distress that develops after tracheal extubation can be due to several issues, including congestive heart failure secondary to residual left-to-right shunts or myocardial dysfunction, phrenic nerve injury with hemidiaphragm paresis, pleural effusion or chylothorax, airway obstruction caused by acquired or congenital anomalies, or pulmonary parenchymal disease. Clinical examination of respiratory pattern, auscultation, and a chest radiograph before reintubation can help to establish the correct diagnosis or guide further investigation.

In some cases, mechanical ventilation becomes an adjunct to cardiovascular therapy and is more prolonged, either electively or because maintenance of adequate gas exchange cannot otherwise be accomplished. Manipulation of $PaCO_2$ has long been a staple of management for patients with pulmonary hypertension, and, as mentioned previously, high $PaCO_2$ can be used to increase cerebral and thus pulmonary blood flow following bidirectional Glenn. Patients with low cardiac output, myocardial dysfunction, residual left-to-right shunts, and pulmonary edema benefit from positive pressure ventilation because it reduces systemic ventricular afterload and can help counteract hydrostatic forces that promote pulmonary blood flow and pulmonary edema. It is important to remember that the lowest pulmonary vascular resistance occurs when end-expiratory lung volumes coincide with functional residual capacity and that high airway pressures in the presence of healthy pulmonary parenchyma are transmitted to the pulmonary vasculature and increase right (pulmonary) ventricular afterload.

This latter situation can be detrimental in the face of right ventricular dysfunction.

Arrhythmias and Pacing

It is essential to determine the cardiac rhythm when the patient returns from the operating room. A multi-lead surface ECG should be performed as soon as possible, and all caregivers must remain alert to the possibility of changes in rhythm. In the early postoperative period, maintenance of AV synchrony is a vital component of maximizing cardiac output and oxygen delivery. In addition to the ECG, other tools that can be used to determine the cardiac rhythm include the bedside monitor and pacing wires, particularly the atrial wires. The bedside monitor is the most readily accessible way to examine cardiac rhythm but may provide the least information. It is reasonably useful for QRS rate and timing, but p-waves are occasionally hard to identify, particularly at faster rates. When the p-wave is not clearly seen or the rhythm is not clear after examination of the surface ECG, an atrial wire recording can be used. This is done by using one or more of temporary atrial pacing wires as a limb lead and allows for the amplified p-wave to be recorded directly from the surface of the heart.

Common arrhythmias following congenital heart surgery and their usual modes of treatment are as follows:

Junctional ectopic tachycardia (JET) is a common tachyarrhythmia that usually occurs in the first 48 hr after surgery, especially after procedures involving closure of a ventricular septal defect and in younger patients [41]. It is generally poorly tolerated, especially in patients with unstable hemodynamics. Junctional ectopic tachycardia impairs hemodynamics because of the loss of AV synchrony and because of the short cycle length at higher rates. Slower junctional rhythms, although not technically JET, may also lead to suboptimal hemodynamics and should be treated. Early recognition of JET and other arrhythmias may be aided by careful surveillance of atrial pressure waveforms; loss of the distinct a and v waves indicating loss of AV synchrony is often the first indication of arrhythmia. Treatment of JET is directed toward the reestablishment of AV synchrony. Pacing, either atrial (if AV conduction is preserved) or AV sequential, is the initial therapy of choice. If the underlying junctional rate is too fast to allow pacing, the goal of pharmacologic therapy is to provide rate control to allow institution of pacing. Although intravenous amiodarone generally is considered the drug of choice [42], induction of hypothermia and procainamide also have been shown to be effective [43]. Junctional ectopic tachycardia may be exacerbated by use of β-adrenergic agonists, so minimizing use of these agents can be helpful, but this strategy is often limited by the impaired hemodynamic state of the patient [41]. In extreme cases, mechanical support may be necessary for refractory tachycardia. Finally, because JET is often a marker of residual hemodynamic problems, its appearance should lead to a thorough evaluation for residual lesions.

Heart block occurs when there is a prolonged PR interval (first degree), progressive prolongation of the PR interval until AV conduction is lost (second degree type I/Wenkebach), AV conduction that occurs in a fixed ratio other than 1:1 (second degree type II), or complete loss of AV conduction (third degree). Heart block may occur after any surgery around the AV node including operations involving ventricular septal defect repair, mitral valve replacement, or enlargement of the left ventricular outflow tract (Konno procedure). Patients with l-looped hearts are at increased risk for heart block. First degree heart block and second degree type I block rarely cause clinical problems although very prolonged AV conduction in the face of tachycardia can have much the same effects as JET, particularly in the immediate postoperative period. Second degree type II block and third degree block require treatment with temporary pacing. Atrial pacing alone is insufficient in heart block, and therefore AV sequential pacing is optimal. When this is not possible, ventricular pacing will prevent ventricular asystole. When the heart block is new following surgery, conduction may return as myocardial edema and inflammation resolve. This most commonly occurs within 7–10 days but has been noted as late as 2 weeks following surgery. If reliable conduction does not return, placement of a permanent pacemaker is generally necessary, even if there is a stable ventricular rhythm.

Atrioventricular reciprocating tachycardia (AVRT) is a reentrant tachycardia that employs both the AV node and an accessory pathway connecting the atria and ventricles. If the accessory pathway is capable of conducting in the antegrade direction during sinus rhythm, the surface ECG may show ventricular preexcitation. Tachycardia in most patients is initiated by a premature atrial beat that conducts antegrade over the AV node and retrograde via the accessory pathway or by a premature ventricular beat that conducts retrograde via the accessory pathway. Most commonly, the tachycardia is orthodromic, with antegrade conduction occurring via the AV node and retrograde conduction via the accessory pathway. Because antegrade conduction occurs down the AV node, QRS complexes are narrow and identical to those seen in sinus rhythm. In rare instances, antegrade conduction occurs over the accessory pathway (antidromic AVRT), leading to a wide QRS complex. Patients with AVRT will manifest a short RP interval with a VA relationship of 1:1. Comparison of the ECG in tachycardia to the preoperative and initial postoperative ECGs may be helpful. The treatment of patients with hemodynamically stable AVRT is adenosine (50–300 μg/kg) or atrial overdrive pacing. If these methods fail to break the tachycardia or are not available rapidly enough to treat an unstable patient, synchronized direct current cardioversion with 0.5–2 Joules/kg should be performed. Recurrent or refractory tachycardia may necessitate treatment with long-acting antiarrhythmic medication.

Atrial flutter is a reentrant tachycardia within the atrium. It may have 2:1 or 3:1 AV conduction and most often displays a narrow QRS complex. This rhythm disturbance is more common in patients with severe right atrial enlargement or after extensive atrial surgery (Ebstein's anomaly, Mustard, Senning, etc.). The typical atrial *sawtooth* flutter waves may be unmasked during treatment with adenosine, a feature that can be helpful in establishing the diagnosis. It is treated with either rapid atrial pacing at a rate greater than the atrial rate (overdrive pacing) or with synchronized direct current cardioversion (0.5–2 Joules/kg). Recurrent episodes may require treatment with amiodarone or other antiarrhythmic agents.

Atrial tachycardia is usually caused by abnormal automaticity at a specific site or sites within the atria. It occurs as a narrow complex tachycardia with a 1:1 VA relationship and may be incessant. Although p-waves are usually identifiable, careful comparison with the preoperative ECG should identify differences in p-wave morphology and axis, although these differences may be subtle, particularly if the ectopic focus originates in the right atrium.

Atrial tachycardia typically has a *warm-up* period but is characterized by little short-term or beat-to-beat variability, distinguishing it from sinus tachycardia. Prolonged atrial tachycardia may lead to cardiac dysfunction. Adenosine, cardioversion, and overdrive pacing do not terminate the tachycardia. Treatment is generally with antiarrhythmic agents; amiodarone is often considered the drug of choice, often in combination with β-blockade or class I antiarrhythmic agents. Digoxin has minimal efficacy, except as a component of treatment for heart failure. Radiofrequency ablation is an option for tachycardia refractory to therapy.

Ventricular tachycardia (VT) is relatively rare after pediatric heart surgery. It is a wide complex tachycardia and is most commonly seen in conjunction with ventricular dysfunction and poor hemodynamics (cardiomyopathy, ventricular surgery, coronary anomalies with ischemia, tamponade, etc.) or in markedly hypertrophied ventricles. An unstable patient with a wide complex tachycardia should be presumed to have VT and treated immediately with direct current cardioversion at 2–4 Joules/kg. Amiodarone and lidocaine may be indicated as well.

Because the use of temporary pacemakers is common in the treatment of postoperative cardiac patients, the intensive care physician needs to be familiar with the use of these devices. The majority of patients who undergo cardiac surgery are returned to the CICU with temporary epicardial pacing wires in situ. The wires are placed in a standard manner with the atrial (A) wires to the patient's right and the ventricular (V) wires to the left, although this may be reversed in dextrocardic patients. If internal temporary pacing wires are not present, emergency electrical access can be obtained with either an esophageal lead for atrial pacing or transcutaneous pads for ventricular pacing. Pacing modes with either temporary or permanent (implanted) pacemakers are based on a standard 3 letter code: P, S, R, where P is the chamber paced, **A**(trium), **V**(entricle), or **D**(ual); S is the chamber sensed, **A**, **V** or **D**; and **R** is the response to sensing, **I**(nhibit), **T**(rigger), or **D**(ual). In general, a pacemaker can be thought of as a series of timers set to a certain cycle length (inversely related to heart rate). During the countdown of the timer, the pacemaker senses for an electrical event, and, if none occurs before the timer reaches zero, a paced event occurs. Commonly used pacing modes and examples of situations in which they might be indicated are as follows:

AAI—Senses the Atrium and paces the Atrium if the sensed rate falls below the set default rate. *Indications: Sick sinus syndrome, sinus bradycardia, junctional ectopic tachycardia (JET).*

AOO—Paces the Atrium at the set default rate with no sensing. *Indication: Junctional ectopic tachycardia (JET).*

VVI—Senses the Ventricle and paces the Ventricle if the sensed rate falls below the set default rate. *Indications: Ventricular backup, usually for sinus rhythm with unreliable AV conduction (such as recovering heart block).*

DDD—Senses the Atrium and paces the Ventricle. Will pace the Atrium if the rate falls below the set default rate. More complex settings can be obtained, such as pacing the Ventricle at a rate lower than the sensed Atrial rate. *Indication: Heart block.*

Pacing thresholds may be checked by decreasing the output until there is loss of electrical capture. Generally, the pacemaker output is set at three times the threshold or at a minimum of 5 mA. For dual chamber pacing, it is also necessary to be aware of the upper rate limit, the AV interval, and the postventricular atrial refractory period (PVARP). The upper rate limit is the fastest atrial rate or the shortest cycle length that can be sensed by the pacemaker and needs to be set appropriately high for the patient and situation. Failure to do this may cause some atrial activity to be not sensed by the pacemaker, leading to inappropriate pacing of either the atrium or the ventricle.

The minimum cycle length that can be sensed or paced is the sum of two components, the AV interval and the PVARP, but can be manually set to an even longer interval than the sum of these two components. The first component of the cycle length, the AV interval, is the amount of time between an atrial event (paced or sensed) and a paced ventricular event. This is analogous to the PR interval on the ECG and should generally be set at a physiologic length. Longer AV intervals may be helpful in giving time for stiff, noncompliant ventricles to fill. The second component of the cycle length is the PVARP. The PVARP is the interval following a ventricular event (paced or sensed) during which sensing in the atrial lead is turned off. The PVARP ensures that the ventricular event will not be sensed by the atrial lead via retrograde conduction, which would set up a pacemaker-mediated tachycardia. Pacemaker-mediated tachycardia is essentially AVRT with the pacemaker serving as the accessory connection.

Sedation, Analgesia, and Muscle Relaxation

Postoperative patients require pain control and often require sedation. The principles of pain management for the postoperative cardiac patient are similar to those for other types of postoperative patients with the primary goals of patient comfort and safety. Occasionally, however, the physiologic or anatomic (delayed sternal closure) state of the patient requires that they remain more or less under general anesthesia. Neonates have been shown to exhibit detrimental hemodynamic effects from high circulating levels of stress hormones, and older patients with limited cardiac output and myocardial reserve may also benefit from treatment that limits their oxygen consumption. High-dose narcotics and benzodiazepines can depress the release of intrinsic catecholamines, and hence decrease systemic vascular resistance and after-load, with an improvement in cardiac output. Furthermore, increasing chest wall compliance with sedation and muscle relaxation may result in improved ventilation, particularly in the face of pulmonary hypertension or parenchymal lung disease. The presumed clinical course of the patient will determine whether a short- or long-acting preparation (e.g., fentanyl vs. morphine) is used and how the drug is administered (bolus vs. continuous infusion). Typically, a combination of both morphine and midazolam is used in the early postoperative period, with the ultimate dose titrated to effect. Fentanyl or morphine infusions are often used when there is the expectation of a prolonged need for anesthesia. Muscle relaxation is used to improve chest wall compliance as described above but may mask the need for higher doses of narcotics or benzodiazepines.

Identification and Treatment of Low Cardiac Output Syndrome

Low cardiac output syndrome (LCOS) is defined as the inability of the heart to provide adequate oxygen delivery to meet the body's metabolic demand. Low cardiac output syndrome in the early postoperative period is due primarily to transient myocardial dysfunction, compounded by acute changes in myocardial loading conditions, including postoperative increases in systemic and/or pulmonary vascular resistance. Residual cardiac abnormalities, even if minor, may further aggravate an underlying low output state. Surgical repair of cardiac malformations exposes the myocardium to periods of ischemia, resulting in transient myocardial stunning or damage. Cardiopulmonary bypass activates the complement and inflammatory cascades [10,12] and also contributes to myocardial injury, alterations in pulmonary and systemic vascular reactivity, and pulmonary dysfunction [13,44–46]. In addition, some repairs require ventriculotomy, which further exacerbates myocardial dysfunction. Although advances in myocardial protection, cardioplegia, and perfusion techniques have dramatically reduced perioperative cardiovascular injury, even relatively simple cardiac procedures are still associated with measurable myocardial dysfunction [47].

Prompt recognition and diagnosis of LCOS is a fundamental component of cardiac intensive care. Optimal postoperative management includes continuous monitoring of pulse oximetry, end-tidal CO_2, atrial and arterial waveforms, and multiple ECG leads [48]. Pulmonary arterial pressure monitoring is useful in selected patients [49]. At present, direct measure of myocardial performance and/or cardiac output in children is primarily a research tool and is not feasible for the routine clinical monitoring of patients in the CICU. Therefore, cardiac output and systemic perfusion are usually assessed indirectly by monitoring vital signs, peripheral perfusion, urine output, and acid–base status. Although postoperative LCOS may cause hypotension, systemic blood pressure is a particularly poor indicator of systemic perfusion in children who can markedly increase their systemic vascular tone. Hypotension and bradycardia tend therefore to be late consequences of LCOS, frequently occurring only minutes before cardiac arrest. Intractable cardiogenic shock results in unrelenting metabolic acidosis and ultimately multiorgan failure, including acute renal failure, gastrointestinal complications, and central nervous system compromise. Because LCOS is magnified in patients with palliated physiology or residual cardiac abnormalities, multiorgan system failure is more likely in such patients.

Low cardiac output after congenital heart surgery is usually caused by related and interacting factors. Although defects in myocardial systolic or diastolic contractile function usually accompany LCOS, myocardial contractile dysfunction should always be considered a diagnosis of exclusion, and other potential causes of LCOS, such as altered ventricular loading and residual cardiac lesions, should be ruled out before initiating therapy with inotropic or lusitropic agents. Changes in ventricular loading are integral to myocardial performance after congenital heart surgery. Ventricular preload is often inadequate because of blood loss, perioperative fluid shifts, changes in diastolic compliance, or physiologic changes resulting from the surgical procedure itself (e.g., Fontan or shunted single ventricle physiology) [50]. Cardiac tamponade, which impairs preload by altering diastolic compliance, should also be considered in patients showing signs of LCOS. Increases in intrathoracic pressure resulting from blood/fluid tamponade or pneumothorax will limit venous return and impede ventricular filling. Myocardial tamponade can result from diffuse intrathoracic fluid accumulation or a localized collection of blood clot or fluid that preferentially limits venous return to one or more chambers of the heart in a selective manner.

Ventricular afterload is often increased after CPB procedures, resulting from CPB-mediated vascular injury and the resultant altered vascular reactivity. Both systemic and pulmonary endothelial dysfunction have been observed following CPB with or without circulatory arrest, presumably resulting from ischemia-reperfusion injury to the endothelium [14,51–54]. Systemic vasoconstriction raises the afterload on the left or systemic ventricle, while pulmonary vasoconstriction increases afterload on the pulmonary or right ventricle. A pulmonary hypertensive crisis causes an acute rise in right ventricular afterload, which shifts the interventricular septum into the systemic ventricle, substantially decreasing the preload of the systemic ventricle. The acute increase in right ventricular afterload and decrease in left ventricular preload can diminish cardiac output dramatically. A pulmonary hypertensive crisis most often presents with acute systemic hypotension and diminished perfusion. Arterial oxygen saturation will decrease only when right-to-left intracardiac shunting can occur.

Residual anatomic or electrophysiologic abnormalities are likely to diminish cardiac output after congenital heart surgery. Uncorrected anatomic defects such as outflow obstruction or valvar insufficiency reduce the effective stroke volume and increase the cardiac workload required to provide adequate systemic blood flow. Similarly, persistence of a left-to-right intracardiac shunt will yield excessive pulmonary blood flow and thus diminish systemic blood flow. Low cardiac output can be exacerbated by arrhythmias that limit ventricular filling and/or compromise AV synchrony. Arrhythmias are relatively common after congenital heart surgery [41,55,56]. It seems likely that a correlation exists between LCOS and certain rhythm disturbances, particularly JET, although this has not been clearly demonstrated. Careful evaluation for residual cardiac abnormalities is indicated in any patient with low cardiac output, especially when patients do not follow their expected postoperative course after heart surgery.

The initial step in management of LCOS is to determine the adequacy of the intravascular volume. Inadequate preload is common in postoperative cardiac surgical patients. Potential causes of postoperative hypovolemia include bleeding, excessive ultrafiltration, and vasodilation from rewarming or afterload reduction [50]. Failure to provide adequate preload cannot be compensated for by using inotropic and vasoactive drugs. Indications that preload is inadequate include tachycardia, dry lips and mucous membranes, sunken fontanel and/or eyes, low blood pressure and filling pressures, and ongoing blood loss. Filling pressures must be interpreted with some caution that hypertrophied ventricles or ventricles with high preoperative filling pressures almost always require higher than normal postoperative filling pressures. Ongoing third space losses of fluid represent a challenge, because these are not readily accounted for by measurement of fluid intake and output and can result in a patient who has excess body edema but intravascular volume depletion. Repletion of intravascular volume with colloid is the most common approach to volume resuscitation in the postoperative pediatric cardiac patient, but crystalloid solutions are used in some institutions. Blood loss should be replaced with blood and blood products as necessary.

Myocardial contractility can be enhanced by using β-adrenergic agonists or phosphodiesterase inhibitors. Low-dose dopamine (≤5 μg/kg/min), dobutamine (5–10 μg/kg/min), and low-dose epinephrine (0.03–0.05 μg/kg/min) all increase contractility via stimulation of myocardial β-adrenergic receptors but do not significantly stimulate vascular α-adrenergic receptors, thereby minimizing associated vasoconstriction. Cardiomyocyte contractility and relaxation occur because of rapid calcium cycling within the cells. During electrical systole calcium is rapidly made available to the contractile apparatus and facilitates the interaction of actin and myosin. During diastole, calcium is actively removed from the cytoplasm, thus facilitating cellular relaxation. β-Adrenergic agonists work by increasing intracellular cyclic adenosine monophosphate (cAMP), which subsequently increases calcium cycling in both systole and diastole. Because cAMP is degraded by phosphodiesterases, phosphodiesterase inhibitors such as milrinone (0.375–0.75 μg/kg/min) also increase cAMP and have many of the same effects as β-adrenergic agonists [57]. One particular advantage of phosphodiesterase inhibition is that it is not receptor dependent and therefore not altered by the type of receptor downregulation that commonly occurs during chronic adrenergic stimulation (either from exogenous or endogenous β-adrenergic stimulation). Milrinone has been shown to prevent LCOS following repair of congenital heart disease [58]. β-Adrenergic receptors also mediate systemic vasodilatation so that another advantage of these drugs is that they promote afterload reduction for the systemic (and perhaps pulmonary) ventricle [59].

Because the goal of management of LCOS is to maintain the best possible perfusion, it is often the case that optimal management is associated with low normal blood pressure. Blood pressure is determined by both the cardiac output and systemic vascular resistance. Furthermore, there is an inverse relationship between systemic vascular resistance and cardiac contractility. Therefore, use of vasodilators for afterload reduction results in an increase in cardiac contractility, cardiac output, and oxygen delivery, albeit often at a lower blood pressure. When vascular tone is high, either intrinsically or secondary to the use of higher doses of adrenergic agonists, and cardiac output is low, pure vasodilating agents can be used to improve oxygen delivery. Sodium nitroprusside (1–3 μg/kg/min), nitroglycerine (1–3 μg/kg/min), and phenoxybenzamine (typically administered as a 0.25 mg/kg loading dose and then as a continuous infusion, administered at a total dose 0.25 mg/kg over 24 hr) are commonly used at many centers for this purpose, particularly in combination with epinephrine or norepinephrine to boost contractility [31,32].

When blood pressure is too low to maintain adequate organ perfusion, it is preferable to maximize preload and contractility before resorting to increasing systemic vascular resistance. Again, this is because of the inverse relationship between afterload and cardiac function and the likelihood that the increase in blood pressure will come at the cost of a further decrease in cardiac output and oxygen delivery. An exception to this relationship occurs when coronary perfusion has become critically low and an increase in blood pressure can improve myocardial function. In this situation, it is sometimes necessary to increase systemic vascular resistance to achieve an acceptable coronary perfusion pressure. This is most common when there are intercurrent issues such as sepsis, but vasodilatory shock has also been reported after CPB. Commonly used vasopressors include epinephrine and norepinephrine (which also have significant β-agonist effects), phenylephrine, and, more recently, arginine vasopressin [60,61]. Persistent hypotension refractory to catecholamines should lead one to consider abnormalities in adrenal or thyroid function [62]. Supplementation with corticosteroids in particular has shown some promise in treating refractory hypotension [63].

Calcium supplementation may also be beneficial in patients with postoperative myocardial dysfunction, particularly for neonates. The neonatal heart has an immature calcium handling system and is more dependent on extracellular calcium for contractility than is the mature heart [64]. Hypocalcemia occurs frequently in the postoperative period and may be pronounced in patients with 22q11 deletion syndrome and in neonates with transient hypoparathyroidism. Transfusion of citrate-treated blood, which chelates calcium, and administration of loop diuretics may exacerbate the hypocalcemia. Ionized calcium, the physiologically active form of calcium, should be monitored frequently in the postoperative period and normal or supernormal levels maintained with supplementation. Many centers routinely use calcium infusions (typically at doses of 10–15 mg/kg/hr) in neonates after CPB to augment and stabilize extracellular ionized calcium, especially in patients with 22q11 deletion syndrome.

Diuretics

Diuretic therapy is usually started on the first postoperative day when changes in cardiovascular status and fluid shifts have stabilized. Diuretics are often necessary to help decrease accumulated lung water that occurs as a consequence of CPB, to treat ongoing pulmonary edema secondary to alterations in ventricular function, or because of sensitization of the kidneys due to preoperative diuretic use. Loop diuretics such as furosemide (1 mg/kg IV every 6–12 hr) are the most commonly used but are often supplemented with thiazide diuretics such as chlorothiazide for synergistic effects. Loop diuretics may be administered as a continuous infusion (0.3–0.5 mg/kg/hr) in patients who become hypotensive as a result of fluid shifts associated with bolus doses. Failure to respond to diuretics should lead to reassessment of the patient's volume status and cardiac output, because hypovolemia and low cardiac output are the main causes of oliguria despite diuretics. Diuretic treatment is associated with predictable metabolic derangements (e.g., hypokalemia, hyponatremia, hypocalcemia, hypomagnesaemia, metabolic alkalosis), which should be accounted for and treated.

Line and Tube Removal

In-dwelling lines, catheters, and pacing wires are removed when they are no longer required. The patient should be observed closely after transthoracic atrial lines are removed because of the risk of bleeding and pericardial tamponade. Pulmonary artery lines have the highest incidence of complications, followed by left atrial lines and finally right atrial lines [49]. Removal of mediastinal and pleural chest tubes should be done with recognition of the risk of pneumothorax. A chest radiograph is usually performed after removal of these tubes to check for the presence of any intrathoracic air collections. Persistent chest tube drainage suggests elevated right-sided filling and central venous pressures or significant venous occlusion.

Lesion-Specific Postoperative Care

One of the most important aspects of intensive care management following surgery for congenital heart disease is the recognition that specific lesions and operations are associated with specific postoperative anatomic and physiologic complications. Despite the lengthy list of potential anatomic types of congenital heart disease and surgical repairs, the types of postoperative complications generally fall into certain categories. The following section briefly reviews some of the more common anatomic and physiologic issues that need to be anticipated following certain operations.

Residual Left-to-Right Shunt

Residual left-to-right shunts can occur after operations that involve repair of septal defects, when preoperative shunts are left unrepaired, or when there are unrecognized or untreated systemic-to-pulmonary artery shunts (such as aortopulmonary collaterals). The mechanisms by which such shunts can be problematic include the development of pulmonary edema secondary to increased pulmonary blood flow, pulmonary hypertension, volume overload of the systemic ventricle, and, in certain circumstances, limitation of systemic cardiac output. Common signs or symptoms include a pulmonary outflow or ventricular septal defect murmur, high systemic atrial pressure, hepatomegaly, and cardiomegaly with increased pulmonary vascularity on chest radiograph. Atrial level shunts are rarely a problem unless they are associated with factors that cause left atrial hypertension, thereby driving the shunt and maintaining high pulmonary artery pressures. Congestive heart failure and pulmonary overcirculation secondary to an atrial left-to-right shunt should therefore lead one to carefully evaluate the patient for mitral stenosis or insufficiency, inadequate systemic ventricular size, poor systemic ventricular function or systemic ventricular outflow tract obstruction with elevated end diastolic pressure.

Making the diagnosis of a residual shunt should lead to discussion regarding the risk/benefit balance of attempting further repair, either surgically or in the catheterization lab. Some lesions are not repairable, and the patient needs to be managed in such a way as to minimize the adverse consequences of the shunt. This may include avoiding therapy that lowers pulmonary resistance or that increases systemic resistance, either of which may aggravate the shunt. Prolonged inotropic support, mechanical ventilation, and relatively large doses of diuretics are often necessary. As the heart recovers from the acute detrimental effects of surgery, the residual shunt may become better tolerated, allowing weaning of support.

Residual Systemic Ventricular Outflow Tract Obstruction

Residual systemic ventricular outflow tract obstruction should be looked for after all surgery to relieve outflow obstruction, such as repair of subaortic stenosis, aortic stenosis, or coarctation of the aorta. Additionally, systemic ventricular outflow obstruction can occur after repair of AV septal defects or after other operations that remove large volume loads from the systemic ventricle when the underlying anatomy includes subvalvar hypertrophy. Signs and symptoms of systemic outflow obstruction include an ejection murmur and elevated systemic atrial pressure. Mild systemic outflow obstruction is usually well tolerated, but more severe lesions can significantly impair cardiac output. Diagnostic studies including Doppler ultrasound and cardiac catheterization should focus on the anatomic features of the outflow tract, because low flow across even a severe obstruction may not produce a large gradient in the face of low cardiac output. Unlike for adults with systemic ventricular outflow obstruction, use of β-adrenergic agonists for children is not usually associated with myocardial ischemia because cardiac output and myocardial oxygen delivery usually improve. Particular caution is necessary, however, when the obstruction is dynamic. Increased contractility can worsen this type of lesion, and inotropic drugs may be contraindicated. Unfortunately, the presence of systemic ventricular outflow obstruction often limits the ability to use vasodilating agents for afterload reduction. In this setting the systemic ventricular afterload is *fixed* at the level of the obstruction. Because of the inability of the

ventricular output to increase, administration of vasodilators will often result in hypotension.

Tricuspid or Mitral Valve Dysfunction

Residual AV valve dysfunction, either insufficiency or stenosis, can occur after any attempted valve repair or when closure of a septal defect unmasks valvar stenosis on one side of the heart. Atrioventricular valve insufficiency is associated with high atrial pressures on the affected side of the heart. If atrial pressure is being directly monitored, there will often be very prominent *v waves* on the tracing, and a regurgitant murmur will be heard. Because of the associated ventricular volume overload, there may be signs or symptoms of ventricular failure. Atrioventricular valve stenosis is also associated with high atrial pressure but with prominent *a waves*. Peripheral (right-sided) or pulmonary (left-sided) edema is common with stenotic lesions, and pulmonary hypertension occurs with mitral stenosis. When severe, either stenosis or insufficiency can limit cardiac output. Medical management of AV valve insufficiency is focused on afterload reduction, with inotropic support when needed. Systemic vasodilators promote antegrade cardiac output in the face of mitral (or even aortic) insufficiency, whereas diuretics may be useful in either stenotic or regurgitant lesions. Atrioventricular valve stenosis is, in general, not particularly amenable to medical management, although its consequences such as pulmonary hypertension may require aggressive treatment.

Right or Left Ventricular Diastolic Dysfunction

Ventricular diastolic dysfunction should be an expected complication of any operation where there is significant ventricular hypertrophy. This most commonly occurs after relief of obstructive lesions or when there is preexisting diastolic dysfunction. Operations that require a right ventriculotomy in an already hypertrophied right ventricle (such as tetralogy of Fallot) are at particularly high risk for postoperative diastolic dysfunction. A ventriculotomy can impair either systolic or diastolic function, and the anterior location of the right ventricle makes myocardial preservation difficult because the right ventricle is relatively exposed to ambient temperature in the operating room.

Diastolic dysfunction is marked by elevated atrial pressure and has many of the same features seen in AV valve disease. The presence of a residual atrial shunt in this setting compounds the adverse effects of left-sided disease by promoting pulmonary overcirculation. An atrial defect can help maintain cardiac output when the right ventricle is noncompliant, although there will be associated cyanosis. The need to maintain high pressure to promote adequate ventricular filling results in hydrostatic pressure favoring extravasation of fluid and leading to pulmonary edema in the case of left-sided problems and third space losses of fluid when there is right ventricular diastolic dysfunction.

In general, the first line of treatment for diastolic dysfunction is to use fluid to maintain adequate preload, although inotropic agents that reduce afterload (such as phosphodiesterase inhibitors) may also improve diastolic function. Fluid administration can be limited by impairment of oxygenation and lung function with progressive pulmonary edema or by complications of peripheral edema and third-spacing of fluid. Right-sided lesions in particular often respond very well to initial fluid boluses, but the hydrostatic forces in combination with diminished lymphatic drainage due to high venous pressure leads to pleural effusions and ascites. As these problems worsen, there is a need for progressively higher airway pressure to compensate for increased abdominal pressure and/or loss of effective lung volume. The high airway pressure is transmitted to the pulmonary vasculature because the pulmonary parenchyma is relatively healthy, and this in turn increases afterload on the already poorly functioning right ventricle. Increased abdominal pressure and low cardiac output also result in decreased renal perfusion and eventually renal failure, further complicating fluid management. A downward spiral develops in which cardiac output cannot be readily restored, and pulmonary gas exchange cannot be adequately maintained. Effective treatment can include drainage of effusions or ascites followed by further fluid resuscitation or mechanical support with a right ventricular assist device or extracorporeal membrane oxygenation. In general, right ventricular diastolic function often improves over several days as the ventricle heals from surgery and becomes more compliant. Left ventricular diastolic dysfunction may similarly resolve, but it is more likely to be associated with prolonged heart failure and/or the need for transplantation.

Pulmonary Hypertension

The incidence of postoperative pulmonary hypertension has decreased as the fields of pediatric cardiology and cardiac surgery have moved toward earlier repairs of the left-to-right shunt lesions most often associated with chronic pulmonary vascular changes. Nevertheless, CPB can provoke pulmonary hypertension in those patients with significant underlying risk [54]. Neonates, patients with pulmonary venous obstruction or mitral valve disease, and those with elevated preoperative pulmonary resistance are at particularly high risk, especially when associated with pain, agitation, suctioning, or hypoventilation. Signs and symptoms of pulmonary hypertension depend on the acuity of the change in resistance and on the underlying anatomy, particularly with regard to the existence of residual shunts. Chronic pulmonary hypertension that is not acutely worsened as a result of CPB can be well tolerated in the postoperative period, whereas acute pulmonary hypertensive crises can precipitate life-threatening symptoms. The presence of a patent foramen ovale, atrial septal defect, ventricular septal defect, or systemic-to-pulmonary artery shunt causes the main clinical consequence of acute elevations in pulmonary vascular resistance to be cyanosis because of an increase in right-to-left shunting. Pulmonary hypertension without shunting can cause acute right ventricular failure and low cardiac output without significant changes in saturation. A sudden fall in either blood pressure or saturation in a patient with known pulmonary vascular disease or with significant risk of postoperative pulmonary hypertension should prompt immediate consideration of this diagnosis and institution of treatment when appropriate. The presence of a pulmonary artery pressure–monitoring catheter can help establish the diagnosis of pulmonary hypertension. Most commonly, the systemic pressure falls while the pulmonary artery pressure remains unchanged. The increased ratio of pulmonary-to-systemic arterial pressure is diagnostic of an increase in pulmonary vascular resistance.

In addition to hypotension or cyanosis, a pulmonary hypertensive crisis in the absence of a right-to-left shunt is usually associated with an acute increase in right atrial pressure, because the increase in right ventricular afterload raises diastolic pressure. This can also result in a shift of the ventricular septum into the left ventricle and a subsequent increase in left atrial pressure despite the decreased filling of the left side of the heart. Other clinical manifestations can include a sudden decrease in lung compliance and/or onset of bronchospasm. Because pulmonary hypertension is exacerbated by hypoxia and hypercarbia, these manifestations can be especially troublesome.

The most effective treatment strategy for those at significant risk of postoperative pulmonary hypertension is prevention. Maintenance of adequate analgesia and sedation, particularly during noxious stimuli such as suctioning, is important. Induction of a respiratory alkalosis can be helpful in an acute pulmonary hypertensive crisis, but maintaining a pH above 7.5 for prolonged periods may have adverse consequences for cerebral perfusion. Therefore, a more practical approach is to avoid common problems that lead to hypoxia and respiratory acidosis, such as pneumothorax, right main bronchus intubation, or mucous plugging, and to maintain a pH between 7.4 and 7.5. It is generally appropriate to try to normalize the pH and reduce sedation on a daily basis while carefully observing the patient for symptoms associated with increased pulmonary artery pressure. Continued problems with pulmonary hypertension for more than 4–7 days suggest important residual lesions or more chronic pulmonary vascular disease.

When prophylactic therapy fails, more aggressive treatment with inhaled nitric oxide, sildenafil, bosentan, or even mechanical support may be helpful. Most studies have shown low doses of nitric oxide (2–20 ppm) are as effective as higher doses (40–80 ppm) but are less likely to be associated with complications such as methemoglobinemia. Sildenafil and bosentan can be used to transition from inhaled nitric oxide to chronic oral therapy for patients with chronic pulmonary vascular disease, because exogenous nitric oxide can lead to inhibition of endogenous production. Numerous other intravenous vasodilators, including calcium channel blockers, nitrovasodilators, and prostaglandins, have been used but are often limited by the occurrence of systemic hypotension because of lack of pulmonary selectivity. Prostacyclin has shown promise as an agent that may reverse pulmonary vascular changes previously thought to be permanent.

Conclusion

The management of the postoperative pediatric cardiac surgical patient requires a comprehensive understanding of the basic principles of oxygen delivery, cardiovascular physiology, and the anatomy and physiology of congenital heart disease. Signs and symptoms of LCOS should be treated aggressively, and diagnostic and therapeutic strategies should address both universal and lesion-specific problems.

References

1. Malviya S, Voepel-Lewis T, Siewert M, Pandit UA, Riegger LQ, Tait AR. Risk factors for adverse postoperative outcomes in children presenting for cardiac surgery with upper respiratory tract infections. Anesthesiology 2003;98(3):628–632.
2. Tait AR, Knight PR. Intraoperative respiratory complications in patients with upper respiratory tract infections. Can J Anaesth 1987; 34(3[Pt 1]):300–303.
3. Jacoby DB, Hirshman CA. General anesthesia in patients with viral respiratory infections: an unsound sleep? Anesthesiology 1991;74(6): 969–972.
4. Dueck R, Prutow R, Richman D. Effect of parainfluenza infection on gas exchange and FRC response to anesthesia in sheep. Anesthesiology 1991;74(6):1044–1051.

5. Khongphatthanayothin A, Wong PC, Samara Y, Newth CJ, Wells WJ, Starnes VA, et al. Impact of respiratory syncytial virus infection on surgery for congenital heart disease: postoperative course and outcome. Crit Care Med 1999;27(9):1974–1981.

6. Swain JA, McDonald TJ, Jr., Griffith PK, Balaban RS, Clark RE, Ceckler T. Low-flow hypothermic cardiopulmonary bypass protects the brain. J Thorac Cardiovasc Surg 1991;102(1):76–84.

7. Newburger JW, Jonas RA, Wernovsky G, Wypij D, Hickey PR, Kuban KC, et al. A comparison of the perioperative neurologic effects of hypothermic circulatory arrest versus low-flow cardiopulmonary bypass in infant heart surgery. N Engl J Med 1993;329(15):1057–1064.

8. Greeley WJ, Kern FH, Ungerleider RM, Boyd JL, 3rd, Quill T, Smith LR, et al. The effect of hypothermic cardiopulmonary bypass and total circulatory arrest on cerebral metabolism in neonates, infants, and children. J Thorac Cardiovasc Surg 1991;101(5):783–794.

9. Myung RJ, Petko M, Judkins AR, Schears G, Ittenbach RF, Waibel RJ, et al. Regional low-flow perfusion improves neurologic outcome compared with deep hypothermic circulatory arrest in neonatal piglets. J Thorac Cardiovasc Surg 2004;127(4):1051–1057.

10. Hall RI, Smith MS, Rocker G. The systemic inflammatory response to cardiopulmonary bypass: pathophysiological, therapeutic, and pharmacological considerations. Anesth Analg 1997;85(4):766–782.

11. Wernovsky G, Wypij D, Jonas RA, Mayer JE Jr, Hanley FL, Hickey PR, et al. Postoperative course and hemodynamic profile after the arterial switch operation in neonates and infants. A comparison of low-flow cardiopulmonary bypass and circulatory arrest. Circulation 1995;92(8):2226–2235.

12. Boyle EM, Jr., Pohlman TH, Johnson MC, Verrier ED. Endothelial cell injury in cardiovascular surgery: the systemic inflammatory response. Ann Thorac Surg 1997;63(1):277–284.

13. Kirshbom PM, Page SO, Jacobs MT, Tsui SS, Bello E, Ungerleider RM, et al. Cardiopulmonary bypass and circulatory arrest increase endothelin-1 production and receptor expression in the lung. J Thorac Cardiovasc Surg 1997;113(4):777–783.

14. Stamler A, Wang SY, Aguirre DE, Johnson RG, Sellke FW. Cardiopulmonary bypass alters vasomotor regulation of the skeletal muscle microcirculation. Ann Thorac Surg 1997;64(2):460–465.

15. Dimopoulou I, Daganou M, Dafni U, Karakatsani A, Khoury M, Geroulanos S, et al. Phrenic nerve dysfunction after cardiac operations: electrophysiologic evaluation of risk factors. Chest 1998;113(1):8–14.

16. Vahasilta T, Saraste A, Kyto V, Malmberg M, Kiss J, Kentala E, et al. Cardiomyocyte apoptosis after antegrade and retrograde cardioplegia. Ann Thorac Surg 2005;80(6):2229–2234.

17. Fischer UM, Klass O, Stock U, Easo J, Geissler HJ, Fischer JH, et al. Cardioplegic arrest induces apoptosis signal-pathway in myocardial endothelial cells and cardiac myocytes. Eur J Cardiothorac Surg 2003;23(6):984–990.

18. Krajewska M, Rosenthal RE, Mikolajczyk J, Stennicke HR, Wiesenthal T, Mai J, et al. Early processing of Bid and caspase-6, -8, -10, -14 in the canine brain during cardiac arrest and resuscitation. Exp Neurol 2004;189(2):261–279.

19. Khan TA, Bianchi C, Voisine P, Feng J, Baker J, Hart M, et al. Reduction of myocardial reperfusion injury by aprotinin after regional ischemia and cardioplegic arrest. J Thorac Cardiovasc Surg 2004;128(4):602–608.

20. Pearl JM, Nelson DP, Schwartz SM, Wagner CJ, Bauer SM, Setser EA, et al. Glucocorticoids reduce ischemia-reperfusion-induced myocardial apoptosis in immature hearts. Ann Thorac Surg 2002;74(3):830–837.

21. Davies MJ, Nguyen K, Gaynor JW, Elliott MJ. Modified ultrafiltration improves left ventricular systolic function in infants after cardiopulmonary bypass. J Thorac Cardiovasc Surg 1998;115(2):361–370.

22. Bando K, Vijay P, Turrentine MW, Sharp TG, Means LJ, Ensing GJ, et al. Dilutional and modified ultrafiltration reduces pulmonary hypertension after operations for congenital heart disease: a prospective randomized study. J Thorac Cardiovasc Surg 1998;115(3):517–527.

23. Huang H, Yao T, Wang W, Zhu D, Zhang W, Chen H, et al. Continuous ultrafiltration attenuates the pulmonary injury that follows open heart surgery with cardiopulmonary bypass. Ann Thorac Surg 2003;76(1):136–140.

24. Duke T, Butt W, South M, Karl TR. Early markers of major adverse events in children after cardiac operations. J Thorac Cardiovasc Surg 1997;114(6):1042–1052.

25. Munoz R, Laussen PC, Palacio G, Zienko L, Piercey G, Wessel DL. Changes in whole blood lactate levels during cardiopulmonary bypass for surgery for congenital cardiac disease: an early indicator of morbidity and mortality. J Thorac Cardiovasc Surg 2000;119(1):155–162.

26. Siegel LB, Dalton HJ, Hertzog JH, Hopkins RA, Hannan RL, Hauser GJ. Initial postoperative serum lactate levels predict survival in children after open heart surgery. Intensive Care Med 1996;22(12):1418–1423.

27. Charpie JR, Dekeon MK, Goldberg CS, Mosca RS, Bove EL, Kulik TJ. Serial blood lactate measurements predict early outcome after neonatal repair or palliation for complex congenital heart disease. J Thorac Cardiovasc Surg 2000;120(1):73–80.

28. Ronco JJ, Fenwick JC, Wiggs BR, Phang PT, Russell JA, Tweeddale MG. Oxygen consumption is independent of increases in oxygen delivery by dobutamine in septic patients who have normal or increased plasma lactate. Am Rev Respir Dis 1993;147(1):25–31.

29. Freed MD, Miettinen OS, Nadas AS. Oximetric detection of intracardiac left-to-right shunts. Br Heart J 1979;42(6):690–694.

30. Taeed R, Schwartz SM, Pearl JM, Raake JL, Beekman RH, 3rd, Manning PB, et al. Unrecognized pulmonary venous desaturation early after Norwood palliation confounds Gp:Gs assessment and compromises oxygen delivery. Circulation 2001;103(22):2699–2704.

31. Tweddell JS, Hoffman GM, Fedderly RT, Berger S, Thomas JP, Jr., Ghanayem NS, et al. Phenoxybenzamine improves systemic oxygen delivery after the Norwood procedure. Ann Thorac Surg 1999;67(1):161–168.

32. Rossi AF, Seiden HS, Gross RP, Griepp RB. Oxygen transport in critically ill infants after congenital heart operations. Ann Thorac Surg 1999;67(3):739–744.

33. Rossi AF, Sommer RJ, Lotvin A, Gross RP, Steinberg LG, Kipel G, et al. Usefulness of intermittent monitoring of mixed venous oxygen saturation after stage I palliation for hypoplastic left heart syndrome. Am J Cardiol 1994;73(15):1118–1123.

34. Trittenwein G, Pansi H, Graf B, Golej J, Burda G, Hermon M, et al. Proposed entry criteria for postoperative cardiac extracorporeal membrane oxygenation after pediatric open heart surgery. Artif Organs 1999;23(11):1010–1014.

35. Hoffman GM, Ghanayem NS, Kampine JM, Berger S, Mussatto KA, Litwin SB, et al. Venous saturation and the anaerobic threshold in neonates after the Norwood procedure for hypoplastic left heart syndrome. Ann Thorac Surg 2000;70(5):1515–1521.

36. Kurth CD, Steven JM, Nicolson SC. Cerebral oxygenation during pediatric cardiac surgery using deep hypothermic circulatory arrest. Anesthesiology 1995;82(1):74–82.

37. Kurth CD, Steven JM, Nicolson SC, Jacobs ML. Cerebral oxygenation during cardiopulmonary bypass in children. J Thorac Cardiovasc Surg 1997;113(1):71–79.

38. Hoffman GM, Ghanayem NS, Stuth EA, Berens RJ, Tweddell JS. NIRS-derived somatic and cerebral saturation difference provides noninvasive real time hemodynamic assessment of cardiogenic shock and anaerobic metabolism [abstr]. Anesthesiology 2004;101:A1448.

39. Dent CL, Spaeth JP, Jones BV, Schwartz SM, Glauser TA, Hallinan B, et al. Brain magnetic resonance imaging abnormalities after the Norwood procedure using regional cerebral perfusion. J Thorac Cardiovasc Surg 2005;130(6):1523–1530.

40. Tortoriello TA, Stayer SA, Mott AR, McKenzie ED, Fraser CD, Andropoulos DB, et al. A noninvasive estimation of mixed venous oxygen saturation using near-infrared spectroscopy by cerebral oximetry in pediatric cardiac surgery patients. Paediatr Anaesth 2005;15(6):495–503.

41. Hoffman TM, Bush DM, Wernovsky G, Cohen MI, Wieand TS, Gaynor JW, et al. Postoperative junctional ectopic tachycardia in children: incidence, risk factors, and treatment. Ann Thorac Surg 2002;74(5): 1607–1611.

42. Raja P, Hawker RE, Chaikitpinyo A, Cooper SG, Lau KC, Nunn GR, et al. Amiodarone management of junctional ectopic tachycardia after cardiac surgery in children. Br Heart J 1994;72(3):261–265.

43. Walsh EP, Saul JP, Sholler GF, Triedman JK, Jonas RA, Mayer JE, et al. Evaluation of a staged treatment protocol for rapid automatic junctional tachycardia after operation for congenital heart disease. J Am Coll Cardiol 1997;29(5):1046–1053.

44. Asimakopoulos G, Smith PL, Ratnatunga CP, Taylor KM. Lung injury and acute respiratory distress syndrome after cardiopulmonary bypass. Ann Thorac Surg 1999;68(3):1107–1115.

45. Burns SA, Newburger JW, Xiao M, Mayer JE, Jr., Walsh AZ, Neufeld EJ. Induction of interleukin-8 messenger RNA in heart and skeletal muscle during pediatric cardiopulmonary bypass. Circulation 1995; 92(9 Suppl):II315–II321.

46. Chai PJ, Williamson JA, Lodge AJ, Daggett CW, Scarborough JE, Meliones JN, et al. Effects of ischemia on pulmonary dysfunction after cardiopulmonary bypass. Ann Thorac Surg 1999;67(3):731–735.

47. Chaturvedi RR, Lincoln C, Gothard JW, Scallan MH, White PA, Redington AN, et al. Left ventricular dysfunction after open repair of simple congenital heart defects in infants and children: quantitation with the use of a conductance catheter immediately after bypass. J Thorac Cardiovasc Surg 1998;115(1):77–83.

48. Perioperative care: management of the infant and neonate with congenital heart disease. In: Castaneda A, Jonas RA, Mayer JE, Hanley FL, eds. Cardiac Surgery of the Neonate and Infant. Philadelphia: WB Saunders; 1994:65–87.

49. Gold JP, Jonas RA, Lang P, Elixson EM, Mayer JE, Castaneda AR. Transthoracic intracardiac monitoring lines in pediatric surgical patients: a ten-year experience. Ann Thorac Surg 1986;42(2):185–191.

50. Burrows FA, Williams WG, Teoh KH, Wood AE, Burns J, Edmonds J, et al. Myocardial performance after repair of congenital cardiac defects in infants and children. Response to volume loading. J Thorac Cardiovasc Surg 1988;96(4):548–556.

51. Schermerhorn ML, Tofukuji M, Khoury PR, Phillips L, Hickey PR, Sellke FW, et al. Sialyl Lewis oligosaccharide preserves cardiopulmonary and endothelial function after hypothermic circulatory arrest in lambs. J Thorac Cardiovasc Surg 2000;120(2):230–237.

52. Schermerhorn ML, Nelson DP, Blume ED, Phillips L, Mayer JE, Jr. Sialyl Lewis oligosaccharide preserves myocardial and endothelial function during cardioplegic ischemia. Ann Thorac Surg 2000;70(3): 890–894.

53. Sellke FW, Tofukuji M, Stamler A, Li J, Wang SY. Beta-adrenergic regulation of the cerebral microcirculation after hypothermic cardiopulmonary bypass. Circulation 1997;96(9 Suppl):II304–II310.

54. Wessel DL, Adatia I, Giglia TM, Thompson JE, Kulik TJ. Use of inhaled nitric oxide and acetylcholine in the evaluation of pulmonary hypertension and endothelial function after cardiopulmonary bypass. Circulation 1993;88(5 Pt 1):2128–2138.

55. Rhodes LA, Wernovsky G, Keane JF, Mayer JE Jr, Shuren A, Dindy C, et al. Arrhythmias and intracardiac conduction after the arterial switch operation. J Thorac Cardiovasc Surg 1995;109(2):303–310.

56. Hoffman TM, Wernovsky G, Wieand TS, Cohen MI, Jennings AC, Vetter VL, et al. The incidence of arrhythmias in a pediatric cardiac intensive care unit. Pediatr Cardiol 2002;23(6):598–604.

57. Bailey JM, Miller BE, Kanter KR, Tosone SR, Tam VK. A comparison of the hemodynamic effects of amrinone and sodium nitroprusside in infants after cardiac surgery. Anesth Analg 1997;84(2):294–298.

58. Hoffman TM, Wernovsky G, Atz AM, Bailey JM, Akbary A, Kocsis JF, et al. Prophylactic intravenous use of milrinone after cardiac operation in pediatrics (PRIMACORP) study. Prophylactic Intravenous Use of Milrinone After Cardiac Operation in Pediatrics. Am Heart J 2002; 143(1):15–21.

59. Chang AC, Atz AM, Wernovsky G, Burke RP, Wessel DL. Milrinone: systemic and pulmonary hemodynamic effects in neonates after cardiac surgery. Crit Care Med 1995;23(11):1907–1914.

60. Argenziano M, Choudhri AF, Oz MC, Rose EA, Smith CR, Landry DW. A prospective randomized trial of arginine vasopressin in the treatment of vasodilatory shock after left ventricular assist device placement. Circulation 1997;96(9 Suppl):II286–II290.

61. Morales DL, Gregg D, Helman DN, Williams MR, Naka Y, Landry DW, et al. Arginine vasopressin in the treatment of 50 patients with postcardiotomy vasodilatory shock. Ann Thorac Surg 2000;69(1):102–106.

62. Portman MA, Fearneyhough C, Karl TR, Tong E, Seidel K, Mott A, et al. The Triiodothyronine for Infants and Children Undergoing Cardiopulmonary Bypass (TRICC) study: design and rationale. Am Heart J 2004;148(3):393–398.

63. Shore S, Nelson DP, Pearl JM, Manning PB, Wong H, Shanley TP, et al. Usefulness of corticosteroid therapy in decreasing epinephrine requirements in critically ill infants with congenital heart disease. Am J Cardiol 2001;88(5):591–594.

64. Schwartz SM, Duffy JY, Pearl JM, Nelson DP. Cellular and molecular aspects of myocardial dysfunction. Crit Care Med 2001;29(10 Suppl): S214–S219.

17

Mechanical Support of the Cardiovascular System: Extracorporeal Life Support/Extracorporeal Membrane Oxygenation and Ventricular Assist Devices

Heidi J. Dalton and Brian W. Duncan

Introduction

As experience and technology have advanced, the use of mechanical circulatory support in infants and children has become more frequent. In many pediatric cardiac surgical centers, the ability to provide extracorporeal life support (ECLS) both before and after cardiac surgery is now considered a mandatory component of the program. Although a variety of implantable ventricular assist devices are available for use in adults with cardiac failure, few have been adapted to the smaller size and physiologic needs of infants and children. Extracorporeal membrane oxygenation (ECMO), also referred to as extracorporeal life support (ECLS), is a technique that historically has been used for respiratory failure, which has proved to be effective for support of refractory cardiac failure as well [1–3]. Although this technique has been used successfully to support over 4,000 children with survival to hospital discharge in nearly 40%, it has some characteristics that make it undesirable as a cardiac support modality. This review describes the use of both ECMO and ventricular assist devices (VADs) to provide circulatory support for children; an important part of this discussion will be the comparison of the two modalities in various clinical settings.

Current Status of Extracorporeal Life Support/ Extracorporeal Membrane Oxygenation for Pediatric Cardiac Disease

Initially adapted from conventional cardiopulmonary bypass practiced in the operating suite, ECMO has been applied to over 30,000 infants, children, and adults (Table 17.1). In recent years, based on the success of ECMO in the neonatal respiratory failure population, ECMO has been expanded to older patients and to those with cardiac dysfunction. To date, ECMO remains the modality that is most easily available for infants and children with cardiac failure, and much of the literature regarding circulatory support of children with cardiac failure is based on ECMO support. Although the majority of patients are postoperative from repair of congenital heart defects, patients with myocarditis, cardiomyopathy, heart transplant, and others have also been successfully supported with ECMO [5,6].

The cannulation techniques and circuit designs used in provision of ECMO have been previously described [7]. Briefly, ECMO consists of draining venous blood from the body through a polypropylene circuit to a roller head or centrifugal pumping device from which blood is advanced to a membrane oxygenator. Here, oxygen is added to the blood, and carbon dioxide is removed. The oxygenated blood is then sent through a heat exchanger that rewarms or cools it to the desired temperature, and it is then returned to the body. The two major forms of ECMO support are venovenous and venoarterial.

Venovenous Support

When used in a venovenous fashion, blood is withdrawn from the venous circulation and then reinfused back into the venous circulation after passing through the extracorporeal circuit (Figure 17.1). Cannulation is typically through the right internal jugular vein to the right atrium or via the femoral vessels [8]. One potential problem with venovenous ECMO is that, because blood drawn into and returned from the ECMO circuit is from the venous circulation, a portion of the oxygenated blood returned to the patient may be immediately drained by the venous ECMO cannula without having a chance to circulate through the patient's body. This is termed *recirculation* [9]. Although the amount of recirculation can be limited by having cannulas separated from each other in the body, by meticulous orientation within the heart, and careful attention to overall blood volume and cardiac output, recirculation of some amount occurs universally. This effect must be appreciated when following the patient's hemodynamics and oxygenation. Venovenous ECMO can provide total carbon dioxide removal but provides less oxygen delivery than venoarterial support. By far the most important aspect of venovenous ECMO for cardiac patients is that it relies on the adequate pumping of the native heart to distribute the extracorporeal volume to the body. Cardiac pump dysfunction

D.S. Wheeler et al. (eds.), *Cardiovascular Pediatric Critical Illness and Injury*,
DOI 10.1007/978-1-84800-923-3_17, © Springer-Verlag London Limited 2009

TABLE 17.1. Extracorporeal life support patient population and outcomes.

Category	No.	Weaned	Survival to discharge
Neonatal respiratory	19,463	16,623 (85%)	14,942 (77%)
Pediatric respiratory	2,883	1,847 (64%)	1,608 (56%)
Adult respiratory	1,025	610 (60%)	542 (53%)
Cardiac	5,902	3,357 (57%)	2,367 (40%)
ECPR	635	338 (53%)	247 (39%)
Total	29,908	22,775 (76%)	19,706 (66%)

Note: ECPR, extracorporeal membrane oxygenation during cardiopulmonary resuscitation.
Source: Data adapted from International Extracorporeal Life Support Organization Registry Report [4], with permission.

is thus a relative contraindication to the use of venovenous ECMO, and, for this reason, it is used in <2% of patients with cardiac disorders.

One potential benefit of venovenous support is that the blood reinfused back into the body from the ECMO circuit is highly oxygenated. This blood flows through the right heart, pulmonary

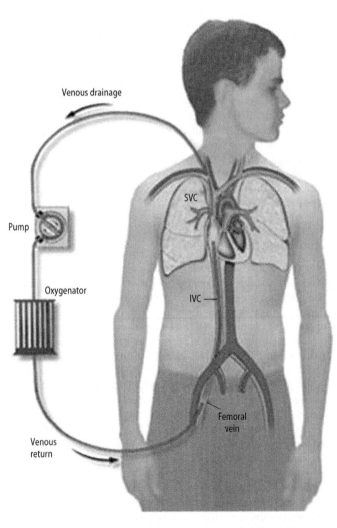

FIGURE 17.1. Venovenous extracorporeal membrane oxygenation circuit with drainage from the atrium and return into the femoral vessel. IVC, inferior vena cava; SVC, superior vena cava.

Venous drainage

Pump

Oxygenator

Venous return

SVC

IVC

Femoral vein

circuit, and back to the left atrium and ventricle. Highly saturated blood ejected from the left ventricle may provide improved oxygen delivery to the coronary vessels and the myocardium, which may enhance cardiac performance. Thus, in some patients with underlying cardiac failure, use of venovenous ECMO has resulted in improvement in cardiac function [10]. However, the majority of these reports involve children with acute respiratory failure who have secondary cardiac dysfunction, which may be the result of the high levels of mechanical ventilatory support required and the relative hypoxemia that the heart has to function with. Once ECMO is begun, ventilatory parameters can be reduced and oxygenation improved. These actions may improve cardiac function and allow successful use of venovenous ECMO. Despite descriptions of immediate improvement in cardiac performance with venovenous ECMO in respiratory failure patients requiring vasoactive infusions before ECMO, few clinicians are so confident of this effect that they will routinely employ venovenous ECMO in cardiac patients. One population in which use of venovenous ECMO seems theoretically plausible are patients with severe hypoxemia following single-ventricle palliation. The improvement in oxygenation that can be obtained with venovenous ECMO may improve overall systemic oxygen delivery to improve hemodynamics and organ perfusion. Unfortunately, the severe degree of myocardial dysfunction that often accompanies hypoxemia in such children has made clinicians reluctant to attempt venovenous support in these fragile patients.

Cannulation in children <10–15 kg body weight can be accomplished using a double-lumen single cannula, which is placed in the right internal jugular vein to the right atrium. Research to develop double-lumen cannulas for older children and adults is currently underway. In larger children or adults, two venous sites must be used to obtain adequate drainage and reinfusion access. Usually, one cannula is placed in the right internal jugular vein to the right atrium and the other in the femoral vein to the inferior vena cava. Bilateral femoral veins can also be used. If adequate oxygenation and hemodynamics are obtained, vasoactive infusions reduced, and adequate cardiac function preserved, venovenous ECMO can provide sufficient support. If this approach does not provide adequate cardiac support, then an arterial cannula can be placed, the venous cannulas or the double-lumen cannula used for venous drainage, and reinfusion accomplished via the arterial cannula.

Venoarterial Support

The majority of pediatric patients with cardiac failure receive venoarterial ECMO (Figure 17.2). In this mode, venous access is obtained via the right internal jugular vein to the right atrium, the femoral vein to the inferior vena cava, or directly into the right atrium via an opened mediastinum. Blood is returned from the ECMO circuit directly into the arterial circulation by way of the right internal carotid artery to the aorta, the femoral artery, or directly into the aorta via the mediastinum. The amount of bypass obtained is primarily regulated by the central venous blood volume and pressure, the length and internal diameter of the access cannulas, correct positioning of the cannulas, the tubing size, and speed of the roller heads in the ECMO pump (assuming a roller head pump is used). Venoarterial ECMO bypasses much of the native cardiopulmonary circuit. Animal work has shown that total limitation of blood flow through the pulmonary circuit can result in lung damage; therefore, total bypass during ECMO is not recommended [11]. Another

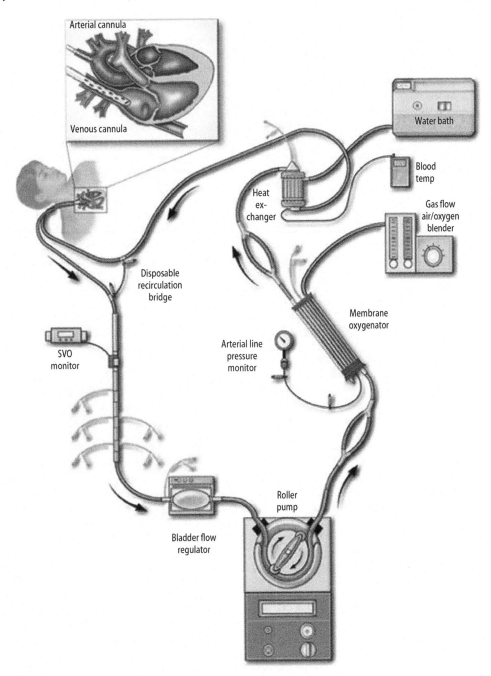

FIGURE 17.2. Venoarterial extracorporeal membrane oxygenation circuit with cervical cannulation.

reason to allow some native blood flow through the heart is that the majority of coronary blood flow has been shown to arise from native left heart ejection instead of from the arterial ECMO return [12,13]. Thus, maintaining some left heart ejection is optimal for improving coronary artery perfusion. Adequate oxygenation of left heart blood can be maintained in most patients by merely providing low concentrations of oxygen to the lungs with mechanical ventilatory support. In children with concomitant respiratory failure and underlying lung disease, the amount of mechanical ventilatory support required may be higher. Care should be taken to limit ventilator-induced lung injury during ECMO primarily for cardiac dysfunction. The goal of bypass during ECMO is to provide

adequate hemodynamics, oxygenation, and perfusion, while optimizing the cardiac milieu for recovery to occur. Careful monitoring of intracardiac filling pressures may be useful as a guide to optimal ECMO bypass as well. Reducing overdistention of the heart improves myocardial blood flow and reduces the risk of arrhythmias. Inability to reduce intracardiac filling pressures to low or normal levels during ECMO support has been described as a poor prognostic factor in some reports [14,15].

One major benefit of venoarterial ECMO in cardiac patients is the ability to reduce or discontinue vasopressor and inotropic agents, which may lessen myocardial work and also reduce secondary organ dysfunction. However, one potentially adverse effect of venoarterial ECMO is that it increases left ventricular afterload, and, in children with severe left heart failure, this increase in afterload may cause the ventricle to fail completely. Under these circumstances, blood flowing through the native right heart and pulmonary circulation, as well as returning via the bronchial and thebesian vessels, accumulates in the left side of the heart. Inability of cardiac contraction to open the aortic valve and eject left ventricular volume may result in a backup of blood and pressure in the left atrium. This can result in acute and severe venous pulmonary hypertension and pulmonary hemorrhage. Although afterload reduction using vasodilators such as sodium nitroprusside, milrinone, or α-blockers may be useful in this situation, they may not be sufficient. Children with severe left ventricular failure often require a left atrial venting line to provide decompression of the left side of the heart [16]. In children with an open mediastinum, the atrial vent is usually placed in the left atrial appendage and is then Y'd into the venous side of the ECMO circuit for drainage. This is easily accomplished in children with an open chest, but it is more difficult in those children with closed chests. In these circumstances, an atrial septostomy can be created in the cardiac catheterization laboratory or at the bedside under fluoroscopic or echocardiographic guidance [17,18]. This allows for decompression of the left atrial blood through the septostomy into the right atrium, where it can be drained into the venous cannula. These considerations should be taken into account when deciding how and where to cannulate the cardiac ECMO patient. Although successful atrial septostomy on ECMO has been well described, it is nonetheless an extremely high-risk procedure. Conversely, failing to identify and treat left atrial hypertension quickly can result in a massive and lethal pulmonary hemorrhage.

Care must also be taken that the arterial ECMO cannula is positioned so that blood flow is not directed at the aortic valve. This may cause aortic insufficiency and contribute to worsening left ventricular failure. If the aortic cannula is placed too distally in the aortic arch, flow to the carotid vessels can be impaired. Optimal positioning is in the high ascending arch just before the take-off of the left carotid artery.

If a left atrial vent or septostomy is used during ECMO, two management issues should be remembered. First, if the patient has normal (or near-normal) respiratory function, the saturation of pulmonary blood returning to the left heart may be high. As this blood will mix with the systemic venous return from the patient, which is usually measured by a device on the ECMO venous return line, artificial elevation of this measured saturation can occur. Therefore, in order to obtain a true mixed venous saturation, which is an indirect measure of the balance between oxygen delivery and extraction in the patient, blood must be obtained from a site away from this mixing area. If the patient has a central venous line in the groin or neck, blood from these sites can provide a more accurate assessment of overall venous saturation than merely following the ECMO venous saturation monitor. Second, during weaning of venoarterial ECMO, the left atrium may continue to be decompressed into the venous drainage of the ECMO circuit to the point where it compromises forward flow into the left ventricle, resulting in limitation of cardiac output to the coronary vessels and the body. Left atrial vents can merely be closed to the ECMO circuit or removed to deal with this potential problem but septostomies usually remain during weaning. As the right atrial pressure rises as ECMO flow is reduced and more native cardiopulmonary circulation occurs, right-to-left shunting can occur through the open

septostomy and decrease arterial saturation. This factor must be remembered when weaning patients with left atrial decompression. If the left atrial vent is turned off for weaning, blood clotting and occlusion are potential problems. If the vent develops a clot and then is embolized into the left side of the heart, this can have major untoward complications.

The major complication in cardiac ECMO patients is bleeding. The large surface area of the ECMO circuit and the membrane oxygenator require more heparinization than some smaller VADs. Bleeding is amplified in patients placed on ECMO directly from cardiopulmonary bypass in the operating suite who may already have coagulation abnormalities. Some authors have found that even a few hours of recovery from cardiopulmonary bypass to fully reverse heparinization and establish some hemostasis helps to limit bleeding and improve outcome in postoperative cardiac ECMO patients. Others, however, have noted that outcome in cardiac patients maintained in a low cardiac output state for hours following surgery is worse than those who require ECMO directly in the operating room. Measures to control bleeding include lowering of heparin and bedside anticoagulation testing parameters, aggressive replacement of coagulation factors and blood products, and administration of antifibrinolytic agents. Persistent hemorrhage mandates surgical exploration to identify potentially controllable bleeding sites. Although there is often reluctance to explore a patient who is heparinized for fear of causing even more bleeding, complications from continued massive resuscitation of hemorrhage outweighs the surgical risks.

ECMO-Lite

One advantage of ECMO over other purely cardiac assist devices is that it also provides adequate gas exchange. In infants and children, concomitant respiratory insufficiency from pulmonary hemorrhage, edema, or other causes is more prominent than in adults with postoperative cardiac failure. As ECMO can provide both adequate cardiac and respiratory support, this may be optimal. However, there is a subset of children in whom the lungs are well functioning, and the gas exchange provided by the membrane oxygenator within the ECMO circuit is not needed. Because the membrane oxygenator is a major site of potential blood clot formation and a major reason that adequate heparinization has to be maintained, removal of this device can result in a lowered need for heparin and potentially reduce bleeding complications. This has been demonstrated as a successful adapted mode of extracorporeal support that is colloquially termed ECMO-lite or NOMO (no oxygenator membrane oxygenation). Use of this form of support has been described in neonates following stage I Norwood palliation of hypoplastic left heart syndrome [19,20]. However, it should be remembered that the oxygenator also serves as a site for air bubble trapping, which is lost when the device is removed from the circuit. The use of specific arterial line filters for air and clots within the ECMO circuit is center specific and not a universal practice.

ECMO During Cardiopulmonary Resuscitation

One extreme form of cardiac support that is proportionally among the fastest expanding population of ECMO is cannulation for cardiac arrest. Designed as a resuscitative tool for patients in refractory cardiac arrest, ECMO during cardiopulmonary resuscitation (ECPR) has been reported in over 600 neonates, children, and adults with an overall survival to discharge rate of 39%. To facilitate expedient access to ECMO support during ECPR, many centers maintain a completely set up roller head ECMO circuit that is kept pre-primed with a crystalloid solution or vacuum primed to shorten the time to priming completion [21,22]. Although this technique works well in many centers, others have concerns over the potential for infection, impaired integrity of the membrane oxygenator when kept *wet* for a prolonged period, and the potential for other adverse effects.

Although few in number, studies of pre-primed circuits have not shown infection when sampled up to 30 days. A recent report also noted no increase in di(2-ethylhexyl)phthalate (DEHP) levels in pre-primed circuits when evaluated up to 14 days [23]. This substance can be leeched from plastic tubing and has been shown to have adverse effects in high levels in animal studies. Another report found no decrease in membrane oxygenator gas exchange when compared with control at 7 or 14 days. This oxygenator was a hollow-fiber device, which does not alleviate concerns over what happens with a solid silicone membrane lung. Scanning electron microscopy of pre-primed silicone membrane oxygenators has shown defects in the past. Other centers use a portable, centrifugal bypass perfusion system that can be primed in 10–20 min or less [24]. Centrifugal systems most often employ a hollow fiber membrane oxygenator, which is less difficult and faster to prime for use than a traditional silicone-coated membrane lung used in routine ECMO. Hollow fiber oxygenators may also be used for roller head set ups. Hollow fiber oxygenators offer many advantages such as less surface area for clotting, the potential to use less heparin to prevent clot formation, low resistance to blood flow (which may reduce trauma to blood elements), and excellent gas exchange. In the past, these devices have been plagued by the development of plasma leak across the porous membrane surface, which limited their life span to several hours to days and required frequent changing of the oxygenator. Newer models of these devices now seem to provide adequate support for many days to weeks. Unfortunately, these oxygenators are currently available only outside the United States. Although use of ECPR is relatively new, initial reports of outcome are encouraging [25].

The ECMO Circuit

The majority of centers provide ECMO with a roller head pump. This device contains steel roller heads enclosed in a box (the pump housing). The heads rotate and push against tubing that is threaded through the box (the raceway). Blood contained in the tubing is thus advanced forward by the motion of the roller heads. The amount of blood advanced from the raceway is dependent on the number of revolutions of the roller heads and the occlusion that occurs when they contact the circuit tubing. Too little contact between the roller heads and the tubing (loose occlusion) will decrease the amount of blood advanced, whereas excessive pressure of the roller heads against the tubing (tight occlusion) will obstruct blood from moving forward and cause excessive wear on the tubing, resulting in rupture. The correct occlusion is set by measuring the displacement of fluid during roller head rotation during set up of the ECMO circuit.

Newer pumps used for ECMO now often incorporate flow probes that display the actual amount of blood flowing through the ECMO circuit. In the past, roller head pumps have been controlled by ser-

voregulating devices that sense when venous return is inadequate and signal the roller heads to stop until venous return is once again sufficient. This on-and-off flow has been shown to cause turbulence in blood flow to the brain in venoarterial ECMO through the carotid artery. Newer circuit and pump designs have eliminated the traditional *bladder box* in favor of a section of collapsible tubing that performs a similar servoregulating function. The changed design of this bladder reduces the potential for clot formation and eliminates one of the most annoying parts of the ECMO circuit (although the new design has some annoying features as well). It also removes a potential site for air trapping, however, which was easily accomplished with the older cylindrical bladder design. In the new systems, as venous return to the ECMO circuit diminishes, the roller heads slow down and then speed up again once adequate venous return is obtained. This may decrease the on/off action of the roller head pump and potentially limit the acute changes in blood flow noted with the older style of servoregulation.

The most important determinants of blood flow via the ECMO circuit remain adequate central venous pressure, proper positioning of large, short cannulas, and proper occlusion of roller heads. As flow generated by the roller heads is under high pressure, occlusion of the post-pump side of the ECMO circuit can result in high arterial line pressure and circuit rupture. This potential for high arterial line pressure and rupture is one of the major safety risks with roller head circuits.

Centrifugal pumps are also used for ECMO support. These pumps are nonocclusive and generate flow via a spinning rotor that is often maintained by magnets within and without the pump head. Blood enters the cone at the apex and is propelled tangentially to the outlet port of the pump head where it is expelled. Active suction is generated at the inlet of the pump head to provide adequate *preload* so that centrifugal pumps do not require gravity drainage or a venous reservoir, although these devices are used in some centers. Loss of preload to the pump head can lead to high negative pressures (up to −700 mm Hg) in the inlet tubing, which can increase hemolysis, cause endothelial damage to cannulated vessels, or result in cavitation of air. Following the flow generated and the revolutions per minute that are displayed on the pump console gives an indication of the adequacy of preload and flow generation. Flows that are widely fluctuating at stable revolutions per minute may indicate that preload is inadequate and that high negative pressure is being produced. As inlet volume to the centrifugal pump will correlate with outlet volume, flow and pressure monitoring are measured on the outlet side of the pump. Unlike a roller head device, obstruction of the outlet side of the centrifugal circuit will not result in high levels of back pressure being generated in the tubing, and rupture is highly unlikely. This is another safety feature of these devices. If forward flow is obstructed, however, blood will remain trapped in the centrifugal head where it will be exposed to further shear stress and heat. Thus, the risk of hemolysis in this situation is high. Most centrifugal systems have an integrated flow probe on the outlet tubing that displays generated flows on a constant basis. Pressure monitoring to provide information regarding venous and arterial line pressures is also available. Although the majority of centrifugal pumps in use today have bearings that fail over time, so that replacement of the pump head is needed on a periodic basis, newer generations of centrifugal pumps have a better design that limits pump head failure and heat generation within the pump head. Improved long-term performance and

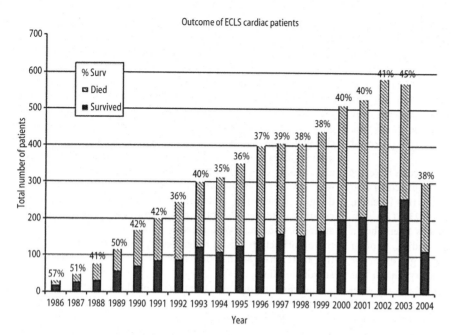

FIGURE 17.3. Overall survival of patients who have received cardiac extracorporeal membrane oxygenation support over time. ECLS, extracorporeal life support.

reduction of blood cell trauma and hemolysis to levels that are lower than those provided with roller head devices or older centrifugal systems may result in an increase in the use of new models of centrifugal pumps in the marketplace. Newer models also contain air bubble detection systems, autoregulation to provide desired blood flows, and even pulsatile flow.

Management of cardiac ECMO patients is often facilitated by the presence of intracardiac pressure lines that provide valuable information regarding intracardiac filling pressures and cardiac function and offer guidance as to the amount of bypass being used. Improvement in pulsatility on the arterial line waveform of the patient and the ability to maintain intracardiac filling pressure within a reasonable range with adequate hemodynamics and organ function as ECMO flow is reduced are markers of cardiac improvement that may be an indication that the child is ready to be weaned off ECMO support. Conversely, lack of improvement in cardiac function after a few days of ECMO support is an indication for cardiac catheterization to determine if any residual defects or surgically correctable abnormalities can be found. Discussion of the potential for heart transplantation in patients without contraindications should also occur within the first week if no recovery is anticipated and the family is interested in this difficult option. Withdrawal of support should also be considered in patients without cardiac recovery who are not surgical or heart transplant candidates. In postoperative cardiac patients, it is rare to have successful recovery of cardiac function that allows removal of ECMO if no cardiac improvement has occurred after 1 week of support. However, successful cardiac recovery has been described after prolonged periods of support in patients with myocarditis or cardiomyopathy. Deciding at what point a child should be listed for transplant is difficult, but, with the prolonged waiting periods to obtain organs, being placed on the transplant list earlier may improve the chances to obtaining a successful transplant. As adequate blood pressure and flow are easily obtained during ECMO, use of other devices to augment organ function such as renal replacement therapy, liver support, or plasmapheresis can also be facilitated by connecting into the ECMO circuit.

Outcome

The overall survival of patients who have received cardiac ECMO support over time is shown in Figure 17.3. Outcomes by diagnosis are shown in Table 17.2; outcomes by age group are shown in Table 17.3. To obtain more specific information regarding cardiac ECMO, an addendum to the Extracorporeal Life Support Organization registry form was developed several years ago. Now in use for about 2 years, this will allow for more specific determination of cardiac ECMO prognostic factors, diagnoses, complications, and outcomes. In a similar fashion, an ECPR addendum to more specifically track data on patient selection, management, and outcome was also recently developed. Careful assessment and analysis of database information is imperative to guide appropriate use of ECMO in diverse patient populations in the future. Long-term outcome studies are also needed to evaluate the neurologic and functional outcome of patients treated with ECMO/ECLS over time.

TABLE 17.2. Outcome of extracorporeal life support cardiac patients by underlying disease.

	Total	Survived	Percent survival
Congenital heart disease	4,299	1,662	39
Cardiac arrest	153	45	29
Cardiogenic shock	145	61	42
Cardiomyopathy	419	212	51
Myocarditis	178	101	58
Other	941	365	39

Source: Data adapted from International Extracorporeal Life Support Organization Registry Report [4], with permission.

TABLE 17.3. Extracorporeal life support for cardiac failure: cardiac runs by diagnosis.

Age groups	Total runs	Survived	Percent survived
0–30 days			
Congenital defect	2,006	719	36
Cardiac arrest	24	5	21
Cardiogenic shock	22	11	50
Cardiomyopathy	72	48	67
Myocarditis	27	11	41
Other	168	74	44
31 Days to <1 year			
Congenital defect	1,318	548	42
Cardiac arrest	25	6	24
Cardiogenic shock	11	4	36
Cardiomyopathy	61	28	46
Myocarditis	33	18	55
Other	155	65	42
1 Year to <16 years			
Congenital defect	740	297	40
Cardiac arrest	49	19	39
Cardiogenic shock	34	11	32
Cardiomyopathy	200	108	54
Myocarditis	96	60	63
Other	260	113	43
16 Years and over			
Congenital defect	42	12	29
Cardiac arrest	43	9	21
Cardiogenic shock	74	34	46
Cardiomyopathy	73	25	34
Myocarditis	14	9	64
Other	297	92	31

Source: Data adapted from International Extracorporeal Life Support Organization Registry Report [4], with permission.

Current Status of Ventricular Assist Devices for Pediatric Cardiac Disease

The use of VADs in children has historically been limited to centrifugal pump systems suitable only for short-term support or adult systems suitable only for larger children, but recent advances suggest pediatric applications of this technology will increase in the future. Although VAD technology has previously seen few advances in pediatrics, recent clinical and research developments suggest that this is an exciting era of significant progress for VAD support in children. New devices and recent advances in pediatric VAD technology as described in the following sections provide evidence for this point.

Centrifugal Pump VADs

Historically, centrifugal pump VADs have been the mainstay of this technology for children. Thuys et al. reported excellent results using the Bio-Pump (Medtronic Bio-Medicus, Minneapolis, MN) in infants and children weighing 6 kg or less [26]. Utilizing this system, the authors supported 34 children (age range 2–258 days and weight range 1.9–5.98 kg); 63% were successfully weaned from VAD support, and 31% of this difficult patient population survived to hospital discharge. Other reports have described the utility of centrifugal VAD to support the entire spectrum of pediatric cardiac

disease [27–33]. Although the Bio-Pump is capable of providing support for the entire range of patients encountered in pediatrics, this technology is not implantable and is capable of providing only short-term support.

Pulsatile Pediatric VAD—Heartmate, Thoratec, and the ABIOMED BVS 5000

Several groups have successfully provided pulsatile mechanical circulatory support for older children utilizing systems designed primarily for adult applications [30,34–36]. Helman et al. described the use of the Heartmate VAD (Thermocardiosystems, Woburn, MA) in 12 adolescent patients, the majority of whom had idiopathic dilated cardiomyopathy [36]. The ages for these patients (range of 11–20 years) and their body surface areas (range of 1.4–2.2 m^2) allowed the use of this device. As in the adult experience with the Heartmate VAD, the majority of patients supported by the vented electric model were discharged home with resumption of normal activities.

McBride et al. [35] and Korfer et al. [36] each described large series utilizing the Thoratec VAD (Thoratec Laboratories Corp., Berkley, CA) with a few implantations in adolescents as young as 11 years of age. Ashton and co-workers employed the ABIOMED BVS 5000 (ABIOMED, Inc., Danvers, MA) in four older children [30]. The ABIOMED device was used to provide temporary circulatory support for patients with a body surface area greater than 1.2 m^2 with flows greater than 2 L/min.

Pulsatile Pediatric VAD—MEDOS HIA VAD and the Berlin Heart

The MEDOS HIA VAD (MEDOS Medizintechnik AG, Stolberg, Germany) and the Berlin Heart VAD (Berlin Heart AG, Berlin, Germany) are two pulsatile VAD systems that are suitable for the entire age range of pediatric patients, including neonates [37,38]. Both are paracorporeal systems that employ pneumatically driven, thin membrane pumps to provide pulsatile flow. Inlet and outlet valves are tri-leaflet and constructed from polyurethane. Both systems are available in a variety of pump sizes (10, 30, 50, and 80 mL), with the smallest pump sizes suitable for infant support (Figure 17.4).

Konertz and co-workers described a series of six children supported by the MEDOS HIA VAD [39]. The range of patient ages in this report was 5 days to 8 years, and patients' weights ranged from 3.1 to 20 kg. Aspirin and intravenous heparin were used for anticoagulation. Four of the six patients in this series (67%) survived to hospital discharge, including two patients who were bridged to transplantation and two patients who had return of ventricular function sufficient for device weaning. The maintenance of the circuit required no trained personnel beyond intensive care unit nursing as opposed to ECMO, which usually requires trained technicians at the bedside for monitoring of the device. Of particular importance, the patients in this report were able to be tracheally extubated, ambulated, and were able to attain some degree of normal daily activities. This resulted in improvement in the physiologic state of these children by the time transplantation occurred. Similar results with the MEDOS system have been reported by other authors [40,41].

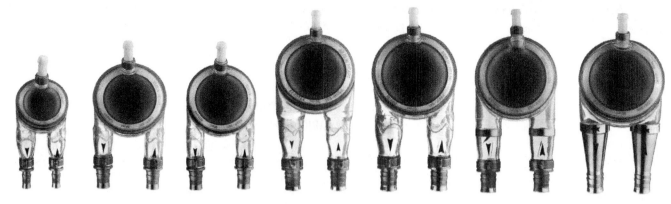

FIGURE 17.4. The Berlin Heart VAD, available in a range of pump sizes from 10 to 80 mL. (Courtesy of Berlin Heart AG, Berlin, Germany, with permission).

Ishino et al. reported 14 children who were supported with the Berlin Heart VAD (age range 2 weeks to 15 years, weight range 3.2–52 kg) [42]. Eleven of these patients were bridged to transplantation, while three were bridged to recovery. Anticoagulation was provided with intravenous heparin, maintaining the activated clotting time at 160–180 sec. Eight of the 11 (73%) bridge to transplant patients were successfully transplanted, with four survivors (36%), and one of the three (33%) bridge to recovery patients survived to hospital discharge. Stiller et al. reported the successful use of the Berlin Heart VAD for the support of four children with myocarditis [43]. All children in this study had admission ejection fractions less than 12%. The duration of support was 11–21 days. Three of the four patients were successfully weaned from support, and one patient was successfully bridged to transplantation. These authors cited fewer bleeding complications with the Berlin Heart than with ECMO because of reduced anticoagulation and less platelet destruction. In addition, this pulsatile paracorporeal system was clearly superior to ECMO for providing moderate to long-term support while awaiting return of ventricular function or as a bridge to transplantation. Several other reports exist detailing the successful use of the Berlin Heart VAD for pediatric patients [38,44,45].

New and Emerging Devices for Pediatric Mechanical Circulatory Support

The MicroMed DeBakey VAD Child

The DeBakey VAD Child (MicroMed Technology, Inc., Houston, TX) was recently granted Humanitarian Device Exemption (HDE) status by the Food and Drug Administration [46]. This device employs the same axial-flow pump used in the adult version with the following modifications: shortened in-flow cannula with a more acute angle for in-flow tubing, shortened plastic outflow graft protector, and reduced size of the flow probe on the outflow graft (Figure 17.5). These design modifications reduce the lateral space requirements for the device in an attempt to produce a VAD that is fully implantable in children. Under the current HDE the VAD Child is used to provide temporary left ventricular support as a bridge to cardiac transplantation for children from 5 to 16 years of age with a body surface area >0.7 m^2 and <1.5 m^2. Although the clinical experience is still limited, this device has been used successfully in a number of children since its introduction.

The Pediatric Circulatory Support Program of the National Heart Lung and Blood Institute

Another important development is the recent Pediatric Circulatory Support initiative from the National Heart, Lung and Blood Institute (NHLBI) of the National Institutes of Health, which made

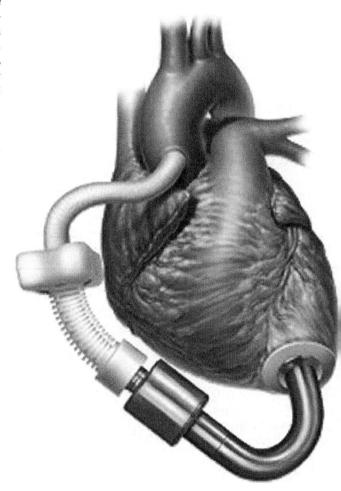

FIGURE 17.5. The MicroMed DeBakey VAD Child. (Courtesy of MicroMed Technology, Inc., Houston, TX, with permission).

TABLE 17.4. Devices and developers supported by the National Heart, Lung and Blood Institute's Pediatric Circulatory Support Program.

Device	Developer
PediaFlow Ventricular Assist Device	The University of Pittsburgh
PediPump™	The Cleveland Clinic Foundation
Pediatric Cardiac Assist System (pCAS)	Ension, Inc.
Pediatric Jarvik 2000 Flowmaker	Jarvik Heart, Inc.
Pediatric Ventricular Assist Device (PVAD)	The Pennsylvania State University

funds available for research into the development of pediatric circulatory support devices. In the spring of 2004, five contracts were awarded by the NHLBI to support preclinical development for a range of pediatric VADs and similar circulatory support systems (Table 17.4). The five projects awarded include an implantable, magnetically suspended mixed-flow turbodynamic VAD (the PediaFlow VAD); an implantable, mixed-flow VAD with a magnetically suspended impeller (the PediPump); a compact integrated pediatric cardiopulmonary assist system (the pCAS); an axial-flow apically implanted pediatric VAD (the Pediatric Jarvik 2000 Flowmaker); and a pulsatile-flow pediatric VAD (PVAD). The Cleveland Clinic PediPump is depicted in Figure 17.6 [47]. Although clinical applications of these devices may not occur for some time, this initiative represents an extremely important point in the developing field of pediatric circulatory support research.

A Comparison of Extracorporeal Membrane Oxygenation Versus Ventricular Assist Device Support for Pediatric Cardiac Disease

Specific Clinical Settings

Despite the fact that ECMO remains the most common form of mechanical circulatory support, the recent rapid expansion of VAD technology as outlined above suggests that expanding clinical applicability of these devices will occur. Adults frequently suffer pure cardiac dysfunction, but children often require both cardiac and respiratory support because of hypoxemia, pulmonary hypertension, and right ventricular failure superimposed on primary cardiac dysfunction. Although VAD may be used in cases of relatively pure ventricular dysfunction, ECMO is a better therapeutic choice when pulmonary hypertension and hypoxemia predominate [6,7]. Anomalous origin of the left coronary artery from the pulmonary artery is a condition encountered in pediatrics with predominant left ventricular failure where VAD support is particularly effective [48]; however, postcardiotomy ventricular dysfunction from any cause may be successfully supported by VAD.

Other considerations exist for the appropriate choice of device for pediatric support. Because of the presence of an oxygenator in the circuit, ECMO can be instituted by peripheral cannulation of cervical or femoral vessels, whereas VAD requires direct cannulation of the heart via sternotomy. In addition, ECMO provides biventricular support with two cannulas, whereas biventricular support with VAD requires four cannulation sites. This is an especially

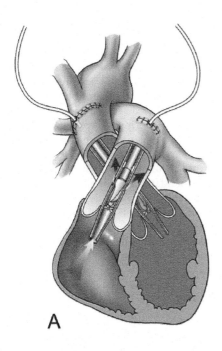

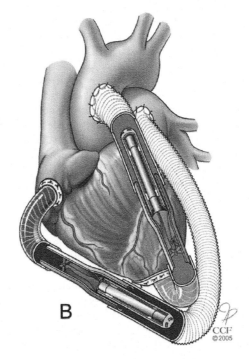

FIGURE 17.6. (A) Intravascular PediPump deployed as a biventricular assist device (BVAD) for patients greater than 15 kg. Pumps are demonstrated placed across both semilunar valves, positioning the inlet below valve level while blood is ejected above the valve to provide biventricular support. **(B)** Extravascular, intracorporeal PediPump deployed as a BVAD for patients less than 15 kg. Biventricular support is provided by inlet cannulation of the right and left ventricles with outlet cannulation of the corresponding great artery. Corresponding left VAD and right VAD deployment of either the intravascular or extravascular versions would be achieved by removing the pump from the unsupported ventricle. (Data from the Cleveland Clinic Foundation. Copyright 2005, with permission.)

TABLE 17.5. Comparison of extracorporeal membrane oxygenation (ECMO) and a ventricular-assist device (VAD).

	ECMO	VAD
Hypoxemia, pulmonary hypertension	+	
ALCAPA		+
Peripheral cannulation	+	
Biventricular support in newborns	+	
Decreased trauma to blood elements		+
Less anticoagulation		+

Note: ALCAPA anomalous origin of the left coronary artery from the pulmonary artery.

important consideration for neonates who require biventricular support where space limitations make the placement of four cannulas difficult. Conversely, the lack of an oxygenator simplifies the VAD circuit, which reduces trauma to blood elements and decreases the need for anticoagulation, which minimizes blood loss if support is instituted in the immediate postoperative period. Table 17.5 summarizes these issues for ECMO and VAD.

Recovery of Ventricular Function

Another important difference between the two devices that has been cited in the past is the likelihood of recovery of ventricular function during support. Some experimental studies have demonstrated increased ventricular wall stress during ECMO support, whereas direct ventricular decompression provided by VAD has been demonstrated to decrease wall stress [49,50]. However, there is substantial evidence supporting the alternative view that ECMO support can be provided without contributing to myocardial injury [12]. For example, avoiding distension injury during ECMO support is especially important to enhance the prospects for myocardial recovery, as discussed earlier. Experimental studies have shown that direct venting of the left atrium during ECMO provides the same ventricular decompression provided by VAD with equivalent likelihood of recovery [17,18,51,52].

To further optimize the chances of ventricular recovery during support, the effect of ECMO on myocardial oxygenation must be appreciated and appropriately managed. With most cannula configurations employed for venoarterial ECMO, retrograde flow of oxygenated blood from the arterial cannula fails to reach the coronary sinuses if there is significant ventricular ejection while coronary arterial blood flow is provided by the left ventricle in these cases [53–55]. If there is significant pulmonary parenchymal disease or mechanical ventilation is withheld during ECMO support, hypoxic blood returning to the left ventricle may provide the sole source of coronary perfusion with deleterious effects on ventricular function and recovery [13]. Provision of oxygenated blood flow to the coronary arteries is easily accomplished by continuing to provide moderate levels of ventilation during ECMO support, which ensures that fully oxygenated pulmonary venous blood returns to the left atrium and serves as the source of coronary perfusion. With these modifications for the conduct of ECMO support, recovery of ventricular function may be anticipated in patients with even the most profound myocardial dysfunction [7,22].

Long-Term Follow-Up Results

The long-term follow-up results of children with cardiac disease who required mechanical circulatory support during a decade of experience at Children's Hospital, Boston, have been analyzed [56,57]. Thirty-seven children (26 ECMO and 11 VAD survivors) were studied for an average of more than 4 years. Only a single patient died in either group for an overall long-term survival rate of 95%. Eighty percent of the patients in both groups were described as exhibiting good to excellent general health. Ninety percent of the patients were in New York Heart Association class I or II, and echocardiographic evaluation of ventricular function was normal in all of the ECMO-supported patients and in 90% of the VAD-supported patients.

These results are reassuring in that children with heart disease who survive to hospital discharge after receiving ECMO or VAD support demonstrate favorable long-term survival and overall general health and cardiac outcomes. However, higher rates of neurologic complications were found in the ECMO-supported group, which may suggest an advantage for VAD support. Possible explanations for this advantage may include decreased anticoagulation needed during VAD support, leading to reduced risk of neurologic complications such as intracranial hemorrhage. However, these results must also be interpreted with the understanding that the ECMO support was used in a higher proportion of critically ill neonates with more complex underlying cardiac conditions [7]. Nevertheless, the potential for greater neurologic risk in ECMO-supported patients should be appreciated, and appropriate management such as carefully avoiding excess anticoagulation should be routine.

Conclusion

Mechanical circulatory support in children will play an increasingly important role in the future practice of congenital cardiac surgery. Aggressive surgical treatment of even the most complex anomalies in infants and older children has led to an expanded role for short-term mechanical circulatory support for postcardiotomy failure. Because of its versatility and familiarity, ECMO or adaptations of this modality will continue to play an important role in providing pediatric mechanical circulatory support in the acute setting. However, it may be anticipated that there will be an increasing need for long-term, implantable VAD systems in pediatrics. For example, an increasing population of adolescents with single-ventricle physiology who have been successfully treated with the Fontan procedure will ultimately develop circulatory failure and may be candidates for chronic circulatory support as a bridge to transplantation or even as destination therapy. Of particular relevance for this patient population are the recent availability of devices such as the MicroMed DeBakey VAD Child and the NHLBI-sponsored research that will hopefully generate new devices designed specifically for pediatric applications.

References

1. Andrews AF, Klein MD, Toomasian JM, Roloff DW, Bartlett RH. Venovenous extracorporeal membrane oxygenation in neonates with respiratory failure. J Pediatr Surg 1983;18:339–346.
2. Heiss KF, Bartlett RH. Extracorporeal membrane oxygenation: an experimental protocol becomes a clinical service. Adv Pediatr 1989;36:117–135.
3. Pennington DG, Merjavy JP, Codd JE, Swartz MT, Miller LL, Williams GA. Extracorporeal membrane oxygenation for patients with cardiogenic shock. Circulation 1984;70:I130–I137.

4. ECLS Registry Report. Ann Arbor, MI: Extracorporeal Life Support Organization; January 2005.

5. Dalton HJ, Siewers RD, Fuhrman BP, et al. Extracorporeal membrane oxygenation for cardiac rescue in children with severe myocardial dysfunction. Crit Care Med 1993;21:1020–1028.

6. Duncan BW. Mechanical circulatory support for infants and children with cardiac disease. Ann Thorac Surg 2002;73:1670–1677.

7. Duncan BW, Hraska V, Jonas RA, et al. Mechanical circulatory support in children with cardiac disease. J Thorac Cardiovasc Surg 1999; 117:529–542.

8. Snider MT, Campbell DB, Kofke WA, et al. Venovenous perfusion of adults and children with severe acute respiratory distress syndrome. The Pennsylvania State University experience from 1982–1987. ASAIO Trans 1988;34:1014–1020.

9. Rais-Bahrami K, Walton DM, Sell JE, Rivera O, Mikesell GT, Short BL. Improved oxygenation with reduced recirculation during venovenous ECMO: comparison of two catheters. Perfusion 2002;17:415–419.

10. Roberts N, Westrope C, Pooboni SK, et al. Venovenous extracorporeal membrane oxygenation for respiratory failure in inotrope dependent neonates. ASAIO J 2003;49:568–571.

11. Kolobow T, Spragg RG, Pierce JE. Massive pulmonary infarction during total cardiopulmonary bypass in unanesthetized spontaneously breathing lambs. Int J Artif Organs 1981;4:76–81.

12. Shen I, Levy FH, Benak AM, et al. Left ventricular dysfunction during extracorporeal membrane oxygenation in a hypoxemic swine model. Ann Thorac Surg 2001;71:868–871.

13. Shen I, Levy FH, Vocelka CR, et al. Effect of extracorporeal membrane oxygenation on left ventricular function of swine. Ann Thorac Surg 2001;71:862–867.

14. Kulik TJ, Moler FW, Palmisano JM, et al. Outcome-associated factors in pediatric patients treated with extracorporeal membrane oxygenator after cardiac surgery. Circulation 1996;94:II63–II68.

15. Undar A, McKenzie ED, McGarry MC, et al. Outcomes of congenital heart surgery patients after extracorporeal life support at Texas Children's Hospital. Artif Organs 2004;28:963–966.

16. Seib PM, Faulkner SC, Erickson CC, et al. Blade and balloon atrial septostomy for left heart decompression in patients with severe ventricular dysfunction on extracorporeal membrane oxygenation. Catheter Cardiovasc Interv 1999;46:179–186.

17. O'Connor TA, Downing GJ, Ewing LL, Gowdamarajan R. Echocardiographically guided balloon atrial septostomy during extracorporeal membrane oxygenation (ECMO). Pediatr Cardiol 1993;14:167–168.

18. Koenig PR, Ralston MA, Kimball TR, Meyer RA, Daniels SR, Schwartz DC. Balloon atrial septostomy for left ventricular decompression in patients receiving extracorporeal membrane oxygenation for myocardial failure. J Pediatr 1993;122:S95–S99.

19. Darling EM, Kaemmer D, Lawson DS, Jaggers JJ, Ungerleider RM. Use of ECMO without the oxygenator to provide ventricular support after Norwood Stage I procedures. Ann Thorac Surg 2001;71:735–736.

20. Jaggers JJ, Forbess JM, Shah AS, et al. Extracorporeal membrane oxygenation for infant postcardiotomy support: significance of shunt management. Ann Thorac Surg 2000;69:1476–1483.

21. del Nido PJ, Dalton HJ, Thompson AE, Siewers RD. Extracorporeal membrane oxygenator rescue in children during cardiac arrest after cardiac surgery. Circulation 1992;86(Suppl II):II300–II304.

22. Duncan BW, Ibrahim AE, Hraska V, et al. Use of rapid-deployment extracorporeal membrane oxygenation for the resuscitation of pediatric patients with heart disease after cardiac arrest. J Thorac Cardiovasc Surg 1998;116:305–311.

23. Han J, Beeton A, Long P, et al. Plasticizer di(2-ethylhexyl)phthalate (DEHP) release in wet-primed extracorporeal membrane oxygenation (ECMO) circuits. Int J Pharm 2005;294:157–159.

24. Jacobs JP, Ojito JW, McConaghey TW, et al. Rapid cardiopulmonary support for children with complex congenital heart disease. Ann Thorac Surg 2000;70:742–750.

25. Morris MC, Wernovsky G, Nadkarni VM. Survival outcomes after extracorporeal cardiopulmonary resuscitation instituted during active chest compressions following refractory in-hospital pediatric cardiac arrest. Pediatr Crit Care Med 2004;5:440–446.

26. Thuys CA, Mullaly RJ, Horton SB, et al. Centrifugal ventricular assist in children under 6 kg. Euro J Cardiothorac Surg 1998;13:130–134.

27. Karl TR. Extracorporeal circulatory support in infants and children. Semin Thorac Cardiovasc Surg 1994;6:154–160.

28. Kesler KA, Pruitt AL, Turrentine MW, Heimansohn DA, Brown JW. Temporary left-sided mechanical cardiac support during acute myocarditis. Journal of Heart and Lung Transplantation 1994;13:268–270.

29. Khan A, Gazzaniga AB. Mechanical circulatory assistance in paediatric patients with cardiac failure. Cardiovasc Surg 1996;4:43–49.

30. Ashton RC, Oz MC, Michler RE, et al. Left ventricular assist device options in pediatric patients. ASAIO J 1995;41:M277–M280.

31. Chang AC, Hanley FL, Weindling SN, Wernovsky G, Wessel DL. Left heart support with a ventricular assist device in an infant with acute myocarditis. Crit Care Med 1992;20:712–715.

32. Ferrazzi P, Glauber M, DiDomenico A, et al. Assisted circulation for myocardial recovery after repair of congenital heart disease. Euro J Cardiothorac Surg 1991;5:419–424.

33. Langley SM, Sheppard SB, Tsang VT, Monro JL, Lamb RK. When is extracorporeal life support worthwhile following repair of congenital heart disease in children? Euro J Cardiothorac Surg 1998;13:520–525.

34. McBride LR, Naunheim KS, Fiore AC, Moroney DA, Swartz MT. Clinical experience with 111 Thoratec ventricular assist devices. Ann Thorac Surg 1999;67:1233–1239.

35. Korfer R, El-Banayosy A, Arusoglu L, et al. Single-center experience with the Thoratec ventricular assist device. J Thorac Cardiovasc Surg 2000;119:596–600.

36. Helman DN, Addonizio LJ, Morales DLS, et al. Implantable left ventricular assist devices can successfully bridge adolescent patients to transplant. J Heart Lung Transplant 2000;19:121–126.

37. Shum-Tim D, Duncan BW, Hraska V, Friehs I, Shin'oka T, Jonas RA. Evaluation of a pulsatile pediatric ventricular assist device in an acute right heart failure model. Ann Thorac Surg 1997;64:1374–1380.

38. Hetzer R, Hennig E, Schiessler A, Friedel N, Warnecke H, Adt M. Mechanical circulatory support and heart transplantation. J Heart Lung Transplant 1992;11:175–181.

39. Konertz W, Hotz H, Schneider M, Redlin M, Reul H. Clinical experience with the MEDOS HIA-VAD system in infants and children. Ann Thorac Surg 1997;63:1138–1144.

40. Sidiropoulos A, Hotz H, Konertz W. Pediatric circulatory support. J Heart Lung Transplant 1998;17:1172–1176.

41. Martin J, Sarai K, Schindler M, Van de Loo A, Yoshitake M, Beyersdorf F. Medos HIA-VAD biventricular assist device for bridge to recovery in fulminant myocarditis. Ann Thorac Surg 1997;63:1145–1146.

42. Ishino K, Loebe M, Uhlemann F, Weng Y, Hennig E, Hetzer R. Circulatory support with paracorporeal pneumatic ventricular assist device (VAD) in infants and children. Euro J Cardiothorac Surg 1997;11:965–972.

43. Stiller B, Dahnert I, Weng Y, Hennig E, Hetzer R, Lange PE. Children may survive severe myocarditis with prolonged use of biventricular assist devices. Heart 1999;82:237–240.

44. Schmitz C, Welz A, Dewald O, Kozlik-Feldmann R, Netz H, Reichart B. Switch from a BIVAD to a LVAD in a boy with Kawasaki disease. Ann Thorac Surg 2000;69:1270–1271.

45. Hetzer R, Loebe M, Potapov EV, et al. Circulatory support with pneumatic paracorporeal ventricular assist device in infants and children. Ann Thorac Surg 1998;66:1498–1506.

46. Morales DL, Dibardino DJ, McKenzie ED, et al. Lessons learned from the first application of the DeBakey VAD Child: an intracorporeal ventricular assist device for children. J Heart Lung Transplant 2005;24:331–337.

47. Duncan BW, Lorenz M, Kopcak MW, et al. The PediPump: a new ventricular assist device for children. Artif Organs 2005;29:527–530.

48. del Nido PJ, Duncan BW, Mayer J, J E, Wessel DL, LaPierre RA, Jonas RA. Left ventricular assist device improves survival in children with left ventricular dysfunction after repair of anomalous origin of the left coronary artery from the pulmonary artery. Ann Thorac Surg 1999;67:169–172.

49. Bavaria JE, Ratcliffe MB, Gupta KB, Wenger RK, Bogen DK, Edmunds LH. Changes in left ventricular systolic wall stress during biventricular circulatory assistance. Ann Thorac Surg 1988;45:526–532.

50. Ratcliffe MB, Bavaria JE, Wenger RK, Bogen DK, Edmunds LH. Left ventricular mechanics of ejecting, postischemic hearts during left ventricular circulatory assistance. J Thorac Cardiovasc Surg 1991;101: 245–255.

51. Eugene J, Ott RA, McColgan SJ, Roohk RV. Vented cardiac assistance: ECMO versus left heart bypass for acute left ventricular failure. ASAIO Trans 1986;32:538–541.

52. Eugene J, McColgan SJ, Roohk HV, Ott RA. Vented ECMO for biventricular failure. ASAIO Trans 1987;33:579–583.

53. Secker-Walker JS, Edmonds JF, Spratt EH, Conn AW. The source of coronary perfusion during partial bypass for extracorporeal membrane oxygenation (ECMO). Ann Thorac Surg 1976;21:138–143.

54. Nowlen TT, Salley SO, Whittlesey GC, et al. Regional blood flow distribution during extracorporeal membrane oxygenation in rabbit. J Thorac Cardiovasc Surg 1989;98:1138–1143.

55. Kato J, Seo T, Ando H, Takagi H, Ito T. Coronary arterial perfusion during venoarterial extracorporeal membrane oxygenation. J Thorac Cardiovasc Surg 1996;111:630–636.

56. Ibrahim AE, Duncan BW. Long-term follow-up of children with cardiac disease requiring mechanical circulatory support. In: Duncan BW, ed. Mechanical Circulatory Support for Cardiac and Respiratory Failure in Pediatric Cardiac Patients. New York: Marcel Dekker; 2001. 205–220.

57. Ibrahim AE, Duncan BW, Blume ED, Jonas RA. Long-term follow-up of pediatric cardiac patients requiring mechanical circulatory support. Ann Thorac Surg 2000;69:186–192.

18

Mechanical Support of the Cardiovascular System: Intraaortic Balloon Pumping in Children

L. LuAnn Minich and John A. Hawkins

Introduction

Resting the injured left ventricle often leads to a dramatic recovery of its function [1–4]. Mechanical devices have been designed to decrease the workload of the left ventricle while maintaining systemic blood flow and mean arterial pressure. These devices allow the injured myocardium to rest while preserving adequate perfusion and oxygen delivery to the remaining organs. Left ventricular assist devices (LVADs), extracorporeal membrane oxygenation (ECMO), and intraaortic balloon pumping (IABP) provide different levels of support, and each has advantages and disadvantages for pediatric use. For example, LVADs may replace ventricular function but have only recently become available for the pediatric population [5–7]. The major experience with LVADs in children has been in European countries. Because ECMO replaces both ventricular and pulmonary function, it may be excessive if the need is for purely left ventricular support. In addition, ECMO is costly, labor intensive, and available only at select centers, access to which often requires transfer of the critically ill and hemodynamically unstable child [8,9].

Unlike LVADs and ECMO, IABP only supports rather than completely replaces left ventricular output and function. Although it is not the appropriate device to use in the most severe phase of heart failure, it is a valuable tool for the treatment of moderate ventricular dysfunction when pharmacology has failed. Despite this, experience with pediatric IABP has been limited to a small number of institutions for several reasons, including the following: (1) limited availability of smaller catheters, (2) difficulties with catheter insertion, (3) technical problems with tracking the rapid heart rates and narrow pulse pressures of children in shock, and (4) controversy regarding the ability to achieve diastolic augmentation and afterload reduction in the compliant pediatric aorta [10–14]. Compared with the other mechanical assist modalities, however, IABP or counterpulsation has the advantage of being the simplest and least expensive device available. In the adult population, IABP is actually the most widely used assist device for managing acute left ventricular dysfunction after myocardial injury or cardiac surgery (1, 2, 4). Its use in children is discussed in this chapter.

Background

The basic principle underlying IABP is synchronization of aortic balloon inflation with aortic valve closure and deflation with aortic valve opening, thereby introducing external energy into the vascular system [15–19]. With the aortic valve closed, the balloon inflates and its volume displaces an equal volume of blood. As a result, both diastolic pressure and coronary artery perfusion increase. When the balloon is deflated, the aortic pressure precipitously drops just before left ventricular ejection, reducing afterload and thereby reducing myocardial oxygen consumption. These effects of reduced left ventricular afterload, reduced myocardial consumption, and increased coronary blood flow combine to maximize oxygen delivery to the heart.

Intraaortic balloon pumping was first validated in an animal model in 1962 [19]. Its clinical efficiency was established for the adult population through a multicenter trial in 1973 [6]. Although theoretically IABP should also be valuable for reducing the workload and enhancing the myocardial contractility of an injured pediatric heart, the first use of IABP in children was not published until 1980 [14]. In that study, Pollock and colleagues successfully treated 6 of 14 patients with ventricular failure after open-heart surgery. The technique became feasible in even smaller children after the miniaturization of balloon catheters, and, in 1983, Veasy and colleagues from Salt Lake City published the results from a series of 15 children, including 4 infants [20]. Despite the commercial availability of pediatric-sized catheters, and in contrast to the adult experience, pediatric IABP has not achieved widespread use. A discussion of the major obstacles to successful pediatric IABP and suggestions to overcome them is included in the following sections.

D.S. Wheeler et al. (eds.), *Cardiovascular Pediatric Critical Illness and Injury*,
DOI 10.1007/978-1-84800-923-3_18, © Springer-Verlag London Limited 2009

Patient Selection and Initiation and Maintenance of Intraaortic Balloon Pumping

Although percutaneous insertion has made the rapid initiation of effective IABP relatively easy in adults, catheter insertion in children is more invasive, frequently requiring a femoral arterial cutdown or insertion through the aortic arch [21]. Therefore, more preparation and planning are required before IABP can be instituted in children. In general, the child with low cardiac output who is unresponsive to vigorous medical management should be evaluated as a candidate for IABP.

Typically, a team that includes the cardiologist, intensivist, and cardiovascular surgeon performs the evaluation. The team attempts to institute therapy at the point where maximal medical management has failed but before the left ventricular dysfunction is so severe that even effective counterpulsation will not provide adequate relief of the myocardial workload to allow the heart to rest. At our institution, the decision is based on an evaluation of peripheral perfusion, mean aortic pressure, persistence of metabolic acidosis, mixed venous PO_2 (<25 torr), oliguria (<1 mL/kg/hr), and, when available, left atrial pressure (>20 mm Hg) [21,22]. The presence of ventricular ectopic activity that develops secondary to poor coronary blood flow or high levels of vasopressor support must also be considered, as the arrhythmia may resolve after IABP is initiated and hemodynamics improve. Indications for pediatric IABP (Table 18.1) include failure to wean from cardiopulmonary bypass, refractory left ventricular dysfunction in the intensive care unit after cardiac surgery, as a bridge to transplantation, before repair of an anomalous left coronary artery, infectious or inflammatory heart disease, sepsis with left ventricular dysfunction, and persistent ventricular arrhythmias [10,11,13,14,21,23–25]. Contraindications are listed in Table 18.2 and essentially include lesions when effective counterpulsation is not possible because of the underlying anatomy [10,13]. If the patient has a residual lesion that can be surgically corrected, IABP should be used to restore adequate cardiac output only long enough to allow the patient to undergo appropriate diagnostic studies and return to the operating room. Patients in the terminal stages of their illness who have no chance of permanent recovery should not be considered candidates.

TABLE 18.1. Reported indications for intraaortic balloon pumping in children.

Surgical
  Preoperative, failure to wean from bypass; postoperative ventricular failure
  Anomalous left coronary artery
  Fontan-type operations
  Closure of atrioventricular septal defects
  Rastelli-type operations
  Tetralogy of Fallot repairs
  Arterial switch operations
  Coronary artery bypass after Kawasaki disease
  Aortic and mitral valve replacements
  Ventricular septal defect repair
Medical
  Kawasaki disease
  Blunt cardiac trauma
  Sepsis
  Hemolytic-uremic syndrome
  Persistent ventricular arrhythmias with ventricular dysfunction
  Myocarditis
  End-stage cardiomyopathy as a bridge to transplantation

TABLE 18.2. Contraindications to intraaortic balloon pumping in children.

Absolute
  Significant aortic regurgitation
  Patent ductus arteriosus
  Recent coarctation or aortic arch repair
  Terminal stage of systemic disease
  Multiorgan failure with unlikely chance of permanent recovery
Relative
  Severe neurologic insult
  Pulmonary artery hypertension leading to isolated right ventricular failure
  Residual lesions amenable to reoperation

Once the decision is made to proceed with IABP, the medical and nursing teams are mobilized. Catheter selection is based on guidelines using both age and weight. The standard pediatric balloon volumes range from 2.5 to 20.0 mL, and balloons are mounted on 4.5–7.0 French catheters. Unlike the adult catheters, pediatric catheters do not contain a lumen for monitoring central aortic pressure. We choose a catheter that has a balloon volume approximating 50% of the normal stroke volume predicted for the individual patient [22]. The surgical team inserts the catheter through a femoral cutdown that is described elsewhere in detail [13,21] and only briefly outlined here (Figure 18.1). After making a small vertically oriented groin incision, the common femoral artery is exposed. The child is heparinized, and then the artery is occluded proximally and distally to isolate a 2-cm segment. The appropriately sized balloon catheter is marked at the groin incision with a silk suture and the tip is positioned at the suprasternal notch, allowing an approximation of how far the catheter should be inserted into the vessel. The catheter is inserted into a 1–2 cm section of expandable polytetrafluoroethylene graft material with a 3.5 or 4.0 mm diameter. To aid in insertion, the surgeon aspirates and wraps the balloon, lubricates the tip with sterile mineral oil, and inserts it with a twisting motion into a longitudinal arteriotomy. The previously placed suture mark is used to determine the distance of catheter insertion. Using 6–0 polypropylene suture, the graft is sewed to the arteriotomy. Intraaortic balloon pumping is then initiated and the tip of the catheter position at the left subclavian artery confirmed using radiography. The catheter is secured by tying it to the graft using a 2–0 or 3–0 suture to prevent bleeding. Further hemostasis is achieved in the wound and the skin closed with a continuous suture. After local hemostasis is secured, the patient is started on a continuous heparin infusion to maintain a partial thromboplastin time of 40–60 sec. Some infants who require IABP are too small to have even the smallest commercially available catheters inserted into the femoral artery. In these instances, aortic arch insertion and catheter placement into the external iliac artery through a flank incision have provided successful alternatives [23,26].

Because of the relatively large catheter/vessel ratio, attention to the distal circulation is particularly important in the pediatric patient. Although the pulse in the involved foot may disappear immediately, the viability of the extremity should never be left in question. Frequently, IABP will improve systemic output enough that the capillary perfusion to the involved extremity is significantly improved even though the pulse is diminished. The care of these patients in the intensive care unit requires two experienced nurses, with one nurse caring for the patient and the other devoting attention to the proper running of the pump. The nurses at our institution have published specific details of care for the child undergoing IABP [27].

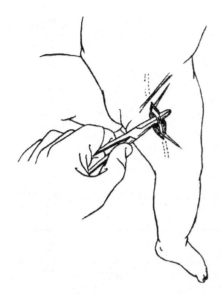

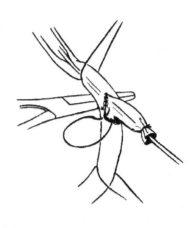

Figure 18.1. The operative technique for femoral artery insertion of the intraaortic balloon pumping catheter involves isolating the femoral artery through a vertical groin incision. The catheter is then inserted through a side-arm graft that is sewn to a longitudinal arteriotomy. (Data from Pinkney et al. [13]. © 2002 with permission from Society of Thoracic Surgeons.)

Timing of Intraaortic Balloon Pumping in the Pediatric Population

For IABP to reduce left ventricular afterload and increase coronary blood flow, inflation and deflation must be precisely synchronized (but 180° out of phase) with the cardiac cycle. Inappropriate timing has been shown to result in either minimal clinical improvement or deterioration of the patient's hemodynamic status [17,28]. Several timing errors may occur: (1) early inflation (before aortic valve closure), resulting in increased afterload; (2) late inflation (well after aortic valve closure), resulting in suboptimal diastolic augmentation and little reduction in afterload; (3) early deflation (well before aortic valve opening), shortening the period of diastolic augmentation and providing a setup for steal from the brachiocephalic and coronary arterial circulations; and (4) late deflation extending into systole, increasing afterload and decreasing left ventricular emptying [17]. Adult animal experiments have shown that an error of 20 msec in deflation time could reduce coronary augmentation by as much as 50% (29).

Most IABP consoles allow operator adjustment of both inflation and deflation points. Conventional balloon timing is accomplished first by electronic tracking of arterial pressure and electrocardiographic signals [16,30–32]. The balloon is inflated at the dicrotic notch on the arterial pressure waveform or at the end of the T wave on the electrocardiogram and deflated just before the upstroke on the arterial waveform or with the R wave on the electrocardiogram. Subtle adjustments are then made to maximize the changes in the arterial waveform that indicate effective afterload reduction and diastolic augmentation [32]. Peripheral arterial pressure and electrocardiographic signals provide only rough estimates of the actual opening and closing of the aortic valve, however, and are inherently associated with error. For example, the variation in the time delay in transmission between aortic valve closure and the appearance of the dicrotic notch on the arterial tracing shown on the monitor is one source of error. This time lag increases as the arterial waveform travels downstream. In adults, the time from aortic valve closure to

the dicrotic notch recorded at the subclavian artery is about 25 msec, at the radial artery about 50 msec, and at the femoral artery about 120 msec [31]. These are estimate, however, as the wave reflection varies with the patient's hemodynamics and degree of shock, making the phase shift unpredictable. Similarly, another source of error lies in assuming a known or constant duration of isovolumetric contraction or relaxation in relation to the R wave of the electrocardiogram. These intervals are difficult to precisely measure and vary widely in the setting of hemodynamic instability. The quality of the arterial pressure tracing provides yet another source of error. When the pediatric patient is in shock, the tracing often has low amplitude and a narrow pulse pressure, making it difficult to track with current IABP equipment [33]. Finally, neither the arterial pressure tracing nor the electrocardiogram has an exact marker for deflating the balloon; rather, attempts are made to deflate before the next arterial upstroke or the R wave on the electrocardiogram.

Because of rapid heart rates, very narrow pulse pressures, and the capability of only peripheral artery monitoring, the margin for error is smaller and the use of the arterial pressure tracing and electrocardiogram for timing even less accurate in children. As a result, most operators of pediatric consoles use the arterial pressure tracing and electrocardiogram only as rough guidelines and arbitrarily adjust timing to produce a presystolic dip on the arterial tracing as described later [11,14,22]. Another common maneuver is to go to 2:1 timing, but this is less than optimal because hemodynamics are compromised by the loss of IABP assistance for every other beat [12,31].

Centers that use conventional timing techniques attempt to deflate the balloon just before systole, during the preejection period. This requires analysis of the augmented pressure tracing (Figure 18.2) for the demonstration of a presystolic dip (balloon-assisted aortic end diastolic pressure less than unassisted end diastolic pressure) to ensure afterload reduction or decreased impedance to ventricular ejection [30,32]. The contours of the tracings, however, vary with changes in aortic compliance, pressure, and shock state. Intraaortic balloon pumping itself alters the left ventricular dP/dT and changes ventriculovascular coupling in

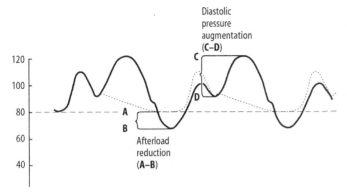

Figure 18.2. Schematic of the ideal arterial pressure tracing demonstrates the presystolic dip as evidence of afterload reduction and the increased pressure in diastole (diastolic augmentation). (Data from Minich et al. [40]. © 2001 with permission from Lippincott Williams & Wilkins.)

ways that are frequently unpredictable and undetectable on the electrocardiogram or arterial pressure tracing. Use of the electrocardiogram and arterial pressure tracing for determining the onset and end of left ventricular ejection is so fraught with error in the pediatric population that IABP may be seen as ineffective in children.

As an alternative to using the electrocardiogram or the arterial pressure trace for pediatric IABP timing, we investigated the use of M-mode echocardiography for this purpose [34]. Because of the rapid sampling rate (>1,000 pulses/min), M-mode echocardiography is ideally suited for demonstrating the precise time points of both aortic valve opening and closure as well as the points of balloon inflation and deflation. By adjusting the standard parasternal short-axis view, both the aortic valve and the balloon in the descending aorta can be visualized (Figure 18.3). Using this two-dimensional image for guidance, the M-mode cursor is placed to allow simultaneous sampling of both aortic valve and balloon motion (Figure 18.4). The exact point of aortic valve closure is

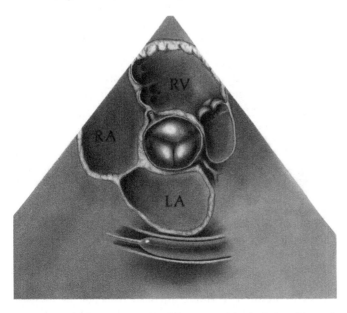

Figure 18.3. Schematic representation of the parasternal short-axis view of the aortic valve and the balloon in the descending aorta posterior to the left atrium (LA). RA, right atrium, RV, right ventricle. (Data from Minich et al. [34]. © 1997 with permission from Excerpta Medica, Inc.)

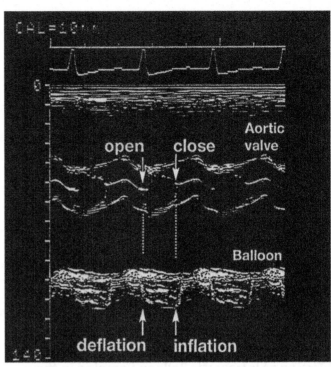

Figure 18.4. M-mode echocardiogram with the cursor placed through both the aortic valve and the intraaortic balloon showing the opening and closing of the valve and the inflation and deflation of the balloon. The vertical dotted lines show that balloon deflation coincides with valve opening and inflation with valve closing. (Data from Minich et al. [37]. © 2001 with permission from International Society for Heart and Lung Transplantation.)

directly compared with that of balloon inflation. Similarly, the exact point of balloon deflation is directly compared with that of aortic valve opening.

To compare conventional timing with the M-mode markers of timing, six patients who underwent IABP between April 1993 and November 1996 were studied, including three with cardiomyopathy and three who failed to wean from cardiopulmonary bypass. An experienced member of the IABP team established counterpulsation using conventional timing. After optimal timing using the conventional method was established, balloon inflation and deflation were assessed using M-mode echocardiography as described earlier. Precise timing was defined as having the balloon deflated during the entire ejection period and inflated during the entire diastolic interval. Systolic error was determined as the percentage of time the balloon was inflated during the ejection period. Diastolic error was determined as the percentage of time the balloon was deflated during the diastolic interval. In this study, systolic error ranged from 6.7% to 80.0%, with five patients having only early inflation and one having both early inflation and late deflation. Diastolic error ranged from 0% to 60%, with five patients having early deflation. The one patient who had both early inflation and late deflation had no diastolic error. Systolic error rates were significantly greater in the smaller patients with the fastest heart rates. Neither patient size nor heart rate had an impact on the diastolic error rates.

To further investigate the accuracy of electrocardiographic markers, arterial pressure waveforms, and M-mode markers for determining the onset of systole and diastole, internal review board approval and informed consent were obtained to study six patients undergoing open-heart surgery [35]. The radial arterial pressure

FIGURE 18.5. The electrocardiogram is recorded simultaneously with the M-mode echocardiogram and the central aortic pressure tracing. The upstroke (U) of the arterial pressure curve coincides with the aortic valve (Ao) opening (O) from the M-mode recording, and the dicrotic notch (D) coincides with aortic valve closure (C). (Data from Minich et al. [36]. © 1998 with permission from Society of Thoracic Surgeons.)

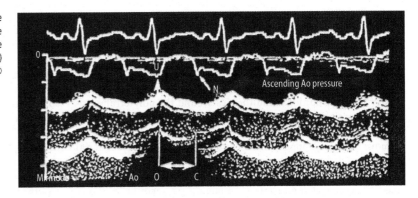

waveform obtained from a fluid-filled system was recorded simultaneously with the aortic root pressure waveform using a high-fidelity catheter, flow waveforms using an ultrasonic transit-time flow probe around the aortic root, electrocardiogram, and the aortic valve M-mode echocardiogram. When compared with the aortic root waveform, the radial arterial dicrotic notch had a variable and unpredictable delay of 107 ± 23 msec after actual aortic valve closure. Similarly, a 92 ± 11 msec delay was found between aortic valve opening and the R wave on the electrocardiogram. In contrast, M-mode echocardiographic timing markers were identical to the markers for aortic valve opening and closing obtained from the high fidelity pressure catheter in the aortic root.

With the use of the currently available balloon catheters that have a central lumen to the tip, central aortic pressure tracings can be used for timing in adults. Unfortunately, the catheter is not sufficiently miniaturized for children to be able to contain a central aortic pressure lumen. Because synchronization of the balloon to aortic valve opening and closing is so important, in the absence of a central pressure recording, another method with precise markers of aortic valve opening and closing would be valuable for improving the results of IABP in children. Therefore, to further validate the use of M-mode echocardiography as such a method, we studied the technique in an immature swine model of congestive heart failure created by disrupting the mitral valve chordae to cause acute severe mitral regurgitation [36]. The piglets were <10 kg to simulate the smallest patients with the fastest heart rates who are the most challenging to pump. The animal investigations resulted in several important findings. First, M-mode echocardiographic markers again corresponded precisely with aortic root pressure markers (Figure 18.5). Second, when the balloon was timed to inflate with aortic valve closure and deflate with valve opening as demonstrated on the M-mode echocardiogram, there was a significant increase in aortic flow and pressure and a significant decrease in left atrial pressure. Interestingly, the diastolic augmentation and presystolic dip seen on the peripheral arterial pressure tracing frequently contradicted what was seen on the simultaneously recorded central aortic pressure tracing. If conventional timing was used, the balloon would have been inflated during much of the ejection time and deflated during much of the diastolic interval. A second series of experiments in this animal model compared M-mode echo-timed IABP with conventionally timed IABP. Echo-timed IABP resulted in significantly greater mean aortic pressure and aortic flow than conventionally timed IABP. In fact, only echo-timed IABP resulted in improvement of the animal's hemodynamic parameters compared with those obtained during the shock state—after mitral valve disruption and before IABP. When conventional timing techniques were used, there was no improvement and even

deterioration in the hemodynamic parameters measured for some animals.

Since 1994, we have used M-mode echocardiography for IABP timing in children. Similar to the experience in the animal model, we have found that the peripherally recorded augmented waveform can be very misleading (Figure 18.6) in the pediatric patient [37]. In this example, the child had evidence of diastolic augmentation and afterload reduction only on the unassisted beat, but the balloon was precisely timed with aortic valve motion as demonstrated with M-mode echocardiography. All adjustments in timing that were made in an attempt to improve the appearance of the pressure waveform resulted in deterioration of the child's hemodynamic status. Therefore, echo-timed IABP was resumed. During the next 24 hr, without further adjustments in the timing of balloon inflation and deflation, hemodynamics improved and the arterial pressure trace gradually changed to reveal the presystolic dip on the assisted beat.

Weaning

The procedure for weaning the pediatric patient from IABP is similar to that for the adult [38,39]. Weaning should take place only when pharmacologic support has been significantly reduced and the child's overall hemodynamic state improved [21]. Echocardiog-

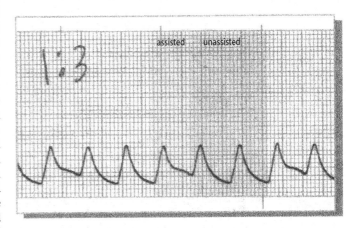

FIGURE 18.6. The intraaortic balloon pump is functioning in 1:3 synchronization to allow analysis of the radial arterial tracing. Note that there is no presystolic dip after the assisted beat, but there are presystolic dips after the unassisted beats. Despite this, the M-mode echocardiogram (see Figure 18.4) shows appropriate timing of intraaortic balloon pumping. (Data from Minich et al. [37]. © 2001 with permission from International Society for Heart and Lung Transplantation.)

raphy should be used to support the clinical and laboratory findings, and the left ventricular shortening and ejection fractions should show some improvement before weaning is attempted. The weaning period often occurs over 24 to 48 hr with the pump assist ratio systematically taken from 1:1 to 1:2 to 1:3 during this time. Once the patient's status appears stable, the groin incision is opened under sterile conditions, and the ties around the polytetrafluoroethylene graft are removed. The pump is discontinued, and the catheter is removed. An embolectomy catheter is routinely used to remove any clot trapped in the common femoral artery. Arterial inflow and distal backflow are confirmed and the graft oversewn, leaving a small length of graft attached to the femoral artery. The method we prefer for insertion through a side-arm graft allows removal without repair of the artery, allowing the lumen size to be preserved. Distal pulses are carefully assessed before closing the incision. If they are weak or absent, further embolectomy is performed.

Diastolic Augmentation in the Compliant Pediatric Aorta

Doubts regarding the ability to effectively provide diastolic augmentation in the highly compliant aorta have also contributed to the perception that IABP is ineffective in children. Left ventricular function depends on both the state of the myocardium and the characteristics of the arterial circulation. Because about 90% of the myocardial oxygen consumption occurs during isovolumetric contraction, the left ventricle must overcome afterload that is mainly determined by aortic compliance and systemic vascular resistance [16]. Clinically, this may be estimated by measuring the left ventricular end diastolic pressure. If the left ventricular end diastolic pressure can be decreased at the same time that peak diastolic pressure is increased, coronary blood flow will increase, and the oxygen supply to the heart will improve. Thus, the effectiveness of diastolic augmentation is at least somewhat dependent on aortic compliance.

Early in vivo studies evaluated the effect of compliance on the amount of volume needed in the balloon for adequate augmentation in two animal models of congestive heart failure [18]. Pressure–volume curves to reflect aortic compliance were developed in both adult dogs and immature calves. The investigators were able to relate balloon volume to compliance and demonstrated that twice the balloon volume was needed to achieve comparable diastolic augmentation in the immature calf, which has the more compliant aorta compared to the adult dog. These findings were supported by clinical studies. The earliest series of IABP from Toronto reported no survivors of children less than 5 years of age compared with an 80% survival rate for children greater than 10 years old [14]. Both the animal and early pediatric data led some investigators to argue that children must be at least 5 years old before their aortic compliance curves are steep enough to provide clinically important diastolic augmentation. The issue remains controversial, however, as other investigators dispute this theory and provide reports of successful IABP even in infants [10,13,20,26].

The selection of balloon catheter size is an important aspect of providing optimal counterpulsation. Generally, to provide adequate diastolic augmentation in a compliant aorta, the largest balloon catheter is used based on the estimated aortic diameter

derived from angiographic studies and the child's height and weigh [22]. As a general rule, the balloon volume should be at least 50% of the normal predicted stroke volume. This is the size that, at leas in theory, provides maximal diastolic augmentation. There are additional considerations, however. The largest catheter size may not be the optimal size if the catheter balloon displaces a volume so large that it results in presystolic flow reversal in the brachiocephalic arteries and compromises cerebral blood flow when it is deflated [15]. There are few objective data in this area, particularly in the pediatric population, and discussions of the magnitude of this risk are ongoing. In a study at our institution, pediatric aortic compliance was determined for six children ranging in age from 9 months to 4 years who were undergoing surgical repair of a cardiovascular lesion [35]. Pressure–volume data using a high-fidelity catheter-tipped pressure transducer in the aortic root and an ultrasonic transit-time flow probe around the proximal aorta were used to generate a range of normal compliance values for children less than five years old. Using these normal values, two test aortas with different compliances that fell within the range were constructed. The effect of IABP for each simulated aorta was then tested using an in vitro pulsatile flow model (Figure 18.7) to simulate pediatric left heart dynamics [40]. IABP resulted in both diastolic augmentation and afterload reduction for both test aortas. Similarly, for both

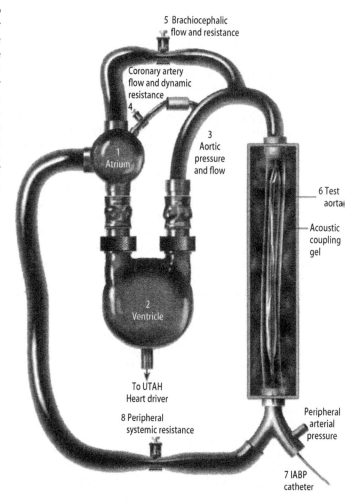

FIGURE 18.7. Schematic of the UTAH-IVAD pulsatile flow simulator used to evaluate the effects of compliance on the effectiveness of IABP. (Data from Minich et al. [40]. © 2001 with permission from Lippincott Williams & Wilkins.)

simulated aortas, IABP resulted in a significant increase in mean aortic pressure as well as a significant increase in both coronary artery and brachiocephalic flow. Flow in the brachiocephalic vessels remained antegrade under all experimental conditions. Although this finding is interesting, it is not conclusive. The antegrade brachiocephalic flow may be a result of stroke volumes always exceeding balloon volumes in the in vitro model. This may not always be the case in the clinical situation, however.

It is also important to note that, despite effective afterload reduction and diastolic augmentation with both simulated aortas, the increase in aortic flow reached statistical significance only for the less-compliant vessel. Although it may have been possible in this in vitro model to use a larger balloon and further increase the ascending aortic flow in the more compliant vessel, realistically, balloon size is limited by the vessel size in vivo. The issue remains unresolved. Evaluation of the relationships among stroke volume, balloon volume, and brachiocephalic and coronary blood flow will need to be performed in an animal model as well as in the clinical setting before the influence of aortic compliance on diastolic augmentation is well understood.

Results of Intraaortic Balloon Pumping in Children

For adults, IABP is a standard therapeutic tool for managing moderate left ventricular dysfunction, with survival rates that approach 80% [38,39]. In contrast, pediatric IABP has been limited to a small number of institutions, and survival rates reflect this limited use. Pollock and colleagues from Toronto successfully pumped 6 of 14 children following cardiac surgery as described in the first report of IABP in the pediatric population [14]. After catheters were miniaturized, the first reports of IABP in infants appeared in 1983, and successful IABP has been described in a 2.0 kg neonate [11,12,14,20,22,26]. These early investigators described overall survival rates ranging from 37% to 45%, with a tendency toward poorer survival for infants. More recently, however, Akomea-Agyin reported 50% long-term survival of infants and 57% of both infants and children after IABP [10].

Intraaortic balloon pumping has been used at our institution, for the most part in the absence of a ventricular assist device or ECMO program, since 1981, giving us a unique opportunity to evaluate the technique in pediatric patients. We reviewed the records of all patients undergoing IABP between 1988 and 2001. Of the total 29 patients undergoing the procedure, 62% were successfully weaned and discharged home [13]. The mean duration of IABP was 4.4 ± 2.9 days, and neither age nor gender was related to survival. Timing of intraaortic balloon pumping using M-mode echocardiography was adopted after 1994. Compared with standard arterial/ECG or conventional-timing, echo-timed IABP improved survival from 46% to 78%. Although not statistically significant at this point, it is encouraging and suggests that IABP with proper timing is a tool that should be utilized for managing moderate left ventricular failure in the pediatric population.

Complications

Complications from IABP (Table 18.3) are similar to those reported for the adult population [38,39,41]. In our series described earlier, one patient developed sepsis while awaiting transplantation, and one patient had evidence of limb ischemia that was transient [13].

TABLE 18.3. Complications of intraaortic balloon pumping in children.

Bleeding and hematoma
Limb, mesenteric, renal, and cerebrovascular ischemia
Wound infection
Sepsis
Balloon leak or rupture
Balloon entrapment
Vessel perforation
Thrombocytopenia
Aortoiliac dissection
Pseudoaneurysm
Emboli

Although neither the incidence nor severity of complications seems to be related to patient age or size, balloon rupture, vessel perforation, thrombocytopenia, dissection of the aorta and mesenteric arteries, and major limb, renal, and cerebrovascular ischemia are problems that have been reported to require particularly close scrutiny for their prevention in the pediatric population [10].

Conclusion

In contrast to its popularity in the adult population, IABP continues to be used in only a few pediatric centers. The greatest experience with this technique seems to be in institutions that do not have well-established ventricular assist device or ECMO programs. In these centers, IABP has been successful for the treatment of moderate shock in children with few complications. Because IABP supports or assists rather than replaces ventricular function, it cannot be used as a last resort, and its use must be anticipated before the child is moribund. Therefore, initiation of IABP should occur when the child is not responding to increases in pharmacologic support and before cardiac output falls below recoverable levels. M-mode echocardiography may be useful for timing balloon inflation and deflation, optimizing both afterload reduction and diastolic augmentation. Further study and more experience are needed to clearly determine the role of IABP in children.

References

1. Christenson JT, Buswell L, Velebit V, Maurice J, Simonet F, Schmuziger M. The intraaortic balloon pump for postcardiotomy heart failure. Experience with 169 intraaortic balloon pumps. Thorac Cardiovasc Surg 1995;43(3):129–133.
2. Kern MJ, Aguirre FV, Tatineni S, Penick D, Serota H, Donohue T, et al. Enhanced coronary blood flow velocity during intraaortic balloon counterpulsation in critically ill patients. J Am Coll Cardiol 1993;21(2):359–368.
3. Pi K, Block PC, Warner MG, Diethrich EB. Major determinants of survival and nonsurvival of intraaortic balloon pumping. Am Heart J 1995;130(4):849–853.
4. Torchiana DF, Hirsch G, Buckley MJ, Hahn C, Allyn JW, Akins CW, et al. Intraaortic balloon pumping for cardiac support: trends in practice and outcome, 1968 to 1995. J Thorac Cardiovasc Surg 1997;113(4):758–769.
5. Goldstein DJ, Oz MC, Rose EA. Implantable left ventricular assist devices. N Engl J Med 1998;339(21):1522–1533.
6. Scheld HH. Mechanical support–benefits and risks. Thorac Cardiovasc Surg 1997;45(1):1–5.
7. Sidiropoulos A, Hotz H, Konertz W. Pediatric circulatory support. J Heart Lung Transplant 1998;17(12):1172–1176.

8. Meliones JN, Custer JR, Snedecor S, Moler FW, O'Rourke PP, Delius RE. Extracorporeal life support for cardiac assist in pediatric patients. Review of ELSO Registry data. Circulation 1991;84(5 Suppl): III168–III172.

9. Walters HL, 3rd, Hakimi M, Rice MD, Lyons JM, Whittlesey GC, Klein MD. Pediatric cardiac surgical ECMO: multivariate analysis of risk factors for hospital death. Ann Thorac Surg 1995;60(2):329–337.

10. Akomea-Agyin C, Kejriwal NK, Franks R, Booker PD, Pozzi M. Intraaortic balloon pumping in children. Ann Thorac Surg 1999; 67(5):1415–14120.

11. Park JK, Hsu DT, Gersony WM. Intraaortic balloon pump management of refractory congestive heart failure in children. Pediatr Cardiol 1993;14(1):19–22.

12. Pennington DG, Swartz MT. Circulatory support in infants and children. Ann Thorac Surg 1993;55(1):233–237.

13. Pinkney KA, Minich LL, Tani LY, Di R, Veasy LG, McGough EC, et al. Current results with intraaortic balloon pumping in infants and children. Ann Thorac Surg 2002;73(3):887–891.

14. Pollock JC, Charlton MC, Williams WG, Edmonds JF, Trusler GA. Intraaortic balloon pumping in children. Ann Thorac Surg 1980; 29(6):522–528.

15. Feola M, Limet RR, Glick G. Direct and reflex vascular effects of intra-aortic balloon counterpulsation in dogs. Am J Physiol 1971;221(3): 748–753.

16. Jaron D, Moore TW, He P. Control of intraaortic balloon pumping: theory and guidelines for clinical applications. Ann Biomed Eng 1985;13(2):155–175.

17. Kantrowitz A, Freed PS, Cardona RR, Gage K, Marinescu GN, Westveld AH, et al. Initial clinical trial of a closed loop, fully automatic intra-aortic balloon pump. ASAIO J 1992;38(3):M617–M621.

18. Lin CY, Galysh FT, Ho KJ, Patel AS. Response to single-segment intraaortic balloon pumping as related to aortic compliance. Ann Thorac Surg 1972;13(5):468–476.

19. Moulopoulos SD, Topaz S, Kolff WJ. Diastolic balloon pumping (with carbon dioxide) in the aorta—a mechanical assistance to the failing circulation. Am Heart J 1962;63:669–675.

20. Veasy LG, Blalock RC, Orth JL, Boucek MM. Intra-aortic balloon pumping in infants and children. Circulation 1983;68(5):1095–1100.

21. Duncan BW, ed. Mechanical Support for Cardiac and Respiratory Failure in Pediatric Patients. New York: Dekker; 2001.

22. Veasy LG, Webster HF, McGough EC. Intra-aortic balloon pumping: adaptation for pediatric use. Crit Care Clin 1986;2(2):237–249.

23. Pozzi M, Santoro G, Makundan S. Intraaortic balloon pump after treatment of anomalous origin of left coronary artery. Ann Thorac Surg 1998;65(2):555–557.

24. Pribble CG, Shaddy RE. Intra-aortic balloon counterpulsation in newborn lambs infected with group B streptococcus. ASAIO Trans 1991;37(1):33–37.

25. Nawa S, Sugawara E, Murakami T, Senoo Y, Teramoto S, Morita K. Efficacy of intra-aortic balloon pumping for failing Fontan circulation. Chest 1988;93(3):599–603.

26. del Nido PJ, Swan PR, Benson LN, Bohn D, Charlton MC, Coles JG, et al. Successful use of intraaortic balloon pumping in a 2-kilogram infant. Ann Thorac Surg 1988;46(5):574–576.

27. Geiger J, Hall T, Breeze E, Davey C, Jones A, Stackhouse D. Intra-aortic balloon pumps in children: a small-nursing-team approach. Crit Care Nurse 1997;17(3):79–86.

28. Smith B, Barnea O, Moore TW, Jaron D. Optimal control system for the intra-aortic balloon pump. Med Biol Eng Comput 1991;29(2):180–184.

29. Barnea O, Moore TW, Dubin SE, Jaron D. Cardiac energy considerations during intraaortic balloon pumping. IEEE Trans Biomed Eng 1990;37(2):170–181.

30. Anella J, McCloskey A, Vieweg C. Nursing dynamics of pediatric intraaortic balloon pumping. Crit Care Nurse 1990;10(4):24–37.

31. Cadwell CA, Quaal SJ. Intra-aortic balloon counterpulsation timing. Am J Crit Care 1996;5(4):254–263.

32. Wojner AW. Assessing the five points of the intra-aortic balloon pump waveform. Crit Care Nurse 1994;14(3):48–52.

33. Webster H, Veasy LG. Intra-aortic balloon pumping in children. Heart Lung 1985;14(6):548–555.

34. Minich LL, Tani LY, McGough EC, Shaddy RE, Hawkins JA. A novel approach to pediatric intraaortic balloon pump timing using M-mode echocardiography. Am J Cardiol 1997;80(3):367–369.

35. Pantalos GM, Minich LL, Tani LY, McGough EC, Hawkins JA. Estimation of timing errors for the intraaortic balloon pump use in pediatric patients. ASAIO J 1999;45(3):166–171.

36. Minich LL, Tani LY, Pantalos GM, Bolland BL, Knorr BK, Hawkins JA. Neonatal piglet model of intraaortic balloon pumping: improved efficacy using echocardiographic timing. Ann Thorac Surg 1998;66(5): 1527–1532.

37. Minich LL, Tani LY, Hawkins JA, Orsmond GS, Di Russo GB, Shaddy RE. Intra-aortic balloon pumping in children with dilated cardiomyopathy as a bridge to transplantation. J Heart Lung Transplant 2001; 20(7):750–754.

38. Cohen M, Urban P, Christenson JT, Joseph DL, Freedman RJ, Jr., Miller MF, et al. Intra-aortic balloon counterpulsation in US and non-US centres: results of the Benchmark Registry. Eur Heart J 2003;24(19): 1763–1770.

39. Ferguson JJ, 3rd, Cohen M, Freedman RJ, Jr., Stone GW, Miller MF, Joseph DL, et al. The current practice of intra-aortic balloon counterpulsation: results from the Benchmark Registry. J Am Coll Cardiol 2001;38(5):1456–1462.

40. Minich LL, Tani LY, Hawkins JA, Bartkowiak RR, Royall ML, Pantalos GM. In vitro evaluation of the effect of aortic compliance on pediatric intra-aortic balloon pumping. Pediatr Crit Care Med 2001;2(2):139–144.

41. Arafa OE, Pedersen TH, Svennevig JL, Fosse E, Geiran OR. Vascular complications of the intraaortic balloon pump in patients undergoing open heart operations: 15-year experience. Ann Thorac Surg 1999;67(3): 645–651.

19
Arrhythmias

Timothy K. Knilans

Introduction

The spectrum of cardiac arrhythmias in the pediatric intensive care unit (PICU) range from those that are immediately life threatening to those with little or no hemodynamic consequences [1]. When a cardiac arrhythmia is suspected or diagnosed in the PICU, the first step should not be to specifically diagnose the rhythm mechanism but rather to determine the effects of the rhythm, some of which may need immediate intervention perhaps without a specific diagnosis. At the other end of the spectrum are rhythms that may initially appear to be benign but may exert subclinical effects before resulting in hemodynamic collapse [2]. Other arrhythmias may never result in hemodynamic collapse, but their effects may prolong the duration of PICU admission or mechanical ventilation [3]. Thus, even rhythm abnormalities that do not initially appear to be of hemodynamic significance should be completely investigated.

Many patients in modern PICU are on continuous electrocardiographic monitoring with *full-disclosure* review [4] with or without *monitor watchers* [5]. Ideally, multiple electrocardiographic leads and other monitoring parameters are reviewable. *Reconstructed* 12-lead electrocardiograms (ECGs) are available without attachment of the standard 10 electrodes in some current commercial systems [6,7], and others allow recording of 12-lead ECGs with standard lead placement using the bedside monitor. These multichannel recordings and *full-disclosure* review greatly aid in establishing heart rhythm diagnoses and reduce the need for traditional ECG machines that have in the past delayed diagnosis and treatment.

In addition to surface electrocardiographic recordings, other parameters are frequently helpful in rhythm diagnosis and assessment. Atrial electrical activity may be directly recorded in patients with recent cardiac surgery with the use of epicardial temporary atrial *pacing* wires [8]. Atrial activity can also be recorded from the esophagus [9] in patients via a bipolar oro- or nasoesophageal catheter or swallowed *pill electrode*. Atrial or central venous pressures and pressure waveforms may also be helpful in arrhythmia diagnosis. Monitoring heart rates with the use of arterial line waveform or pulse oximetry deflections may also be important, especially when artifact is present in the ECG recording (Figure 19.1). In pacemaker-dependent patients, the algorithm of a monitoring system may interpret the artifact of an electronic pacing spike as a QRS complex and not trigger an alarm if capture failure occurs. Heart rate monitors based on secondary indicators that require pacemaker capture, such as pulse oximetry or arterial pressure, will notify personnel immediately should capture failure occur.

Interpretation of Electrocardiograms

The ECG remains the primary modality for diagnosis of cardiac rhythm abnormality. In most cases and for most interpreters, printing the ECG on paper aids in the analysis of the heart rhythm. If full-disclosure review is available, identifying the points of initiation, termination, and any spontaneous perturbations of the arrhythmia and printing them in as many recorded leads as available should be done.

Identification of atrial activity is the most helpful first step in arrhythmia analysis. Marking the location of visible P waves with pen on paper can help in the identification of a pattern of atrial activity. Measuring calipers can also be quite useful. The atrial mechanism is often regular, and, if it is dissociated from ventricular activity, caliper measurements can identify the probable timing of P waves that are concealed by QRS complexes or T waves. When readily available from postoperative epicardial wires placed at the time of recent cardiac surgery, recording of an ECG with augmented atrial recording with the use of the wires can easily identify previously concealed atrial activity. Ideally this recording is performed with a separate amplifier channel recording a unipolar or bipolar atrial electrogram separate from, but on the same recording paper as, the surface ECG (Figure 19.2). When such recording equipment is not available, atrial augmentation can be achieved by attaching the atrial epicardial wire to the left arm lead. When this is done, recording from leads I and III will show atrial electrogram augmentation, while lead II recorded simultaneously will show a normal nonaugmented ECG (Figure 19.3). Similar atrial electrogram recordings can be performed with a greater degree of

D.S. Wheeler et al. (eds.), *Cardiovascular Pediatric Critical Illness and Injury*,
DOI 10.1007/978-1-84800-923-3_19, © Springer-Verlag London Limited 2009

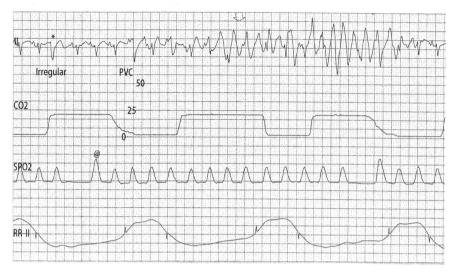

FIGURE 19.1. Recording from monitor showing full-disclosure review of an infant. Recorded is electrocardiogram (ECG) lead II, end-tidal CO_2, pulse oximeter waveform, and chest impedance respirometer. The rhythm is sinus, with the third beat being a premature ventricular contraction (*). The pulse oximeter waveform does not show a waveform from the PVC but shows an accentuated pulse from the post extrasystolic beat (@). The ECG recording subsequently develops significant artifact, which was initially interpreted as polymorphic ventricular tachycardia. The pulse oximeter shows a regular pattern throughout with another pause, suggesting a second premature ventricular contraction, and confirms, but confirms artifact in the ECG recording rather than ventricular arrhythmia.

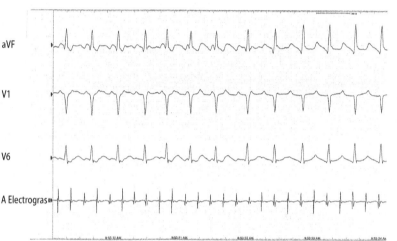

FIGURE 19.2. Recording of surface electrocardiogram lead aVF, V1, and V6 with the simultaneous recording of an atrial electrogram with a separate amplifier. Rapid regular atrial activity identifies an atrial tachycardia with variable atrioventricular conduction and confirms atrial activity, which is more difficult to identify on the surface electrocardiogram.

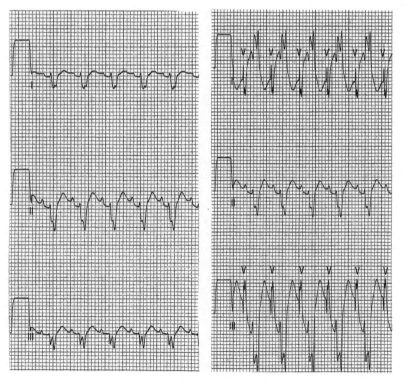

FIGURE 19.3. Recording of surface electrocardiogram leads I, II, and III in the left panel and the same recording in the right panel with placement of an epicardial atrial wire under the left arm electrode. The rhythm in both cases is sinus rhythm conducted with aberration. In the right panel, augmentation of atrial activity (arrowheads) is evident in leads I and III, but lead II is unaffected.

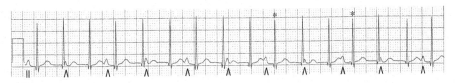

FIGURE 19.4. Accelerated junctional rhythm in a child with retrograde block to the atrium. P waves that are dissociated from QRS complexes are labeled with arrowheads. Atrioventricular conduction is evident by advancement of the QRS complex when atrial activity occurs at an opportune time (*).

difficulty using an esophageal electrode recording. More complex arrhythmias or those where atrial pacing may be useful in termination of a tachycardia or treatment of a bradycardia favor this technique when epicardial wires are not available [10].

Once all atrial activity has been identified and marked, the atrial rate can be determined. If the atrial rate is the same as the ventricular rate, there is likely to be atrioventricular (AV) conduction, ventriculoatrial (VA) conduction, or both (AV reentrant rhythm). If the atrial rate exceeds the ventricular rate, there is AV block of higher than first degree (see Figure 19.2) or nonconducted atrial ectopy. If the ventricular rate exceeds the atrial rate, there is an abnormal ventricular mechanism, which, depending on the ventricular rate itself, may be due to an inappropriately slow atrial rate or to an abnormally fast ventricular rate with some degree of VA block (Figure 19.4).

The P wave axis and morphology and the QRS axis, duration, and morphology should be inspected and if possible compared with the P waves during sinus rhythm and QRS complexes conducted from atrial activity from previous ECG recordings on the same patient if they are available. The performance of a multilead ECG on all patients immediately before interventions anticipated to result in potential intraprocedural or postprocedural arrhythmia is strongly advised for this purpose. P waves with a morphology and axis identical to sinus rhythm seen during a tachycardia suggest sinus tachycardia or sinus node reentrant tachycardia, but some automatic atrial tachycardias may have very similar P waves, and careful review in all leads, especially leads V1 and V2 should be undertaken. P waves that are upright in the inferior leads during a tachycardia are inconsistent with AV nodal reentrant tachycardia and unlikely to be seen in accessory pathway-mediated tachycardias such as orthodromic AV reentrant tachycardia.

Narrow QRS complexes during a tachycardia most often indicate a supraventricular mechanism, but ventricular tachycardia in children may have QRS complexes that have a duration less than the upper limits of normal for age (Figure 19.5). If the QRS complex during a tachycardia is identical in morphology and duration to that seen during sinus rhythm, the tachycardia is supraventricular in mechanism. Care must be taken to review the QRS morphology in several leads, as it may appear similar or even identical in some leads but quite different in others.

Supraventricular tachycardia may occur with wide QRS morphology caused by aberrant conduction (Figure 19.6) or ventricular preexcitation. Aberrant conduction may be caused by preexisting conduction system abnormality or block in the conduction system related to a rate faster than the refractory period of a portion of the His-Purkinje system, so-called rate-dependent aberrant conduction. Ventricular preexcitation may be caused by conduction over an accessory AV connection or less commonly a connection between the AV node and a fascicle of the conduction system or the ventricular myocardium [11,12]. Conduction with aberration can usually be distinguished from preexcited conduction by the pres-

ence of a sharp high-frequency depolarization during the first 40 msec of the QRS complex (Figure 19.7). This represents normal activation of the ventricle over the functional portion of the conduction system, while the terminal portion of the QRS complex is delayed. Preexcited conduction will generally show a low-frequency, slurred pattern at the beginning of the QRS complex because of activation of ventricular myocardium by the accessory pathway (Figure 19.8). This pattern may not be present if the accessory pathway inserts into a fascicle of the conduction system, thereby resulting in rapid depolarization of ventricular myocardium by specialized conduction fibers. If aberrant conduction or ventricular preexcitation is seen on previous ECG from the same patient during sinus rhythm, the pattern may be extremely helpful in diagnosis of the tachycardia. Again, the availability of multiple leads for comparison may be critical.

On rare occasion, ventricular preexcitation and aberrant conduction may be seen in the same patient. This is especially true for patients with Ebstein's anomaly of the tricuspid valve in which right-sided accessory AV connections are common and right bundle branch block is frequently seen. In this scenario, the right-sided accessory pathway may function as a surrogate for the right bundle branch and result in normalization of conduction [13].

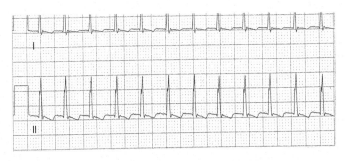

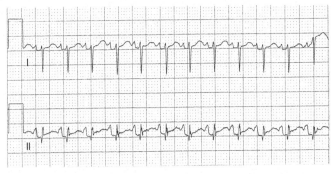

FIGURE 19.5. Narrow QRS complex ventricular tachycardia in a child is shown in electrocardiogram leads I and II in the upper panel. The QRS duration is normal for age, but the QRS morphology is substantially different from that seen during sinus rhythm in the same leads in the bottom panel.

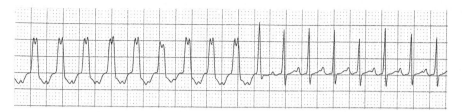

Figure 19.6. Atrial tachycardia conducted with aberrati is seen in the left side of the panel, resulting in a wide Q complex tachycardia. The aberrant conduction resolves the middle of the recording, and the tachycardia develops narrow QRS complex. P waves are more easily seen duri the narrow QRS complex tachycardia but, in retrospect, c also be seen during the wide QRS complex tachycardia.

Basic Mechanisms of Cardiac Arrhythmias

Heart rhythms can be classified as bradycardia, tachycardia, or normal based on their rate. Normal heart rates vary by age and physiologic state. Typically when classifying a rhythm by rate, the physiologic state is discounted. As such, it is recognized that *tachycardia* may be normal under conditions of stress and that *bradycardia* may be normal during sleep. Normal resting heart rate ranges are listed in Table 19.1.

Bradycardia Mechanisms

Bradycardia results from improper impulse formation in the sinus node or from failure of the impulse to propagate from the sinus node to the atrium (SA exit block) or from the atrium to the ventricle (AV block). Failure of adequate impulse formation in the sinus node may be the result of intrinsic abnormalities of the node. These include congenital abnormality of cardiac ion channels [14] or improper or absent sinus node development and damage to the node from autoantibodies, inflammation, or surgical intervention. It can also occur because of extrinsic factors such as parasympathetic stimulation or metabolic disturbance. The severity of the abnormality may range from a sinus rate that is slightly less than normal to sinus arrest (complete absence of impulse formation). Failure of propagation of the impulse from the sinus node to the atrium clinically can be difficult to differentiate from failure of adequate impulse formation as sinus node activity cannot be directly seen on the surface ECG. It may result from congenital or acquired abnormalities, and from a practical standpoint differentiation is usually not important as these problems are typically treated in the same way [15].

Abnormalities in propagation of the impulse from the atrium to the ventricle (AV block) are similar to those seen in the sinus node and occur related to intrinsic abnormality of the AV node or extrinsic factors identical to those that cause sinus node dysfunction. Conduction abnormality may occur at the level of the AV node, the common bundle of His, or the right or left bundle branches or their ramifications. In the case of severe prolongation of the QT interval, the impulse conduction may fail because of functional inexcitability of the His-Purkinje system [16] or the ventricle itself. The PR interval (measuring from the beginning of the P wave to the begin ning of the QRS complex) measures the conduction time throug the atrium, the AV node, the bundle branches, and the Purkin fibers. When all atrial impulses are conducted, but the PR interva is longer than normal for age, criteria for first degree AV block ar satisfied (Figure 19.9). The range of normal PR intervals are liste in Table 19.1. As first degree AV block does not reduce the relativ frequency of ventricular activity compared with atrial activity, will not result in bradycardia. When some but not all atrial impulse are conducted from the atrium to the ventricle, there is secon degree AV block (Figure 19.10). When no atrial impulses are con ducted to the ventricle there is third degree or complete AV bloc (Figure 19.11).

Second degree AV block occurs in three forms, Mobitz types and II and 2:1. In Mobitz type I, also referred to as Wenckebac conduction, there is progressive prolongation of the PR interva before conduction block occurs (see Figure 19.10). This electrocar diographic pattern is most commonly observed when the conduc tion abnormality is occurring in the AV node [17]. In Mobitz typ II there is a constant PR interval preceding a nonconducted P wav (Figure 19.12). This pattern is most commonly seen when the His Purkinje conduction system is abnormal [18]. Because of this, ther is usually a bundle branch block or intraventricular conductio delay pattern (wide QRS complex) accompanying Mobitz type II A block. In 2:1 AV conduction there is conduction of every othe atrial complex (Figure 19.13). This eliminates the ability to deter mine whether or not there is PR prolongation. Most individual with 2:1 AV block will have either Mobitz type I or II AV block a other times, and thus the expected level of conduction block ma be inferred from the associated type of block. AV block occurring in the AV node is considered to be better in prognostic significanc in pediatric patients [19]. The presence of intact conduction from the AV junctional subsidiary pacemaker to the ventricle would be expected to protect the patient from sudden asystole in the even of sudden AV nodal block. The presence of adequate subsidiary pacemakers below the level of His-Purkinje conduction block is les likely, and thus sudden AV block at this level is more dangerous.

From a practical standpoint, in the PICU the anatomic level o AV block is rarely important. These patients are typically on con tinuous monitoring, and, if sudden AV block occurs, rapid treat-

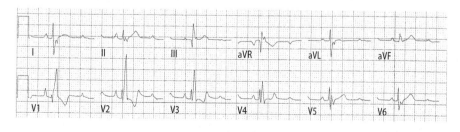

Figure 19.7. The appearance of a wide QRS complex related to conduction with aberration. A sharp high-frequency depolarization is seen in the first 40 msec of the QRS complex.

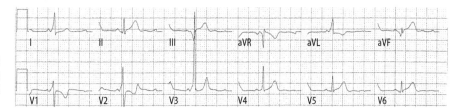

FIGURE 19.8. The appearance of a wide QRS complex related to ventricular preexcitation. In addition to the shorter PR interval, the QRS complex shows a low-frequency, slurred pattern in the first 40 msec of the QRS complex.

TABLE 19.1. Normal ranges for pediatric heart rhythm intervals.

Age	Heart rate (beats/min)	PR interval (msec)	QRS duration (msec)
0–1 day	93–155	79–161	21–76
1–3 days	91–158	81–139	22–67
3–7 days	90–166	73–136	21–68
7–30 days	106–182	72–138	22–79
1–3 months	120–179	72–130	23–75
3–6 months	106–186	73–146	22–79
6–12 months	108–169	72–157	23–76
1–3 years	90–151	81–148	27–75
3–5 years	72–138	83–161	30–72
5–8 years	64–132	90–163	32–79
8–12 years	62–130	88–171	32–85
12–16 years	61–120	92–176	34–88

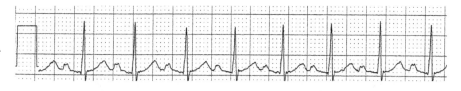

FIGURE 19.9. Sinus rhythm with first degree atrioventricular block is demonstrated by a PR interval of 190 msec, above the upper limits of normal for a child.

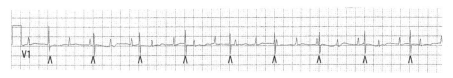

FIGURE 19.10. Sinus rhythm with second degree atrioventricular block, Mobitz type I (Wenckebach) is demonstrated with progressive PR interval prolongation followed by a nonconducted sinus P wave marked with an arrowhead.

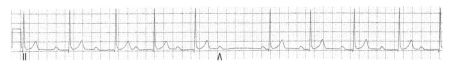

FIGURE 19.11. The atrial mechanism is sinus at a rate of 125/min as evidenced by large P waves with a regular pattern. There is complete atrioventricular block as evidenced by a slower regular ventricular rhythm at a rate of 60/min, with narrow QRS complexes marked with arrowheads. The narrow QRS complex suggests a junctional mechanism.

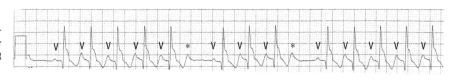

FIGURE 19.12. Sinus rhythm with second degree atrioventricular block, Mobitz type II is demonstrated, with a regular atrial mechanism (marked with arrowheads), a constant PR interval, and sudden nonconducted P waves (asterisks).

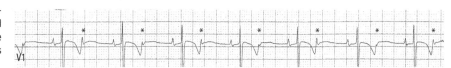

FIGURE 19.13. Sinus rhythm with second degree atrioventricular block 2:1 is demonstrated with a regular atrial mechanism, with every other P wave not conducting to the ventricle (asterisks). Note that the nonconducted P waves may be somewhat concealed within the previous T wave.

TABLE 19.2. Bradycardic rhythms.

	Mechanism	Causes	ECG appearance
Slow atrial rate	Sinus node dysfunction	Mechanical damage to sinus node; congenital ion channel, metabolic, or autonomic abnormality resulting in slow sinus rate or atrial inexcitability	Slow sinus rate or absence of sinus activity with ectopic atrial escape or atrial standstill
	Sinus node exit block	Congenital or acquired mechanical abnormality; congenital ion channel abnormality	Same as sinus node dysfunction if first or third degree; definable pattern of atrial depolarization if second degree
Atrial rate faster than ventricular rate	Second degree AV block, Mobitz type I (Wenckebach)	Most commonly AV nodal block; congenital, mechanical, or autoantibody damage; congenital ion channel abnormality; autonomic abnormality	Partial AV association: progressive increase in PR interval followed by nonconducted P wave
	Second degree AV block, Mobitz type II	Most commonly His-Purkinje system block: mechanical damage to conduction system, myocardial infarction	Partial AV association: constant PR interval followed by sudden nonconducted P wave; usually with wide QRS, often bifascicular block pattern
	Second degree AV block, 2:1	Usually associated with Mobitz type I or type II	Partial AV association: two P waves for every QRS complex, constant PR interval of conducted P wave
	Complete (third degree) AV block	Same as causes of second degree AV block types I and II	AV dissociation with faster atrial than ventricular rate; regular ventricular mechanism: narrow QRS complex if junctional escape, wide QRS if ventricular escape

Note: AV, atrioventricular; ECG, electrocardiogram.

ment with chest compressions followed by external, transvenous, or epicardial pacing can be instituted. The level of block is far more important for patients no longer in intensive care areas and not on continuous cardiac monitoring. The potential for unsuccessfully resuscitated bradycardic arrest is substantially higher in this setting. Third degree or complete AV block may occur at either of the anatomic levels described for second degree AV block. There may be an escape rhythm from a subsidiary pacemaker in the AV junction or the ventricle, or there may be no escape rhythm. If there is no escape rhythm of acceptable rate, immediate treatment is necessary, usually in the form of cardiac pacing. The causes and electrocardiographic appearances of clinical bradycardic rhythms are summarized in Table 19.2.

Tachycardia Mechanisms

Tachycardia is generally thought to be caused by one of three basic mechanisms: reentry, automaticity, and triggered automaticity. Reentry requires a circular movement of propagated impulses over either a large (macro-reentry) or small (micro-reentry) area of the myocardium. Automaticity occurs when cardiac myocytes have regular spontaneous depolarization to reach threshold and activate surrounding cells. Triggered automaticity is a spontaneous depolarization that occurs in response to a preceding depolarization.

Reentry may take place in the atrium, the ventricle, the normal conduction system, the sinus node, or combinations of these. Reentrant rhythms typically initiate following a premature depolarization and have characteristics of sudden onset and termination.

Multiple reentrant circuits that are active simultaneously may be responsible for rather disordered rhythms such as polymorphic ventricular tachycardia and atrial and ventricular fibrillation [20].

Automatic rhythms may also originate in any area of the heart. Automatic tachycardia from the sinus node is usually a normal phenomenon, but automatic tachycardias from other cardiac cells result from abnormal automaticity. Automatic rhythms tend to have gradual onset and offset or *warming-up* and *cooling-down* periods. Triggered automatic rhythms are most commonly recognized in ventricular myocardium but probably also result in tachycardia in atrial tissue as well. They are implicated in tachyarrhythmia related to digitalis toxicity and congenital and acquired QT prolongation.

Clinically tachycardias are usually divided into narrow and wide QRS complex tachycardias. Narrow QRS complex tachycardias are those that activate the ventricle via the normal AV conduction system. They most commonly occur with 1:1 AV relationship but can have faster atrial than ventricular rates and vice versa. When a 1:1 AV relationship exists, the tachycardias are the result of automatic mechanisms in the atria or AV junction or reentrant mechanisms in the atria or the AV node or utilizing the AV node and accessory AV connection (Figure 19.14). Some patients with complex congenital heart disease will have duplication of the AV conduction system or *twin AV nodes* and have an AV reentrant tachycardia utilizing the two conduction systems [21]. Rare ventricular tachycardias may have QRS duration that is normal for age, generally because the ventricular mechanism activates the conduc-

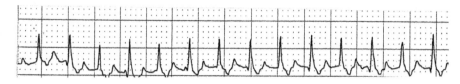

FIGURE 19.14. Orthodromic atrioventricular (AV) reentrant tachycardia is demonstrated by a regular narrow QRS complex tachycardia with 1:1 AV relationship and atrial activity following the QRS, with an RP interval of 100 msec.

TABLE 19.3. Regular narrow QRS complex tachycardia with atrial rate equal to ventricular rate.

Mechanism	Causes	ECG appearance	Adenosine response	Cardioversion response
Automatic atrial tachycardia	Congenital, myocarditis, metabolic, autonomic	RP > PR, P wave morphology different from sinus, rate may vary slightly	Transient AV nodal block then continuation of tachycardia; atrial rate may slow, rarely terminates	Usually none, autonomic response may accelerate the tachycardia rate
Reentrant atrial tachycardia	Congenital or postcardiac surgical reentrant circuit	RP > PR, P wave different from sinus, rate usually fixed	Transient AV nodal block then continuation of tachycardia; atrial rate constant, occasionally terminates	Terminates, may reinitiate
Orthodromic AV reentrant tachycardia	Congenital accessory AV connection	RP < PR, P wave usually negative in inferior leads, may have ventricular preexcitation in sinus rhythm	Slowing of tachycardia with increase in PR and termination with last event being a P wave	Terminates, may reinitiate
Permanent form of "junctional" reciprocating tachycardia (PJRT)	Congenital accessory AV connection with slow pathway conduction	RP > PR, P wave negative in inferior leads, tachycardia is usually incessant	Slowing of tachycardia with increase in PR and termination with last event being a P wave	Terminates, usually reinitiates
Typical AV nodal reentrant tachycardia (AV over slow pathway, VA over fast pathway)	Congenital or acquired dual AV nodal pathways	Nearly simultaneous P and QRS, P may be visible slightly before or after QRS, always negative in inferior leads	Slowing and termination of tachycardia	Terminates, may reinitiate
Atypical AV nodal reentrant tachycardia (AV over fast pathway, VA over slow pathway)	Congenital or acquired dual AV nodal pathways	RP > PR, P waves always negative in inferior leads	Slowing and termination of tachycardia	Terminates, may reinitiate
Junctional automatic tachycardia with conduction to atrium	Congenital, postcardiac surgical	Nearly simultaneous P and QRS	Transient AV dissociation with faster ventricular rate, continuationm of tachycardia	Usually none, autonomic response may accelerate the tachycardia rate
Ventricular tachycardia with narrow QRS complex and conduction to atrium	Usually congenital	RP < PR, QRS morphology different from that during sinus rhythm	Transient AV dissociation with faster ventricular rate, usually continuation of tachycardia, may terminate tachycardia	Usually terminates

Note: AV, atrioventricular; ECG, electrocardiogram; PR, PR interval (time interval from beginning of the P wave to the beginning of the next QRS complex); RP, RP interval (time interval from beginning of the QRS complex to the beginning of the next P wave); VA, ventriculoatrial.

tion system in some way, resulting in more rapid ventricular depolarization (see Figure 19.5). These ventricular tachycardias may have 1:1 conduction to the atrium over the AV node. Regular narrow QRS complex tachycardias with a 1:1 AV relationship, their causes, ECG appearances, and responses to adenosine and cardioversion are summarized in Table 19.3.

When a narrow QRS complex tachycardia occurs with a faster atrial rate than ventricular rate, the mechanism is an automatic or reentrant mechanism in the atrium or AV node with variable or no conduction to the ventricle (Figure 19.15). These clinical tachycardias and their ECG appearances and adenosine and cardioversion responses are summarized in Table 19.4. Rarely, narrow QRS complex tachycardias are seen with a faster ventricular rate than atrial rate. Most commonly this is automatic junctional tachycardia, which occurs in a familial congenital form as well as following

cardiac surgery. There may be some degree of conduction to the atrium or complete VA block (see Figure 19.4). Narrow QRS complex ventricular tachycardia can also occur with retrograde conduction to the atrium. These rhythms are summarized in Table 19.5.

Wide QRS complex tachycardia represents either supraventricular tachycardia with aberrant [22] or preexcited conduction [23] or ventricular tachycardia [24]. The causes and responses to adenosine and cardioversion for these rhythms are the same as their narrow QRS complex counterparts. Wide QRS complex supraventricular tachycardia may offer important insights into the mechanism of the tachycardia. When a narrow QRS complex tachycardia is seen to progress directly into a wide QRS complex tachycardia or vice versa, the mechanism of both tachycardias is likely common. If the wide QRS complex tachycardia is occurring because of rate-dependent aberrant conduction and the RP interval is longer during

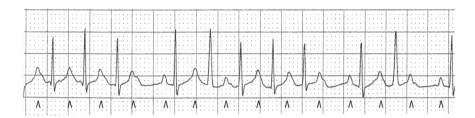

FIGURE 19.15. An atrial tachycardia with variable atrioventricular (AV) conduction is demonstrated by a regular atrial mechanism (marked with arrowheads) the rate of which exceeds that of the ventricular mechanism. The QRS complexes are related in a pattern consistent with second degree AV block Mobitz type I (Wenckebach) with prolongation of the PR interval before a nonconducted P wave.

TABLE 19.4. Regular narrow QRS complex tachycardia with atrial rate faster than ventricular rate.

Mechanism	ECG appearance	Adenosine response	Cardioversion response
Automatic atrial tachycardia with second or third degree AV block	Regular atrial rhythm with P wave morphology different from sinus P wave; irregular ventricular response with pattern of type I or type II second degree AV block or regular ventricular response if complete AV block with junctional rhythm	Atrial rate may slow transiently and rarely terminate; degree of AV block may increase if second degree; no effect on ventricular rate if complete AV block already present	Usually none, autonomic respons may accelerate the atrial rate enhance AV nodal conduction
Reentrant atrial tachycardia with second or third degree AV block	Regular atrial rhythm with P wave morphology different from sinus P wave; irregular ventricular response with pattern of type I or type II second degree AV block or regular ventricular response if complete AV block with junctional rhythm	Atrial rate remains constant and occasionally terminates; degree of AV block may increase if second degree; no effect on ventricular rate if complete AV block already present	Terminates, may reinitiate
AV nodal reentrant tachycardia with AV block below AV node or His bundle	Regular atrial rhythm, usually with 2:1 AV relationship, P waves always negative in inferior leads, one P wave usually nearly simultaneous with QRS complex	Tachycardia usually slows and terminates; rarely AV nodal conduction is affected in such a way that 1:1 AV conduction develops	Terminates, may reinitiate

Note: AV, atrioventricular; ECG, electrocardiogram.

the wide than the narrow QRS complex tachycardia, the mechanism of the tachycardias is likely to be orthodromic AV reentrant tachycardia utilizing an accessory pathway that is ipsilateral to the side of the bundle branch block causing the aberrant conduction.

The pattern of the QRS complexes in a wide QRS complex tachycardia may also be helpful in differentiating a supraventricular versus ventricular mechanism [25,26]. A typical right or left bundle branch block pattern favors supraventricular tachycardia, whereas atypical bundle branch block patterns or bundle branch block with an opposite QRS axis (e.g., right bundle branch block with left axis deviation) favor ventricular tachycardia. Likewise, a concordant pattern of QRS complexes in the precordial leads (all leads showing either a positive or negative deflection) favors ventricular tachycardia [27].

Mechanisms of Arrhythmia with Normal Heart Rate

Many arrhythmias occur with heart rates that are within the range of normal for the patient's age. First degree AV block is rarely of clinical significance, but, in patients with marginal hemodynamic status, providing a normal atrial to ventricular mechanical contraction sequence may reduce the need for other support. In most circumstances the invasive intervention required to provide such support is prohibitive. For patients who have had immediately preceding cardiac surgery and have postoperative atrial and ventricular epicardial pacing wires, ventricular pacing tracking atrial activity is relatively simple. Isolated atrial and ventricular ectopy do not usually result in alteration of the heart rate from normal.

Frequent premature atrial complexes that are nonconducted alternating with sinus complexes that are conducted (atrial bigeminy) may result in a ventricular bradycardia [28]. Frequent premature ventricular complexes in a bigeminal pattern will result in a normal ventricular rate but may result in an effective bradycardia hemodynamically as the premature contraction is rather ineffective because of a limited ventricular filling tim preceding it. Atrial tachyarrhythmias that are conducted with second or third AV block may result in a normal ventricular rate Ectopic atrial rhythm and accelerated junctional and ventricula rhythms also occur within normal heart rate ranges but hav abnormal mechanisms and may potentially be hemodynamicall compromising.

Treatment of Bradyarrhythmia

Immediate treatment of hemodynamically significant bradycardi includes chest compressions, administration of supplementa oxygen and mechanical ventilation to mitigate the metabolic effect of the slow heart rate, and administration of epinephrine and atro pine. If bradycardia persists, cardiac pacing is indicated. Trans cutaneous pacing is increasingly available in the PICU, ofter incorporated into devices that are used for defibrillation and car dioversion. Transcutaneous pacing that occurs above the threshol for stimulation results in ventricular contraction and may also result in simultaneous atrial contraction [29] or atrial depolariza tion from retrograde conduction [30]. Without instantaneous bloo

TABLE 19.5. Regular narrow QRS complex tachycardia with ventricular rate faster than atrial rate.

Mechanism	ECG appearance	Adenosine response	Cardioversion response
Junctional automatic tachycardia with second or third degree VA block	Narrow QRS complex tachycardia with AV dissociation; P waves may be negative in inferior leads and have relationship to QRS if second degree VA block, sinus P waves if complete VA block	None on ventricular rate; may increase degree of VA block if second degree	Usually none; autonomic response may accelerate the atrial and/or ventricular rate
Ventricular tachycardia with narrow QRS complex with second or third degree VA block	QRS morphology different from that during sinus rhythm; P waves may be negative in inferior leads and have relationship to QRS if second degree VA block, sinus P waves if complete VA block	May slow or terminate tachycardia and increase degree of VA block if second degree	Usually terminates

Note: AV, atrioventricular; ECG, electrocardiogram; VA, ventriculoatrial.

pressure monitoring, it may be difficult to assess the patient for adequate ventricular capture. The application of transcutaneous pacing is tolerated for only limited periods because of skeletal muscle stimulation and skin irritation. If the patient's bradycardia is secondary to isolated sinus node dysfunction, which is rare, esophageal atrial pacing may be utilized for longer periods, but it is still quite uncomfortable in a nonanesthetized patient. If AV node dysfunction is present, transvenous pacing with a balloon-tipped catheter introduced from the subclavian vein or jugular vein can provide safe and stable pacing for a longer period in most pediatric patients. Occasionally placement of a lead from a femoral venous approach with the use of fluoroscopy may be needed. Temporary dual-chamber transvenous pacing is rarely performed in pediatric patients. Epicardial atrial and ventricular pacing is common in patients following cardiac surgery when pairs of temporary epicardial wires can be placed [31,32]. In principle, the patient with exclusively sinus node dysfunction benefits the most from atrial pacing alone, as normal AV conduction is preferential to ventricular pacing in the mechanical activation sequence of the ventricle. The critically ill patient with AV block requires ventricular pacing. If sinus node function is intact, ventricular pacing tracking native atrial activity is preferred. For the patient with right bundle branch block, pacing the right ventricle tracking native atrial activity, or an atrial-paced rhythm with an appropriate AV delay, may be beneficial in allowing for simultaneous right and left ventricular contraction and providing *resynchronization* with a single pacing lead.

Temporary cardiac pacing, as mentioned, can be performed with either epicardial or transvenous endocardial pacing leads or for shorter periods with esophageal atrial pacing, esophagogastric ventricular pacing [33], or transcutaneous pacing [34]. Regardless of the specific method, some general principles apply. Pacing capture and sensing thresholds exist for the given patient, pacing arrangement, physiologic circumstance, and time. The capture threshold is the amount of energy required to effectively stimulate the heart. In temporary pacing devices, the current is generally adjustable and the pulse width (duration of stimulation) is fixed but in some instances may be adjustable. A longer pulse width will achieve capture with a lower current than a shorter pulse width, and, if the pulse width is adjustable, varying the current and pulse width may result in optimal cardiac pacing but minimize skeletal muscle stimulation. Longer pulse widths are required for esophageal and transcutaneous pacing applications.

To determine the capture threshold, the pulse width should be maintained and the current adjusted until a cardiac depolarization is seen following each spike artifact from pacing. As previously mentioned, the wider pulse width and skeletal muscle response to transcutaneous pacing can make assessment of capture with an electrocardiographic recording difficult [34], and secondary indicators such as an arterial pressure waveform may be needed. Once the capture threshold has been determined, the output current should be set at least twice the capture threshold. The sensing threshold is the voltage from a cardiac depolarization that an electrical signal must exceed to be considered by the pacemaker as intrinsic cardiac activity. The sensitivity is programmed in millivolt units. The higher the setting in millivolts, the less sensitive the pacemaker will be to cardiac activity. To determine the sensing threshold, the pacing rate should be programmed to lower than the patient's intrinsic rate, and the pacemaker sensitivity should be adjusted to an insensitive or asynchronous mode. The sensitivity setting should then be gradually increased (to a lower millivolt

setting) until the device indicates sensing of cardiac activity by an indicator light or by inhibition of cardiac pacing. The sensitivity should then be set to a millivolt setting of one-half the sensing threshold. In patients with severely inadequate intrinsic rhythms, the ventricular sensing threshold may not be able to be practically determined, and sensing can be programmed to a nominal setting (usually 2 mV). Care should be taken to avoid setting the sensitivity to such a highly sensitive setting that extraneous electrical noise or skeletal muscle artifact is sensed as intrinsic cardiac activity and inhibits cardiac pacing. As previously mentioned, if AV nodal conduction is intact and sinus node rate inadequate, atrial pacing is preferred.

The rate of pacing can be adjusted to optimize measurable hemodynamic parameters. If sinus node rate is appropriate, but AV block is present, ventricular pacing tracking atrial activity is preferred. The lower rate limit of the pacemaker should be set to a rate slower than the sinus rate and the upper rate set to a value as high as desired. In pediatric pacing the desired upper rate limit is generally greater than 200 beats per minute unless an atrial tachycardia is present. The AV interval (maximal interval from paced or sensed atrial activity to sensed or paced ventricular activity) can also be adjusted to achieve the best hemodynamic benefit. The postventricular atrial refractory period (PVARP) is the time after a paced or sensed ventricular event during which the atrial channel of the pacemaker will not sense atrial activity. The primary purpose of this interval in a temporary pacemaker is to prevent the device from sensing the ventricular pacing spike or ventricular electrical activity as intrinsic atrial activity and to prevent *pacemaker-mediated* tachycardia. Pacemaker-mediated tachycardia occurs when paced ventricular activity is conducted to the atrium (usually retrograde over the AV node) and is sensed by the atrial channel of the pacemaker, triggering ventricular pacing and resulting in an artificial form of reentrant tachycardia. This form of tachycardia usually initiates with a premature ventricular contraction and can be terminated with brief cessation of ventricular pacing. Programming of the PVARP to a higher value will prevent this form of tachycardia but will limit the fastest rate at which the pacemaker can pace the ventricle tracking atrial activity. In practical application, the PVARP can be programmed to its lowest possible value (usually between 150 and 180 msec) and adjusted to a higher value only if inappropriate sensing on the atrial channel or pacemaker-mediated tachycardia occurs.

Patients with permanent cardiac pacemakers and implanted defibrillators require special consideration in the PICU. Electrical noise associated with medical devices, especially electrocautery, may be sensed by the device [35] and result in inhibition of output, triggered pacing, or an inappropriate shock. Proper management of the device before placing the patient in such an environment is critical. Metabolic changes and effects of medications in critically ill patients may result in an increase in the pacing capture threshold and failure of pacing. The defibrillation threshold for defibrillation with an implanted defibrillator may also be elevated by medications or metabolic imbalance. Regular analysis of the device while the patient is in the PICU and appropriate adjustment of the device output and sensitivity is important. Monitoring should be used that responds to pacing failure with an appropriate alarm. Algorithms for detection of a QRS complex on a monitor may not be adequate to differentiate a pacing spike without capture from a QRS complex. As such a secondary method such as measurement of heart rate from an arterial line tracing or pulse oximeter is helpful as an adjunct.

Treatment of Tachyarrhythmia

Immediate Treatment, Cardioversion, Defibrillation, and Pacing

If a tachyarrhythmia is accompanied by poor perfusion and suspected hemodynamic compromise, and demonstrates a wide QRS complex, immediate cardioversion is indicated. If a narrow QRS complex is seen, application of vagal maneuvers or adenosine administration may be applied as long as they do not result in a delay of cardioversion if they are unsuccessful [36]. Rarely, adenosine administration may result in ventricular fibrillation [37]. Availability of a defibrillator should be confirmed before its administration. Cardioversion should be performed with paddles, electrical conductive jelly, and adequate pressure to the chest wall to maximize skin contact with the paddles and minimize impedance. When available, skin patches are preferred, as they allow for more effective application of chest compressions between shocks and, as mentioned previously, may also allow for transcutaneous pacing in the event of cardioversion or defibrillation to a bradycardic or asystolic rhythm.

Placement of the paddles or patches in an anteroposterior orientation in neonates and infants is frequently preferred to avoid any contact between them. Anteroposterior orientation may also be preferable for older patients with palliated congenital heart disease, especially when cardioversion of atrial arrhythmias is being performed. For other patients a sternoapical position is acceptable and does not require raising the patient from the supine position.

Synchronization of the shock to the cardiac rhythm is always preferred, if it can be performed. An asynchronous shock delivered during ventricular repolarization and vulnerability may convert a stable rhythm to ventricular fibrillation. On the other hand, attempts to deliver a synchronous shock when there is no rhythm for synchronization (ventricular fibrillation) will result in the unnecessary delay of a shock. For this reason, most defibrillators start and reset to an asynchronous mode after each shock. If a synchronous mode is desired, it must be initially activated and reactivated after each shock. Care should be taken to be certain that the device is appropriately synchronizing on a QRS complex each time. The leads may need to be adjusted if synchronization is not appropriate. Shock advisories, an outgrowth of automated external defibrillators, are increasingly available on inhospital defibrillators in the PICU. These advisories on many devices have been shown to have excellent sensitivity and specificity for identifying "shockable" rhythms in the pediatric population. They may help to guide the novice in delivering an appropriate shock but should never dissuade an experienced physician from delivering what is thought to be an appropriate shock. When a first shock is not successful, subsequent shocks should be administered, as successive shocks reduce chest wall impedance and increase the likelihood for subsequent successful cardioversion or defibrillation.

Tachycardia accompanied by adequate perfusion, good pulses, and suspected hemodynamic stability allow for a more considered approach. Diagnostic studies, including multilead ECG and atrial electrogram recordings, can be performed in an attempt to determine a mechanism for the tachycardia and choose a specific treatment. Rapid adenosine administration during the recording of a multilead ECG, preferentially with an atrial electrogram, is often diagnostic for the cause of the tachyarrhythmia and may be therapeutic as well [38,39]. Adenosine is more likely to be diagnostic than vagal maneuvers, which tend to result in patient movement artifact and lead disconnection of the ECG [40]. If adenosine is diagnostic of an atrial tachycardia, showing continuation of the atrial mechanism with AV nodal block, consideration can be given to atrial pacing with an esophageal, transvenous, or epicardial lead. As previously mentioned, atrial reentrant mechanisms will be likely to be terminated with a brief period of atrial pacing at a faster rate. Once a tachycardia has been terminated, the subsequent bradycardia and pauses may result in recurrence of tachycardia. Atrial or ventricular pacing may help to prevent this tachycardia recurrence.

Junctional automatic tachycardia is a rhythm that may benefit from atrial pacing at a faster rate. The benefit provided by AV synchrony may offset the negative effects of a somewhat faster heart rate. This rhythm is exacerbated by hemodynamic instability resulting in increased endogenous catecholamines and administration of exogenous catecholamines, and as such management with atrial pacing may reduce the need for more aggressive therapies.

Antiarrhythmic Medications

As previously mentioned, adenosine is frequently diagnostic when administered during ECG and atrial electrogram recording. By causing transient AV nodal block it is also therapeutic for AV nodal–dependent supraventricular tachycardias such as AV reentrant tachycardia and AV nodal reentrant tachycardia, common in pediatric patients. Intravenous amiodarone has recently assumed a rather wide role in treatment of tachyarrhythmia in the PICU. It is a highly effective medication when given in an appropriate dosage in appropriate situations. Amiodarone has effects on cardiac sodium, potassium, and calcium channels as well as β-adrenergic blocker effects. It is effective for supraventricular and ventricular tachyarrhythmias of both reentrant and automatic mechanisms. Adverse effects of intravenous amiodarone are common and most frequently include hypotension, bradycardia, and AV block [41]. The hypotensive response frequently requires administration of intravenous fluids, and supplemental calcium is also frequently helpful. Bradycardia can be managed by cardiac pacing, and, unless the use of amiodarone is in a resuscitation setting, plans for cardiac pacing as outlined earlier should be considered before administration of the drug. Nausea and vomiting also occur frequently.

Procainamide and lidocaine are the only sodium channel blocking (Vanghan-Williams class I) drugs currently available in the United States for intravenous administration. Procainamide has potassium channel blocking effects as well and prolongs the action potential duration. It can be effective for supraventricular and ventricular arrhythmias of both automatic and reentrant mechanisms. Although never compared blindly to amiodarone in a study, it seems less effective than amiodarone for most arrhythmias. Procainamide also results in hypotension, cardiac depression, and bradycardia. Support is frequently needed for these associated problems. Nausea and vomiting are also commonly seen. Lidocaine shortens the action potential and ventricular refractory period and is effective for some ventricular arrhythmias. It is ineffective for supraventricular tachycardias and may be detrimental for some atrial tachycardia mechanisms. It has minimal hemodynamic effects, and most adverse effects are the result of central nervous system impairment. Compared in adults undergoing cardiac resuscitation for ventricular arrhythmia, intravenous amiodarone has been shown to be more effective than lidocaine.

β-adrenergic blockade can be extremely helpful in the PICU for control of tachycardia. It can terminate and prevent reinitiation of eentrant tachyarrhythmia. It is also helpful in slowing AV nodal conduction during atrial tachyarrhythmias, thereby reducing the ventricular rate. Hypotension, bradycardia, and AV block are also seen with β-blockade. Esmolol, a β-adrenergic blocker with a half-life of approximately 10 min, is particularly suited to the PICU. The dose may be titrated to effect or toxicity. If toxic effects predominate, the drug can be discontinued without prolonged effects. If it is effective, a continuous infusion can be given, or the drug can be transitioned to propranolol, which has a longer half life.

Calcium channel blockade is less commonly used in the PICU. Neonates have limited ability to store calcium in the cardiac sarcoplasmic reticulum, and calcium channel blockers can result in hemodynamic collapse. In older children, verapamil and diltiazem can slow AV nodal conduction and terminate and prevent reinitiation of AV nodal–dependent tachycardia. They can also be used to control the conducted rate of atrial tachycardias but should be used with great caution if in combination with β-adrenergic blockade.

Digoxin is now less commonly used than it was in the past, but it is still a helpful drug in the PICU. It slows the sinus rate and AV nodal conduction and increases the refractory period of the AV node. It is administered intravenously in small amounts, and inappropriate administration has resulted in serious consequences for many pediatric patients. Determination of the correct dose should be performed in milligram amount, microgram amount, and milliliters of the drug and checked by another individual before administration. Measurement of the drug should be done with an appropriate syringe (usually a properly marked 1 mL syringe). Overdosage of digoxin when accompanied by arrhythmia should be managed with digoxin-specific Fab antibodies. The drug is effective for AV nodal–dependent tachycardias and may also be effective for some atrial tachyarrhythmias, and it slows the rate of conduction of atrial tachycardia. Digoxin use is relatively contraindicated for individuals with ventricular preexcitation, as it may enhance rapid accessory pathway conduction during atrial fibrillation and result in life-threatening arrhythmia. This would be unlikely in infants and young children with low likelihood of atrial fibrillation, and some individuals continue to use the drug in this setting.

Special Circumstances Involving Arrhythmia in the Pediatric Intensive Care Unit

Electrolyte Imbalance

The imbalance of serum electrolytes is common in patients in the PICU for many reasons. Potassium is the electrolyte with the greatest propensity to cause cardiac rhythm abnormality [42]. Hyperkalemia results in electrocardiographic changes at serum potassium levels far lower than those that cause arrhythmia. With modest hyperkalemia, the T wave will become peaked and narrow. Pediatric patients with faster resting heart rates tend to have narrower T waves, and, depending on the electrocardiographic leads that are monitored, the peaking of T waves may not be immediately evident. With higher levels of serum potassium, the QRS widens. Sinus tachycardia with wide QRS complexes from hyperkalemia is frequently mistaken for ventricular tachycardia, and antiarrhythmic drugs are administered (Figure 19.16). This frequently will exacerbate the cardiac toxicity of the elevated serum potassium. In situations when hyperkalemia is anticipated, the presence of regular wide QRS complex rhythms should be suspected to be sinus tachycardia. Full-disclosure electrocardiographic review when available will show little change in heart rate and gradual increase in the QRS duration in this circumstance and can be very helpful in diagnosing and appropriately treating the electrolyte abnormality. With extreme elevation of serum potassium, ventricular tachycardia and fibrillation will ultimately occur. Hypokalemia results in prominent U waves and prolongation of the QT-U interval. Although the arrhythmogenic potential of hypokalemia is typically less than that of hyperkalemia, it may ultimately result in polymorphic ventricular tachycardia and ventricular fibrillation. Imbalance of serum calcium in isolation is rare and, even when it occurs, does not frequently result in significant arrhythmia. Serum magnesium imbalance in isolation has little effect on the electrocardiogram or heart rhythm. Administration of serum magnesium has been shown to be particularly effective in the treatment of arrhythmia, especially torsades de pointes ventricular tachycardia associated with prolonged QT interval.

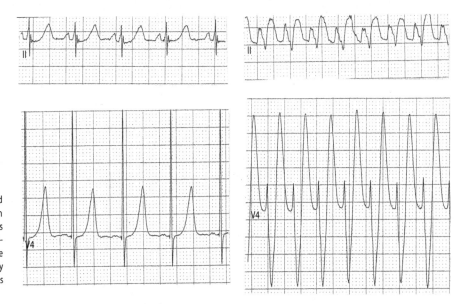

FIGURE 19.16. The left panels demonstrate ECG leads II and V4 in an infant with hyperkalemia (serum potassium 6.8 mmol/L). The T waves are peaked, but the QRS remains narrow. The right panels demonstrate the same lead recordings in the same patient with a serum potassium level above 9 mmol/L. The QRS complexes are wide, and atrial activity cannot be clearly seen, but the rhythm likely remains sinus rhythm.

Thermal Imbalance

Mild hypothermia slows the rate of sinus rhythm. More significant hypothermia results in the development of a deflection in the terminal portion of the QRS termed an Osborn wave. This is accompanied by QT interval prolongation. Even more profound hypothermia results in AV block and subsequently ventricular arrhythmia and fibrillation [43]. Mild hyperthermia results in sinus tachycardia. In susceptible individuals, fever may increase the likelihood of automatic and reentrant arrhythmia. This is especially true with postoperative automatic junctional tachycardia, which is significantly exacerbated by fever and can be treated with mild hypothermia.

Endocrine Imbalance

Thyroid imbalance is the most significant known endocrine imbalance to affect cardiac rhythm. Relative hypothyroid state is not uncommon in the PICU patient and may result in sinus bradycardia and AV block. Evaluation of thyroid state is important in patients with sinus node or AV node dysfunction before intervention with permanent pacing devices [44]. Hyperthyroidism is less common and is associated with sinus tachycardia and more rarely atrial fibrillation.

Central Nervous System Injury

Injury to the central nervous system frequently results in significant electrocardiographic changes. These are most characteristically ST segment and T wave changes and QT interval prolongation. These frequently simulate findings of cardiac ischemia. Cardiac rhythm disturbance is less common and includes a gamut of brady- and tachyarrhythmias.

Infection

Systemic infection may result in a reflex sinus tachycardia from an increase in metabolic demand. Endocarditis near the normal conduction system may result in AV block caused by direct mechanical damage to the conduction system. Myocarditis is associated with atrial and ventricular tachyarrhythmia, and treatment of suspected or biopsy proven myocarditis with antiinflammatory medications may treat the associated tachyarrhythmias more successfully than antiarrhythmic agents. Rheumatic heart disease may result in transient or permanent AV block and sinus node dysfunction. Lyme disease is also known to result in AV block and other cardiac conduction abnormalities [45].

Toxins

Many toxic agents are associated with cardiac rhythm in the PICU. These include toxins consumed by patients before their admission and those administered in the course of therapy. Those consumed before admission include drugs of abuse, with cocaine resulting in the most significant arrhythmias. Ventricular arrhythmia is most common and is related to coronary vasoconstriction in combination with sinus tachycardia, increased myocardial oxygen demand, and increased afterload. The most common prescribed medications with cardiac arrhythmia risk in the pediatric population include psychostimulants for attention deficit and hyperactivity. Less commonly prescribed but more likely to cause arrhythmia are

tricyclic antidepressants and neuroleptic agents [46]. These agents produce cardiac effects similar to sodium channel blocking antiarrhythmic drugs. Newer selective serotonin reuptake inhibitor antidepressants and *atypical* antipsychotic agents have been introduced in the last decade. Although these newer agents seem to have a more benign side-effect profile than their predecessors, they have been shown in some individuals to prolong the QT interval and result in significant myocardial depression [47].

Drugs commonly administered in the PICU with significant potential proarrhythmic effects include exogenous catecholamines, digoxin, and antiarrhythmic drugs. Although the arrhythmic effects of exogenous catecholamines are usually immediately recognized and must be balanced against their beneficial effects, digoxin toxicity may be more insidious. Alteration in renal function in a critically ill patient and administration of medications known to alter digoxin metabolism or excretion are common occurrences. The decreased frequency of administration of digoxin in favor of other more effective agents in the PICU has decreased the likelihood of its toxicity but has also decreased the recognition of the problem in treated patients. Digitalis toxicity can result in nearly any arrhythmia and frequently results in several types of tachyarrhythmia in short order. Treatment of digitalis toxicity has been simplified with the availability of digoxin-immune Fab antibody therapy. Adverse effects are few, and this treatment should be considered for all children with documented arrhythmias associated with digoxin toxicity. When renal failure is present, the bound drug will not be excreted, and repeated doses may be necessary. Toxicity with other antiarrhythmic drugs has become less frequent. Quinidine is rarely used and the use of procainamide is also waning. Intravenous amiodarone use has increased substantially in the PICU for both cardiac arrest situations the elective treatment of tachyarrhythmia. Immediate adverse effects of intravenous amiodarone are common, but rarely include tachyarrhythmia. Bradycardia and AV block are more common.

References

1. Reinelt P, Karth GD, Geppert A, Heinz G. Incidence and type of cardiac arrhythmias in critically ill patients: a single center experience in a medical-cardiological ICU. Intensive Care Med 2001;27:1466–1473.
2. Balaji S, Ellenby M, McNames J, Goldstein B. Update on intensive care ECG and cardiac event monitoring. Card Electrophysiol Rev 2002;6:190–195.
3. Brown KL, Ridout DA, Goldman AP, Hoskote A, Penny DJ. Risk factors for long intensive care unit stay after cardiopulmonary bypass in children. Crit Care Med 2003;31:28–33.
4. Kotar SL, Gessler JE. Full-disclosure monitoring: a concept that will change the way arrhythmias are detected and interpreted in the hospitalized patient. Heart Lung 1993;22:482–489.
5. Peterson MC, Whetten DK, Renlund DG, Coletti A. Sensitivity of rhythm disturbance detection by community hospital telemetry. Ann Noninvasive Electrocardiol 2002;7:219–221.
6. Nelwan SP, Kors JA, Meij SH, van Bemmel JH, Simoons ML. Reconstruction of the 12-lead electrocardiogram from reduced lead sets. J Electrocardiol 2004;37:11–18.
7. Drew BJ, Pelter MM, Brodnick DE, Yadav AV, Dempel D, Adams MG. Comparison of a new reduced lead set ECG with the standard ECG for diagnosing cardiac arrhythmias and myocardial ischemia. J Electrocardiol 2002;35(Suppl):13–21.
8. Mantle JA, Strand EM, Wixson SE. Atrial electrogram monitoring in a cardiac care unit. Med Instrum 1978;12:289–292.

9. Prochaczek F, Jerzy G, Stopczyk MJ. A method of esophageal electrogram recording for diagnostic atrial and ventricular pacing. Pacing Clin Electrophysiol 1990;13:1136–1141.

10. Twidale N, Roberts-Thomson P, Tonkin AM. Transesophageal electrocardiography and atrial pacing in acute cardiac care: diagnostic and therapeutic value. Aust N Z J Med 1989;19:11–15.

11. Schoen WJ, Fujimura O. Variant preexcitation syndrome: a true nodoventricular Mahaim fiber or an accessory atrioventricular pathway with decremental properties? J Cardiovasc Electrophysiol 1995; 6:1117–1123.

12. Hluchy J. Mahaim fibers: electrophysiologic characteristics and radiofrequency ablation. Z Kardiol 2000;89:136–143.

13. Lau EW, Green MS, Birnie DH, Lemery R, Tang AS. Preexcitation masking underlying aberrant conduction: an atriofascicular accessory pathway functioning as an ectopic right bundle branch. Heart Rhythm 2004;1:497–499.

14. Benson DW, Wang DW, Dyment M, Knilans TK, Fish FA, Strieper MJ, Rhodes TH, George AL. Congenital sick sinus syndrome caused by recessive mutations in the cardiac sodium channel gene (SCN5A). J Clin Invest 2003;112:1019–1028.

15. Oberhoffer R, von Bernuth G, Lang D, Gildein HP, Weismuller P. [Sinus node dysfunction in children without heart defect.] Z Kardiol 1994; 83:502–506.

16. van Hare GF, Franz MR, Roge C, Scheinman MM. Persistent functional atrioventricular block in two patients with prolonged QT intervals: elucidation of the mechanism of block. Pacing Clin Electrophysiol 1990;13:608–618.

17. Wogan JM, Lowenstein SR, Gordon GS. Second-degree atrioventricular block: Mobitz type II. J Emerg Med 1993;11:47–54.

18. Markel ML, Miles WM, Zipes DP, Prystowsky EN. Parasympathetic and sympathetic alterations of Mobitz type II heart block. J Am Coll Cardiol 1988;11:271–275.

19. Shaw DB, Gowers JI, Kekwick CA, New KH, Whistance AW. Is Mobitz type I atrioventricular block benign in adults? Heart 2004;90:169–174.

20. Oral H. Mechanisms of atrial fibrillation: lessons from studies in patients. Prog Cardiovasc Dis 2005;48:29–40.

21. Epstein MR, Saul JP, Weindling SN, Triedman JK, Walsh EP. Atrioventricular reciprocating tachycardia involving twin atrioventricular nodes in patients with complex congenital heart disease. J Cardiovasc Electrophysiol 2001;12:671–679.

22. Pollack ML, Chan TC, Brady WJ. Electrocardiographic manifestations: aberrant ventricular conduction. J Emerg Med 2000;19:363–367.

23. Nelson JA, Knowlton KU, Harrigan R, Pollack ML, Chan TC. Electrocardiographic manifestations: wide complex tachycardia due to accessory pathway. J Emerg Med 2003;24:295–301.

24. Lau EW, Ng GA. The reliable electrocardiographic diagnosis of regular broad complex tachycardia: a holy grail that will forever elude the clinician's grasp? Pacing Clin Electrophysiol 2002;25:1756–1761.

25. Levy S. Differentiating SVT from VT—a personal viewpoint. Eur Heart J 1994;15(Suppl A):31–38.

26. Hudson KB, Brady WJ, Chan TC, Pollack M, Harrigan RA. Electrocardiographic manifestations: ventricular tachycardia. J Emerg Med 2003;25:303–314.

27. Drew BJ, Scheinman MM. ECG criteria to distinguish between aberrantly conducted supraventricular tachycardia and ventricular tachycardia: practical aspects for the immediate care setting. Pacing Clin Electrophysiol 1995;18:2194–2208.

28. Gaudio C, Di Michele S, Ferri FM, Mirabelli F, Franchitto S, Alessandri N. A case of non-conducted atrial bigeminy simulating a second-degree atrioventricular block. A Holter ECG diagnosis. Eur Rev Med Pharmacol Sci 2004;8:169–171.

29. Altamura G, Toscano S, Bianconi L, Lo Bianco F, Montefoschi N, Pistolese M. Transesophageal cardiac pacing: evaluation of cardiac activation. Pacing Clin Electrophysiol 1990;13:2017–2021.

30. Falk RH, Ngai ST, Kumaki DJ, Rubinstein JA. Cardiac activation during external cardiac pacing. Pacing Clin Electrophysiol 1987;10:503–506.

31. Elmi F, Tullo NG, Khalighi K. Natural history and predictors of temporary epicardial pacemaker wire function in patients after open heart surgery. Cardiology 2002;98:175–180.

32. Kallis P, Batrick N, Bindi F, Mascaro G, Chatzis A, Keogh BE, Parker DJ, Treasure T. Pacing thresholds of temporary epicardial electrodes: variation with electrode type, time, and epicardial position. Ann Thorac Surg 1994;57:623–626.

33. McEneaney DJ, Cochrane DJ, Anderson JA, Adgey AA. Ventricular pacing with a novel gastroesophageal electrode: a comparison with external pacing. Am Heart J 1997;133:674–680.

34. Beland MJ, Hesslein PS, Finlay CD, Faerron-Angel JE, Williams WG, Rowe RD. Noninvasive transcutaneous cardiac pacing in children. Pacing Clin Electrophysiol. 1987;10:1262–1270.

35. Levine PA, Balady GJ, Lazar HL, Belott PH, Roberts AJ. Electrocautery and pacemakers: management of the paced patient subject to electrocautery. Ann Thorac Surg 1986;41:313–317.

36. Blomstrom-Lundqvist C, Scheinman MM, Aliot EM, et al. ACC/AHA/ESC Guidelines for the management of patients with supraventricular arrhythmias. Circulation 2003;108:1871–1909.

37. Gupta AK, Shah CP, Maheshwari A, Thakur RK, Hayes OW, Lokhandwala YY. Adenosine induced ventricular fibrillation in Wolff-Parkinson-White syndrome. Pacing Clin Electrophysiol 2002; 25:477–480.

38. Bakshi F, Barzilay Z, Paret G. Adenosine in the diagnosis and treatment of narrow complex tachycardia in the pediatric intensive care unit. Heart Lung 1998;27:47–50.

39. Rossi AF, Steinberg LG, Kipel G, Golinko RJ, Griepp RB. Use of adenosine in the management of perioperative arrhythmias in the pediatric cardiac intensive care unit. Crit Care Med 1992;20:1107–1111.

40. Ralston MA, Knilans TK, Hannon DW, Daniels SR. Use of adenosine for diagnosis and treatment of tachyarrhythmias in pediatric patients. J Pediatr 1994;124:139–143.

41. Saul JP, Scott WA, Brown S, et al. Intravenous amiodarone for incessant tachyarrhythmias in children. Circulation 2005;112:3470–3477.

42. Schaefer TJ, Wolford RW. Disorders of potassium. Emerg Med Clin North Am 2005;23:723–747.

43. Mattu A, Brady WJ, Perron AD. Electrocardiographic manifestations of hypothermia. Am J Emerg Med 2002;20:314–326.

44. Biondi B, Palmieri EA, Lombardi G, Fazio S. Effects of subclinical thyroid dysfunction on the heart. Ann Intern Med 2002;137:904–914.

45. Lo R, Menzies DJ, Archer H, Cohen TJ. Complete heart block due to Lyme carditis. J Invasive Cardiol 2003;15:367–369.

46. Reilly JG, Ayis SA, Ferrier IN, Jones SJ, Thomas SH. QTc-interval abnormalities and psychotropic drug therapy in psychiatric patients. Lancet 2000;355:1048–1052.

47. Pacher P, Kecskemeti V. Cardiovascular side effects of new antidepressants and antipsychotics: new drugs, old concerns? Curr Pharm Des 2004;10:2463–2475.

20

Inflammatory Diseases of the Heart and Pericardium: Infective Endocarditis and Kawasaki Disease

Michael H. Gewitz and Gary M. Satou

Infective Endocarditis

Infective endocarditis (IE) remains an important cause of morbidity and mortality in the pediatric population despite substantial increases in the tools used to diagnose and treat this condition. In fact, as the epidemiology of cardiovascular disease continues to evolve, the clinician involved with children's health care must be increasingly diligent in the suspicion for infective endocarditis when confronted with this possibility in a sick child. Congenital heart diseases remain the focus of attention for the clinical background of children who develop IE in the United States and other developed countries [1]. In contrast, rheumatic heart disease (Table 20.1), which remains prevalent in many of the world's less advantaged populations, is the most common substrate for IE in those areas. Completely corrective heart surgery eliminates added risks for IE in many, but this is true only when there is no residual defect at all, and for some patients cardiac surgery itself is an associated risk factor for IE [2]. As more infants and young children undergo cardiovascular surgical procedures and succeed at growing up with subtotal palliation for substantial cardiovascular structural problems, ever-increasing numbers of candidates for the development of IE will be added to the epidemiologic pool. Finally, an increasingly recognized group of pediatric patients who develop IE are neonates who survive the rigors of prematurity and other complex medical and surgical problems, even *without* the added risk of congenital heart disease. These babies are managed with increasing use of invasive technology, including long-standing indwelling central catheters, and are subject to prolonged courses of multiple, late-generation antibiotics; they have become increasingly diagnosed with IE. Table 20.2 lists some of the conditions recognized by the American Heart Association as having the highest risks for the development of IE [3].

Pathogenesis

Infective endocarditis occurs at sites of endothelial alteration that develop from either direct or indirect trauma or from abnormal development. Intact endothelium can be disrupted during intracardiac surgical intervention or from abnormal shear stresses associated with flow disturbances created by structural congenital heart disease. Additionally, intracardiac prostheses, such as nontissue valves and conduits, that do not develop complete endothelial layering can be sites for IE localization. Animal models of IE have demonstrated that these areas of disrupted or deficient endothelium induce thrombogenesis with aggregation of fibrin, platelets, and red blood cells (RBCs), which lead to the accumulation of a noninfected thrombotic lesion, called *nonbacterial thrombotic endocarditis* (NBTE). When bacteremia is present it is this NBTE lesion to which circulating bacteria adhere and from which the hallmark lesion of IE, the *vegetation*, emerges. In addition, certain bacteria, such as Gram-positive cocci, express individual virulence factors that allow them to overcome protective antibody resistance and to promote propagation of the vegetation.

These recently elucidated pathogenetic mechanisms help to explain why certain organisms, such as staphylococci, predominate in the diagnosis of IE and why certain clinical circumstances, such as complex cyanotic congenital heart disease treated with a surgically placed intravascular conduit, are high on the list of predisposing conditions. Correspondingly, a lesion such as a secundum atrial septal defect, which is usually associated with low velocity intracardiac shunting, is not considered a risk factor for IE development.

Etiologic Agents

Table 20.3 reviews the more important microorganisms associated with IE [1]. Viridans group streptococci remain the most frequent causative organisms in childhood IE. Staphylococci are particularly associated with indwelling foreign bodies, such as central catheters and prosthetic valves, and are not uncommon agents in neonatal endocarditis. Gram-negative bacilli are much less frequent culprits for IE in children than they are in adults, but fungal endocarditis caused principally by *Candida* species is not uncommon in neonates, especially those on prolonged intravenous alimentation regimens.

Diagnosis

Clinical Features

Nonspecific clinical findings include an aggregation of symptoms that can connote any of a number of disease processes; thus, sus-

D.S. Wheeler et al. (eds.), *Cardiovascular Pediatric Critical Illness and Injury*,
DOI 10.1007/978-1-84800-923-3_20, © Springer-Verlag London Limited 2009

TABLE 20.1. Diagnostic criteria for rheumatic heart disease (Jones criteria 1992 revision).

Major manifestations
  Carditis
  Polyarthritis
  Chorea
  Erythema marginatum
  Subcutaneous nodules
Minor manifestations
  Clinical findings
    Arthralgia
    Fever
  Laboratory findings
    Elevated acute phase reactants (erythrocyte sedimentation rate, C-reactive protein)
    Prolonged PR interval on electrocardiogram
  Supporting evidence of antecedent group A streptococcal infections
    Positive throat culture or rapid streptococcal antigen test (on throat swab)
    Elevated or rising streptococcal antibody titer

Note: If supported by evidence of an antecedent group A streptococcal infection, the presence of two major manifestations or of one major and two minor manifestations is highly suggestive of acute rheumatic fever.

picion must be high, and the clinical context is crucial to establish the diagnosis of IE in children. Generalized fatigue, muscle weakness, rigor, myalgias, arthralgias, and inappropriate diaphoresis in association with prolonged low-grade fever are often part of the litany of complaints expressed by parents of young children or by older children themselves. Subacute IE is characterized by this type of history, which can also include weight loss and anorexia as well. The clinical signs also are often generalized. In particular, although the infection is primarily cardiac, extracardiac findings can be diagnostically critical and clinically crucial with regard to outcome. These clinical markers are related to central pathogenetic developments—the presence of bacteremia, the progression of cardiac inflammation including valvulitis, the occurrence of embolic complications, and the development of host-related immunologic responses. Thus, skin and conjunctival lesions (Roth spots, Janeway lesions, Osler nodes) should be sought for, abdominal visceromegaly (notably splenomegaly) should be palpated for, and renal findings (immune complex–mediated nephritis) should be tested for. Emboli can strike anywhere but in particular should be looked for with examination of the abdominal viscera, the joints, the retina, and the central nervous system. Early clinical diagnosis of emboli is crucial for designing an effective management strategy and maximizes chances for a favorable outcome.

TABLE 20.2. Cardiac conditions and endocarditis.

Highest risk category
  Prosthetic cardiac valves, including bioprosthetic and homograft valves
  Previous bacterial endocarditis
  Complex cyanotic congenital heart disease (eg, single-ventricle states, transposition of the great arteries, tetralogy of Fallot)
  Surgically constructed systemic-pulmonary shunts or conduits
Moderate-risk category
  Most other congenital cardiac malformations (other than above and below)
Acquired valvular dysfunction (e.g., rheumatic heart disease)
Hypertrophic cardiomyopathy
Mitral valve prolapse with valvular regurgitation and/or thickened leaflets

Source: Modified from Dajani et al. [3].

TABLE 20.3. Principal pathogenic bacterial agents.

Microorganism	Johnson et al.[18] (N = 149)	Martin et al.[19] (N = 76)	Stockheim et al.[20] (N = 111)
Viridans group streptococci	43	38	32
Staphylococcus aureus	33	32	27
Coagulase-negative staphylococci	2	4	12
Streptococcus pneumoniae	3	4	7
HACEK	N/A	5	4
Enterococcus species	N/A	7	4
Culture negative	6	7	5

Note: Values are percentages of patients in the series. HACEK, Haemophilus species, Actinobacillus (Haemophilus) actinomycetemcomitans, Cardiobacterium hominis, Eikenella species, and Kingella kingae.
Source: Modified from Dajani et al. [3].

Similar to the variability of the extracardiac findings, the cardiac examination is also widely changeable. The type of underlying heart disease and the specific area of cardiac involvement are keys to the cardiac findings. Children in whom valvar pathology is created by IE can manifest new murmurs associated with new-onset valve regurgitation. On the other hand, children who have depended on a surgically created systemic-pulmonary artery shunt to palliate a cyanotic condition may have a declining murmur, or no change in murmur at all, if the infection involves the graft with obstruction to flow as a result. In these children, new exacerbation of arterial desaturation may be a presenting finding. Irregularities of heart rhythm may also be present if myocardial extension of infection develops.

Laboratory Diagnosis

The sine qua non for diagnosis of IE is a positive blood culture. All patients with a history of structural heart disease and a fever not associated with an overtly obvious cause (e.g., acute streptococcal pharyngitis) should have blood cultures obtained before initiation of an antibiotic regimen. This is true also for children who have had a history of endocarditis or in whom a pathologic murmur is heard de novo with a febrile presentation. Usually, three blood cultures obtained through separate venipunctures will suffice to yield the two positive cultures on samples drawn >12hr apart that are called for in the Duke Criteria [4] for the diagnosis of IE (Table 20.4). In general, more than five blood cultures over 2 days are considered unnecessary for patients who have not been on antibiotics before the workup has begun. Empiric therapy for an acutely ill patient in whom IE is seriously suspected can be initiated once at least three separate cultures are taken. Even if only a short time period has elapsed since initial presentation, the duration of untreated IE can be critical for outcome in an acute setting.

As much sample volume as is practical is preferred, but, for young infants, as little as 1–3 mL may be adequate. For older children, 5–7 mL is optimal. During the course of treatment, the microbiology laboratory is an important aid to successful outcome. Minimum inhibitory concentration (MIC) testing of the chosen antibiotic for the bacterial agent is required in order to select the appropriate antibiotic and to sustain proper therapy. In addition, infectious disease consultation should be considered to add insight and perspective for accurate diagnosis.

TABLE 20.4. Duke criteria for the diagnosis of infective endocarditis (IE).

Major criteria

I. Positive blood culture for IE
   A. Typical microorganism consistent with IE from 2 separate blood cultures as noted below:
      i. Viridans streptococci,* *Streptococcus bovis,* or HACEK group or
      ii. Community-acquired *Staphylococcus aureus* or enterococci, in the absence of a primary focus or
   B. Microorganisms consistent with IE from persistently positive blood cultures defined as
      i. ≥2 Positive cultures of blood samples drawn >12 hr apart or
      ii. All of 3 or a majority of ≥4 separate cultures of blood (with first and last sample drawn ≥1 hr apart)
II. Evidence of endocardial involvement
   A. positive echocardiogram for IE defined as
      i. Oscillating intracardiac mass on valve or supporting structures, in the path of regurgitant jets, or on implanted material in the absence of an alternative anatomic explanation or
      ii. Abscess or
      iii. New partial dehiscence of prosthetic valve or
   B. New valvular regurgitation (worsening or changing of preexisting murmur not sufficient)

Minor criteria

I. Predisposition: predisposing heart condition or intravenous drug use
II. Fever: temperature ≥38°C
III. Vascular phenomena: major arterial emboli, septic pulmonary infarcts, mycotic aneurysm, intracranial hemorrhage, conjunctival hemorrhages, and Janeway lesions
IV. Immunologic phenomena: glomerulonephritis, Osler nodes, Roth spots, and rheumatoid factor
V. Microbiologic evidence: positive blood culture but does not meet a major criterion as noted above or serologic evidence of active infection with organism consistent with IE
IV. Echocardiographic findings: consistent with IE but do not meet a major criterion as noted above

Definite IE

Pathologic criteria
   Microorganisms: demonstrated by culture or histology in a vegetation, a vegetation that has embolized, or an intracardiac abscess or
   Pathologic lesions: vegetation or intracardiac abscess present, confirmed by histology showing active endocarditis
Clinical criteria as defined above
   2 major criteria or
   1 major criterion and 3 minor criteria or
   5 minor criteria

Possible IE

Findings consistent with IE that fall short of "definite" but not "rejected"

Rejected

Firm alternative diagnosis for manifestations of endocarditis or
Resolution of manifestations of endocarditis with antibiotic therapy for ≥4 days or
No pathologic evidence of IE at surgery or autopsy, after antibiotic therapy for ≥4 days

*Includes nutritionally variant strains (*Abiotrophia* species).
Excludes single positive cultures for coagulase-negative staphylococci and organisms that do not cause endocarditis.
Note: HACEK, *Haemophilus* species, *Actinobacillus* (*Haemophilus*) *actinomycetemcomitans,* *Cardiobacterium hominis, Eikenella* species, and *Kingella kingae.*
Source: Modified from Durack et al. [4].

In addition to blood cultures, a few selected other laboratory tests may be helpful. A complete blood count should be obtained as leukocytosis, particularly with a shift toward immature cells, is usually, but not invariably, present. Either thrombocytosis or thrombocytopenia can be present, depending on clinical circumstances, such as the presence of immune complex renal disease. Acute phase reactants should be assayed as well (erythrocyte sedimentation rate and C-reactive protein), and urinalysis, looking for hematuria and/or RBC casts, should be part of the initial assessment.

Cardiac Imaging

No evaluation for IE is adequate without performance of cardiac ultrasound, as echocardiography results are considered important aspects of the major criteria for establishing the diagnosis of IE with the Duke criteria (see Table 20.4). A complete echocardiogram can delineate the presence, size, and mobility of vegetation (Figure 20.1), indicate the extent of cardiac involvement, and quantitatively measure cardiac performance. All of these findings are highly important not only for diagnosis but also for planning therapy and for monitoring results of treatment and the need for change in course. Although for adults transesophageal echocardiography (TEE) is considered more sensitive than transthoracic echocardiography (TTE) for detecting vegetations, TTE can detect very small lesions, and this is particularly true for children in whom

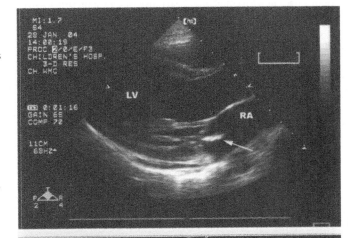

A

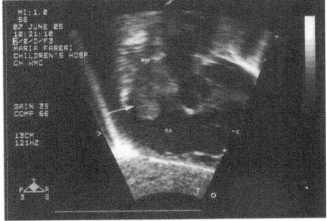

B

FIGURE 20.1. (A) Two-dimensional echo image of vegetation (arrow) localized to mitral valve and protruding into left atrium. LV, left ventricle. **(B)** Vegetation (arrow) stemming from superior vena cava (SVC) and extending into the right atrium (RA) in a newborn infant.

high levels of sensitivity [5] have been reported. Nevertheless, when the suspicion for IE is high yet the TTE study is negative, a TEE study should be strongly considered. For pediatric patients in whom thoracic imaging windows are compromised (pulmonary disease, post-thoracic surgical patients, etc.), TEE may be the more reliable method to employ. However, even with the best imaging technique, echocardiography cannot be considered universally definitive. Ironically, patients with complex congenital heart disease are less likely to have diagnostic echocardiographic findings than are those with isolated valvar abnormalities or structurally normal hearts, because acoustic interference from prosthetic valves, conduits, and other devices frequently used in these patients may interfere with interpretation of the findings.

Echocardiography, particularly TEE, is also extremely important for delineating complications that can influence treatment decisions. For example, extension of infection from the aortic valve can be grave, and TEE diagnosis of such a turn in events can lead to life-saving intervention. In general, certain echocardiographic findings have been associated with the need for surgical intervention in the treatment of IE (Table 20.5) [6]. Finally, even in the most experienced laboratories, echocardiographic studies can have limited value. A negative echocardiographic study, even TEE, does not alone rule out IE. Furthermore, defining the specific nature of echocardiographic densities in the setting of possible IE in a patient with congenital heart disease can sometimes be very difficult.

Duke Criteria

As referenced earlier, a criteria-based system has been advocated as a utilitarian tool in the diagnosis of IE. The original clinical criteria were expanded recently to include echographic results (see Table 20.4) and have been verified as useful in pediatric populations as well as in adults [7]. Under the best circumstances, however, these criteria should be considered only as a clinical guide to diagnose IE and as a help in decision analysis for difficult diagnostic situations. As elsewhere in medicine, the clinical judgment of the practitioner directly involved with the case at hand should trump artificial scoring systems.

Management

Recent comprehensive reviews are available that detail the specific of antibiotic therapies for IE depending on the clinical circumstance and the specific microbial organism [8]. Certain generic principles are applicable in most cases and need to be emphasized (1) bactericidal antibiotics are preferable to bacteriostatic drugs; (2) intravenous therapy is preferable to other routes in most circumstances; (3) a prolonged course of therapy is a requirement (never less than 2 weeks; usually 4 weeks or longer); (4) ready access to appropriate medical and surgical care is required particularly early in the treatment course; and (6) serial monitoring studies, serologic and echocardiographic, are vital to successful outcomes.

Attention to these principles will help to avoid complications in the first place and allow prompt response should they nevertheless occur. In IE management, under the best of conditions, complications can ensue, but these guidelines afford the practitioner some possibility for anticipatory treatment and preventing a complication from becoming a disaster. Tables 20.6, 20.7, and 20.8 offer management recommendations from the American Heart Association [1] for the more typical clinical situations involving IE.

Complications

Certain clinical circumstances are associated with a higher likelihood for complications, and these are reviewed in Table 20.9. When they occur, complications of IE (Table 20.10) require prompt attention and often result in the decision to change course from medical to surgical therapy. For example, the development of either congestive heart failure or a septic embolus while on antibiotic treatment is considered an urgent turn in which appropriate, prompt surgery can be life-saving. Surgery may be required before a complete course of antibiotics has been administered. Indications for consideration of surgery are listed in Table 20.5 [1].

Prophylaxis

There continues to be ongoing controversy about the indications for and value of the use of prophylactic antibiotics to prevent the development of IE. To date, no controlled prospective trial has ever been implemented to yield an evidence basis for this practice. In view of the lack of supportive data and in concert with general concerns over the long-term impact of the widespread use of antibiotics, The American Heart Association has progressively modified the recommendations it publishes on measures to prevent endocarditis, and a substantial new modification is currently in preparation, with anticipated publication in 2006–2007.

Although the specifics are still, as of this writing, being developed, it is clear that certain general principles will remain as part of any new recommendations: (1) there are particular subgroups of patients who are either at greatest statistical risk for the develop-

---

TABLE 20.5. Echocardiographic features suggesting potential need for surgical intervention.

Vegetation
    Persistent vegetation after systemic embolization:
        Anterior mitral leaflet vegetation, particularly with size >10 mm*
        ≥1 Embolic event during first 2 weeks of antimicrobial therapy*
        ≥2 Embolic events during or after antimicrobial therapy*
    Increase in vegetation size after 4 weeks of antimicrobial therapy[†,‡]
Valvular dysfunction
    Acute aortic or mitral insufficiency with signs of ventricular failure[‡]
    Heart failure unresponsive to medical therapy[‡]
    Valve perforation or rupture[‡]
Perivalvular extension
    Valvular dehiscence, rupture, or fistula[‡]
    New heart block[‡]
    Large abscess or extension of abscess despite appropriate antimicrobial therapy[‡]

*Surgery may be required because of risk of recurrent embolization.
[†]Surgery may be required because of risk of embolization.
[‡]Surgery may be required because of heart failure or failure of medical therapy.
Source: Modified from Bayer et al. [6].

TABLE 20.6. Regimens for therapy of native valve infective endocarditis caused by viridans group streptococci, *Streptococcus bovis*, or enterococci.*

Microorganism	Antimicrobial agent	Dosage (per kg per 24 hr)	Frequency of administration	Duration of therapy (weeks)
Penicillin-susceptible streptococci (MIC ≤0.1 µg/mL)[†]	Penicillin G[‡] or	200,000 U IV	q 4–6 hr	4
	ceftriaxone	100 mg IV	q 24 hr	4
	Penicillin G[‡] or	200,000 U IV	q 4–6 hr	2
	ceftriaxone or	100 mg IV	q 24 hr	2
	Ceftriaxone plus	100 mg IV	q 24 hr	2
	gentamicin	3 mg IM or IV	q 8 hr[‡]	2
Streptococci relatively resistant to penicillin (MIC >0.1–0.5 µg/mL)	Penicillin G[‡] or	300,000 U IV	q 4–6 hr	4
	Ceftriaxone plus	100 mg IV	q 24 hr	4
	gentamicin	3 mg IM or IV	q 8 hr[†]	2
Enterococci,[§] nutritionally variant viridans streptococci, or high-level penicillin-resistant streptococci (MIC >0.5 µg/mL)	Penicillin G[‡] plus	300,000 U IV	q 4–6 hr	4–6[¶]
	gentamicin	3 mg IM or IV	q 8 hr[∥]	4–6[¶]

*Dosages suggested are for patients with normal renal and hepatic function. Maximum dosages per 24 hr: penicillin, 18 million units; ampicillin, 12 g; ceftriaxone, 4 g; gentamicin, 240 mg. The 2-week regimens are not recommended for patients with symptoms of infection >3 months in duration or for those with extracardiac focus of infection, myocardial abscess, mycotic aneurysm, or infection with nutritionally variant viridans streptococci (*Abiotrophia* sp).

[†]Ampicillin 300 mg/kg per 24 hr in 4–6 divided dosages may be used as alternative to penicillin.

[‡]Studies in adults suggest gentamicin dosage may be administered in single daily dose. If gentamicin is administered in 3 equally divided doses per 24 hr, adjust dosage to achieve peak and trough concentrations in serum of ≈3.0 and <1.0 µg of gentamicin per 1 mL, respectively.

[§]Studies in adults suggest that 4 weeks of therapy is sufficient for patients with enterococcal infectious endocarditis with symptoms of infection of <3 months' duration; 6 weeks of therapy is recommended for patients with symptoms of infection of >3 months' duration.

[∥]Adjust gentamicin dosage to achieve peak and trough concentrations in serum of ≈3.0 and >1.0 µg of gentamicin per 1 mL, respectively.

[¶]For enterococci resistant to penicillins, vancomycin, or aminoglycosides, treatment should be guided by consultation with a specialist in infectious diseases (cephalosporins should not be used to treat enterococcal endocarditis regardless of in vitro susceptibility).

Note: For treatment of patients with prosthetic cardiac valves or other prosthetic materials, see text. IM, intramuscular; IV, intravenous; MIC, minimum inhibitory concentration of penicillin.

Source: Modified from Ferrieri et al. [1].

ment of IE or for whom morbidity and mortality rates from IE exceed others (see Tables 20.2 and 20.9), and it is for these patients that any effort at prophylaxis should be concentrated; (2) although prevention is desirable, it is not always achievable despite best efforts; (3) events of daily life may have a greater role in the development of IE than is often recognized, adding to the difficulty of prevention regimens; (4) for children at risk, maintenance of good oral health should be a key element of any prophylaxis strategy. It is likely that in selected patients, even more carefully delimited than before, the current single-dose regimens will still be applicable, but the reader is cautioned to follow the literature for changes in even this aspect of prevention strategy.

TABLE 20.7. Treatment regimens for therapy of infectious endocarditis caused by viridans group streptococci, *Streptococcus bovis*, or enterococci in patients unable to tolerate a β-lactam.*

Microorganism	Antimicrobial agent	Dosage (per kg per 24 hr)	Frequency of administration	Duration of therapy (weeks)
Native valve (no prosthetic material)				
Streptococci	Vancomycin	40 mg IV	q 6–12 hr	4–6
Enterococci[†] or nutritionally variant viridans streptococci	Vancomycin plus gentamicin	40 mg IV 3 mg IM or IV	q 6–12 hr q 8 hr[‡]	6 6
Prosthetic devices				
Streptococci	Vancomycin plus gentamicin	40 mg IV 3 mg IM or IV	q 6–12 hr q 8 hr[‡]	6 2
Enterococci[†] or nutritionally variant viridans streptococci	Vancomycin plus gentamicin	40 mg IV 3 mg IM or IV	q 6–12 hr q 8 hr[‡]	6 6

*Dosages suggested are for patients with normal renal function. Maximum daily dose per 24 hr of gentamicin is 240 mg.

[†]For enterococci resistant to vancomycin or aminoglycosides, treatment should be guided by consultation with a specialist in infectious diseases.

[‡]Dosage of gentamicin should be adjusted to achieve peak and trough concentration in serum of ~3.0 and <1.0 µg of gentamicin per mL respectively.

Note: IM, intramuscular; IV, intravenous.

Source: Modified from Ferrieri et al. [1].

Table 20.8. Treatment regimens for endocarditis caused by staphylococci.*

Microorganism	Antimicrobial agent	Dosage (per kg per 24 hr)	Frequency of administration	Duration of therapy (week
Native valve (no prosthetic material)				
Methicillin susceptible	Nafcillin or oxacillin with or without gentamicin[†]	200 mg IV 3 mg IM or IV[‡]	q 4–6 hr q 8 hr	6 3–5 days
β-Lactam allergic	Cefazolin[§] with or without gentamicin[†] or Vancomycin	100 mg IV 3 mg IM or IV[‡] 40 mg IV	q 6–8 hr q 8 hr q 6–12 hr	6 3–5 days 6
Methicillin resistant	Vancomycin	40 mg IV	q 6–12 hr	6
Prosthetic devices or other prosthetic materials				
Methicillin susceptible	Nafcillin or oxacillin or cefazolin[§] plus rifampin[‖] plus gentamicin[†]	200 mg IV 100 mg IV 20 mg PO 3 mg IM or IV[‡]	q 4–6 hr q 6–8 hr q 8 hr q 8 hr	≥6 ≥6 ≥6 2
Methicillin resistant	Vancomycin plus rifampin[‖] plus gentamicin[†]	40 mg IV 20 mg PO 3 mg IM or IV[‡]	q 6–12 hr q 8 hr q 8 hr	≥6 ≥6 2

*Dosages suggested are for patients with normal renal and hepatic function. Maximum daily doses per 24 hr: oxacillin or nafcillin, 12 g; cefazolin, 6 g; gentamicin, 240 mg; rifampi 900 mg.

[†]Gentamicin therapy should be used only with gentamicin-susceptible strains.

[‡]Dosage of gentamicin should be adjusted to achieve peak and trough concentrations in serum of ≈3.0 and <1.0 μg of gentamicin per 1 mL, respectively.

[§]Cefazolin or other first-generation cephalosporin in equivalent dosages may be used in patients who do not have a history of immediate type hypersensitivity (urticaria, angioedem anaphylaxis) to penicillin or ampicillin.

[‖]Dosages suggested for rifampin are based on results of studies conducted in adults and should be used only with rifampin-susceptible strains.

Note: IM, intramuscular; IV, intravenous; PO, by mouth.

Source: Modified from Ferrieri et al. [1].

Kawasaki Disease

Epidemiology and Pathogenesis

Kawasaki disease (KD), initially known as *mucocutaneous lymph node syndrome*, was first described in Japan by Dr. Tomosaku Kawasaki in 1967. To this day, it continues to be a regularly seen inflammatory disorder with an unclear etiology and potentially life-threatening cardiac complications. In the United States, KD has become the most common acquired heart disease of childhood [9]. Despite this, continued advances in the care of children afflicted by this syndrome have resulted in a reduction in both morbidity and mortality. The general clinical presentation of Kawasaki disease (Table 20.11) consists of fever for at least several days' duration accompanied by varying degrees of conjunctivitis, exan-

them, oral–mucosal and extremity changes, cervical lymphade nopathy, and associated clinical and laboratory features (Table 20.12 and 20.13).

The incidence of KD in the United States ranges from 9.1 to 17. cases/100,000 children <5 years old [10]. Worldwide, Japan contin ues to have the highest prevalence, with an annual incidence o approximately 112 cases/100,000 children <5 years old [11]. Th disease occurs more frequently in winter and spring and has proclivity for specific demographic subgroups. The majority o patients are under 5 years of age (~80%), and boys are affected 1.! times as often as girls. In addition, Asian and African-America children are affected more frequently than Caucasian or Hispani children in the United States.

The inciting etiologic agent underlying the clinical phenomen of KD is speculated to be infectious, but this remains unprover

Table 20.9. Clinical situations constituting high risk for complications of infective endocarditis.

Prosthetic cardiac valves
Left-sided infective endocarditis
Infective endocarditis caused by *Staphylococcus aureus*
Infective endocarditis caused by fungal disease
Previous history of infective endocarditis
Prolonged clinical symptoms (>3 months)
Cyanotic congenital heart disease
Systemic-to-pulmonary shunts
Poor clinical response to antimicrobial therapy

Source: Modified from Bayer et al. [6].

Table 20.10. Complications of infectious endocarditis.

Congestive heart failure
Embolic events (cerebral, pulmonary, renal, coronary)
Periannular extension of abscess
Arrhythmia development
New heart block
Prosthetic device dysfunction
Valvar dehiscence
Graft or shunt occlusion
Persistent bacteremia or fungemia
Metastatic infection; mycotic aneurysms
Glomerulonephritis/renal failure

Source: Modified from Ferrieri et al. [1].

TABLE 20.11. Classical clinical features of Kawasaki disease.

Fever of at least 5 days' duration* *and* presence of at least four of the below principal features:
Bilateral bulbar conjunctival injection (nonpurulent)
Oral mucosal changes: erythema, cracked lips, strawberry tongue, pharyngeal injection
Polymorphous exanthema
Extremity changes
    Acute: palmar/sole erythema, edema of hands and/or feet
    Subacute: periungual peeling of digits
Cervical lymphadenopathy (usually unilateral and diameter >1.5 cm)

*Recent guidelines include acceptance of less than 5 days of fever when diagnosis is established by an experienced clinician or in the presence of more than four of the principal criteria. Also, less than four principal criteria are accepted when coronary artery changes are detected by echocardiography (or angiography).

TABLE 20.13. Laboratory findings.

Leukocytosis (neutrophilia)
Elevated erythrocyte sedimentation rate
Elevated c-reactive protein
Anemia (normochromic/normocytic)
Hypoalbuminemia
Hyponatremia
Thrombocytosis (after 1 week)
Sterile pyuria
Elevated serum transaminases

Multiple agents have previously been suspected but never proven to be etiologic, including bacteria (e.g., streptococci and staphylococci), rickettsia, various viral agents, and even dust mite antigens. Pathogenesis is thought to involve an immune-mediated response against a suspected infectious agent that leads to activation and/or increased production of monocytes, macrophages, T cells, B lymphocytes, and immunoglobulins. Increased cytokine release also occurs, including release of interleukins and tumor necrosis factor-α. Activation of the vascular endothelium also has been demonstrated, with increased expression of intercellular adhesion molecules, vascular endothelial growth factor, and platelet-derived growth factor, especially during the active stages of disease.

Cardiovascular pathology has been well described (Table 20.14) [12] and occurs in a staged fashion. An initial phase of microvasculitis occurs, followed by myocarditis and possibly valvulitis. Inflammation of the walls of medium and large arteries, primarily coronary arteries, can occur and lead to aneurysm formation. When present, aneurysms are most often found in the proximal vessels and also at vessel branching points, thought possibly to be caused by increased wall stress at these sites. Most often, the lesions occur in the left main coronary artery or in proximal portions of the left anterior descending and right coronary arteries. The circumflex coronary artery is uncommonly involved. Aneurysms can be different in shape (e.g., saccular, fusiform, cylindrical), and, when they are 8 mm or greater in diameter, they are defined as *giant*

and are associated with an increased risk of myocardial infarction. In addition to coronary artery involvement, dilation or aneurysms can develop in other vessels, such as the subclavian, axillary, or brachial arteries, as well as femoral vessels or the abdominal aorta. Aortic root dilation has also been described as well as aortic valvulitis. Mitral valve papillary muscle dysfunction and mitral regurgitation are also not uncommon sequelae.

Diagnosis

Clinical Features

To this day, KD remains a clinical diagnosis based on a constellation of symptoms and laboratory data. No specific diagnostic test exists. The diagnosis classically depends on the presence of 5 or more days of fever and at least four of the five principal clinical features (see Table 20.10), including nonpurulent conjunctivitis, changes in the lips and oral cavity, *strawberry* tongue, edema and/or erythema of the hands and feet, an erythematous rash, and cervical lymphadenopathy. The various clinical findings do not always occur at the same time and frequently evolve over days.

There is frequently an acute phase, for the first week or two, in which a number of these findings develop, and a secondary, subacute phase. The fever, starting at the onset of the acute phase, is usually high and spiking and persists for over a week if untreated. When properly treated (see below), it usually remits within 2 days. The bilateral conjunctival injection is usually bulbar and

TABLE 20.12. Features associated with Kawasaki disease.

Cardiovascular
    Myocarditis, pericarditis, valvulitis, congestive heart failure
    Coronary artery changes/aneurysms
    Noncoronary arterial changes
Musculoskeletal
    Arthritis
    Arthralgia
Gastrointestinal
    Diarrhea/vomiting
    Hepatic dysfunction
    Hydrops of gallbladder
Central nervous system
    Irritable disposition
    Aseptic meningitis
    Sensorineural hearing loss
Genitourinary
    Urethritis

TABLE 20.14. Stages of cardiovascular pathology.

Stage 1 (0–9 days)
    Microvascular angitis
    Acute endarteritis and perivasculitis of major coronary arteries
    Pericarditis, valvulitis, and endocarditis
    Myocarditis, including atrioventricular conduction system
    Causes of death: heart failure and dysrhythmia
Stage 2 (12–25 days)
    Panvasculitis of major coronary arteries with aneurysms and thrombus formation
    Intimal proliferation of coronary arteries
    Myocarditis, endocarditis, and pericarditis
    Causes of death: same as in stage 1; also myocardial infarction, aneurysm rupture
Stage 3 (28–31 days)
    Granulation of coronary arteries
    Marked intimal thickening
    Disappearance of microvascular angitis
    Cause of death: myocardial infarction
Stage 4 (40 days–4 years)
    Scaring, stenosis, calcification, and recanalization of major coronary arteries
    Fibrosis of myocardium and endocardium
    Cause of death: myocardial infarction

nonpurulent. It most often develops shortly after fever onset and resolves soon after treatment. The changes affecting the lips and oral mucosal include a generalized and diffuse erythema without focal lesions or exudates. The lips are often dry and cracked. Extremity changes include erythema of the palms and/or soles and can be painful. In the subacute phase, several weeks after onset, there is typically desquamation and peeling of the skin, which typically initiates from the nail beds. The rash in KD is variable in presentation and usually is present within the first week of fever. Most commonly, the rash is maculopapular and involves the trunk and extremities. At times, it may be limited solely to the groin area. Finally, unilateral (greater than 1.5 cm) cervical lymphadenopathy, although less common than the other findings, can occur and is nonfluctuant and often nontender. On occasion, however, the node can be quite inflamed and tender, resembling cervical adenitis.

Cardiovascular physical examination findings at the initial acute phase include tachycardia and a hyperdynamic precordium. There may be a murmur, either flow related or from valvular insufficiency. A gallop rhythm may be present, and less frequently, when significant left ventricular dysfunction exists, children may present with low cardiac output or shock.

Laboratory Findings

During the acute phase of KD, serology reveals an elevated white blood cell count (leukocytosis), anemia, and elevated acute phase reactants, specifically erythrocyte sedimentation rate and C-reactive protein. Serum transaminase levels may be elevated, and sterile pyuria is often present. Into the second week of the illness, thrombocytosis is usually seen, with counts ranging from 500,000 to >1 million. Thrombocytopenia is rare, although, interestingly, a low platelet count on presentation is a risk factor for coronary artery aneurysms. If drawn, blood cultures are negative. Serum albumin can be reduced, and some have found a low albumin level to be a marker for cardiovascular complications.

Cardiac Imaging

The fundamental cardiovascular diagnostic tool in the evaluation of KD and its potential cardiovascular complications is echocardiography. Chest radiography is usually normal, and electrocardiography may be normal or demonstrate the general findings of sinus tachycardia or nonspecific ST/T wave changes. Echocardiography demonstrates detailed anatomy and provides quantitative measurements of the heart, valves, and, most importantly, the coronary arteries (Figure 20.2). These include internal coronary artery diameter measures, which need to be carefully measured, and best practices include correspondence with body surface area and published standard deviation graphs (z-score system) (Figure 20.3) [13].

Incomplete Kawasaki Disease

Recently, an algorithm was developed (Figure 20.4) to help clinicians evaluate and manage patients with *incomplete* KD [9]. This term is utilized to describe the subcategory of children who have some features of KD but who do not satisfy the conventional clinical criteria for diagnosis. Incomplete KD is more often seen in young infants. The laboratory findings are similar to those seen in conventional cases. Integral to the new algorithm is the use of echocardiography to describe abnormal cardiac changes such as

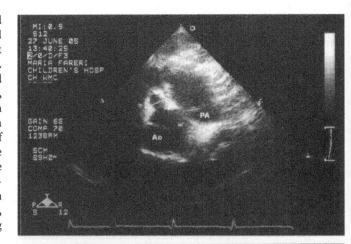

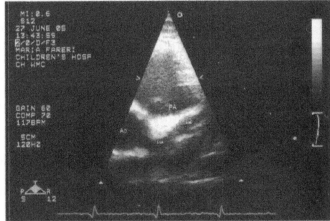

FIGURE 20.2. (A) Two-dimensional echo image of right coronary artery aneurysm (−) dimension. Ao, aortic root; PA, pulmonary. **(B)** Two-dimensional echo image of left anterior descending (LAD) dilation. LCA, left coronary artery.

coronary *ectasia, perivascular brightness*, or left ventricular dysfunction. The goal of structuring an approach to the patient with incomplete KD is not only to reduce overdiagnosis but also, importantly, to screen young infants who may be at increased risk for developing coronary abnormalities and to promote early treatment in these cases.

Management

Administration of intravenous immune gamma globulin (IVIG) has become the mainstay of KD therapy. Aspirin is also still considered a mainstay of therapy by most, as it plays both antiinflammatory and antiplatelet roles. It is administered initially at 80–100 mg/kg per day divided into four doses. This is generally reduced to the *low-dose* aspirin regimen of 3–5 mg/kg per day once the child is afebrile for 48–72 hr. With the majority of patients (i.e., when no coronary changes have occurred), aspirin is discontinued at 6–8 weeks after the onset of illness. This overlaps with the time at which the highest incidence of coronary artery aneurysm formation occurs. Despite the theoretical association of Reye syndrome and aspirin therapy, it is very rarely experienced in the current era, but Reye syndrome is still a caveat of therapy that requires attention and the diligence of the supervising physician.

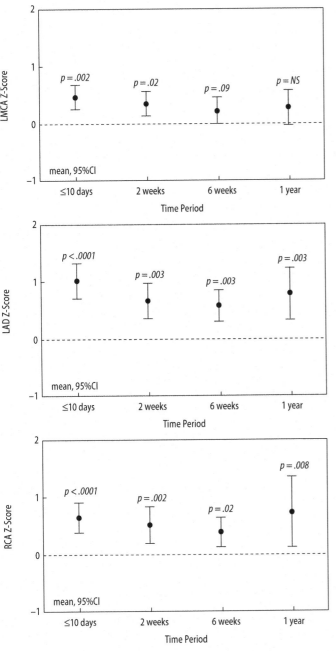

Figure 20.3. Z-score graph for coronary artery dimensions as developed by DeZorzi et al. [12] and used to determine coronary artery dimension abnormalities.

Concurrent with the initiation of high-dose aspirin is administration of IVIG. Although the mechanism of action remains somewhat unclear (other than a general antiinflammatory effect), its efficacy in reducing the prevalence of coronary artery changes is well documented [14]. Dosing is usually 2 g/kg in a single infusion usually over 12 hr. When given within the first 10 days of illness, only ~5% of children with KD will still experience coronary artery changes. When given after 10 days, IVIG efficacy regarding coronary changes may be reduced, but it is still appropriate to administer the medication as long as fever or evidence of persistent systemic inflammation exists. In the small percentage of patients who do not defervesce upon IVIG administration, the current

recommendation is to provide an additional infusion, given at least 36 hr following the first infusion. The dosing regimen is the same. In the very rare event that two infusions of IVIG are ineffective, a third may be considered along with a 1–3 day course of pulsed methylprednisolone (30 mg/kg). Various studies in the past utilizing corticosteroids or agents other than aspirin and IVIG for the initial treatment of KD have demonstrated mixed and sometimes conflicting results. A multicenter randomized, placebo-blind trial reevaluating the efficacy of steroid therapy in the treatment of children with KD is currently underway.

In patients with evidence of coronary artery changes, additional levels of care depend on the degree of abnormality. When mild forms of coronary artery dilation are present, clinicians will often utilize, in addition to continued aspirin therapy, additional antiplatelet agents such as clopidogrel or dipyridamole or oral anticoagulation with coumadin. When aneurysms are large or rapidly expanding, there is an increased risk of thrombosis, and intravenous heparin infusion may be appropriate. Once patients with coronary artery abnormalities are on coumadin, typically the International Normalized Ratio (INR) is used to monitor therapy with the goal to maintain INR in the 2.0–2.5 range.

Coronary thrombosis in children with KD is fortunately unusual, and thus management needs to be individualized and is not based on data obtained from randomized, controlled trials. Thus, typical approaches often mimic treatment strategies utilized in adult acute coronary syndromes, even though the underlying model (plaque

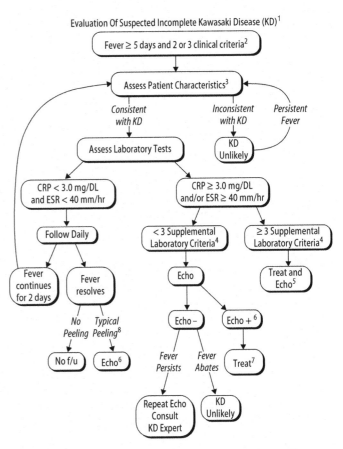

Figure 20.4. Algorithm for evaluation of patients with suspected *incomplete* Kawasaki disease (see text) (Data from Newberger et al. [9], with permission. © 2004 by the American Heat Association.)

rupture/inflammation vs. thrombosis) is different. Experience with thrombolytic therapy (via intravenous bolus and subsequent infusion) includes the use of streptokinase, tissue plasminogen activator, and urokinase [15]. As well, there may be promise in the use of glycoprotein IIb/IIIa inhibitors, such as abciximab.

The indications for transvascular or surgical revascularization are also not evidence based at this time. The most frequent surgical approach is internal mammary bypass grafting, which has demonstrated better long-term patency than saphenous vein grafting. Results have generally been successful, with the majority of patients demonstrating patency up to 10 years following bypass. The number of children with KD and coronary artery occlusion who have undergone transcatheter balloon angioplasty, rotational ablation, and/or stenting is relatively small and has mostly occurred outside of the United States, particularly in Japan. Reported results are encouraging in the small series reported to date [16].

Prognosis

Long-term prognosis for children with KD depends on the specific nature of the coronary artery involvement. The large majority of children, in whom coronary artery changes do not occur (or in whom only mild, transient dilation is present), will continue to demonstrate normal caliber coronaries without aneurysms. In more recent years, limited data suggest that subtle endothelial dysfunction or enhanced arterial stiffness may be present in these patients as well as possible accelerated adult atherosclerotic coronary disease [17]. Because of this, it is now recommended that these children be evaluated every 3–5 years for *tracking* purposes and cardiovascular risk factor evaluation.

For children with coronary aneurysms, the likelihood of regression over time appears to correlate with the initial lesion size, with the smaller lesions more likely to demonstrate complete resolution. Approximately 50% of all aneurysmal coronary segments will demonstrate regression on angiography, often within the first year or two. Other factors influencing aneurysm regression include age at presentation, proximal versus distal location, and morphology of the aneurysm (i.e., saccular vs. fusiform). Stenotic coronary segments can be progressive and must be followed carefully. Children with giant aneurysms (8 mm or greater) demonstrate the greatest chance of thrombotic occlusion secondary to stasis of flow, associated with stenosis and lumen narrowing. This can lead to myocardial infarction and death. The highest risk of myocardial infarction in this small subset of patients is within the first year after presentation.

Follow-up evaluations for these children with coronary artery abnormalities occur on a regular basis and are tailored individually for each child. When age appropriate, exercise stress testing and myocardial perfusion imaging are considered typical parts of the follow-up protocol. Cardiac catheterization with selective coronary angiography is indicated for children with large coronary artery aneurysms or stenoses or suspected multiple sites of coronary involvement. Intense investigation into the fundamental etiologic mechanisms of KD is currently underway worldwide and hopefully will lead to not only enhanced diagnostic acumen but also more selective and specific treatment regimens.

References

1. Ferrieri P, Gewitz MH, Gerber MA, et al. Unique features of infecti endocarditis in childhood. Circulation 2002;105:2115–2127.
2. Morris CD, Keller MD, Menashe VD. Thirty year incidence of infecti endocarditis after surgery for congenital heart defect. JAMA 1998;27 599–603.
3. Dajani AS, Taubert KA, Wilson W, et al. Prevention of bacterial end carditis: recommendations by the American Heart Association. J A Dent Assoc 1997;128:1142–1151.
4. Durack DT, Lukes AS, Bright DK. New criteria for diagnosis of infecti endocarditis: utilization of specific echocardiographic findings. Am Med 1994;96:200–209.
5. Kavery RE, Frank DM, Byron CJ, et al. Two-dimensional echocardi graphic assessment of infective endocarditis in children. Am J D Child 1983;137:851–856.
6. Bayer A, Bolger AF, Taubert, KA et al. Diagnosis and management infective endocarditis and its complications. Circulation 1998;9 2936–2948.
7. Stockheim JA, Chadwich EG, Kessler S, et al. Are the Duke criter superior to the Beth Israel criteria for the diagnosis of infective end carditis in children? Clin Infect Dis 1998;27:1451–1456.
8. Baddour LM, Wilson WR, Bayer AS, et al. Infective endocarditis: dia nosis, antimicrobial therapy, and management of complications: statement for healthcare professionals from the committee on rhe matic fever, endocarditis, and Kawasaki disease, Council on Cardi vascular Disease in the Young, and the Councils on Clinical Cardiolog Stroke, and Cardiovascular Surgery and Anesthesia, American Hea Association–Executive Summary. Circulation 2005;111:3167–3184.
9. Newburger JW, Takahashi M, Gerber MA, Gewitz MH, et al. Diagnosi treatment and long-term management of Kawasaki disease. Circula tion 2004;110:2747–2771.
10. Holman RC, Carns AT, Belay ED, Steiner CA, Schonberger L Kawasaki syndrome hospitalizations in the United States, 1997 an 2000. Pediatrics 2003;112:495–501.
11. Yanagawa H, Nakamura Y, Yashiro M, Oki I, Hirata S, Zhang Kawasaki T. Incidence survey of Kawasaki disease in 1997 and 1998 i Japan. Pediatrics 2001;107:E33.
12. Fujiwara H, Mamashima Y. Pathology of the heart in Kawasaki disease Pediatrics 1968;61:1001–131.
13. DeZorzi A, Colan SD, Gavreau K, Baker AL, Smidel RP, Newburger JW Coronary artery dimensions may be classified as normal in Kawasak disease. J Pediatr 1998;133:254–158.
14. Newburger JW, Takahashi M, Burns JC, et al. The treatment o Kawasaki syndrome with intravenous gamma 13 globulin. N Eng Med 1986;314:341–347.
15. Kato H, Inchinose E, Inoue O, Akagi T. Intracoronary thrombolyti therapy in Kawasaki disease: treatment and prevention acute myocar dial infarction. Prog Clin Biol Res 1987;250:445–454.
16. Ino T, Akimoto K, Ohkubo M. et al. Application of percutaneous trans luminal coronary angiography to coronary arterial stenosis i Kawasaki disease. Circulation 1996;93:1709–1715.
17. Dhillon R, Clarckson P, Donald AE, et al. Endothelial dysfunction lat after Kawasaki disease. Circulation 1996;96:2103–2106.
18. Johnson DH, Rosenthal A, Nadas AS. A forty-year review of bacteria endocarditis in infancy and childhood. Circulation 1975;51:581–588.
19. Martin JM, Neches WH, Wald ER. Infective endocarditis: 35 years o experience at a children's hospital. Clin Infect Dis 1997;24:669–675.
20. Stockheim JA, Chadwick EG, Kessker S. Amer M, Abdel-Hag N, Dajan AS, Shulmin ST. Are the Duke criteria superior to Beth Israel criteri for diagnosis of infective endocarditis in children? Clin Infact Di 1998;27:1451–1456.

Inflammatory Diseases of the Heart and Pericardium: Dilated Cardiomyopathy and Myocarditis

Henry B. Wiles, Neil W. Kooy, and Derek S. Wheeler

Dilated Cardiomyopathy

Definition and Epidemiology

Treatment of congestive heart failure (CHF) in the pediatric intensive care unit (PICU) is a common occurrence. The numbers of diseases that lead to decreased cardiac function are innumerable and are discussed in this chapter and elsewhere in this textbook (Table 21.1). The final common pathway for any of these conditions is dysfunction of the sarcomere, the contractile element of the myocyte. This section reviews the presentation, diagnosis, pathophysiology, and treatment of two causes of CHF: primary dilated (congestive) cardiomyopathy and myocarditis.

The World Health Organization (WHO) in 1995 classified cardiomyopathies into dilated, hypertrophic, restrictive, arrhythmogenic right ventricular, and unclassified types [1]. The dilated form is characterized as dilatation and impaired contraction of the left ventricle or both ventricles. Inflammatory cardiomyopathy is a specific subset of dilated cardiomyopathy and is defined as myocarditis, as diagnosed by histologic, immunologic, and immunohistochemical criteria, that occurs in association with cardiac dysfunction. Both of these conditions result in some degree of CHF, depending on their severity, from myocardial pump failure. They are often interrelated, although their complete association, or cause and effect, is not known.

Dilated cardiomyopathy may be caused by many agents and is a structural and/or a functional derangement of myocardial muscle. This definition generally excludes causes of myocardial dysfunction such as hypertension, congenital heart disease, cardiac valvular disease, and pulmonary vascular disease [2]. Ischemic cardiomyopathy is a common condition in adults and meets the definition of dilated cardiomyopathy, but the incidence of this subtype in children is low. Pharmacologic treatment of ischemic cardiomyopathy in the child, as caused by either anomalous left coronary artery from the pulmonary artery (ALCAPA) or in association with Kawasaki disease (discussed in Chapter 20), is similar to other forms of dilated cardiomyopathy. A special category of dilated cardiomyopathy is peripartum cardiomyopathy, which occurs in the last trimester of a pregnancy or in the first 6 months postpartum.

The incidence of dilated cardiomyopathy in children is low and variable. The Pediatric Cardiomyopathy Registry found an incidence of 1.13 cases per 100,000 children for all forms of cardiomyopathy [3]. The registry data also noted a regional difference—1.44 cases per 100,000 in New England and 0.98 cases per 100,000 in the central Southwest. The incidence of dilated cardiomyopathy was higher in certain groups, namely, African Americans, infants, and males. In a prospective study of cardiomyopathy in children in one medium-sized state (population 3.5 million), the number of newly diagnosed cases each year (over a 12 year period) ranged from 0 to 10 cases per year (H. Wiles, unpublished data). In the past, the largest single class of dilated cardiomyopathy was idiopathic, with the largest identified cause being myocarditis (usually viral) [4]. Now there is recognition that many cases are familial or genetic in origin, perhaps as many as 30% of cases [5]. Although dilated cardiomyopathy more frequently occurs in families or in those with a genetic mutation, the exact cause or structural abnormality is still not known. Recognition of familial occurrence or genetic markers does not yet provide any meaningful therapeutic options.

Pathophysiology

Following the initiation of myocardial injury, whether from viral-mediated inflammation (discussed later), autoimmunity, genetic factors, or unknown etiology, the injury-related reduction in cardiac output initiates a cascade of events that ultimately may prove detrimental to the myocardium. Paramount in these events is (1) the activation of the neural and humoral sympathetic nervous system, (2) the activation of the renin–angiotensin–aldosterone pathway, and (3) humoral release of vasodilatory substances such as atrial natriuretic peptides, prostaglandins, and nitric oxide.

Activation of the sympathetic nervous system results in release of the catecholamines epinephrine and norepinephrine, which originate from two separate components of the sympathetic nervous system: the humoral system, consisting of adrenal medullary cells that, in response to physiologic stress, release primarily epinephrine into the systemic circulation; and sympathetic adrenergic nerve fibers, which travel along arteries within the adventitia and, upon stimulation, release norepinephrine. Under normal physiologic conditions, the majority of norepinephrine released from nerve terminals is reabsorbed and subsequently recycled or metabolized, while a small amount diffuses into the circulation. However,

D.S. Wheeler et al. (eds.), *Cardiovascular Pediatric Critical Illness and Injury*,
DOI 10.1007/978-1-84800-923-3_21, © Springer-Verlag London Limited 2009

TABLE 21.1. Partial list of causes of dilated cardiomyopathy.

Idiopathic
Postmyocarditis
Alcoholic
Peripartum
Neuromuscular
   Muscular dystrophy
   Myotonic dystrophy
Metabolic
   Carnitine deficiency
   Thyroid dysfunction
   Hypocalcemia
   Uremia
   Catecholamine cardiomyopathy
Connective tissue disorder
   Systemic lupus erythematosus
   Rheumatoid disease
   Polyarteritis
Nutritional
   Beriberi
   Kwashiorkor
   Selenium deficiency
Glycogen storage disease
Toxins
   Cobalt
   Lead
   Arsenic
Doxorubicin hydrochloride
Infiltrative
   Amyloid
   Hemochromatosis
   Sarcoid
Inherited
   Fabry disease
   Gaucher disease
   X-linked familial
Supraventricular tachycardia
Anomalous coronary artery anatomy

under conditions of physiologic stress, the amount of norepinephrine entering the circulation may increase dramatically.

The effects of circulating epinephrine and norepinephrine on myocardial and vascular function are mediated through α- and β-adrenergic receptor activation. As the serum epinephrine concentration increases, there is an increase in heart rate and systolic blood pressure as a consequence of myocardial β_1-adrenoreceptor activation. As serum epinephrine concentrations continue to increase, α-adrenoreceptor–mediated vasoconstriction begins to predominate, with a significant increase in systemic vascular resistance and left ventricular afterload. Similar to epinephrine, circulating norepinephrine has β_1- and α-adrenoceptor–mediated effects on the myocardium and systemic vascular beds but binds more avidly to α-adrenoceptors, causing a more robust increase in systemic vascular resistance and increased left ventricular afterload. Therefore, under physiologic stress, modest serum concentrations of epinephrine serve to increase cardiac output through the predominance of β_1-adrenoreceptor–mediated increased inotropy. However, with further stress, higher serum concentrations of epinephrine and norepinephrine may result in a profound increase in left ventricular afterload, further diminishing function of the compromised myocardium.

Decreased renal perfusion leads to the renal release of renin with a subsequent increase in circulating angiotensin II. Angiotensin II has a direct effect on renal tubular reabsorption of sodium and water and secondarily stimulates aldosterone biosynthesis and secretion by the adrenal cortex. Moreover, angiotensin II also stimulates the release of vasopressin from the posterior pituitary resulting in increased reabsorption of free water in the distal collecting tubule. The increase in intravascular volume exerted by the direct renal activity of angiotensin II, and the secondary release of aldosterone and vasopressin, results in an increase in ventricular preload as a mechanism to maintain cardiac output. Paradoxically, however, direct stimulation of the vascular smooth muscle by angiotensin II results in potent vasoconstriction of the splanchnic and renal vasculature beds. In addition, angiotensin II also stimulates norepinephrine synthesis and release from the sympathetic nervous system and epinephrine release from the adrenal medulla. The increase in systemic vascular resistance mediated by the direct activity of angiotensin II and the secondary activation of the neural and humoral sympathetic nervous system engenders increased left ventricular afterload, again diminishing function of the compromised myocardium.

Progressive and sustained increases in left ventricular afterload as may occur with chronic stimulation of the sympathetic nervous system and the renin–angiotensin–aldosterone pathway, result in an inability for the heart to maintain an adequate stroke volume in response to the increased preload, and, ultimately, the ventricle undergoes dilatation. Because ventricular afterload may be defined as the sum of maximal ventricular wall stress, which is characterized by Laplace's law,

$$\text{Wall stress} = \frac{\text{Intraventricular pressure} \times \text{Intraventricular radius}}{2 \times \text{Ventricular wall thickness}}$$

the increase in intraventricular radius and decrease in ventricular wall thickness associated with ventricular dilatation results in a further increase in ventricular afterload, setting up a perpetual and deleterious cycle of worsening myocardial function. In addition to the mechanical compromise, ventricular dilatation also results in an alteration in the papillary muscles and atrioventricular valve apparatus with consequent mitral valve regurgitation, further adding to the decreased cardiac output and myocardial function.

Further changes in ventricular morphology not related to volume overload are termed *myocardial remodeling* and involve two independent mechanisms of myocardial cell death, namely, necrosis and apoptosis, or programmed cell death. Angiotensin II, aldosterone, catecholamines, endothelins, mechanical stretch, and ischemia have all been identified as promoters of myocardial necrosis via the secondary release of inflammatory mediators such as bradykinin, prostaglandins, platelet-derived growth factor, and the interleukins. Myocardial necrosis results in myocardial fibrosis, primarily at the site of injury but also at sites remote from the site of injury. As a result of myocardial fibrosis, compliance of the ventricle decreases, resulting in initial diastolic and subsequent systolic dysfunction. Factors that promote myocardial necrosis may also induce myocardial apoptosis, a process of programmed cell death that occurs without fibrosis or the promotion of inflammation but does result in the continuing loss of cardiac myocytes and decreased myocardial performance. Remodeling of the peripheral vasculature also plays a critical role in determining the hemodynamics and progression of CHF in dilated cardiomyopathy. In addition to the direct vasoconstriction induced by angiotensin II, epinephrine, norepinephrine, and vasopressin, secondary effects on the vasculature include abnormalities in endothelium-dependent vasodilation, including impaired release of nitric oxide, or increased metabolism of nitric oxide to deleterious reactive nitrogen species, such as peroxynitrite.

Clinical Manifestations

The child who presents with dilated cardiomyopathy will have some degree of symptoms of congestion, i.e., CHF, which may be subtle or overt. Conversely, severely depressed cardiac function may result in cardiogenic shock. Physical symptoms and signs of CHF include tachypnea, fatigue, malaise, tachycardia, and hepatomegaly. Chest radiography often shows cardiomegaly with or without pulmonary congestion (Figure 21.1). Dilated cardiomyopathy must be considered in the differential diagnosis for any child who presents with signs and symptoms of CHF with no other identified cause (e.g., unexplained cardiomegaly, unexplained abdominal pain, or abnormal ventricular ectopy) [4]. Echocardiography is the diagnostic test of choice. The heart is enlarged with increased chamber dimensions, thin walls, and reduced systolic function. Mitral and/or tricuspid regurgitation may be present. In the infant with this presentation, cardiac catheterization is often necessary to confirm the absence of an anomalous left coronary artery from the pulmonary artery (ALCAPA), as the sensitivity and specificity of echocardiographic diagnosis of this condition are low enough to warrant cardiac catheterization in the appropriate scenario.

Serum markers such as B-type natriuretic peptide, a hormone secreted by the left ventricle in response to volume overload and excessive ventricular stretching (whether caused by increased volume or pressure) may be sensitive, although not necessarily specific for, dilated cardiomyopathy [11,12]. An endomyocardial biopsy for the diagnosis and management of dilated cardiomyopathy is controversial, but many cardiologists believe it provides useful information. The myocardial cells will almost always show diffuse but nonspecific histologic changes such as myocyte hypertrophy, enlarged and bizarrely shaped nuclei, increased interstitial

edema, and scarring [13,14]. The most common diagnostic finding is myocardial inflammation (i.e., myocarditis). In experienced hands endomyocardial biopsy procedures can usually be safely performed in a child at any age, and, the sooner the biopsy procedure can be performed, the more useful the information. Table 21.2 outlines a comprehensive approach to the diagnosis of dilated cardiomyopathy in children.

Classification and staging of the severity of CHF is often helpful for both management and prognosis. The New York Heart Association (NYHA) classification is widely used for grading the severity of CHF in adults (Table 21.3), although its applicability to infants and children is relatively limited. The Ross classification (Table 21.4) [15] was specifically developed for use in children and is currently used by both the Canadian Cardiovascular Society [15] and the International Cardiomyopathy Registry [16]. Several other scoring systems have been proposed [review in 17] as well. One particular weakness of both the NYHA and Ross classifications is that both scores describe the current symptomatology and do not discriminate between stable and decompensating stages of CHF. In response to this criticism, the American College of Cardiology

TABLE 21.2. Suggested diagnostic approach to the child with dilated cardiomyopathy.

History and physical examination (with attention to recent viral illnesses)
Chest x-ray
Echocardiogram
Electrocardiogram
Laboratory evaluation
   CBC/white blood cell differential, platelet count
   Complete metabolic panel
   Erythrocyte sedimentation rate
   Urinalysis
   Serum carnitine level and acylcarnitine profile
   Urine carnitine level
   Urine organic acid profile
   Serology (generally, acute and convalescent serum obtained at least 2 weeks apart)
      Epstein-Barr virus
      Cytomegalovirus
      Herpes simplex virus
      Toxoplasma gondii
      Coxsackie virus A, B1–B6
      Influenza types A and B
      Mumps
      Poliovirus types 1–3
      Adenovirus
   Thyroid function studies
   Serum cholesterol and triglycerides
   Viral cultures (nasopharyngeal, rectal swabs for enterovirus)
24-Hour Holter (heart rate variability)
Cardiac catheterization with endomyocardial biopsy procedure

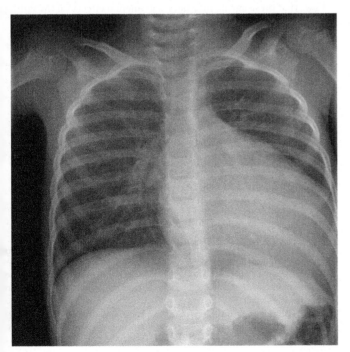

FIGURE 21.1. Characteristic chest x-ray of a child with dilated cardiomyopathy. Note the markedly increased size of the cardiac silhouette.

TABLE 21.3. New York Heart Association staging criteria for congestive heart failure.

Stage	Description
I	No limitation of physical activity. Ordinary physical activity does not cause undue fatigue, palpitation, or dyspnea (shortness of breath).
II	Slight limitation of physical activity. Comfortable at rest, but ordinary physical activity results in fatigue, palpitation, or dyspnea.
III	Marked limitation of physical activity. Comfortable at rest, but less than ordinary activity causes fatigue, palpitation, or dyspnea.
IV	Unable to carry out any physical activity without discomfort. Symptoms of cardiac insufficiency at rest. If any physical activity is undertaken, discomfort is increased.

TABLE 21.4. Ross classification for congestive heart failure in infants and children (modified from 15, 17).

Score	Criteria for infants	Criteria for older children
I	Asymptomatic	Asymptomatic
II	Mild tachypnea or diaphoresis with feeding	Dyspnea on exertion in older children
III	Marked tachypnea or diaphoresis with feeding in infants; prolonged feeding times with growth failure because of congestive heart failure	Marked dyspnea on exertion
IV	Symptoms such as tachypnea, retractions, grunting, or diaphoresis at rest	Symptoms at rest

(ACC)/American Heart Association (AHA) proposed a staging system for the severity of CHF in infants and children that has been recommended by a recent consensus group for widespread use (Table 21.5) [17,18].

Management

The treatment of dilated cardiomyopathy depends on the severity of the ventricular dysfunction, the severity of symptoms, and the underlying cause, if identified. When severity of symptoms requires admission to the PICU, many treatment modalities are available to the physician to provide support for cardiac function and output. There are several guidelines available to assist physicians with the management of CHF in adults, although, given the unique differences between adults and children with CHF, these guidelines are likely not very applicable to the management of pediatric dilated cardiomyopathy. Until relatively recently, there were no published guidelines for children. Practice guidelines have recently been developed and published by the International Society for Heart and Lung Transplantation for the management of CHF in children [17].

When the severity of CHF causes borderline or overt cardiogenic shock, management of the airway, breathing, and circulation is paramount. In addition to supporting cardiac output, reducing metabolic demands and stresses on the heart through the judicious use of sedation, neuromuscular blockade, and mechanical ventilation is also important. However, sedative agents such as midazolam and morphine frequently cause hypotension and should be used cautiously in this scenario. Mechanical ventilatory support also reduces left ventricular afterload and often improves cardiac output as well (see Chapter 3).

TABLE 21.5. ACC/AHA Congestive heart failure (CHF) staging for infants and children.

A	Infants and children with increased risk of developing chf, but who have normal cardiac function and no evidence of cardiac chamber volume overload (e.g., history of exposure to cardiotoxic agents, family history of inherited cardiomyopathy, single-ventricle physiology)
B	Infants and children with abnormal cardiac morphology or cardiac function, with no signs and symptoms of CHF, past or present
C	Infants and children with underlying structural or functional heart disease and past or current signs and symptoms of CHF
D	Infants and children with end-stage CHF requiring continuous infusion of inotropic agents, mechanical cardiac support, cardiac transplantation, or hospice care

Source: Modified from Rosenthal et al. [17] and Hunt et al. [18].

Pharmacologic Agents

Digoxin

A hallmark of therapy for CHF is support of the systolic function of the heart. Digoxin is widely used for the treatment of CHF in infants and children [17], but very limited data exist to suggest any real benefit for either improving hemodynamics or reducing morbidity and mortality. Digoxin is 80% bioavailable and has an onset of action of 0.5–2.0 hr, with a peak effect 2–6 hr following ingestion. With normal renal function, digoxin's half-life is 30–45 hr. Digoxin inhibits Na/K-ATPase, thereby decreasing the transmembrane sodium gradient and increasing intracellular sodium. The transporter also moves potassium out of the extracellular space. Without this driving force for Na^+/Ca^{2+} transport, intracellular calcium accumulates, increasing cardiac contractility. Digoxin also decreases sinoatrial and atrioventricular nodal conduction and increases automaticity of cardiac tissue. Hypokalemia decreases Na/K-ATPase activity and compounds toxicity from all the cardiac glycosides. Dosing recommendations are shown in Table 21.6.

If data are abstracted from the adult literature, digoxin appears to relieve symptoms, although again there are no data to suggest any survival benefit [reviewed in 17]. The study by Rathore et al. [19], in fact, found that higher digoxin blood levels in patients with CHF had higher morbidity than subjects taking placebo. The International Society of Heart and Lung Transplantation, therefore, recommends the use of digoxin only for symptomatic CHF (i.e., stage C) in children.

Inotropes

Inotropic support was previously believed to be the mainstay of therapy for children with end-stage CHF, and, in many cases, children were frequently admitted to the PICU for a brief respite (or *tune-up*) on intravenous inotropic agents such as dobutamine (G. Benzing, personal communication). More recent evidence, however, shows that these agents may have detrimental effects on the failing

TABLE 21.6. Digoxin dosage recommendations for infants and children.*

Age	Total digitalizing dose (μg/kg)[†]		Daily maintenance dose (μg/kg)[‡]	
	PO	IV or IM	PO	IV or IM
Neonates				
Preterm	20–30	15–25	5–7.5	4–6
Full-term	25–35	20–30	6–10	5–8
Infants and Children				
1 month to 2 years	35–60	30–50	10–15	7.5–12
2–5 years	30–40	25–35	7.5–10	6–9
5–10 years	20–35	15–30	5–10	4–8
>10 years	10–15	8–12	2.5–5	2–3
Adults	0.75–1.5 mg	0.5–1 mg	0.125–0.5 mg	0.1–0.4 mg

*Based on lean body weight and normal renal function for age. Decrease maintenance dose for patients with decreased renal function, and decrease total digitalizing dose by 50% in end-stage renal disease.
[†]Give one-half of the total digitalizing dose (TDD) in the initial dose, and then give one-fourth of the TDD in each of two subsequent doses at 6- to 12-hr intervals. Obtain electrocardiogram 6 hr after each dose to assess potential toxicity.
[‡]Divided every 12 hr for infants and children <10 years of age. Given once daily to children >10 years of age and to adults.
Note: IM, intramuscular; IV, intravenous; PO, by mouth.

myocardium. Not only will these agents reduce the number and sensitivity of adrenergic receptors (through β-adrenergic receptor downregulation) [20], but they may also cause damage to the connections between sarcolemma and sarcomere through increased stress on contractile proteins, especially dystrophin [21,22]. In addition, inotropic agents are arrhythmogenic and may precipitate life-threatening arrhythmias in children with dilated cardiomyopathy. Finally, these agents, especially epinephrine and dopamine, may increase myocardial oxygen consumption, thereby worsening cardiac function! However, inotropic support remains the mainstay of treatment for infants and children with severely depressed systolic function (i.e., stage D CHF) or cardiogenic shock. Dobutamine (5–10 μg/kg/min) should be used in the lowest possible doses and for the shortest possible time to minimize these effects. An important adjunct to the acute treatment of CHF in the child with dilated cardiomyopathy is the phosphodiesterase inhibitor milrinone. This bipyridine compound selectively inhibits cyclic nucleotide phosphodiesterase, which leads to increased intracellular cAMP (and therefore increased contractility). Milrinone also decreases afterload and is called an *inodilator* for this reason. In children it has been shown to lower filling pressures and both systemic and pulmonary vascular resistance and pressure, thereby increasing cardiac output without increasing myocardial oxygen consumption (even despite a slight increase in heart rate) [23].

β-Adrenergic Receptor Antagonists (β-Blockers)

Studies in adults suggest that modulation of the normal neurohormonal response to worsening cardiac function with β-adrenergic antagonists is associated with improving left ventricular systolic function and reduced mortality [reviewed in 17,24–26]. The most commonly used drugs for this scenario are carvedilol and metoprolol. Several small case series and cohort studies suggest that β-blockade in children with chronic CHF may also be beneficial [26–33]. Although this therapy is mostly used as a chronic outpatient therapy, its use in the PICU should be considered, especially before discharge, as the potential negative inotropic effects on initiation of these drugs can be closely monitored in the intensive care setting. There are no studies with children looking at the use of intravenous β-blockers in the acute treatment of dilated cardiomyopathy, and these agents should generally be avoided for children with markedly depressed systolic function (stage D) CHF [17]. The International Society for Heart and Lung Transplantation did not make any firm recommendations as to the use of β-blockers in children with stage B or C CHF given the lack of available evidence. An ongoing multicenter, randomized, placebo-controlled trial of carvedilol in children with cardiomyopathy will hopefully address some of these questions and concerns.

Afterload Reduction

If the child's blood pressure can tolerate it, afterload reduction is critically important in the management of CHF in the PICU. Decreased afterload increases cardiac output and reduces myocardial work and therefore myocardial oxygen demand. Sodium nitroprusside (1–3 μg/kg/min) has been used for many years in this scenario. It is a potent afterload reducing agent and requires careful monitoring with indwelling arterial catheters. Its short-half life makes it ideal for the desired effect.

Angiotensin-Converting Enzyme Inhibitors

Angiotensin-converting enzyme (ACE) inhibitors also play a significant role in the treatment of CHF. When viewed in context with the known pathophysiology of CHF, the rationale for using ACE inhibitors in this setting certainly makes sense. Increased activation of the renin–angiotensin–aldosterone neurohormonal axis in children with CHF may be beneficial acutely but over the long term result in progression of symptoms and worsening cardiac function. Treatment with either ACE inhibitors (e.g., enalaprilat, which is administered parenterally, and enalapril, captopril, and lisinopril, which are administered orally) or angiotensin receptor blockers (ARB, e.g., losartan), which competitively inhibit the angiotensin receptor, are associated with significant improvement in symptoms and cardiac function in adults with CHF. For example, two large multicenter trials in adults, the HOPE trial [34] and SOLVD trial [35], demonstrated significantly improved survival in patients taking adequate doses of ACE inhibitors. Again, there are very few data regarding children, although the use of these agents in children with CHF is probably justified [reviewed in 17]. Numerous small observational studies have demonstrated some benefit with the use of ACE inhibitors [17,36–41], although ARB use in children has only been reported in a small series of children with hypertension [42].

Diuretics

One of the single most beneficial acute treatments for CHF is reduction in preload and elimination of the excessive total body water associated with the neurohormonal response to decreased cardiac output. The loop diuretics, including furosemide and ethacrynic acid, are the mainstay of treatment. They inhibit reabsorption of sodium, potassium, and chloride in the thick portion of the ascending limb of the loop of Henle. This results in a net increase in the excretion of water along with potassium and chloride. Care must be taken about the consequence of a contraction metabolic alkalosis when these drugs are used in high or prolonged doses. In addition, excessive diuresis will reduce preload and worsen cardiac function.

Another class of diuretic is the aldosterone antagonist spironolactone. Spironolactone produces its effects in the distal tubule by blocking sodium reabsorption caused by aldosterone. Spironolactone has a mild diuretic effect, but it has major additional advantages from its effects on potassium sparing and blockage of the neurohormonal renin–angiotensin–aldosterone axis. It produces positive effects in patients with dilated cardiomyopathy beyond its diuretic properties and has been recommended by the International Society for Heart and Lung Transplantation despite relatively few studies with children [17].

Arrhythmia Control

Children with dilated cardiomyopathy are at significant risk for abnormal atrial and ventricular rhythm disturbances [4,43]. One rare but treatable cause of dilated cardiomyopathy in children is incessant supraventricular tachycardia [44]. Treatment of this arrhythmia may be all that is necessary to produce resolution of the cardiomyopathy. The management of arrhythmias is covered elsewhere in this textbook.

Immunosuppression

The use of immunosuppressive agents in the treatment of idiopathic dilated cardiomyopathy has no known clinical benefit and is not currently justified by the available evidence [17,45,46]. Immunosuppression in the context of myocarditis is discussed in detail later in this chapter.

Anticoagulation

There is no study that has scientifically investigated the use of anticoagulation in dilated cardiomyopathy; therefore, there are no data to support their use to improve outcome or survival. Warfarin is generally limited to children who have either a previous neurologic embolic event (stoke) or a documented mural thrombus. The International Normalized Ratio level should be maintained between 2 and 3. Aspirin has also not been investigated. Its use is based on individual clinical style. If used, an antiplatelet dose of 6 mg/kg/day is appropriate. The risks and side effects of these drugs should be carefully considered before starting therapy. The International Society of Heart and Lung Transplantation does not currently recommend routine anticoagulation in children with dilated cardiomyopathy [17].

Other Agents

Nesiritide is a recombinant human B-type natriuretic peptide produced through recombinant DNA technology. Nesiritide causes a dose-dependent arterial and venous dilation for both preload and afterload reduction, rapidly decreasing left ventricular filling pressure. It has both diuretic and natriuretic properties. It also affects aldosterone levels and may be beneficial in regulating the neurohormonal axis of congestive heart failure. It should not be used when the patient's blood pressure, vascular resistance, preload, or cardiac output is too low to tolerate the effects of nesiritide. Again, there is no randomized study of children using this drug.

Mechanical Support

The use of mechanical support is appropriate to use in children with dilated cardiomyopathy who have poor clinical progression. These devices are often used as bridges to transplantation and are discussed at length elsewhere in this textbook (see Chapter 17).

Surgery

The hallmark surgery for dilated cardiomyopathy is cardiac transplantation. Recent attempts at improving outcome in patients with end-stage dilated cardiomyopathy by removing a wedge of wall from the left ventricle, left ventriculectomy, also referred to as a Batista procedure [47], have not confirmed its usefulness. The theory is to reduce left ventricular wall stress by reducing left ventricular size because wall stress is directly proportional to the radius of the chamber. It is not currently an option for children.

Dilated cardiomyopathy is the most common indication for transplantation in children. Transplantation is considered for any child with end-stage heart failure who is not likely to live more than 6 months and with no other standard surgical therapy available. An extensive pretransplantation evaluation is necessary to assess both medical necessity and medical acceptability. Although this evaluation is comprehensive, it can be performed in a short time when necessary. A pretransplantation evaluation can take less than 24 hr when the patient's medical condition is critical. Survival for children is 85%–89% at 1 year, 74%–84% at 3 years, and 71%–76% at 5 years (Organ Procurement and Transplantation Network Heart Kaplan-Meier Patient Survival Rates For Transplants Performed: 1995–2002. Based on OPTN data obtained as of May 27, 2005; http://

www.optn.org). Infants have the lowest survival rate at all follow up periods, whereas children between ages 6 and 10 years at transplantation have the highest survival rate. Cardiac transplantation is discussed in greater detail in Chapter 24.

Outcome

The prognosis of dilated cardiomyopathy is variable depending on the population examined. Mortality rate may be as high as 25%–100% depending on age in some series [39]. Outcome from idiopathic dilated cardiomyopathy generally follows the *rule of thirds*: approximately one third of affected children die (or require cardiac transplantation), one third have persistent cardiomyopathy, and one third apparently completely recover [4]. No one clinical feature serves as a consistent predictor of outcome, but several reported features associated with prognosis include age at presentation, arrhythmia, left ventricular hypertrophy on presenting electrocardiogram, family history, and presence of inflammation on endomyocardial biopsy [4,48].

Myocarditis

The subject of myocarditis raises many controversial issues. It is defined as inflammation of heart muscle with cardiac dysfunction. The child with myocarditis who presents to the PICU will most certainly have either significant myocardial dysfunction (CHF) or rhythm disturbances. The issues discussed in the section on dilated cardiomyopathy are therefore similarly pertinent to the child with myocarditis and CHF.

Incidence

The true incidence of inflammatory cardiomyopathy has been difficult to ascertain for a number of reasons [49]. First, the clinical manifestations of myocardial inflammation represent a broad spectrum of disease, with the distinct probability that the majority of cases remain asymptomatic and, therefore, generally undiagnosed. Second, because of the lack of specificity and sensitivity of the endomyocardial biopsy, the diagnosis of clinically apparent myocardial inflammation has been made on clinical grounds without the benefit of a unifying definition. Finally, the proposed definition for inflammatory cardiomyopathy [50] requires histologic, immunologic, and immunohistochemical evidence for myocardial inflammation, yet these criteria are not specifically characterized and are based on endomyocardial biopsy, the specificity and sensitivity of which is generally lacking as a diagnostic tool [51–57]. Nevertheless, myocardial inflammation has been demonstrated in nearly 20% of postmortem studies of young adults who experienced sudden death [58–61] and in 16% of infants who died from sudden infant death syndrome [62]. Although inflammation of the heart is a relatively nonspecific finding on postmortem examination, these studies suggest that myocardial inflammation may be relatively common and play an important associative role in mortality.

Etiology

Although myocardial inflammation may occur in response to systemic disease and toxins, it is clear from polymerase chain reaction (PCR) data that infections, specifically viral infections, are the most common cause of myocarditis in North America and Europe, whereas *Trypanosoma cruzi* (Chagas disease) and *Corynebacterium diphtheriae* (diphtheria) remain common etiologic factors in some underdeveloped countries [53,63]. Various viruses have been demonstrated as etiologic factors in myocarditis, with adenovirus and coxsackie virus B generally considered as the most common pathogens [64–81].

Pathogenesis and Pathophysiology

Recently, a greater comprehension of the pathogenesis of viral myocarditis has been gained from animal models of the disease. Although viral infection mediates a degree of direct myocyte injury, more importantly, viral invasion and replication initiate the host immune response, which ultimately serves as the principle mediator of myocardial injury and dysfunction [66,82,83]. Based on animal studies, the pathogenesis of myocardial injury in response to viral infection has been divided into three temporal stages: the acute phase, the subacute phase, and the chronic phase [83,85]. Correspondingly, Liu et al. [83] introduced the concept that viral myocarditis represents a continuum of three distinct disease processes: viral infection, secondary immune response and autoimmunity, and dilated cardiomyopathy, although the transition from one stage to the next may be indistinct. Accordingly, the pathogenesis, diagnosis, and management at each individual stage differ considerably.

The Acute Phase (Viral Infection)

The acute phase, days 1–3 following infection, is characterized by direct viral cytotoxicity and focal myofibrillary necrosis. In human disease, viral infection is most frequently associated with coxsackie virus B and adenovirus infections, raising the question of the apparent cardiac tropism demonstrated by these two viruses. The coxsackie virus–adenovirus receptor (CAR), a member of the immunoglobulin superfamily of receptors mapped to chromosome 2q11.2 [66,85,86], appears to mediate the attachment and internalization of the coxsackie virus and adenovirus genome [85–87]. In addition, the complement deflecting protein decay accelerating factor (DAF, CD55) is an important co-receptor in the internalization of coxsackie virus B, whereas other cell surface adhesion molecules serve this role in the internalization of adenoviruses [88–91]. It is certainly conceivable that the individual expression of these receptors could play a primary role in determining individual susceptibilities to the development of myocarditis.

The Subacute Phase (Secondary Immune Response and Autoimmunity)

The subacute phase, days 4–14 following infection, is characterized by the host immune response to viral invasion, replication, and proliferation, which, if unregulated, may contribute to additional myocardial injury as a principal determinant of pathogenesis. This phase is heralded by tissue macrophage activation and the consequent production of inflammatory cytokines, such as interleukin (IL)-1β, IL-2, tumor necrosis factor (TNF)-α, and interferon (IFN)-γ, leading to the recruitment of natural killer cells and cytotoxic T lymphocytes, which play an important role in eliminating virally infected myocytes and limiting viral replication. In addition to this classic cellular immunity, humoral immunity is also important during this phase, with titers of neutralizing antibodies closely correlating with viral elimination. Moreover, the cytokine-induced activation of nuclear factor (NF)-κB results in the transcription

and translation of the inducible isoform of nitric oxide synthase, leading to the production of nitric oxide in high concentration. Although nitric oxide appears to be beneficial in viral elimination [92–96], in murine models of autoimmune myocarditis, nitric oxide synthase inhibition results in reduced inflammation and mortality [97,98], suggesting a potential detrimental role for nitric oxide in mediating cellular injury. Finally, in addition to the release of inflammatory cytokines, there is also increased expression of anti-inflammatory cytokines, such as IL-10 and IL-12, with consequent protection against immune-mediated cellular injury, suggesting a complex interplay between proinflammatory and antiinflammatory cytokines during this phase of myocarditis [99–103]. The pattern of cytokine activation may be instrumental in differentiating a T_H1 versus T_H2 type of T-cell response, with T_H1 cells producing proinflammatory cytokines and contributing primarily to cell-mediated immunity and T_H2 cells contributing primarily to the augmentation of humoral immunity.

The Chronic Phase (Dilated Cardiomyopathy)

The chronic phase, days 15–90 following viral infection, is characterized by diffuse myocardial fibrosis and the development of dilated cardiomyopathy. There is a growing body of evidence suggesting that viral myocarditis and idiopathic dilated cardiomyopathy represent a continuum of disease [82,84,104,105], yet the pathogenetic mechanisms leading to the transition from acute myocarditis to dilated cardiomyopathy remain obscure. Sustained activation of T cells may occur in response to the persistence of viral RNA in myocardial tissue [82–84,106], or recurrence of infection may elicit a T-cell response, causing additional myocardial damage via autoimmune mechanisms [82–84,107]. Additionally, apoptosis, or *programmed cell death* of myocardial cells, may occur in response to viral infection [82–84,108]. Whether any of these mechanisms of pathogenesis from myocarditis to dilated cardiomyopathy are important, or whether an as yet unidentified mechanism is predominant pathophysiologically, remains to be determined. Nevertheless, consistent with animal models, there appears to be a genetic predisposition for the development of dilated cardiomyopathy [109–112], suggesting that certain individuals are predisposed to the transition from acute viral myocarditis to dilated cardiomyopathy.

Clinical Presentation and Diagnosis

Often preceded by a viral prodrome, the clinical presentation of myocarditis varies considerably, from asymptomatic in the majority of cases, to mild lethargy and malaise, to dysrhythmias, fulminant heart failure, and death. The variability and nonspecificity of the clinical presentation emphasizes that no symptomatology is pathognomonic for myocarditis. Moreover, because any cause of myocardial dysfunction or congestive heart failure may mimic myocarditis, the differential diagnosis is largely encompassing. Signs and symptoms of congestive heart failure, including respiratory distress, diaphoresis, poor feeding, irritability, gallop rhythm, decreased peripheral pulses, and hepatomegaly, are common. The chest x-ray typically demonstrates evidence of cardiomegaly, increased pulmonary vascular markings, and increased interstitial fluid, with or without pleural effusions. The electrocardiogram classically demonstrates sinus tachycardia with low-voltage QRS complexes and ST-T wave flattening. A variety of dysrhythmias, occasionally as the primary clinical manifestation, have been described in children, contributing significantly to morbidity and mortality [53,113–117]. Echocardiography frequently demonstrates globally reduced ventricular function—most notably in, but not restricted to, the left ventricle, increased ventricular cavity dimensions, ventricular wall thinning, atrioventricular valve regurgitation, segmental wall motion abnormalities, and pericardial effusion.

Selected laboratory tests may provide additional information in the evaluation of children with suspected viral myocarditis. The MB fraction of creatine kinase [53,63,84,118] and cardiac troponin levels [53,63,84,119–122] are relatively specific markers of myocardial injury that may be elevated in children with myocarditis. In conjunction with a suspicious clinical scenario, an increased serum C-reactive protein and an increased lymphocyte-predominant, peripheral white blood cell count may serve as additional markers for myocarditis [53,63,123], whereas traditionally, a fourfold rise in acute and convalescent viral antibody titers has been used to establish a diagnosis of viral myocarditis [82,84]. Experimental markers of acute myocarditis appear promising as well, including serum levels of soluble Fas and soluble Fas ligand, myosin antibodies, and adenine nucleotide translocator antibodies [63,84,124–126].

The endomyocardial biopsy is still considered by many to be the *gold standard* for the diagnosis of viral myocarditis; however, the specificity and sensitivity of histologic criteria remain unacceptable as a mode of diagnosis [127–129]. The Dallas criteria, established in 1986 by consensus among a group of pathologists and later revised by the World Health Organization panel, were developed to unify the histologic criteria for the diagnosis of myocarditis (Table 21.7). Under this system of classification, biopsy specimens demonstrating light microscopic evidence of infiltrating lymphocytes and necrosis are considered diagnostic for active myocarditis; specimens demonstrating only lymphocyte infiltration in the absence of necrosis are classified as borderline myocarditis; and specimens showing absence of both lymphocyte infiltration and necrosis are classified as negative for myocarditis. Pathologists' interpretations of endomyocardial biopsy specimens using the Dallas criteria, however, have remained highly variable and controversial [51–57]. Moreover, even if pathologist consensus were achievable, the areas of myocardial inflammation and necrosis are erratically dispersed throughout the myocardium and are therefore frequently missed in endomyocardial biopsy specimens (spatial variability) [130]. Furthermore, endomyocardial biopsy specimens

obtained late in the course of disease may demonstrate fibrosis and chronic inflammation that will also be misinterpreted by the Dallas criteria (temporal variability) [130].

Finally, the risk of endomyocardial biopsy may be prohibitively high for critically ill children with suspected myocarditis, particularly those weighing less than 10 kg [129]. Nevertheless, advanced molecular biology techniques, such as PCR, may increase the diagnostic sensitivity and specificity of the endomyocardial biopsy. Utilizing this technique, it is possible to detect evidence of viral infection in endomyocardial biopsy specimens obtained even in the late stages of myocarditis, when histologic evidence is often equivocal [53,127,131,132]. Polymerase chain reaction techniques, however, may obviate the need for endomyocardial biopsy, as evidence of viral infection in extracardiac tissues or secretions may provide evidence for the diagnosis of viral myocarditis. For example, in a series of seven patients with suspected myocarditis, PCR analysis of tracheal aspirates yielded identical results to PCR analysis of endomyocardial biopsy specimens, suggesting a possible corroborative role for this less invasive diagnostic method [133].

Management

The most important aspect for treatment of the child with viral myocarditis is appropriate early diagnosis, allowing for early intervention and prevention of further deterioration in myocardial structure and function. Ideally, critically ill children with viral myocarditis should be managed in a pediatric referral center with critical care, cardiology, and cardiothoracic surgery capabilities. Supportive care remains the mainstay of therapy, with treatment goals falling into three categories: (1) reduction of high ventricular preload, (2) reduction of ventricular afterload, and (3) optimization of tissue oxygen delivery.

Supportive Care

Children presenting with signs and symptoms of CHF should be managed aggressively with the institution of inotropic support, afterload reduction, and diuresis. When utilizing inotropic agents such as dopamine and epinephrine, care must be employed to avoid excessive α-adrenoreceptor–mediated vasoconstriction with the consequent increase in left ventricular afterload. Placement of an indwelling arterial catheter for continuous arterial blood pressure observation and arterial blood gas assessment is an important aspect of cardiorespiratory monitoring. Moreover, placement of a central venous catheter in the superior vena cava (internal jugular or subclavian vein) allows for monitoring of central venous pressure and assessment of superior vena cava oxygen saturations, which correlate with mixed venous oxygen saturations, permitting assessment of oxygen delivery adequacy [134,135]. Although placement of a pulmonary artery catheter has not been shown to improve outcome in randomized, controlled trials in critically ill adults, the added information, including mixed venous oxygen saturation, pulmonary capillary wedge pressure, cardiac output, systemic vascular resistance, oxygen delivery, and oxygen consumption, available from a pulmonary artery catheter may prove invaluable in the titration of supportive care and should be given due consideration.

Children with cardiogenic shock resulting from viral myocarditis display varying degrees of respiratory distress, often with impending respiratory failure. For multiple reasons, positive pressure mechanical ventilation proves to be therapeutic and should be

TABLE 21.7. Dallas criteria for myocarditis.

Myocarditis
  Inflammatory infiltrate of the myocardium (mild, moderate, severe; focal, confluent, diffuse):
    Lymphocytic
    Eosinophilic
    Neutrophilic
    Giant cell
    Granulomatous
    Mixed
and
  Necrosis and/or degeneration of adjacent myocytes (not typical of ischemic damage):
    Frank necrosis
    Myocyte vacuolization
    Irregular cellular outlines
    Cellular disruption with lymphocytes closely applied to the sarcolemma
Borderline myocarditis
  Sparse infiltrate and/or no myocyte damage

instituted early in the course of this disease, preferably before the onset of complete cardiovascular collapse. Mechanical ventilatory support eliminates the work of breathing, reducing respiratory muscle oxygen consumption and lactate production, and optimizing the oxygen consumption/oxygen delivery relationship. More importantly, positive pressure mechanical ventilation augments left ventricular ejection, reducing left ventricular afterload and left ventricular stroke work, thereby improving hemodynamics. Furthermore, as lung compliance is reduced in the presence of pulmonary edema, positive pressure mechanical ventilation allows for optimal lung recruitment toward normal functional residual capacity. Because pulmonary vascular resistance, hence right ventricular afterload, is optimal at normal functional residual capacity, positive pressure mechanical ventilation may also reduce right ventricular stroke work.

Immunosuppressive Therapy

Although there is consensus acknowledgement that the host immune response is primarily responsible for the myocardial injury and dysfunction associated with myocarditis, the use of immunosuppressive treatment regimens remains highly controversial. To date, the two most studied and utilized regimens include the use of intravenous immunoglobulin (IVIG) and systemic corticosteroids. Used extensively and successfully in the treatment of children with myocardial inflammation associated with Kawasaki disease [136,137], IVIG has been poorly studied in patients with documented viral myocarditis. In the only pediatric study published to date [138], children with presumed viral myocarditis treated with 2 g/kg IVIG over 24 hr were more likely to achieve normal left ventricular function during the 12 months of follow up and had a higher likelihood of survival when compared with historical controls. However, patients in the treated group were also more likely to have received intravenous inotropic support during the acute phase of their illness and acute and chronic therapy with systemic afterload reduction. This is particularly important, because left ventricular function was assessed echocardiographically using the shortening fraction, an afterload-dependent measure of ventricular function, raising considerable questions regarding the validity of the findings. Moreover, in a randomized, placebo-controlled study in adults with recent-onset dilated cardiomyopathy, IVIG failed to demonstrate any benefit in left ventricular function [46]. Nevertheless, despite a lack of good clinical data for children or adults, IVIG is still considered by some as standard therapy for the treatment of acute viral myocarditis [53,63,84].

To date, no large, placebo-controlled studies utilizing corticosteroids in the treatment of myocarditis have been performed with children. However, in the first randomized, controlled study utilizing corticosteroids [139], adults with idiopathic dilated cardiomyopathy were randomly assigned to treatment with either prednisone or placebo. Patients were classified as either *reactive* or *nonreactive* based on results of endomyocardial biopsy utilizing a modification of the Dallas criteria. Although patients with both reactive and nonreactive cardiomyopathy in the prednisone group showed statistically significant improvement in left ventricular function at 3 months when compared to the control group, this improvement disappeared by 9 and 15 months follow-up, respectively. Furthermore, close inspection of the data suggests a possible deleterious effect of prednisone treatment.

These findings are substantially corroborated in subsequent adult studies utilizing corticosteroids alone or in combination with other immunosuppressive agents, such as cyclosporine and azathioprine [140,141]. Several small, uncontrolled studies utilizing various combinations of immunosuppressive agents, including prednisone, OKT3, cyclosporine, and azathioprine, have shown benefit in the treatment of viral myocarditis in children. However, a well-designed, placebo-controlled, prospective trial has yet to be performed [142–144]. Alternatively, some studies in animal models have suggested that the use of immunosuppressive regimens for the treatment of viral myocarditis may increase mortality. [53,145]. The answer to this apparent conundrum may simply be a matter of timing. For example, immunosuppression during the acute phase may be contraindicated, as it may impair viral clearance and lead to persistence of infection and worsened myocardial injury, whereas immunosuppression during the subacute phase may limit autoimmune injury and improve recovery. The difficulty with this concept, however, lies in the fact that in many cases there is no clear distinction between these disease phases.

Antiviral Agents

The continued improvement in diagnostic techniques may usher in an era of effective treatment of myocarditis with antiviral agents, with several experimental agents for the treatment of enteroviral infection being currently available [146], including pleconaril, a drug that inhibits coxsackieviral entry and replication [53]. In addition, several studies have suggested that those patients with myocarditis secondary to either coxsackie virus and adenovirus may benefit from ribavirin if started early in the disease course [147,148]. The initial presentation in the majority of cases of viral myocarditis, however, is probably during the subacute or secondary immune response and autoimmunity stage at a time when antiviral therapy will most likely be of limited therapeutic benefit.

Nonconventional Support

Although supportive care and maximal medical therapy are usually sufficient in the care and management of children with myocarditis, a subset of patients may require nonconventional therapeutic measures. Given the overall prognosis for recovery, mechanical extracorporeal life support (ECLS) with extracorporeal membrane oxygenation (ECMO) or transthoracic placement of a left or biventricular assist device (LVAD/BVAD) should be instituted when more conventional measures fail. Although the choice of mechanical support ultimately will depend on local institutional experience, both methods of ECLS have been used in children with acute myocarditis and severe heart failure. Venoarterial ECMO requires cannulation of the carotid artery and internal jugular vein, whereas cannulation for VAD requires a midline sternotomy and cardiotomy. The most common complication of ECLS is hemorrhage; VAD may be more advantageous in this regard, as this method of ECLS requires less systemic anticoagulation than ECMO. Mechanical complications are also less frequent with VAD than with ECMO. An additional method of mechanical cardiopulmonary support that has had widespread use in the adult population is the intraaortic balloon pump (IABP). However, experience with this method in children is limited. Furthermore, isolated left ventricular failure is more commonly encountered in adults than in children, and IABP will not support the right ventricle and lungs.

Heart Transplantation

Heart transplantation is the final option for the management of children with severe heart failure secondary to myocarditis.

Patients with rapidly progressive cardiac failure and cardiogenic shock may benefit from mechanical cardiopulmonary support, which can serve as an effective bridge to heart transplantation [149,150]. However, as patients with fulminant myocarditis generally have an excellent long-term prognosis [144,151,152], these children should be given a sufficient period of time to demonstrate recovery before consideration for transplantation. The 5-year survival rate following heart transplantation in the Pediatric Heart Transplant Study was approximately 70% [153], and, with the development of newer immunosuppressants, heart transplantation is becoming a more viable alternative for the treatment of children with severe heart failure following myocarditis.

Prognosis

The clinical course of fulminate myocarditis may lead to early death, but the overall prognosis of myocarditis in children appears to be better than that for idiopathic dilated cardiomyopathy. Survival may approach 80%–100% [144]. In addition, the long-term cardiac function of children with myocarditis is excellent; long-term follow-up studies of 14 of 15 children who survived biopsy-proven myocarditis showed that all had normal global left ventricular function and no clinical symptoms (H. Wiles, unpublished data). None of these children has developed chronic dilated cardiomyopathy.

References

1. Richardson P, McKenna W, Bristow M, et al. Report of the 1995 World Health Organization International Society and Federation of Cardiology Task Force on the Definition and Classification of Cardiomyopathies. Circulation 1996;93:841–842.
2. Denfield SW, Gajarski RJ, Towbin JA. Cardiomyopathies. In: Garson A, Bricker JT, Fisher DJ, Neish SR, (eds). The Science and Practice of Pediatric Cardiology, 2nd ed. Baltimore, MD: Williams & Wilkins; 1998:1851–1883.
3. Lipshultz SE, Sleeper LA, Towbin JA, et al. The incidence of pediatric cardiomyopathy in two regions of the United States. N Engl J Med 2003;348:1647–1655.
4. Wiles HB, McArthur PD, Taylor AB, et al. Prognostic features of children with idiopathic dilated cardiomyopathy. Am J Cardiol 1991;68:1372–1376.
5. Towbin JA, Solaro RJ. Genetics of dilated cardiomyopathy: more genes that kill. J Am Coll Cardiol 2004;44:2041–2043.
6. Towbin JA, Bowles NE. Sarcoglycan, the heart, and skeletal muscles: new treatment, old drug? J Clin Invest 2001;107:153–154.
7. Berko BA, Swift M. X-Linked dilated cardiomyopathy. N Engl J Med 1987;316:1186–1191.
8. Towbin JA, Hejtmancik JF, Brink P, et al. X-linked dilated cardiomyopathy: molecular genetic evidence of linkage to the Duchenne muscular dystrophy (dystrophin) gene at the Xp21 locus. Circulation 1993;87:1854–1865.
9. Feng J, Yan J, Buzin CH, Towbin JA, Sommer SS. Mutations in the dystrophin gene are associated with sporadic dilated cardiomyopathy. Mol Genet Metab 2002;77:119–126.
10. Schlant RC, Sonnenblick EH. Pathophysiology of heart failure. In: Hurst JW, Logue RB, Rackley CE, et al. (eds). The Heart, Arteries and Veins, 6th ed. New York: McGraw-Hill; 1986:319–345.
11. Westerlind A, Wahlander H, Lindstedt G, Lundberg PA, Holmgren D. Clinical signs of heart failure are associated with increased levels of natriuretic peptide types B and A in children with congenital heart defects or cardiomyopathy. Acta Paediatr 2004;93:340–345.
12. Nasser N, Perles Z, Rein AJ, Nir A. NT-proBNP as a marker for persistent cardiac disease in children with history of dilated cardiomyopa-

thy and myocarditis. Pediatr Cardiol 2005;25, www.springerlink.cor online publication (early release).
13. Wiles H, Lambiotte C, Gillette P, Sens M, Nicholson J. Morphometri analysis of endomyocardial biopsy specimen from children wit ventricular tachycardia. Pace 1991;14:656.
14. Wiles HB, Gillette PC, Upshur JK, Harley RA. Endomyocardial biops diagnosis of myocarditis/cardiomyopathy in children presenting wit incessant ventricular ectopy. Circulation 1990;82:III223.
15. Ross RD, Daniels SR, Schwartz DC, Hannon DW, Shukla R, Kaplan S Plasma norepinephrine levels in infants and children with congestiv heart failure. Am J Cardiol 1987;59:911–914.
16. Johnstone DE, Abdulla A, Arnold JM, et al. Diagnosis and manage ment of heart failure. Canadian Cardiovascular Society. Can J Cardio 1994;10:613–631.
17. Rosenthal D, Chrisant MR, Edens E, et al. International Society fo Heart and Lung Transplantation: practice guidelines for managemen of heart failure in children. J Heart Lung Transplant 2004;23 1313–1333.
18. Hunt SA, Baker DW, Chin MH, et al. ACC/AHA guidelines for th evaluation and management of chronic heart failure in the adul executive summary. A report of the American College of Cardiology American Heart Association Task Force on Practice Guidelines (Com mittee to revise the 1995 Guidelines for the Evaluation and Manage ment of Heart Failure). J Am Coll Cardiol 2001;38:2101–2113.
19. Rathore SS, Curtis JP, Wang Y, Bristow MR, Krumholz HM. Associa tion of serum digoxin concentration and outcomes in patients with heart failure. JAMA 2003;289:871–878.
20. Smiley RM, Kwatra MM, Schwinn DA. New developments in cardio vascular adrenergic receptor pharmacology: molecular mechanism and clinical relevance. J Cardiothorac Vasc Anesth 1998;12:80–95.
21. Vatta M, Stetson SJ, Perez-Verdia A, et al. Molecular remodelling o dystrophin in patients with end-stage cardiomyopathies and reversa in patients on assistance-device therapy. Lancet 2002;359:936–941.
22. Vatta M, Stetson SJ, Jimenez S, et al. Molecular normalization of dys trophin in the failing left and right ventricle of patients treated with either pulsatile or continuous flow-type ventricular assist devices. J Am Coll Cardiol 2004;43:811–817.
23. Chang AC, Atz AM, Wernovsky G, Burke RP, Wessel DL. Milrinone systemic and pulmonary hemodynamic effects in neonates after cardiac surgery. Crit Care Med 1995;23:1907–1914.
24. Clark AL, Cleland JG. The control of adrenergic function in heart failure: therapeutic intervention. Heart Fail Rev 2000;5:101–114.
25. Fonarow GC. When to initiate beta-blockers in heart failure: is it ever too early? Curr Heart Fail Rep 2005;2:94–99.
26. Ross RD. Medical management of chronic heart failure in children. Am J Cardiovasc Drugs 2001;1:37–44.
27. Bruns LA, Canter CE. Should beta-blockers be used for the treatment of pediatric patients with chronic heart failure? Paediatr Drugs 2002;4:771–778.
28. Bruns LA, Christant MK, Lamour JM, et al. Carvedilol as therapy in pediatric heart failure: an initial multicenter experience. J Pediatr 2001;138:505–511.
29. Azeka E, Franchini Ramires JA, Valler C, Aclides Bocchi E. Delisting of infants and children from the heart transplantation waiting list after carvedilol treatment. J Am Coll Cardiol 2002;40:2034–2038.
30. Laer S, Mir TS, Behn F, et al. Carvedilol therapy in pediatric patients with congestive heart failure: a study investigating clinical and pharmacokinetic parameters. Am Heart J 2002;143:916–922.
31. Williams RV, Tani LY, Shaddy RE. Intermediate effects of treatment with metoprolol or carvedilol in children with left ventricular systolic dysfunction. J Heart Lung Transplant 2002;21:906–909.
32. Giardini A, Formigari R, Bronzetti G, et al. Modulation of neurohormonal activity after treatment of children in heart failure with carvedilol. Cardiol Young 2003;13:333–336.
33. Rusconi P, Gomez-Marin O, Rossigque-Gonzalez M, et al. Carvedilol in children with cardiomyopathy: 3-year experience at a single institution. J Heart Lung Transplant 2004;23:832–838.

34. Yusuf S, Sleight P, Pogue J, Bosch J, Davies R, Dagenais G. Effects of an angiotensin-converting-enzyme inhibitor, ramipril, on cardiovascular events in high-risk patients. The Heart Outcomes Prevention Evaluation Study Investigators. N Engl J Med 2000;342:145–153.

35. Anonymous. Effect of enalapril on survival in patients with reduced left ventricular ejection fractions and congestive heart failure. The SOLVD Investigators. N Engl J Med 1991;325:293–302.

36. Bengur AR, Beekman RH, Rocchini AP, Crowley DC, Schork MA, Rosenthal A. Acute hemodynamic effects of captopril in children with a congestive or restrictive cardiomyopathy. Circulation 1991;83:523–527.

37. Leversha AM, Wilson NJ, Clarkson PM, et al. Efficacy and dosage of enalapril in congenital and acquired heart disease. Arch Dis Child 1994;70:35–39.

38. Seguchi M, Nakazawa M, Momma K. Effect of enalapril on infants and children with congestive heart failure. Cardiol Young 1992;2:14–19.

39. Stern H, Weil J, Genz T, Vogt W, Buhlmeyer K. Captopril in children with dilated cardiomyopathy: acute and long-term effects in a prospective study of hemodynamic and hormonal effects. Pediatr Cardiol 1990;11:22–28.

40. Schiffman H, Gawlik L, Wessel A. Treatment effects of captopril in neonates, infants, and young children with congestive heart failure. Z Kardiol 1996;85:709.

41. Lewis AB, Chabot M. The effect of treatment with angiotensin-converting enzyme inhibitors on survival of pediatric patients with dilated cardiomyopathy. Pediatr Cardiol 1993;14:9–12.

42. Marino MR, Vachharajani NN. Pharmacokinetics of irbesartan are not altered in special populations. J Cardiovasc Pharmacol 2002;40:112–122.

43. Friedman RA, Moak JP, Garson A, Jr. Clinical course of idiopathic dilated cardiomyopathy in children. J Am Coll Cardiol 1991;18:152–156.

44. Lashus AG, Case CL, Gillette PC. Catheter ablation treatment of supraventricular tachycardia-induced cardiomyopathy. Arch Pediatr Adolesc Med 1997;151:264–266.

45. O'Connell JB. Immunosuppression for dilated cardiomyopathy. N Engl J Med 1989;321:1119–1121.

46. McNamara DM, Holubkov R, Starling RC, et al. Controlled trial of intravenous immune globulin in recent-onset dilated cardiomyopathy. Circulation 2001;103:2254–2259.

47. Gorcsan J, III, Feldman AM, Kormos RL, Mandarino WA, Demetris AJ, Batista RJ. Heterogeneous immediate effects of partial left ventriculectomy on cardiac performance. Circulation 1998;97:839–842.

48. Griffin ML, Hernandez A, Martin TC, et al. Dilated cardiomyopathy in infants and children. J Am Coll Cardiol 1988;11:139–144.

49. Tobin JA. Myocarditis. In: Allen HD, Gutgesell HP, Clark EB, Driscoll DJ, eds. Moss and Adams' Heart Disease in Infants, Children, and Adolescents Including the Fetus and Young Adult, 6th ed. Philadelphia: Lippincott, Williams & Wilkins, 2001:1197–1215.

50. Richardson P, McKenna W, Bristow M, et al. Report of the 1995 World Health Organization/International Society and Federation of Cardiology Task Force on the Definition and Classification of cardiomyopathies. Circulation 1996;93:841–842.

51. Billingham ME. Acute myocarditis: a diagnostic dilemma. Br Heart J 1987;58:6–8.

52. Chow LH, Sears TD, McManus BM. Insensitivity of right ventricular endomyocardial biopsy in the diagnosis of myocarditis: whither the gold standard [abstr]? J Am Coll Cardiol 1989;13(Suppl A):253A.

53. Levi D, Alejos J. Diagnosis and treatment of pediatric viral myocarditis. Curr Opin Cardiol 2001;16:77–83.

54. Lie JT. Myocarditis and endomyocardial biopsy in unexplained heart failure: a diagnosis in search of a disease. Ann Intern Med 1998;109:525–528.

55. Peters NS, Poole-Wilson PA. Myocarditis, continuing clinical and pathological confusion. Am Heart J 1991;121:942–946.

56. Pisani B, Taylor DO, Mason JW. Inflammatory myocardial disease and cardiomyopathies. Am J Med 1997;102:459–469.

57. Shanes JG, Gahli J, Billingham ME, et al. Interobserver variability in the pathologic interpretation of endomyocardial biopsy results. Circulation 1987;75:401–405.

58. Drory Y, Turetz Y, Hiss Y, et al. Sudden unexpected death in persons less than 40 years of age. Am J Cardiol 1991;68:1388–1392.

59. McCaffrey FM, Braden DS, Strong WB. Sudden cardiac death in young athletes: a review. Am J Dis Child 1991;145:177–183.

60. Phillips M, Robinowitz M, Higgins JR, Boran KJ, Reed T, Virmani R. Sudden cardiac death in Air Force recruits: a 20-year review. JAMA 1986;256:2696–2699.

61. Wesslen L, Pahlson C, Lindquist O, et al. An increase in sudden unexpected cardiac deaths among young Swedish orienteers during 1979–1992. Eur Heart J 1996;17:902–910.

62. Rasten-Almqvist P, Eksborg S, Rajs J. Heart weight in infants: a comparison between sudden death infant syndrome and other causes of death. Acta Paediatr 2000;89:1062–1067.

63. Batra AS, Lewis AB. Acute myocarditis. Curr Opin Pediatr 2001;13:234–239.

64. Ainger LE, Lawyer NG, Fitch CW. Neonatal rubella myocarditis. Br Heart J 1966;28:691–697.

65. Barbaro G, Di Lorenzo G, Grisorio B, et al. Incidence of dilated cardiomyopathy and detection of HIV in myocardial cells of HIV-positive patients. N Engl J Med 1998;339:1093–1099.

66. Bowles KR, Gibson J, Wu J, et al. Genomic organization and chromosomal localization of the human coxsackievirus B–adenovirus receptor gene. Hum Genet 1999;105:354–359.

67. Chaundry S, Jaski BE. Fulminant mumps myocarditis. Ann Intern Med 1989;110:569–570.

68. Fishman W, Kraus ME, Zabkar J, et al. Infectious mononucleosis and fatal myocarditis. Chest 1977;72:535–538.

69. Fraisse A, Pout O, Zandotti C, et al. Epstein-Barr virus: an unusual cause of acute myocarditis in children. Arch Pediatr 2000;7:752–755.

70. Fukae S, Ashzawa N, Morikawa S, et al. A fatal case of fulminant myocarditis with human herpesvirus infection. Intern Med 2000;39:632–636.

71. Grumbach IM, Heim A, Pring-Akerbloml I, et al. Adenoviruses and enteroviruses as pathogens in myocarditis and dilated cardiomyopathy. Acta Cardiol 1999;54:83–88.

72. Hirschman ZS, Hammer SG. Coxsackie virus myopericarditis: a microbiological and clinical review. Am J Cardiol 1974;34:224–232.

73. Lipshultz SE, Easley KA, Orav EJ, et al. Left ventricular structure and function in children infected with human immunodeficiency virus: the prospective P2C2 HIV Multicenter Study. Circulation 1998;97:1246–1256.

74. Lorber A, Zonis A, Maisuls E, et al. The scale of myocardial involvement in varicella myocarditis. Int J Cardiol 1988;20:257–262.

75. Martin AB, Webber S, Fricker FJ, et al. Acute myocarditis: rapid diagnosis by PCR in children. Circulation 1994;90:330–339.

76. Matsumori A, Yutani C, Ikeda Y, et al. Hepatitis C virus from the hearts of patients with myocarditis and cardiomyopathy. Lab Invest 2000;80:1137–1142.

77. Nigro G, Bastianon V, Colloridi V, et al. Human parvovirus B19 infection in infancy associated with acute and chronic lymphocytic myocarditis and high cytokine levels: report of 3 cases and review. Clin Infect Dis 2000;31:65–69.

78. Okabe M, Fukuda K, Arakawa K, Kikuchi M. Chronic variant myocarditis associated with hepatitis C virus infection. Circulation 1997;96:22–24.

79. Proby CM, Hackett S, Gupta S, et al: Acute myopericarditis in influenza A infection. Q J Med 1986;60:887–892.

80. Schonian U, Crombach M, Maser S, et al. Cytomegalovirus associated heart muscle disease. Eur Heart J 1995;16(Suppl O):46–49.

81. Schwonengerdt KO, Ni J, Denfield SW, et al. Parvovirus B19 as a cause of myocarditis and cardiac allograft rejection: diagnosis using the polymerase chain reaction (PCR). Circulation 1997;96:3549–3554.

82. Kawai C. From myocarditis to cardiomyopathy: mechanisms of inflammation and cell death. Learning from the past for the future. Circulation 1999;99:1091–1100.

83. Liu P, Aitken K, Kong YY, et al: Essential role for the tyrosine kinase p56lck in coxsackievirus B3 mediated heart disease. Nat Med 2000;6:429–434.

84. Feldman AM, McNamara D: Myocarditis. N Engl J Med 2000;343:1 388–1398.

85. Bergelson JM. Receptors mediating adenovirus attachment and internalization. Biochem Pharmacol 1999;57:975–979.

86. Bergelson JM, Cunningham JA, Droguett G, et al. Isolation of a common receptor for Coxsackie B viruses and adenoviruses 2 and 5. Science 1997;275:1320–1323.

87. Martino T, Petric M, Weingartl H, et al. The coxsackievirus–adenovirus receptor (CAR) is used by reference strains and clinical isolates representing all 6 serotypes of coxsackievirus group B, and by swine vesicular disease virus. J Virol 2000;271:99–108.

88. Chapman PR, Weiss RA. Spoilt for choice of co-receptors. Nature 1997;388:230–231.

89. Martino T, Petric M, Brown M, et al. Cardiovirulent coxsackieviruses and the decay-accelerating factor (CD55) receptor. Virology 1998;244: 302–314.

90. Rolvink PW, Mi Lee G, Linfeld DA, et al. Identification of a conserved receptor-binding site on the fiber proteins of CAR-recognizing Adenoviridae. Science 1999;286:1568–1571.

91. Tracy S, Wiegand V, McManus B, et al. Molecular approaches to enteroviral diagnosis in idiopathic cardiomyopathy and myocarditis. J Am Coll Cardiol 1990;15:1688–1694.

92. Hiraoka Y, Kishimoto C, Takada H, et al. Nitric oxide and murine coxsackievirus B3 myocarditis: aggravation of myocarditis by inhibition of nitric oxide synthase. J Am Coll Cardiol 1996;28:1610–1615.

93. Lowenstein CJ, Hill SL, Lafond-Walker A, et al. Nitric oxide inhibits viral replication in murine myocarditis. J Clin Invest 1996;97: 1837–1843.

94. Mikami S, Kawashima S, Kanazawa K, et al. Expression of nitric oxide synthase in a murine model of viral myocarditis induced by coxsackievirus B3. Biochem Biophys Res Commun 1996;220:983–989.

95. Mikami S, Kawashima S, Kanazawa K, et al. Low-dose N^ω-nitro-L-arginine methyl ester treatment improves survival rate and decreases myocardial injury in a murine model of viral myocarditis induced by coxsackievirus B3. Circ Res 1997;81:504–511.

96. Zaragoza C, Ocampo C, Saura M, et al. The role of inducible nitric oxide synthase in the host response to coxsackievirus myocarditis. Proc Natl Acad Sci USA 1998;95:2469–2474.

97. Hirono S, Islam O, Nakazawa M, et al. Expression of inducible nitric oxide synthase in rat experimental autoimmune myocarditis with special reference to changes in cardiac hemodynamics. Circ Res 1997;80:11–20.

98. Ishiyama S, Hiroe M, Nishikawa T, et al. Nitric oxide contributes to the progression of myocardial damage in experimental autoimmune myocarditis in rats. Circulation 1997;95:489–496.

99. Damas JK, Aukrust P, Ueland T, et al. Monocyte chemoattractant protein-1 enhances and interleukin-10 suppresses the production of inflammatory cytokines in adult rat cardiomyocytes. Basic Res Cardiol 2001;96:345–352.

100. Gluck B, Schmidtke M, Merkle I, Stelzner A, Gemsa D: Persistent expression of cytokines in the chronic stage of CVB3-induced myocarditis in NMRI mice. J Mol Cell Cardiol 2001;33:1615–1626.

101. Hofmann P, Schmidtke M, Stelzner A, Gemsa D. Suppression of proinflammatory cytokines and induction of IL-10 in human monocytes after coxsackievirus B3 infection. J Med Virol 2001;64: 487–498.

102. Nishio R, Matsumori A, Shioi T, et al. Treatment of experimental viral myocarditis with interleukin-10. Circulation 1999;100:1102–1108.

103. Seko Y, Takahashi N, Yagita H, Okumura K, Yazaki Y. Expression of cytokine mRNAs in murine hearts with acute myocarditis caused by coxsackievirus b3. J Pathol 1997;183:105–108.

104. Dec GW, Fuster V. Idiopathic dilated cardiomyopathy. N Engl J M 1994;331:1564–1575.

105. Fujioka S, Kitaura Y, Ukimura A, et al. Evaluation of viral infecti in the myocardium of patients with idiopathic dilated cardiomyop thy. J Am Coll Cardiol 2000;36:1920–1926.

106. Martino TA, Liu O, Sole MJ. Viral infection and the pathogenesis dilated cardiomyopathy. Circ Res 1994;74:182–188.

107. Klingel K, Hohenadl C, Canu A, et al. Ongoing enterovirus-induc myocarditis is associated with persistent heart muscle infectio quantitative analysis of virus replication, tissue damage, and inflam mation. Proc Natl Acad Sci U S A 1992;89:314–318.

108. Sole MJ, Liu P. Viral myocarditis: a paradigm for understanding t pathogenesis and treatment of dilated cardiomyopathy. J Am Co Cardiol 1993;22(Suppl A):99A–105A.

109. Baig MK, Goldman JH, Caforio ALP, Coonar AS, Keeling PJ, McKenn WJ. Familial dilated cardiomyopathy: cardiac abnormalities a common in asymptomatic relatives and may represent early diseas J Am Coll Cardiol 1998;31:195–201.

110. Caforio ALP, Keeling PJ, Zachara E, et al. Evidence from family studi for autoimmunity in dilated cardiomyopathy. Lancet 1994;34 773–777.

111. Limas C, Limas CJ, Boudoulas H, et al. T-cell receptor gene polymo phisms in familial cardiomyopathy: correlation with anti-β-recept autoantibodies. Am Heart J 1992;124:1259–1263.

112. Michels VV, Moll PP, Rodeheffer RJ, et al. Circulating heart autoant bodies in familial as compared with nonfamilial idiopathic dilate cardiomyopathy. Mayo Clin Proc 1994;69:24–27.

113. Cunningham R, Silbergleit R. Viral myocarditis presenting wit seizure and electrocardiographic findings of acute myocardi infarction in a 14-month-old child. Ann Emerg Med 2000;3 618–622.

114. Hornung TS, Bernard EJ, Howman-Giles RB, et al. Myocardial infar tion complicating neonatal enterovirus myocarditis. J Pediatr Chil Health 1999;35:309–312.

115. Huang M, Bigos D, Levine M. Ventricular arrhythmia associate with respiratory syncytial viral infection. Pediatr Cardiol 1998;1 498–500.

116. Shah SS, Hellenbrand WE, Gallagher PG. Atrial flutter complicatin neonatal Coxsackievirus B2 myocarditis. Pediatr Cardiol 1998;19:185 186.

117. Tai YT, Lau CP, Fong PC, et al. Incessant automatic ventricular tach cardia complicating acute coxsackievirus B myocarditis. Cardi 1992;80:339–344.

118. Bachmaier K, Mair J, Offner F, Pummerer C, Neu N. Serum cardia troponin T and creatine kinase-MB elevations in murine autoimmun myocarditis. Circulation 1995;92:1927–1932.

119. Briassoulis G, Papadopoulos G, Zavras N, et al. Cardiac tropon I in fulminant myocarditis treated with a 24-hour infusion o high-dose intravenous immunoglobulin. Pediatr Cardiol 2000;2 391–394.

120. Checchia PA, Appel HJ, Kahn S, et al. Myocardial injury in childre with respiratory syncytial virus infection. Pediatr Crit Care Me 2000;1:146–150.

121. Lauer B, Niederau C, Kuhl U, et al. Cardiac troponin T in patients wit clinically suspected myocarditis. J Am Coll Cardiol 1997;30:1354 1359.

122. Smith SC, Ladenson JH, Mason JW, Jaffe AS. Elevations of cardia troponin I associated with myocarditis: experimental and clinica correlates. Circulation 1995;95:163–168.

123. Kaneko K, Kanda T, Hasegawa A, et al. C-reactive protein as a prog nostic marker in lymphocytic myocarditis. Jpn Heart J 2000;41 41–47.

124. Fuse K, Kodama M, Okura Y, et al. Predictors of disease cours in patients with acute myocarditis. Circulation 2000;102:2829 2835.

125. Lauer B, Schwannwell M, Kuhl U, et al. Antimyosin autoantibodie are associated with deterioration of systolic and diastolic lef

ventricular function in patients with chronic myocarditis. J Am Coll Cardiol 2000;35:11–18.

126. Schultheiss HP, Schulze K, Domer A. Significance of the adenine nucleotide translocator in the pathogenesis of viral heart disease. Mol Cell Biochem 1996;163/164:319–327.

127. Angelini A, Crosato M, Boffa GM, et al. Active versus borderline myocarditis: clinicopathologic correlates and prognostic implications. Heart 2002;87:210–215.

128. Parillo JE: Inflammatory cardiomyopathy (myocarditis). Which patients should be treated with anti-inflammatory therapy? Circulation 2001;104:4–6.

129. Pophal SG, Sigfusson G, Booth KL. Complications of endomyocardial biopsy in children. J Am Coll Cardiol 1999;34:2105–2110.

130. Hauck AJ, Kearney DL, Edwards WD. Evaluation of postmortem endomyocardial biopsy specimens from 28 patients with lymphocytic myocarditis: implications for role of sampling error. Mayo Clin Proc 1989;63:1235–1245.

131. Kandolf R, Ameis D, Kirschner P, et al. In situ detection of enteroviral genomes in myocardial cells by nucleic acid hybridization: an approach to the diagnosis of viral heart disease. Proc Natl Acad Sci USA 1987;84:6272–6276.

132. Tracy S, Wiegand V, McManus B, et al. Molecular approaches to enteroviral diagnosis in idiopathic cardiomyopathy and myocarditis. J Am Coll Cardiol 1990;15:1688–1694.

133. Noorullah A, Jiyuan N, Stromberg D, et al. Tracheal aspirate as a substrate for polymerase chain reaction detection of viral genome in childhood pneumonia and myocarditis. Circulation 1999;99:2011–2018.

134. Hoffman GM, Ghanayem NS, Kampine JM, et al. Venous saturation and the anaerobic threshold in neonates after the Norwood procedure for hypoplastic left heart syndrome. Ann Thorac Surg 2000;70:1515–1521.

135. Thayssen P, Klarholt E: Relation between caval and pulmonary artery oxygen saturation in children. Br Heart J 1980;43:574–578.

136. Newburger JW, Sanders SP, Burns JC, Parness IA, Beiser AS, Colan SD. Left ventricular contractility and function in Kawasaki syndrome: effect of intravenous gamma globulin. Circulation 1989;79:1237–1246.

137. Newburger JW, Takahashi M, Burns JC, et al. The treatment of Kawasaki syndrome with intravenous gamma globulin. N Engl J Med 1986;315:341–347.

138. Drucker NA, Colan SD, Lewis AB, et al. γ-Globulin treatment of acute myocarditis in the pediatric population. Circulation 1994;89:252–257.

139. Parillo JE, Cunnion RE, Epstein SE, et al. A prospective, randomized, controlled trial of prednisone for dilated cardiomyopathy. N Engl J Med 1989;321:1061–1068.

140. Mason JW, O'Connell JB, Herskowitz A, et al. A clinical trial of immunosuppressive therapy for myocarditis. N Engl J Med 1995;333:269–275.

141. Wojnicz R, Nowalany-Kozielska E, Wojciechowska C, et al. Randomized, placebo-controlled study for immunosuppressive treatment of inflammatory dilated cardiomyopathy: two-year follow-up results. Circulation 2001;104:39–45.

142. Ahdoot J, Galindo A, Alejos JC, et al. Use of OKT3 for acute myocarditis in infants and children. J Heart Lung Transplant 2000;19:1118–1121.

143. Kleinert S, Weintraub RG, Wilkinson JL, Chow CW. Myocarditis in children with dilated cardiomyopathy: incidence and outcome after dual therapy immunosuppression. J Heart Lung Transplant 1997;16:1248–1254.

144. Lee KJ, McCrindle BW, Bohn DJ. Clinical outcomes of acute myocarditis in childhood. Heart 1999;82:226–233.

145. Matoba Y, Matsumori A, Okada I, et al. The effect of cyclosporine on the immunopathogenesis of viral myocarditis in mice. Jpn Circ J 1991;55:407–416.

146. Rotbart HA. Antiviral therapy for enteroviral infections. Pediatr Infect Dis J 1999;18:632–633.

147. Kishimoto C, Crumpacker CS, Abelmann WH, et al. Ribavirin treatment of coxsackie B3 myocarditis with analysis of lymphocyte subsets. J Am Coll Cardiol 1988;12:1334–1341.

148. Matsumori A, Wang H, Abelmann WH, et al. Treatment of viral myocarditis with ribavirin in an animal preparation. Circulation 1985;71:834–839.

149. Duncan BW, Bohn DJ, Atz AM, French JW, Laussen PC, Wessel DL. Mechanical circulatory support for the treatment of children with acute fulminant myocarditis. J Thorac Cardiovasc Surg 2001;122:440–448.

150. Shekerdemian L. Nonpharmacologic treatment of acute heart failure. Curr Opin Pediatr 2001;13:240–246.

151. Lieberman EB, Hutchins GM, Herskowitz A, Rose NR, Baughman KL. Clinicopathologic description of myocarditis. J Am Coll Cardiol 1991;18:1617–1626.

152. McCarthy III RE, Boehmer JP, Hruban RH, et al. Long term outcome of fulminant myocarditis as compared with acute (nonfulminant) myocarditis. N Engl J Med 2000;342:690–695.

153. Morrow RW. Cardiomyopathy and heart transplantation in children. Curr Opin Cardiol 2000;15:216–223.

22
Diseases of the Pericardium

Michael H. Gewitz, Gary M. Satou, and Derek S. Wheeler

Introduction

Illnesses affecting the pericardium can be categorized into three general categories. *Pericarditis* is a nonspecific term denoting an inflammatory process and is usually not a medical emergency. *Pericardial effusion*, the term utilized for the description of more than the normal amount of fluid in the pericardial space, requires careful evaluation but may or may not require intervention. *Cardiac tamponade* is a true medical emergency resulting in decreased cardiac output secondary to a restrictive process that impairs ventricular filling (diastole), and it requires immediate attention. Cardiac tamponade may be secondary to a large pericardial effusion or caused by thickening of the pericardium itself, with or without fluid accumulation (see later).

Pericarditis

Table 22.1 [1] reviews the principal causes of pericarditis in the pediatric population. When considering the cause of pericardial disease or other systemic diseases in which the pericardium is involved, it is important to remember that the pericardium is not only adjacent to the heart but is also in continuity with the surrounding intrathoracic structures. Thus, any inflammatory condition or process in which the heart, pleura, mediastinal structures, or the diaphragm are involved may affect the pericardium as well. Infectious diseases are the most common etiologic source of pericarditis in childhood. Although viral agents are often thought to be causative, a majority of cases will not have an actual viral pathogen confirmed. In recent years, advances in polymerase chain reaction (PCR) technology have helped to increase the yield of confirmatory etiologies, particularly for coxsackie (group B) and other enteroviruses. Other viruses traditionally thought to play a role include adenovirus, influenza, Ebstein-Barr virus, rubella, and mumps. Cardiac tamponade physiology is a less common occurrence with a viral etiology of pericarditis.

Purulent pericarditis, on the other hand, can be a medical emergency secondary to its association with cardiac tamponade. Up to 30% of these cases involve children under the age of 6 years [2]. The principal agents responsible for pyogenic pericarditis include *Staphylococcus aureus, Neisseria meningitides, Streptococcus pneumoniae*, and other streptococci. *Haemophilus influenzae* pericarditis, once a major concern, is less commonly seen in the current era of immunizations. *Mycobacterium tuberculosis* is another causative organism, particularly in children from underdeveloped countries. The presence of associated infections in children undergoing evaluation for pericarditis, such as respiratory tract disease, osteomyelitis, or pyogenic arthritis, can be helpful in elucidating the potential organism. Staphylococcal pericarditis has been shown to be associated with sites often distant anatomically from the pericardium, such as osteomyelitis, whereas cases of *H. influenzae* pericarditis are found in association with concurrent respiratory tract infections. Meningococcemia is associated with pericardial involvement in approximately 5% of cases.

Noninfectious pericarditis can occur in children as well and is usually found in the setting of *postpericardiotomy syndrome*, whereby postoperative cardiac patients demonstrate a constellation of findings associated with pericardial inflammation [3]. This usually includes pericardial effusion, fever, leukocytosis, and an elevated erythrocyte sedimentation rate. On average, postpericardiotomy syndrome manifests from 1 to 4 weeks following cardiac surgery. It usually is limited to cardiac surgical patients who have undergone open heart procedures where the pericardium has been entered and is estimated to affect approximately 10%–15% of these patients [3]. However, it can develop in *closed* procedures such as pulmonary artery banding and palliative shunt procedures (e.g., Blalock-Taussig shunt). Less common forms of noninfectious pericardial inflammation include those occurring in association with collagen vascular and oncologic diseases, particularly lymphomas of the mediastinum. Rheumatic fever and Kawasaki disease remain other important inflammatory diseases with pericardial involvement as one of the cardiovascular manifestations.

Diagnosis

The clinical manifestations of pericarditis are variable, but often the child complains of chest pain or shortness of breath. An upright position is described to be most comfortable. The chest pain may change in intensity, particularly with body positioning. Persistent respiratory difficulties, often after resolution of a prior upper respiratory illness, may be a clue toward pericardial involvement. Not

D.S. Wheeler et al. (eds.), *Cardiovascular Pediatric Critical Illness and Injury*,
DOI 10.1007/978-1-84800-923-3_22, © Springer-Verlag London Limited 2009

TABLE 22.1. Causes of diseases of the pericardium.

Infectious
    Bacterial
    Viral
    Fungal
    Parasitic
    Tuberculous
Noninfectious/inflammatory
    Acute rheumatic fever
    Systemic lupus erythematosus
    Uremia
    Radiation
    Juvenile rheumatoid arthritis
    Drug induced
Traumatic
    Postpericardiotomy syndrome
    Chest wall injury
    Foreign body contact with the heart
Oncologic
    Leukemia
    Lymphoma
    Cardiac tumors (rhabdosarcoma)
Chronic
    Constrictive pericarditis
    Subacute effusive pericarditis
    Blood dyscrasias

infrequently, abdominal pain is described, particularly in young children. In the presence of a substantial pericardial effusion and/or restrictive cardiac filling, there may be cardiac findings similar to those seen in congestive heart failure, including tachycardia, tachypnea, pallor, and cool extremities. The elevated heart rate is a compensatory mechanism to augment cardiac output when stroke volume is decreased. The respiratory symptoms arise secondary to elevated pulmonary venous pressure and decreased pulmonary compliance. Elevated right heart pressures transmit higher pressure to the systemic veins, leading to the potential for venous distension in the neck and hepatomegaly. More chronically, there can be protein loss through the gastrointestinal tract or in the urine.

Cardiac auscultation findings depend on the degree of fluid accumulated in the pericardium. A friction rub, which is a *scratching* sound heard throughout the cardiac cycle, may be heard when there is only a modest amount of fluid in the pericardium and is usually absent when the fluid collection is large. Quiet or muffled heart sounds and a weakened apical impulse are common when there is substantial fluid accumulation. These findings, in association with the symptoms previously described, should alert the clinician to the possibility of cardiac tamponade [4]. The hallmark bedside finding in cardiac tamponade is pulsus paradoxus (see later). The finding of a paradoxical pulse greater than 10–15 mm Hg is direct evidence of restrictive cardiac filling and cardiac compromise.

Management

Pericarditis without pericardial effusion does not usually require more than pharmacologic therapy, and symptomatic therapy is indicated while an etiologic work-up is undertaken. This often involves pain management and antiinflammatory therapy. An arbitrarily chosen course of one to several weeks of oral nonsteroidal

antiinflammatory agents (NSAIDs) is often sufficient. Caref█ evaluation initially is indicated to rule out the associated develo█ ment of myocarditis, pericardial effusion, or cardiac tampona█ Depending on etiology, most initial symptomatic treatment strat█ gies are successful. When a significant pericardial effusion █ present, a more definitive approach is needed. Careful recording vital signs and ruling out pulsus paradoxus is important and nee█ to be followed closely. These children often require close observ█ tion and monitoring in the pediatric intensive are unit settin█ Echocardiography is also capable of describing restrictive fillin█ properties noninvasively. Diagnostic and/or therapeutic pericar█ ocentesis is often electively required and may be emergently ind█ cated in the setting of cardiac tamponade. If a purulent pericardi█ process is suspected, drainage and initiation of antibiotic thera█ is certainly indicated (Table 22.2), but an open drainage procedu█ may often be needed in order to avoid long-term sequelae such █ constrictive pericarditis and consequent myocardial compromi█ [5]. Although large amounts of intrapericardial fluid are surpri█ ingly well tolerated when developed over a long period of time, a█ acute pericardial fluid collection is much less well tolerated, an█ patients with rapidly changing pericardial fluid dynamics can pr█ cipitously become threatened. They require maximum clinic█ vigilance and closely supervised care.

Although the underlying condition certainly influences outcom█ in most young patients pericardial disease resolves without lon█ term sequelae. However, the outcome is not entirely predictab█ from the initial presentation and the results of early managemen█ Thus serial assessment even after resolution of the initial proces█ is an important component of effective management.

Cardiac Tamponade

Physiology of Cardiac Tamponade

The pericardium is relatively noncompliant such that the accumu█ lation of a small amount of fluid (usually less than 200 mL) i█ sufficient to produce cardiac tamponade. However, chronic accu█ mulation of fluid may occur with little to no hemodynamic derange█ ments as the pericardium slowly stretches to accommodate th█ excess volume. Tamponade is therefore determined by the compli█ ance of the pericardium (Figure 22.1). As pericardial fluid accumu█ lates acutely, the pericardial tissue stretches to accommodate th█ additional volume such that the increase in intrapericardial pres█

TABLE 22.2. Purulent pericarditis: management.

1. Ensure adequate ventilation and cardiac output
2. Administer oxygen
3. Provide cardiorespiratory monitoring
4. Obtain laboratory studies (simultaneous with step 5): complete blood count, platelet count, electrolytes, blood urea nitrogen, creatine, glucose, arterial blood gas, blood culture, chest radiograph, electrocardiography, echocardiography
5. Establish venous access
6. Perform pericardiocentesis (usually with ultrasound guidance): send specimen for laboratory studies: cultures, viral titers, antinuclear antibody, Gram stain, cytology, cell count and differential, chemical profile
7. Administer antibiotics*: oxacillin (150–200 mg/kg/day) or nafcillin or methicillin and chloramphenicol (100 mg/kg/day); aminoglycoside (immunocompromised patient or until cultures/sensitivities available)

*Select antimicrobials to cover *Staphylococcus aureus*.

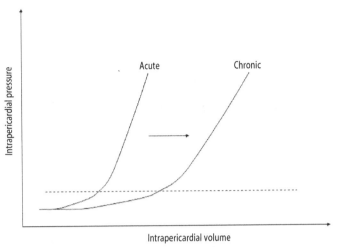

FIGURE 22.1. Pericardial compliance curves: acute (left) and chronic (right) accumulation of pericardial fluid. The rapid accumulation of pericardial fluid is compensated at first by expansion of the pericardium. However, once a critical threshold is attained (dotted line), there is a rapid, steep increase in intrapericardial pressure for a given increase in pericardial volume at which time signs and symptoms of cardiac tamponade are observed. The slow accumulation of fluid allows passive stretch of the pericardium such that the increase in intrapericardial pressure is less significant for any given increase in pericardial volume.

sure for a given increase in intrapericardial volume is small (flat portion of the compliance curve). However, once a certain threshold is attained, a small change in intrapericardial volume results in a steep increase in intrapericardial pressure (*J-shaped* compliance curve). Conversely, a slow increase (over days to weeks) in intrapericardial volume is compensated as the compliance curve is shifted to the right and the slope of the compliance curve flattens. Therefore, the rise in intrapericardial pressure for a given change in volume is much less. The therapeutic implications of an acute versus chronic pericardial fluid accumulation are also important. For example, removal of even a small volume of pericardial fluid from an acute effusion or hemopericardium will decrease the intrapericardial pressure significantly and relieve symptoms of cardiac tamponade. Conversely, because of the change in compliance curves, a large volume of pericardial fluid from a symptomatic, chronic effusion will need to be removed to attain comparable relief of tamponade.

Cardiac tamponade is produced by compression of the heart by accumulation of pericardial fluid beyond a certain threshold (i.e., the steep, J-shaped portion of the pericardial compliance curve). The true *filling pressure* of the heart is represented by the myocardial transmural pressure (i.e., intracardiac pressure minus intrapericardial pressure). Therefore, as intrapericardial pressure rises, the filling pressure of the heart decreases and stroke volume falls. The body attempts to compensate for the increase in intrapericardial pressure (and hence transmural pressure) by increasing systemic central venous pressure and pulmonary venous pressure so that the left and right ventricular filling pressures are higher than the intrapericardial pressure. Left atrial and right atrial pressures increase and equilibrate with the rising intrapericardial pressure—this equalization of pressures is the hallmark of cardiac tamponade [6,7]. Despite the subsequent fall in stroke volume, cardiac output is, at least temporarily, preserved due to the body's compensatory mechanisms.

Clinical Manifestations

Initial signs and symptoms of cardiac tamponade are readily identified in older children and include tachycardia, tachypnea, and hypotension. A pericardial friction rub is frequently noted on auscultation of the heart (see earlier). *Beck's triad*, described initially in 1935 and consisting of jugular venous distension, muffled heart sounds, and hypotension, is classically present with acute cardiac tamponade [8]. However, in neonates and infants, tachycardia may be the only presenting sign. Chest radiographs may show cardiomegaly (*water bottle–shaped heart*) in the absence of pulmonary edema (Figure 22.2). A 12-lead electrocardiogram typically shows sinus tachycardia, a relatively nonspecific finding. However, low-voltage QRS complexes or electrical alternans (Figures 22.3 and 22.4) are more specific for cardiac tamponade. The central venous pressure waveform is characterized by a rapid X descent and a blunted Y descent because of the inability of the heart to fill during diastole (Figure 22.5).

A key diagnostic finding is the presence of a pulsus paradoxus (over a 10 mm Hg change in systolic blood pressure between inspiration and expiration). The pulsus paradoxus was first defined by Adolf Kussmaul in 1873 [9]. Kussmaul described these changes as *paradoxic* because he was unable to palpate a radial pulse during inspiration despite a palpable heart beat. Gauchat and Katz further described the pulsus paradoxus as *a rhythmic pulse occurring in natural breathing, which shows a waxing and waning in size during respiration, evident on palpation in all accessible arteries* in 1924 [10]. Although the exact mechanisms underlying this phenomenon are quite complex, the essence of pulsus paradoxus relies on the fact that right-sided heart filling is favored during inspiration, whereas left-sided heart filling is favored during expiration (Figure 22.6). Under normal cardiac physiologic conditions, there is a small, less than 10 mm Hg, decrease in systolic blood pressure with inspiration. During normal inspiration, negative intrathoracic pressure (relative to atmospheric pressure) causes an increase in systemic venous return. However, there is an even greater increase in the pulmonary vascular capacitance such that there is a decrease

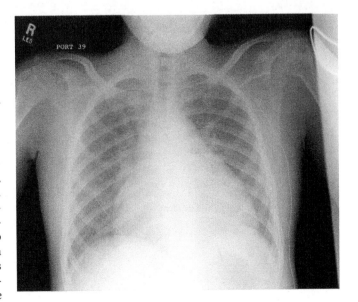

FIGURE 22.2. Chest radiograph demonstrating that classic findings of cardiomegaly in the absence of pulmonary edema (*water bottle-shaped heart*) in a child with a pericardial effusion.

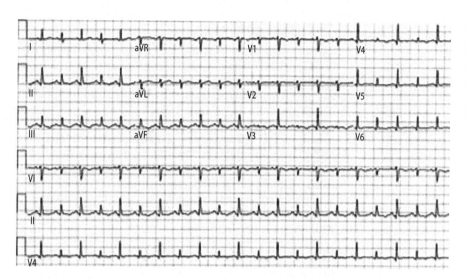

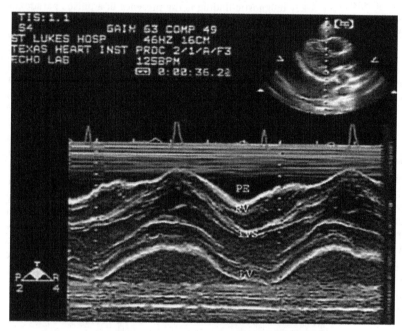

FIGURE 22.3. Electrical alternans. Alternation of QRS complexes, usually in a 2:1 ratio, on electrocardiogram findings is called *electrical alternans*. This is caused by movement the heart in the pericardial space. (Data from Lau TK, Civitello AB, Hernandez A, Coulter SA. Cardiac tamponade and electrical alternans. Tex Heart Inst J 2002;29:66–67, with permission of the Texas Heart Institute. © 2002 Texas Heart Institute with permission.)

FIGURE 22.4. An M-mode echocardiographic image in the parasternal long axis view shows cardiac tamponade. Note the alternating cardiac position in the pericardial effusion. IVS, interventricular septum; LV, left ventricle; PE, pericardial effusion; RV, right ventricle. (Data from Lau TK, Civitello AB, Hernandez A, Coulter SA. Cardiac tamponade and electrical alternans. Tex Heart Inst J 2002;29:66–67, with permission of the Texas Heart Institute. © 2002 Texas Heart Institute with permission.)

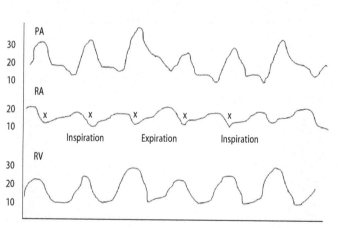

FIGURE 22.5. Central venous pressure tracing from a child with cardiac tamponade showing equalization of right atrium (RA), pulmonary artery (PA) diastolic and right ventricular (RV) diastolic pressures at 15 mm Hg. Also note that there is marked attenuation of the *y* descent on the RA tracing.

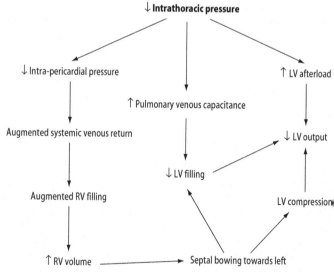

FIGURE 22.6. Mechanism of pulsus paradoxus (see text for explanation). LV, left ventricular; RV, right ventricular.

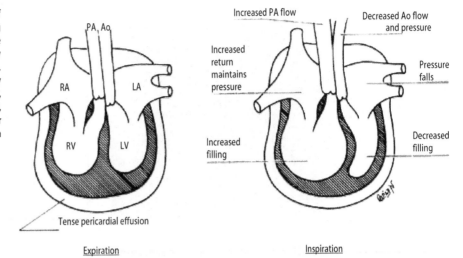

FIGURE 22.7. Line drawing demonstrating the effect of inspiration in the setting of pericardial effusion. During inspiration (right), right heart filling is enhanced at the expense of systemic output, which is diminished secondary to a decrease in left atrial pressure and left ventricular filling. RA, right atrium; RV, right ventricle; PA, pulmonary artery; LA, left atrium; LV left ventricle. (Data from Darsee JR, Braunwald E. Diseases of the pericardium. In: Braunwald E, ed. Heart Disease: a Textbook of Cardiovascular Medicine. New York: WB Saunders; 1980:1535–1582, with permission.)

in filling of the left ventricle. Concurrently, diaphragmatic excursion exhibits a traction effect on the heart, limiting filling and ejection. Hence, left-sided cardiac output is decreased, resulting in a normal decrease in systolic blood pressure during inspiration (less than 10 mm Hg under normal conditions). Finally, under normal conditions, intrathoracic pressure and intrapericardial pressure vary almost equally during the respiratory cycle. However, in cardiac tamponade physiology, intrapericardial pressures remain elevated relative to intrathoracic pressure. As right ventricular filling is augmented during inspiration, intrapericardial pressure increases further and compresses the left ventricle via ventricular interdependence, thereby accentuating the fall in cardiac output during inspiration (Figure 22.7).

Pulsus paradoxus may be measured noninvasively using a standard blood pressure cuff or invasively using an indwelling arterial catheter. For example, noninvasive measurement for detection of pulsus paradoxus starts with establishing the baseline blood pressure and then repeating the blood pressure measurement by inflating the sphygmomanometer cuff several mm Hg above the baseline systolic blood pressure followed by slow deflation of the cuff. As the pressure falls, the Korotkoff sounds disappear with each inspiration. At the point at which they cease to disappear, becoming equal to that auscultated during expiration, the measured blood pressure is recorded. The pulsus paradoxus is the difference between the initial maximum systolic blood pressure and this final measurement. Tamburro et al. [11] eloquently describe the use of the pulse oximetry waveform as a noninvasive measure of the pulsus paradoxus in children with large pericardial effusions (Figures 22.8 and 22.9).

Notably, pulsus paradoxus may also occur with status asthmaticus, tension pneumothorax, profound shock, pulmonary embolism, and restrictive cardiomyopathy. Cardiac tamponade may also occur in the absence of a pulsus paradoxus [4,12,13] in a number of situations. For example, extreme hypotension, as occurs in shock, can eliminate any perceptible differences in blood pressure secondary to respiratory variation. In addition, cardiac tamponade in the face of hypovolemia will dampen any perceptible differences in blood pressure caused by respiratory variation as well. In the latter scenario, commonly called *low-pressure tamponade*, a fluid challenge will often lead to signs and symptoms of classic tamponade [4,12,13]. Local, usually postsurgical, changes can cause pericardial adhesions, leading to a highly localized compression of the

heart in what is commonly called *regional cardiac tamponade*. The regurgitant flow produced by severe aortic regurgitation, with or without left ventricular dysfunction, will dampen any respiratory variations in blood flow and pressure. Inspiratory venous return is balanced by shunting to the left atrium in children with atrial level shunting (i.e., through a patent foramen ovale or surgically created atrial septal defect). Finally, excessive right-sided resistances to flow, as occurs in children with right ventricular hypertrophy or pulmonary hypertension, will also dampen any respiratory variations in blood flow and pressure.

Echocardiography is the principal modality for diagnosing the presence of a pericardial effusion. However, cardiac tamponade remains a clinical diagnosis, and definitive treatment should not be delayed while waiting for echocardiography. A circumferential fluid layer in the presence of right atrial collapse during diastole is diagnostic of cardiac tamponade (Figure 22.10). Right atrial

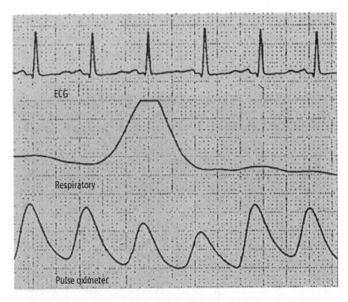

FIGURE 22.8. Simultaneous electrocardiographic tracing and respiratory and pulse oximetry waveforms during a single respiratory cycle. The highest value of the upper plethysmographic peak of the pulse oximetry waveform falls dramatically with inspiration. (Data from Tamburro et al. [11].)

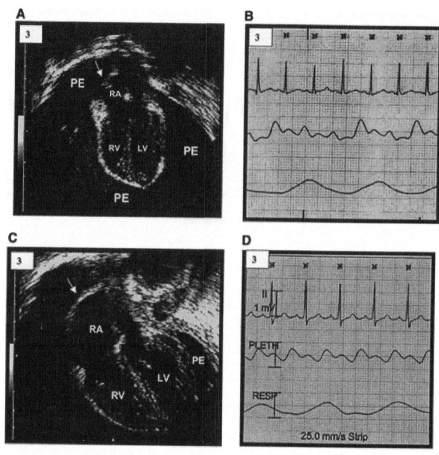

Figure 22.9. Echocardiographic findings and associated pulse oximetry waveform findings. **(A)** Echocardiogram before pericardiocentesis. PE designates the large circumferential pericardial effusion. The arrow highlights considerable flattening of the right atrial (RA) wall during diastole, a sign of compromised cardiac filling. LV, left ventricle; PE, large circumferential pericardial effusion; RV, right ventricle. **(B)** Simultaneous (from top to bottom) electrocardiogram, pulse oximetry, and respiratory tracings demonstrate a marked decrease in the highest value of the upper plethysmographic peak of the pulse oximetry waveform upon inspiration before pericardiocentesis. **(C)** Echocardiogram aft pericardiocentesis. The circumferential pericardial effusion (PE), although still present, smaller. The right atrial (RA) wall (arrow) remains convex during diastole, indicating ree pansion of this chamber after the procedure. LV, left ventricle; RV, right ventricle. (**▶** Simultaneous tracings document that the highest value of the upper plethysmograph peak of the pulse oximetry waveform (PLETH) is well maintained on inspiration after th procedure. (Data from Tamburro et al. [11].)

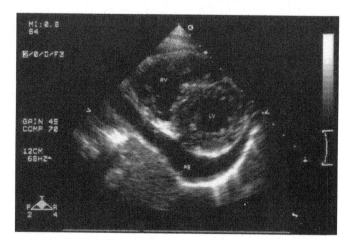

Figure 22.10. Two-dimensional echocardiogram, short axis view, of pericardial effusion (PE) in a child with viral pericarditis. LV, left ventricle; RV, right ventricle.

diastolic collapse consists of an inward collapse of the free wall o the atria, starting at the end of atrial systole and continuing int early ventricular systole [14,15]. Although less commonly observe than right atrial collapse, the presence of right ventricular collaps appears to be more specific for cardiac tamponade than the pres ence of a pulsus paradoxus [16]. Echocardiographic diagnosis o pericardial effusions is discussed further in Chapter 4.

Management

Pericardiocentesis is the life-saving procedure of choice for chil dren with cardiac tamponade. Medical stabilization with fluid resuscitation and inotropic support is controversial and temporary at best. However, fluid resuscitation may precipitate (i.e., in th case of low-pressure tamponade) or worsen tamponade physiology especially in children who are either normovolemic or hypervol emic. In the latter scenario, fluid administration will increas intracardiac pressures further, hence increasing intrapericardia pressures and worsening tamponade [16–18]. Animal studies suggest that naloxone counteracts the hypotensive effects of cardiac tamponade, although the use of this therapeutic modality in the clinical setting has not been attempted [19]. Mechanical ventilatory support may worsen tamponade physiology, although, if unavoidable (e.g., cardiac tamponade in the postoperative setting), excessive swings in intrathoracic pressure with high airway pressures are best avoided [1,4]. Chest compressions in this setting may have limited efficacy, as there is very little room for additional filling of the heart. In addition, even if systolic pressure rises, diastolic pressure falls and worsens coronary perfusion [1,4].

Closed-needle pericardiocentesis via the subxiphoid is the preferred approach for removal and drainage of a pericardial effusion. The subxiphoid approach minimizes the risk of pleural or coronary artery laceration, although complications are further minimized when using echocardiographic guidance [20–22]. Another option is to use the probing needle as an electrocardiographic lead and monitor for an *injury* current (e.g., ST segment elevation), indicating contact with either the ventricular or atrial epicardium. A pericardial pigtail catheter may be placed via the Seldinger technique and left in place for drainage of chronic effusions for a period of up to 5–7 days [23]. Reported complications of needle pericardiocentesis include myocardial laceration with hemopericardium [20–22,24–28], pneumothorax [20–22], dysrhythmias [20–22], pulmonary edema [29–32], and right ventricular volume overload [33].

References

1. Gewitz MH, Votter VL. Cardiac emergencies. In: Fleisher GR, Ludwig SK, eds. Textbook of Pediatric Emergency Medicine, 4th ed. Philadelphia: Lippincott, Williams & Wilkins; 2000:659–700.
2. Van Reken D, Strauss A, Hernandez A, et al. Infectious pericarditis in children. J Pediatr 1974;85:165–169.
3. Engle MA, Zabriskie JB, Senterfit LB, Ebert PA. Post-pericardiotomy syndrome. A new look at an old condition. Mod Concepts Cardiovasc Dis 1975;44:59–64.
4. Spodick DH. Acute cardiac tamponade. N Engl J Med 2003;349:684–690.
5. Hirschmann JV. Pericardial constriction. Am Heart J 1978;96:110–122.
6. Shabetai R, Fowler NO, Guntheroth WG. The hemodynamics of cardiac tamponade and constrictive pericarditis. Am J Cardiol 1970;26:480–489.
7. Reddy PS, Curtiss EI, Uretsky BF. Spectrum of hemodynamics changes in cardiac tamponade. Am J Cardiol 1990;66:1487–1491.
8. Sternback G. Claude Beck: Cardiac compression triads. J Emerg Med 1988;6:417–419.
9. Bilchick KC, Wise RA. Paradoxical physical findings described by Kussmaul: Pulsus paradoxus and Kussmaul's sign. Lancet 2002;359:1940–1942.
10. Gauchat H, Katz LN. Observations on pulsus paradoxus. Arch Intern Med 1924;33:371–393.
11. Tamburro RF, Ring JC, Womback K. Detection of pulsus paradoxus associated with large pericardial effusions in pediatric patients by analysis of the pulse-oximetry waveform. Pediatrics 2002;109:673–677.
12. Shabetai R. Pericardial effusion: Haemodynamic spectrum. Heart 2004;90:255–256.
13. Spodick DH. Pulsus Paradoxus. New York: Dekker; 1997.
14. Singh S, Wann LS, Schuchard GH. Right ventricular and right atrial collapse in patients with cardiac tamponade—a combined echocardiographic and hemodynamic study. Circulation 1984;70:966–971.
15. Singh S, Wann LS, Klopfenstein HS. Usefulness of right ventricular diastolic collapse in diagnosing cardiac tamponade and comparison to pulsus paradoxus. Am J Cardiol 1986;57:652–656.
16. Cogswell TL, Bernath GA, Keelan J, M.H., Wann LS, Klopfenstein HS. The shift in the relationship between intrapericardial fluid pressure and volume induced by acute left ventricular pressure overload during cardiac tamponade. Circulation 1986;74:173–180.
17. Gascho JA, Martins JB, Marcus ML, Kerber RE. Effects of volume expansion and vasodilators in acute pericardial tamponade. Am J Physiol 1981;240:H49–H53.
18. Hashim R, Frankel H, Tandon M, Rabinovici R. Fluid resuscitation-induced cardiac tamponade. J Trauma 2002;53:1183–1184.
19. Klopfenstein HS, Mathias DW. Influence of naloxone on response to acute cardiac tamponade in conscious dogs. Am J Physiol 1990;259:H512–H517.
20. Callahan JA, Seward JB, Tajik AJ. Cardiac tamponade: Pericardiocentesis directed by two dimensional echocardiography. Mayo Clin Proc 1985;60:344–347.
21. Tsang TS, El-Najdawi EK, Seward JB, Hagler DJ, Freeman WK, O'Leary PW. Percutaneous echocardiographically guided pericardiocentesis in pediatric patients: evaluation of safety and efficacy. J Am Soc Echocardiogr 1998;11:1072–1077.
22. Vayre F, Lardoux H, Pezzano M, Bourdarias JP, Dubourg O. Subxiphoid pericardiocentesis guided by contrast two-dimensional echocardiography in cardiac tamponade: experience of 110 consecutive patients. Eur J Echocardiogr 2000;1:66–71.
23. Lock JE, Bass JL, Kulik TJ. Chronic percutaneous drainage with modified pigtail catheters in children. Am J Cardiol 1984;53:1179–1182.
24. Sobol SM, Thomas HM, Jr., Evans RW. Myocardial laceration not demonstrated by continuous electrocardiographic monitoring occurring during pericardiocentesis. N Engl J Med 1975;292:1222–12223.
25. Duvernoy O, Borowiec J, Helmius G, Erikson U. Complications of percutaneous pericardiocentesis under fluoroscopic guidance. Acta Radiol 1992;33:309–313.
26. Hsia HH, Kander NH, Shea MJ. Persistent ST-segment elevation following pericardiocentesis: caution with thrombolytic therapy. Intensive Care Med 1988;14:77–79.
27. Souza LS, Mesquita AA, Chula ED, Lima GA. Iatrogenic left ventricular pseudoaneurysm. Ann Thorac Surg 2001;72:1388–1389.
28. Dabbah S, Fischer D, Markiewicz W. Pericardiocentesis ending in the superior vena cava. Cathet Cardiovasc Intervent 2005;64:492–494.
29. Vandyke WHJ, Cure J, Chakko CS, Gheorghiade M. Pulmonary edema after pericardiocentesis for cardiac tamponade. N Engl J Med 1983;309:595–596.
30. Newman B, Park SC, Oh KS. Coexistent transient pulmonary edema and pericardial effusion. Pediatr Radiol 1988;18:455–458.
31. Downey RJ, Bessler M, Weissman C. Acute pulmonary edema following pericardiocentesis for chronic cardiac tamponade secondary to trauma. Crit Care Med 1991;19:1323–1325.
32. Chamoun A, Cenz R, Mager A, Rahman A, Champion C, Ahmad M, et al. Acute left ventricular failure after large volume pericardiocentesis. Clin Cardiol 2003;26:588–590.
33. Armstrong WF, Feigenbaum H, Dillon JC. Acute right ventricular dilation and echocardiographic volume overload following pericardiocentesis for relief of cardiac tamponade. Am Heart J 1984;107:1266–1270.

Management of Hypertension in the Pediatric Intensive Care Unit

Marianne N. Majdalani and Neil W. Kooy

Introduction

Acutely elevated blood pressure in the pediatric patient, resulting from a complex interaction of blood volume, vascular compliance, cardiac output, and systemic arteriolar resistance, generally constitutes a medical emergency that can result in significant morbidity, including hypertensive encephalopathy [1,2], renal failure [3,4], and congestive heart failure [5,6], and mortality. Prompt recognition of the clinical manifestations of systemic hypertension, a thorough understanding of the potential pathophysiologic mechanisms, and a comprehensive understanding of antihypertensive pharmacology are, therefore, of the utmost importance.

Definitions

In contrast to the adult population, for whom hypertension is defined as a systolic pressure greater than 140 mm Hg and/or a diastolic pressure greater than 90 mm Hg, in children blood pressure will vary, requiring that evaluation be based on age-, gender-, and height-appropriate norms. Values that are available for healthy children from several epidemiologic studies provide a starting point for evaluation of blood pressure in critically ill children, wherein hypertension is defined as a systolic or diastolic pressure of greater than the 95th percentile for age, gender, and body size, and *severe* hypertension is defined as a systolic or diastolic blood pressure greater than the 99th percentile (Tables 23.1 and 23.2) [7–9].

Hypertensive crises are commonly divided into *hypertensive urgencies*, wherein severe hypertension occurs without evidence of new or worsening end-organ injury [10,11], and *hypertensive emergencies*, wherein severe hypertension is associated with signs and symptoms of new or progressive end-organ impairment [10–13]. Hypertensive emergencies have been further categorized into *accelerated hypertension*, which is defined by the presence of marked systemic hypertension associated with grade III Keith-Wagener retinopathy, and *malignant hypertension*, defined as the presence of marked hypertension in association with grade IV Keith-Wagener retinopathy [13]. Hypertensive encephalopathy is the most common severe manifestation of uncontrolled blood pressure in children.

Determinants of Blood Pressure

General Considerations

The pathogenesis of acute hypertension is related to the complex interaction of blood volume, vascular compliance, cardiac output, and total peripheral vascular resistance. In a static system without flow, the pressure within a blood vessel is directly related to the intravascular volume and inversely related to the vascular compliance:

$$\text{Pressure} = \text{Volume/Compliance}$$

In a pulsatile, dynamic system, in addition to intravascular volume and vascular compliance, pressure is also directly related to blood flow and vascular impedance, the opposition to flow in a system confined to oscillatory motions:

$$\text{Pressure} = \text{Volume/Compliance} + \text{Flow} \times \text{Impedance}$$

The complexity of impedance measurements makes its routine use impractical. However, vascular resistance, the measure of opposition to flow in nonoscillatory systems, may be used as a reasonable approximation of impedance:

$$\text{Pressure} = \text{Volume/Compliance} + \text{Flow} \times \text{Resistance}$$

Resistance is determined by Poiseuille's law:

$$R = \frac{8\eta l}{\pi r^4}$$

where η is blood viscosity, l is vessel length, and r is vessel radius. This inverse relationship of resistance to the fourth power of the vessel radius demonstrates the fundamental importance of vasoconstriction and vasorelaxation in the regulation of arterial blood pressure. Because it ignores the complexity of interaction between the various components for the determination of blood pressure, equation 3 above is clearly an oversimplification; however, it

D.S. Wheeler et al. (eds.), *Cardiovascular Pediatric Critical Illness and Injury*,
DOI 10.1007/978-1-84800-923-3_23, © Springer-Verlag London Limited 2009

TABLE 23.1. 90th and 95th percentiles of blood pressure for boys aged 1–17 years by percentiles of height.

Age (years)	Blood pressure percentile	Systolic blood pressure by percentile of height (mm Hg)							Diastolic blood pressure by percentile of height (mm Hg)						
		5%	10%	25%	50%	75%	90%	95%	5%	10%	25%	50%	75%	90%	95
1	90th	94	95	97	98	100	102	102	50	51	52	53	54	54	5
	95th	98	99	101	102	104	106	106	55	55	56	57	58	59	5
2	90th	98	99	100	102	104	105	106	55	55	56	57	58	59	5
	95th	101	102	104	106	108	109	110	59	59	60	61	62	63	6
3	90th	100	101	103	105	107	108	109	59	59	60	61	62	63	6
	95th	104	105	107	109	111	112	113	63	63	64	65	66	67	6
4	90th	102	103	105	107	109	110	111	62	62	63	64	65	66	6
	95th	106	107	109	111	113	114	115	66	67	67	68	69	70	7
5	90th	104	105	106	108	110	112	112	65	65	66	67	68	69	6
	95th	108	109	110	112	114	115	116	69	70	70	71	72	73	7
6	90th	105	106	108	110	111	113	114	67	68	69	70	70	71	7
	95th	109	110	112	114	115	117	117	72	72	73	74	75	76	7
7	90th	106	107	109	111	113	114	115	69	70	71	72	72	73	7
	95th	110	111	113	115	116	118	119	74	74	75	76	77	78	7
8	90th	107	108	110	112	114	115	116	71	71	72	73	74	7	7
	95th	111	112	114	116	118	119	120	75	76	76	77	78	79	8
9	90th	109	110	112	113	115	117	117	72	73	73	74	75	76	7
	95th	113	114	116	117	119	121	121	76	77	78	79	80	80	8
10	90th	110	112	113	115	117	118	119	73	74	74	75	76	77	78
	95th	114	115	117	119	121	122	123	77	78	79	80	80	81	82
11	90th	112	113	115	117	119	120	121	74	74	75	76	77	78	78
	95th	116	117	119	121	123	124	125	78	79	79	80	81	82	83
12	90th	115	116	117	119	121	123	123	75	75	76	77	78	78	79
	95th	119	120	121	123	125	126	127	79	79	80	81	82	83	83
13	90th	117	118	120	122	124	125	126	75	76	76	77	78	79	80
	95th	121	122	124	126	128	129	130	79	80	81	82	83	83	84
14	90th	120	121	123	125	126	128	128	76	76	77	78	79	80	80
	95th	124	125	127	128	130	132	132	80	81	81	82	83	84	85
15	90th	123	124	125	127	129	131	131	77	77	78	79	80	81	81
	95th	127	128	129	131	133	134	135	81	82	83	83	84	85	86
16	90th	125	126	128	130	132	133	134	79	79	80	81	82	82	83
	95th	129	130	132	134	136	137	138	83	83	84	85	86	87	87
17	90th	128	129	131	133	134	136	136	81	81	82	83	84	85	85
	95th	132	133	135	136	138	140	140	85	85	86	87	88	89	89

does serve as a suitable framework for understanding the pathogenesis of acute hypertension resulting from a variety of etiologies (Table 23.3).

Renin–Angiotensin–Aldosterone System

Regulation of the renin–angiotensin–aldosterone system is an extremely complex process that involves interactions among a number of hormones to influence fluid and electrolyte balance and arterial blood pressure. In general, there are three major mechanisms leading to the release of renin:

Baroreceptors: Baroreceptors located within the juxtaglomerular cells of the renal afferent arteriole sense small changes in the transmural pressure gradient, with the resultant regulation of renin release being inversely related to changes in the pressure gradient. For example, as the renal perfusion pressure decreases, there is decreased stretch exerted on the baroreceptors, resulting in decreased stimulation and increased renin release. Correspondingly, as the renal perfusion pressure increases, the increased stretch exerted on the baroreceptors results in a decrease in renin release [14–16].

Macula densa: The macula densa, specialized epithelial cells within the distal collecting tubule adjacent to the juxtaglomerular cells, acts as a sensor of the chloride content of the distal tubular fluid to regulate renin release. A decrease in the chloride content of the tubular fluid is indicative of decreased tubular sodium and a decrease in intravascular volume, resulting in an increase in renin release from the juxtaglomerular cells [17–19].

Renal sympathetic nerves: Under conditions of physiologic or pathologic stress, release of norepinephrine from sympathetic neurons stimulates β-receptors on the juxtaglomerular cells resulting in the release of renin [20,21].

Renin is a proteolytic enzyme that acts on angiotensinogen, an α_2-globulin produced in the liver, to generate angiotensin I. Biologically inactive angiotensin I is subsequently cleaved to form biologically active angiotensin II via the activity of angiotensin-converting enzyme in the lungs [22,23]. In addition to cleaving angiotensin I, angiotensin-converting enzyme also inactivates bradykinin, an endothelium-dependent vasodilator, secondarily mediating control of systemic vascular tone [24]. Angiotensin II engenders an increase in systemic blood pressure through two separate and distinct mechanisms: (1) contraction of the vascular smooth muscle resulting in an increase in systemic vascular resistance and (2) sodium and water retention resulting in increased intravascular volume. Through direct stimulation of the vascular smooth muscle, angiotensin II is a potent vasoconstrictor of the

TABLE 23.2. 90th and 95th percentiles of blood pressure for girls aged 1 to 17 years by percentiles of height.

Age (years)	Blood pressure percentile	Systolic blood pressure by percentile of height (mm Hg)							Diastolic blood pressure by percentile of height (mm Hg)						
		5%	10%	25%	50%	75%	90%	95%	5%	10%	25%	50%	75%	90%	95%
1	90th	97	98	99	100	102	103	104	53	53	53	54	55	56	56
	95th	101	102	103	104	105	107	107	57	57	57	58	59	60	60
2	90th	99	99	100	102	103	104	105	57	57	58	58	59	60	61
	95th	102	103	104	105	107	108	109	61	61	62	62	63	64	65
3	90th	100	100	102	103	104	105	106	61	61	61	62	63	63	64
	95th	104	104	105	107	108	109	110	65	65	65	66	67	67	68
4	90th	101	102	103	104	106	107	108	63	63	64	65	65	66	67
	95th	105	106	107	108	109	111	111	67	67	68	69	69	70	71
5	90th	103	103	104	106	107	108	109	65	66	66	67	68	68	69
	95th	107	107	108	110	111	112	113	69	70	70	71	72	72	73
6	90th	104	105	106	107	109	110	111	67	67	68	69	69	70	71
	95th	108	109	110	111	112	114	114	71	71	72	73	73	74	75
7	90th	106	107	108	109	110	112	112	69	69	69	70	71	72	72
	95th	110	110	112	113	114	115	116	73	73	73	74	75	76	76
8	90th	108	109	110	111	112	113	114	70	70	71	71	72	73	74
	95th	112	112	113	115	116	117	118	74	74	75	75	76	77	78
9	90th	110	110	112	113	114	115	116	71	72	72	73	74	74	75
	95th	114	114	115	117	118	119	120	75	76	76	77	78	78	79
10	90th	112	112	114	115	116	117	118	73	73	73	74	75	76	76
	95th	116	116	117	119	120	121	122	77	77	77	78	79	80	80
11	90th	114	114	116	117	118	119	120	74	74	75	75	76	77	77
	95th	118	118	119	121	122	123	124	78	78	79	79	80	81	81
12	90th	116	116	118	119	120	121	122	75	75	76	76	77	78	78
	95th	120	120	121	123	124	125	126	79	79	80	80	81	82	82
13	90th	118	118	119	121	122	123	124	76	76	77	78	78	79	80
	95th	121	122	123	125	126	127	128	80	80	81	82	82	83	84
14	90th	119	102	121	122	124	125	126	77	77	78	79	79	80	81
	95th	123	124	125	126	128	129	130	81	81	82	83	83	84	85
15	90th	121	121	122	124	125	126	127	78	78	79	79	80	81	82
	95th	124	125	126	128	129	130	131	82	82	83	83	84	85	86
16	90th	122	122	123	125	126	127	128	79	79	79	80	81	82	82
	95th	125	126	127	128	130	131	132	83	83	83	84	85	86	86
17	90th	122	123	124	125	126	128	128	79	79	79	80	81	82	82
	95th	126	126	127	129	130	131	132	83	83	83	84	85	86	86

splanchnic and renal vasculature. Moreover, angiotensin II also stimulates norepinephrine synthesis and release from the sympathetic nervous system and epinephrine release from the adrenal medulla, thereby resulting in secondary catecholamine-induced vasoconstriction and increased systemic blood pressure [25]. Pathologic states the result in increased renin production may beget a vicious cycle of angiotensin II–mediated vasoconstriction, impairment of renal perfusion, increased renin production, and further escalation of circulating angiotensin II.

Angiotensin II has a direct effect on renal tubular reabsorption of sodium and water and secondarily stimulates aldosterone biosynthesis and secretion by the adrenal cortex [26,27]. Aldosterone stimulates the active reabsorption of sodium from the distal tubular urine. Because water is passively reabsorbed with the sodium, there is little increase in serum sodium concentration, and extracellular fluid volume expands in an isotonic fashion. Moreover, angiotensin II also stimulates the release of vasopressin (antidiuretic hormone) from the posterior pituitary resulting in increased reabsorption of free water in the distal collecting tubule [25]. The increase in intravascular volume exerted by the direct renal activity of angiotensin II, and the secondary release of aldosterone and vasopressin, results in an increase in systemic blood pressure (Figure 23.1).

Circulating Catecholamines

The circulating catecholamines, epinephrine and norepinephrine, originate from two separate components of the sympathetic nervous system. Derived from embryonic neural crest cells, adrenal medullary chromaffin cells are postganglionic sympathetic nervous system effectors, receiving innervation from corresponding preganlionic cholinergic sympathetic nerve fibers. In response to physiologic stress, the preganglionic release of acetylcholine stimulates chromaffin cell release of epinephrine (80%) and norepinephrine (20%) into the systemic circulation. Moreover, the primary source for circulating norepinephrine is release from vascular sympathetic nerve terminals. Under normal physiologic conditions, the majority of norepinephrine released from nerve terminals is reabsorbed by the preganglionic nerve fibers, where it is subsequently recycled or metabolized, while a small amount diffuses into the circulation. However, under conditions of physiologic stress, where there is increased sympathetic nerve activation, the amount of norepinephrine entering the circulation may increase significantly.

The effects of circulating epinephrine and norepinephrine on blood pressure and blood flow are mediated through α- and β-adrenergic receptor activation. The basal level of circulating epi-

TABLE 23.3. Etiologies of severe hypertension in the pediatric population.

Renal	Head trauma
Acute glomerulonephritis	Dysautonomia
Postinfectious	Guillian-Barré syndrome
Henoch-Schönlein purpura	Spinal cord lesions
Systemic lupus erythematosus	
IgA nephropathy	**Neoplasia**
Chronic glomerulonephritis	Pheochromocytoma
Focal and segmental glomerulosclerosis	Neuroblastoma
Membranoproliferative glomerulonephritis	Neurofibromatosis
Hemolytic uremic syndrome	Wilms tumor
Congenital malformations	Adrenal adenoma
Dysplasia	
Hypoplasia	**Medications**
Polycystic kidney disease	Steroids
Pyelonephritis	Cyclosporine A
Obstructive uropathy	Sympathomimetics
Renal tranplantation	Oral contraceptives
	Amphetamines
Cardiovascular	Cocaine
Coarctation of the aorta	Phencyclidine
Renovascular disease	Theophylline
Renal artery stenosis	Caffeine
Renal artery thromboemboli	Lead poisoning
Takayasu arteritis	
	Trauma
Endocrine	Burns
Cushing syndrome	Immobilization
Hyperthyroidism	Perirenal hematoma
Congenital adrenal hyperplasia	
Hyperaldosteronism	**Miscellaneous**
Hyperparathyroidism	Intravascular volume overload
	Hypercalcemia
Central nervous system	Hypernatremia
Increased intracranial pressure	Anxiety/algesia
Seizures	

nephrine is 25–75 pg/mL. As the serum epinephrine concentration increases to 75–125 pg/mL, there is an increase in heart rate and systolic blood pressure as a consequence of myocardial β_1-adrenoreceptor activation. Diastolic blood pressure, however, decreases up to a serum concentration of 200 pg/mL as a consequence of β_2-adrenorector–mediated vasodilation, primarily in the somatic vascular bed. As a result, the mean arterial pressure changes very little, but the overall effect is an increase in cardiac output with redistribution of blood flow from the splanchnic and renal vascular beds and to the somatic muscle. As serum epinephrine concentrations continue to increase, α-adrenoreceptor–mediated vasoconstriction begins to predominate, with potential compromise of organ blood flow to the cutaneous, splanchnic, and renal vascular beds. Similar to epinephrine, circulating norepinephrine has β_1- and α-adrenoceptor–mediated effects on the myocardium and systemic vascular beds; however, norepinephrine lacks the β_2-adrenoceptor–mediated vasodilator effect of epinephrine and therefore raises systolic, diastolic, and mean arterial pressure primarily through increases in systemic vascular resistance. Owing to this increase in vascular resistance, although norepinephrine stimulates myocardial β_1-adrenoreceptors, heart rate may slow as a consequence of reflex baroreceptor feedback.

Vasopressin (Antidiuretic Hormone)

The primary function of vasopressin, a peptide hormone released from the posterior pituitary, is to regulate extracellular fluid volume by affecting renal handling of free water [28]. Consonant with this role in water metabolism, the secretion of vasopressin is primarily regulated by osmotic and intravascular volume stimuli. Located within cell bodies of the hypothalamus, osmoreceptors are extremely sensitive, detecting increases in serum osmolality as small as 1% [29,30]. Osmoreceptor activation generates a nerve impulse that travels from cell bodies within the hypothalamus to the pituitary, producing neurosecretory vesicle depolarization and the consequent release of vasopressin. A fall in effective circulating volume can also trigger release of vasopressin, even at low or normal serum osmolality. However, the recognition of alterations in blood volume is less sensitive, requiring a decrease in blood volume of 10% or greater to trigger vasopressin release. Less severe reductions in circulating volume shift the osmolar set point such that a lower osmotic threshold is required to trigger vasopressin release during states of volume depletion [31–33]. Specialized stretch receptors within the atria and vena cavae decrease their firing rate when there is a fall in atrial or central venous pressure decreasing sympathetic afferent inhibition and thereby increasing vasopressin release.

Vasopressin has two principal sites of action: the kidneys and blood vessels. Mediated by the activation of V_2 receptors located on the peritubular side of the collecting duct epithelium, the most important physiologic action of vasopressin is the selective enhancement of free water permeability, permitting reabsorption and maintenance of intravascular volume [34,35]. Vasopressin may also mediate effects on blood pressure through the activation of V receptors located on the vascular smooth muscle, leading to vasoconstriction; however, this effect of vasopressin requires very high serum levels and is generally not considered important in the maintenance of blood pressure under normal physiologic conditions. This pressor effect may, however, gain importance in the maintenance of blood pressure during acute hypovolemia or states of pathophysiologic vasodilation (Figure 23.2) [36,37].

Nitric Oxide

Nitric oxide is a ubiquitous signal transduction molecule formed from the amino acid L-arginine via the activity of nitric oxide synthase. Within the vasculature, endothelial cells contain a constitutively active form of the enzyme whose activity can be humorally regulated by acetylcholine, histamine, bradykinin, or adenosine. More importantly, however, nitric oxide release is regulated by shear forces exerted on the luminal surface of the vascular endothelium; increased flow velocity stimulates intracellular calcium release and increased nitric oxide synthase activity. The released nitric oxide acts in a paracrine fashion, activating soluble guanylate cyclase in the vascular smooth muscle, leading to an increase in intracellular cyclic GMP, smooth muscle relaxation, and vasodilation. Other important functions mediated by nitric oxide within the cardiovascular system include inhibition of platelet and leukocyte adhesion to the vascular wall [38].

Endothelin

Released primarily by the vascular endothelium, endothelin is a 21 amino acid polypeptide that acts in a paracrine fashion by binding to endothelin receptors on the vascular smooth muscle leading to the G-protein–mediated increase in intracellular calcium, smooth muscle contraction, and vasoconstriction. Endothelin release is

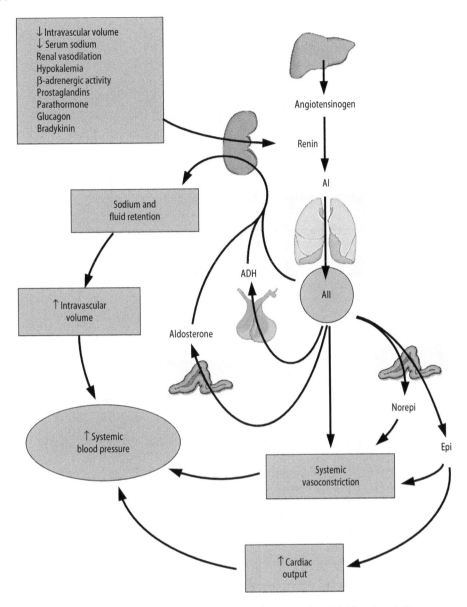

FIGURE 23.1. The rennin–angiotensin–aldosterone system. AI, angiotensin I; AII, angiotensin II.

positively controlled by angiotensin II, vasopressin, thrombin, and shear forces acting on the luminal side of the vascular endothelium, and it is negatively controlled by nitric oxide, prostacyclin, and atrial natriuretic peptide. In addition to vasoconstriction, endothelin stimulates aldosterone secretion and produces positive inotropy and chronotropy in the heart [39].

Eicosanoids

The eicosanoids are a large family of oxygenated metabolites of arachidonic acid released from cell membranes via the activity of phospholipase A_2. Of the three major pathways of eicosanoid production within the vasculature, the cyclooxygenase pathway, the lipoxygenase pathway, and the NADPH-dependent cytochrome P-450 epoxygenase pathway, the endothelium predominantly metabolizes arachadonic acid through the cyclooxygenase pathway, resulting in the formation of prostacyclin (PGI_2). Prostacyclin synthesis is stimulated by many humoral and inflammatory mediators and by shear forces exerted on the luminal surface of the vascular endothelium. Similar to nitric oxide, prostacyclin released from the endothelium acts in a paracrine fashion, activating adenylate cyclase within the vascular smooth muscle, leading to an increase in intracellular cyclic AMP, smooth muscle relaxation, and vasodilation. In addition, prostacyclin act as an inhibitor of platelet adhesion to the vascular wall [40,41]. Thromboxane synthesis is limited within the vascular epithelium but is most pronounced within platelets. Although chemically closely related to prostacyclin, thromboxane acts as a potent vasoconstrictor and platelet aggregator [40].

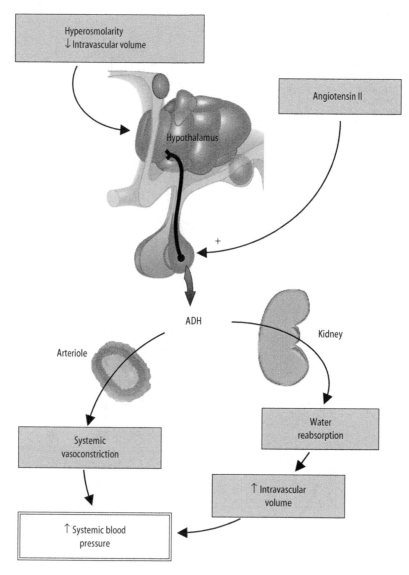

Figure 23.2. Vasopressin-mediated effects on systemic blood pressure.

Blood Pressure Monitoring

Many methods are available for the determination of blood pressure, but, because of the frequency of blood pressure monitoring in the critically ill, only two methods of blood pressure monitoring prove practical in the intensive care unit: noninvasive oscillometric methods and invasive indwelling arterial catheters.

Oscillometric Methods

Noninvasive oscillometric methods are similar to manual auscultatory sphygmomanometry with the exception of directly measuring systolic and mean arterial pressures while calculating the diastolic pressure, which is therefore the least accurate. As with manual auscultatory sphygmomanometry, accuracy in blood pressure determination is predicated on proper cuff size selection: the cuff

size should have a bladder width that is approximately 40% of the arm circumference at a point midway between the olecranon and the acromion and should cover 80%–100% of the arm circumference [8,42]. Although oscillometric devices provide consistent readings that can be used to follow trends over time, significant differences exist between manufacturers with variable deviation from invasively determined blood pressure, with the greatest deviations being reported for critically ill neonates. Recently oscillometric blood pressure standards were published for one manufacturer (Dinamap, Model 8100) in an effort to more accurately assess abnormal blood pressures based on oscillometric determinations [43–45]. Ulnar neuropathy and venostasis may occur if blood pressure cycling is too frequent. Therefore, for a critically ill children receiving continuous vasoactive infusions, it is recommended that blood pressure be monitored invasively [46,47].

Arterial Catheters

Indwelling arterial catheters allow for the continuous monitoring of arterial blood pressure and provide the "gold standard" for blood pressure determination. Although theoretically any accessible artery can be used for cannulation, the vessel must be large enough to reflect accurately the true systemic blood pressure with the provision of adequate collateral blood flow to maintain tissue viability should the cannulated vessel become thrombosed. Adequate collateral circulation is normally present for the radial, ulnar, posterior tibial, and dorsalis pedis arteries, making them the preferred sites of cannulation. Adequacy of collateral circulation, however, should not be presumed, and assessment of limb perfusion following compression of the proposed artery for cannulation should be performed prior to cannulation (e.g., modified Allen test). For those patients who present with severely compromised peripheral pulses, the femoral or axillary arteries may be utilized, however, the brachial artery, due to its relatively small size and lack of collateral circulation should be avoided.

The major problems encountered when utilizing direct blood pressure measurement via an arterial catheter are imprecise zeroing, zero drift, and inaccurate calibration. Proper zeroing of the pressure monitoring system is of the highest importance, as small errors may convey vital erroneous information with significant impact upon clinical management. Therefore, pressure monitoring systems should be zeroed frequently and always prior to initiating treatment changes based upon changes in the pressure data. Indwelling arterial catheters can result in serious vascular complications, such as arterial thrombosis and circulatory insufficiency. A limb with an arterial catheter should be carefully observed and the catheter should be removed if there are any signs of vascular compromise.

Etiology and Pathogenesis

Renal Parenchymal Disease

Because renal perfusion and function are fundamental to the control of intravascular volume and hormonal control of vascular tone, renal parenchymal disease is the most common cause of acute and chronic hypertension in children. Acute, severe hypertension is most frequently associated with acute glomerulonephritis, predominantly acute poststreptococcal glomerulonephritis, where diminution in glomerular filtration rate, sodium retention, and intravascular volume expansion are primarily responsible for the acute rise in blood pressure [48,49].

Hypertension in chronic glomerulonephritis, such as occurs with focal and segmental glomerulosclerosis and membranoproliferative glomerulonephritis, is closely related to the severity of glomerular injury, and its pathogenesis is generally multifactorial, including sodium retention, expanded intravascular volume, increased cardiac output resulting from anemia, and peripheral vasoconstriction resulting from increased renin release [50,51]. During the acute phase of hemolytic uremic syndrome, hypertension, the severity of which is related to the severity of disease, occurs in the majority of cases, is usually labile and easily controlled, and resolves before discharge from the hospital. The hypertensive pathogenesis is unclear; however, it is not related to an elevation in renin activity but may occur in response to an elevation in circulating endothelin levels [52,53]. With progression of the disease and the development of oliguric renal failure, sodium retention and expansion of the intravascular volume may acutely and significantly increase the blood pressure, resulting in hypertensive crises.

Hypertension may also result from congenital renal anomalies, such as dysplasia, hypoplasia, and polycystic kidney disease, or from acquired renal scarring from chronic pyelonephritis, most commonly occuring as a result of vesicoureteral reflux or obstructive uropathy. Increased renin release from the affected kidney accounts for the hypertension.

Cardiovascular Disease

With hypertension as a cardinal feature, coarctation of the aorta is the most common cause of hypertension in infancy and is occasionally seen during childhood into adolescence. Although it is assuredly an oversimplification to attribute mechanical obstruction as the sole etiology for the incidence of hypertension, determinations of plasma renin activity fail to consistently demonstrate activation of the renin–angiotensin system [54–56]. Activation of the renin–angiotensin–aldosterone system in a manner analogous to the one-kidney model of Goldblatt may provide an explanation for this apparent conundrum. According to this model, diminished pulsatile renal blood flow results in upregulation of the renin–angiotensin–aldosterone system, development of hypertension, and improved renal perfusion related to an increase in circulating intravascular volume. Maintenance of the increased intravascular volume and improved renal perfusion results in the stabilization of plasma renin activity at near-normal levels in a new hypertensive steady state [56]. In addition to the renin–angiotensin–aldosterone system, elevated vasopressin and lowered atrial natriuretic factor levels may also contribute to the development of hypertension in coarctation of the aorta [57].

Hypertension associated with renal artery stenosis is usually the result of fibromuscular dysplasia and may occur in as many as 8%–10% of children who have severe hypertension. Renal artery stenosis may be an isolated finding but more frequently occurs in the presence of neurofibromatosis, Williams syndrome, Marfan syndrome, Turner syndrome, or the autoimmune vasculitides. Hypertension results from activation of the renin–angiotensin–aldosterone system in response to diminished renal blood flow distal to the stenosis.

Endocrine Disease

Hypertension may result from Cushing syndrome (glucocorticoid excess), hyperthyroidism, or congenital adrenal hyperplasia (mineralocorticoid excess), where the etiology is relatively manifest because of the multiple diagnostic characteristics of these disease processes [58–61]. Other rare endocrine causes of hypertension include hyperaldosteronism, which should be considered in the presence of hypokalemia, renin-secreting tumors, primary or secondary hyperparathyroidism, and hypercalcemia [62–66].

Central Nervous System Disease

Increased intracranial pressure resulting from any cause, including central nervous system neoplasia, hydrocephalus, intracranial hemorrhage, meningoencephalitis, or trauma, may result in hypertension, bradycardia, and bradypnea (Cushing's triad) as a physiologic response to maintain adequate cerebral perfusion [67]. When central nervous system pathology is present, and systemic hypertension is important for the maintenance of cerebral perfusion, clinical interventions to lower the blood pressure may be detrimental and should be avoided. Clinical scenarios in which the presence of increased intracranial pressure may be readily inferred pose little challenge to this assertion; however, the presence of hypertension in an obtunded child may be the result of central nervous system pathology, or the cause of hypertensive encephalopathy, where prompt lowering of the blood pressure is essential, creating a significant clinical dilemma.

In addition to intracranial pathology, head trauma may also cause hypertension as a result of hypothalamic stimulation of the sympathetic nervous system, causing excessive catecholamine release, where tachycardia, rather than bradycardia is the general rule [68]. The same mechanism may lead to hypertension during acute seizure activity but is usually transient, persisting only until the seizure activity ceases, and it may result in bradycardia because of parasympathetic stimulation [69].

Neoplasia

Pheochromocytoma, a catecholamine-secreting tumor of the adrenal medulla, may cause remittent, intermittent, or sustained hypertension in the absence of additional abnormal physical findings. A thorough review of systems generally reveals other symptomatology associated with catecholamine excess, including flushing, sweating, anxiety, palpitations, chest pain, abdominal pain, nausea, vomiting, weight loss, and fatigue [70]. Like pheochromocytomas, neuroblastomas may also cause hypertension via the direct secretion of catecholamines [71]. Alternatively, neuroblastoma may secondarily cause hypertension via extrinsic compression of the renal artery and increased activation of the renin–angiotension–aldosterone system resulting from decreased renal perfusion [72], as is also the case for neurofibromas [73]. Hypertension is present in approximately 60% of patients presenting with Wilms tumor (nephroblastoma), the pathogenesis of which appears to be mediated via the renin–angiotensin–aldosterone system as a result of neoplastic hypersecretion of renin [74–77].

Management of Hypertension

Although historical information may often differentiate the potential etiologies, in patients with neurologic signs and symptoms, every effort should be made to distinguish hypertensive encephalopathy from hypertension resulting from primary intracranial pathology. A brain computed tomographic scan should be acquired and other intracranial pathology ruled out before the initiation of antihypertensive therapy, because (1) lowering the systemic blood pressure in the face of increased intracranial pressure will lower the cerebral perfusion pressure and potentially result in focal or global cerebral ischemia; (2) the use of nitroprusside, a first-line agent for the acute treatment of hypertension (see later) can worsen intracranial pressure via vasodilation of cerebral arterioles; and (3) the radiologic pattern of abnormalities resulting from hypertensive encephalopathy has a characteristic distribution [78] if the clinical circumstances are not clear. For acute hypertension, although some estimate of etiology can be useful in selecting an appropriate pharmacologic therapy, except when hypertension is related to increased intracranial pressure, the determination of etiology is less essential than immediate blood pressure control. As such, once increased intracranial pressure has been eliminated as a clinical concern, the performance of complex diagnostic studies or transport of the patient from

the intensive care unit to other departments for evaluation should avoided until the blood pressure is suitably controlled.

The chronicity of systemic hypertension dictates the rapidi and extent of blood pressure reduction. In children with acu hypertension complicated by hypertensive encephalopathy, blo pressure reduction should be achieved as rapidly as possib Sudden lowering of blood pressure in a child with chronic hype tension, however, may incur cerebral hypoperfusion because of t failure of cerebral autoregulation to adapt to lower systemic blo pressures. Because gradual blood pressure reduction obviates aut regulatory failure, blood pressure reduction in chronically hype tensive children lacking acute symptomatology should accomplished over hours to days. Overall, the potential benefi associated with prompt blood pressure reduction must be weighe against the potential risk of brain injury resulting from hypoperfu sion. In general, the goal of antihypertensive therapy is to redu the blood pressure to below the 95th percentile for age, gender, an body size.

Acute, symptomatic blood pressure elevations usually manda the use of potent, short-acting parenteral pharmaceuticals rapidly and predictably titrate blood pressure reduction. Titratic of therapy should be continuously monitored by direct intraarteri measurement of blood pressure. The overall effectiveness of therap must be determined by the reversal of hypertension-induced sym tomatology, which should be assessed frequently and in a seri manner, for example, neurologic assessment in children presentin with hypertensive encephalopathy or cardiovascular assessment children presenting with congestive heart failure.

Direct Vasodilators

Sodium Nitroprusside

As a potent vaso- and venodilator with rapid onset and short dura tion of action, sodium nitroprusside is the consensus drug of choic for hypertensive emergencies (Table 23.4). The short duration c action enables precise blood pressure titration and necessitate administration via continuous infusion, which should be introduce at a low dose (0.5 µg/kg/min) and increased cautiously to achieve th desired level of blood pressure control. Continuous blood pressur monitoring via arterial catheterization should be employed to ensur safety and efficacy. Because nitroprusside is a nonselective organi nitrate that is metabolized to nitric oxide, it reduces blood pressur by decreasing systemic vascular resistance (vasodilation) and b decreasing cardiac output as a result of decreased preload (venodila tion) [79]. Therefore, caution must be used to prevent precipitou falls in blood pressure with resultant tissue ischemia.

Nitroprusside induces vasodilation in cerebral resistance an capacitance vessels and therefore may increase cerebral bloo volume and intracranial pressure [80,81]. In the setting of increase intracranial pressure, further compromise in cerebral perfusio and ischemic complications may occur [82]. Therefore, nitroprus side must be administered cautiously and with close neurologi monitoring in all patients with potential intracranial patholog Any deterioration in the neurologic examination, particularly decrease in the level of consciousness, should prompt a change i the antihypertensive agent or continuous monitoring of intracra nial pressure.

In addition to the release of nitric oxide, metabolism of nitro prusside by erythrocytes results in the release of cyanide, which is detoxified by rhodanase in the liver to thiocyanate and subse-

TABLE 23.4. Pharmaceutical agents for the treatment of hypertensive emergencies in children.

Class	Agent	Route of administration	Dosage	Onset of action	Duration of action	Adverse effects
Direct vasodilators	Nitroprusside	Continuous IV	0.5–6 μg/kg/min	Immediate		Tachycardia Thiocyanate toxicity Cyanide toxicity Intracranial hypertension
	Diazoxide	Intermittent IV	1–3 mg/kg/dose (max 150 mg/dose) q 5–15 min	1–5 min	3–12 hr	Hypotension Hyperglycemia Hyperuricemia Sodium and water retention
	Hydralazine	Intermittent IV	0.1–0.2 mg/kg/dose (max 20 mg/dose) q 4–6 hr	5–30 min	4–12 hr	Tachycardia Sodium and water retention Lupus-like syndrome
Calcium channel blockers	Nicardipine	Continuous IV	1–3 μg/kg/min	1–2 min	40 min	Thrombophlebitis Tachycardia
	Nifedipine	PO or sublingual	0.25–0.5 mg/kg/dose (max 10 mg/dose) q 4–6 hr	1–5 min 20–30 min	3–4 hr	Flushing Palpitations Fatigue
Adrenoceptor antagonists	Labetalol	Intermittent bolus or continuous IV	0.25–0.5 mg/kg/dose (max 10 mg/dose) q 6 hr 0.25–3.0 mg/kg/hr	5–10 min	2–4 hr	Bronchoconstriction Dizziness Fatigue Nausea Pruritis
	Esmolol	Continuous IV	0.5–1.0 mg/kg/min	Immediate	2–16 min	Bronchoconstriction Nausea Bradycardia
	Phentolamine	Intermittent bolus or continuous IV	0.05–0.1 mg/kg/dose (max 5 mg/dose) repeated to effect 1–4 μg/kg/min	Immediate	15–30 min	Tachycardia Nausea Headache
ACE inhibitors	Enalaprilat	Intermittent bolus	5–10 μg/kg/dose q 6 hr	15–30 minutes	4–6 hr	Hyponatremia Hyperkalemia Diarrhea Anemia Cough Angioedema

Note: ACE, angiotensin-converting enzyme; IM, intramuscular; IV, intravenous; PO, by mouth.

quently excreted by the kidneys. Particularly prevalent in renal failure, thiocyanate accumulation constitutes the principal toxicity of nitroprusside, resulting in metabolic acidosis, tachycardia, flushed skin, altered consciousness, decreased reflexes, dilated pupils, and methemoglobinemia [79].

Diazoxide

Diazoxide is a potent vasodilator that has been extensively used in children for the treatment of hypertensive emergencies. Diazoxide produces direct arteriolar dilation, resulting in decreased systemic vascular resistance, decreased blood pressure, reflex tachycardia, and increased cardiac output. The dosing range for diazoxide is 1–3 mg/kg to a maximum of 150 mg/dose when administered by rapid infusion over a period of 30 sec or less, with dosing repeated every 5–15 min until the blood pressure is decreased to an acceptable level [7,83]. Despite having a rapid onset of action (1–5 min) and excellent efficacy, the use of diazoxide is limited by a long duration of action (3–12 hr), difficulty of dose titration, and the propensity to cause significant hypotension in both degree and duration [84]. Other adverse effects of diazoxide include inhibition of insulin release and resultant hyperglycemia, rashes, hyperuricemia, sodium and water retention requiring the concomitant use of a diuretic, skin flushing, and headaches. Therefore, diazoxide, once commonly used for hypertensive emergencies, has been generally supplanted by newer therapies.

Hydralazine

One of the oldest vasodilators utilized for the treatment of hypertensive emergencies, hydralazine is a direct vasodilator that acts primarily on arterioles to decrease systemic vascular resistance. The usual dose is 0.1–0.2 mg/kg/dose up to a maximum dose of 20 mg every 4–6 hr. Onset of action occurs within 5–30 min after intravenous administration with a prolonged duration of action (4–12 hr). Adverse effects include significant reflex tachycardia, for which its use is usually paired with a β-blocker, skin flushing, sodium and water retention, and a lupus-like syndrome. Like diazoxide, hydralazine has generally been replaced by more rapid and efficacious antihypertensive agents.

Calcium Channel Blockers

Nicardipine

The only dihydropyridine calcium channel blocker available for intravenous administration, nicardipine reduces peripheral vascular resistance by inhibiting the movement of calcium into vascular smooth muscle cells, thereby inhibiting vasoconstriction with little effect on myocardial inotropy [85]. At a starting dose of 5 μg/kg/min via continuous intravenous infusion followed by 1–3 μg/kg/min maintenance dosing, the onset of action is rapid (1–2 min) with a relatively short duration of action (approximately 40 min). As such, precise titration to a desired blood pressure may be easily achieved with little risk of significant hypotension when performed with continuous blood pressure monitoring. Should hypotension occur, however, it may be readily reversed by the administration of calcium.

Although no large clinical trials have been performed in the pediatric population, the safety and efficacy of nicardipine for the treatment of hypertension has been demonstrated in several small series and case reports involving a variety of patient populations [85–91], including preterm infants, cardiothoracic surgical patients, and patients with renal disease. Reported adverse effects include local thrombophlebitis with peripheral administration, skin flushing, and tachycardia. In adult trials, the efficacy and safety of nicardipine compares favorably with nitroprusside [93,94]; however, unlike nitroprusside, to which rapid tachyphylaxis develops, nicardipine maintains its efficacy for a minimum of 10 days [91].

Nifedipine

Nifedipine is a dihydropyridine calcium channel blocker that can be administered orally or sublingually for the treatment of hypertension in children who are relatively asymptomatic. The onset of action occurs within 1–5 min if administered sublingually, 20–30 min if administered orally, with duration of action of approximately 3–4 hr. The recommended dosage range is 0.25–0.5 mg/kg with a maximum of 10 mg/dose. Minor adverse effects consist of flushing, palpitations, and fatigue.

Adrenoreceptor Antagonists

Labetalol

As a competitive inhibitor of peripheral α_1-adrenergic receptors, labetalol reduces blood pressure by inhibiting catecholamine-induced increases in peripheral vascular resistance. Because of competitive inhibition of β_1-adrenergic receptors, reflex tachycardia is not observed, yet cardiac output and stroke volume are preserved [95]. Intravenous administration may be via continuous infusion, starting at 0.25–1.5 mg/kg/hr to a maximum of 3 mg/kg/hr; or intermittent bolus, 0.2–1 mg/kg/dose to a maximum of 20 mg [96]. Time to onset of action is 5–10 min, with an activity duration of 2–4 hr, making it somewhat more difficult to titrate to effect than either sodium nitroprusside or nicardipine. Metabolism is via glucuronide conjugation in the liver, the products of which are then excreted in the urine and bile. Elimination, however, is not altered by renal or hepatic insufficiency [95]. Adverse effects include dizziness, fatigue, nausea and vomiting, pruritus, tingling, rash, and nasal congestion. Because labetalol competitively inhibits β_2-adrenergic receptors, it should be avoided by patients with asthma, as it may induce significant bronchospasm. Labetalol is also contraindicated for patients with myocardial dysfunction and chronic lung disease [95].

Esmolol

As a cardioselective β-adrenergic blocking agent, esmolol reduces blood pressure by decreasing heart rate, inotropy, stroke volume, and cardiac output; therefore, in pediatrics, esmolol has been used on a limited basis for the treatment of hypertensive crises associated with the repair of congenital heart disease [97–99]. The onset of action is nearly immediate, with duration of action of 2–16 min, requiring administration via continuous intravenous infusion [100]. Initial dosing should be 300 μg/kg/min, with

50–100 μg/kg/min incremental increases every 10 min to a maximum of 1,000 μg/kg/min [101]. Adverse effects associated with esmolol administration include bronchospasm, nausea and vomiting, and bradycardia.

Phentolamine

Phentolamine is an α-adrenergic receptor antagonist that blocks the vasoconstricting effects of circulating epinephrine and norepinephrine, and it is therefore indicated for the treatment of hypertensive emergencies associated with pheochromocytoma or other catecholamine-secreting tumors. When administered intravenously, the onset of action is nearly immediate, and the duration of action is 15–30 min. Intravenous dosing ranges from 0.05 to 0.1 mg/kg/dose to a maximum of 5 mg/dose. Repeated doses may be administered as necessary to maintain blood control. Based on its immediate onset and short duration of action, phentolamine has also been administered via continuous intravenous infusion (1–4 μg/kg/min) [102]. Adverse effects include tachycardia, nausea and vomiting, and headaches.

Angiotensin-Converting Enzyme Inhibitors

Enalaprilat

Enalaprilat is an intravenous preparation of the angiotensin-converting enzyme inhibitor enalapril and as such inhibits the conversion of angiotensin I to angiotensin II, preventing the vasoconstrictive and salt-retaining effects of angiotensin II and aldosterone. The use of enalaprilat for the treatment of hypertensive emergencies has variable efficacy depending on the patient's intravascular volume status and plasma renin level. Following intravenous dosing, the onset of action is within 15–30 min, limiting its value during a true hypertensive emergency, and its duration is 4–6 hr, making precise titration somewhat difficult [103]. The pediatric dose is 5–10 μg/kg every 6 hr [104]. It is 60%–80% eliminated via the kidney and therefore requires dosing adjustment in the patient with renal failure. For critically ill adults, enalaprilat has been shown to be efficacious when used as a continuous infusion [105–107]. The use of enalaprilat, like all angiotensin-converting enzyme inhibitors, is contraindicated in bilateral renovascular disease, where renal function is dependent on an intact renin–angiotensin–aldosterone system. Adverse effects include hyponatremia, hyperkalemia, diarrhea, anemia, cough, and angioedema.

Diuretics

Once the mainstay for treatment of hypertension, the use of diuretics in the treatment of hypertension has diminished with the development of newer, more focused therapies. Diuretics exert antihypertensive effects through fluid and salt excretion, resulting in decreased intravascular volume. As such, diuretics are particularly beneficial in those hypertensive states characterized by an increased intravascular volume. In addition, diuretics may be useful as adjuncts to overcome the fluid and salt-retaining properties of other antihypertensive agents.

Loop Diuretics

Furosemide and bumetanide act by blocking the Na-K-2Cl cotransporter in the ascending loop of Henle. These agents are particularly useful when rapid diuresis is desired and generally maintain effectiveness during states of renal insufficiency. For furosemide, intravenous dosing may be via intermittent bolus, 1 mg/kg/dose up to 10 mg/kg/day; or continuous infusion, 0.1–0.4 mg/kg/hr. For critically in children, continuous infusion of furosemide has been associated with more controlled diuresis and greater hemodynamic stability than intermittent dosing [108,109]. For bumetanide, intravenous dosing is via intermittent bolus, 0.015–0.1 mg/kg/dose up to 10 mg/day [110]. Although continuous infusion of bumetanide has been reported for adults, there are currently no reports of continuous infusion for children [111]. Adverse effects of the loop diuretics include hypokalemia, alkalosis, hypocalcemia, hypercalciuria with resultant development of nephrocalcinosis, and ototoxicity. It should be noted that continuous infusion of bumetanide in adults is associated with significant musculoskelatal symptomatology [111].

Thiazide Diuretics

Thiazide diuretics inhibit the Na—Cl contransporter in the distal tubule, preventing the reabsorption of sodium, resulting in natriuresis and diuresis. These agents provide a less vigorous but more sustained diuresis than do the loop diuretics. Adverse effects include hypokalemia, alkalosis, glucose intolerance, and adverse effects on lipid profiles.

References

1. Pavlakis SG, Frank Y, Chusid R. Hypertenisve encephalopathy, reversible occipitoparietal encephalopathy, or reversible posterior leukoencephalopathy: three names for an old syndrome. Child Neurol 1999;14:277–281.
2. Singhi P, Subramanian C, Jain V, Singhi S, Ray M. Reversible brain lesions in childhood hypertension. Acta Paediatr 2002;9:1005–1007.
3. Mattern WD, Sommers SC, Kassirer JP. Oliguric acute reanl failure in malignant hypertension. Am J Med 1972;52:187–197.
4. Wollam GL, Gifford RW Jr. The kidney as a target organ in hypertension. Geriatrics 1976;31:71–79.
5. Artman M, Graham TP. Congestive heart failure in infancy: recognition and management. Am Heart J 1982;103:1040–1055.
6. McConigle LF, Beaudry MA, Coe JY. Recovery from neonatal myocardial dysfunction after treatment of acute hypertension. Arch Dis Child 1987;62:614–615.
7. Porto I. Hypertensive emergencies in children. J Pediatr Health Care 2000;14:312–317.
8. Report of the Second Task Force on Blood Pressure in Children—1987. Pediatrics 1987;79:1–25.
9. Update on the 1987 Task Force Report on High Blood Pressure in Children and Adolescent: a Working Group Report from the National High Blood Pressure Education Program. Pediatrics 1996;98:649–658.
10. Houston M. Hypertensive emergencies and urgencies: pathophysiology and clinical aspects. Am Heart J 1986;111:205–210.
11. Cherney D, Straus S. Management of patients wtih hypertensive urgencies and emergencies: a systematic review of the literature. J Gen Inten Med 2002;17:937–945.
12. Bales A. Hypertensive crisis: how to tell if it's an emergency or an urgency. Postgrad Med 1999;105:119–126.
13. Fivush B, Neu A, Furth S. Acute hypertensive crisis in children: emergencies and urgencies. Curr Opin Pediatr 1997;9:233–236.
14. Churchill PC, Malvin RL, Opava SC. Evidence for baroreceptor control of renin release. Nephron 1974;13:382.
15. Zehr JE, Kurz KD, Seymour AA, Schultz HD. Mechanisms controlling renin release. Adv Exp Med Biol 1980;130:135–170.
16. Thrasher TN. Baroreceptor regulation of vasopressin and renin secretion: low-pressure versus high-pressure receptors. Front Neuroendocrinol 1994;15:157–196.
17. Briggs JP, Schnermann J. Macula densa control of renin secretion and glomerular tone: evidence for common cellular mechanisms. Ren Physiol 1986;9:193–203.
18. Skott O, Griggs JP. Direct demonstration of macula densa–mediated renin secretion. Science 1987;237:1618–1620.
19. Lorenz JN, Weihprecht H, Schnermann J, Skott O, Briggs JP. Renin release from isolated juxtaglomerular apparatus depends on macula densa chloride transport. Am J Physiol 1991;260:F486–F493.
20. Johnson JA, Davis JO, Gotshall RW, Lohmeier TE, Davis JL, Braverman B, Tempel GE. Evidence for an intrarenal beta receptor in control of renin release. Am J Physiol 1976;230:410–418.
21. Osborn JL, DiBona GF, Thames MD. Beta-1 receptor mediation of renin secretion elicited by low-frequency renal nerve stimulation. J Phamacol Exp Ther 1981;216:265–269.
22. Peart WS. Renin–angiotensin system. N Engl J Med 1975;292:302–306.
23. Hall JE. Historical perspective of the renin–angiotensin system. Mol Biotechnol 2003;24:27–39.
24. Sheikh IA, Kaplan AP. Mechanisim of digestion of bradykinin and lysylbradykinin (kallidin) in human serum. Role of carboxypeptidase, angiotensin-converting enzyme and determination of final degradation products. Biochem Pharmacol 1989;38:993–1000.
25. Reid IA. Actions of angiotensin II on the brain: mechanisms and physiologic role. Am J Physiol 1984;246:F533–F543.
26. Hsueh WA. Components of the renin system. An update. Am J Nephrol 1983;3:109–117.
27. Reid IA. The renin–angiotensin system and body function. Arch Intern Med 1985;145:1425–1479.
28. Rocha AS, Kokko JP. Permeability of medullary nephron segments to urea and waer: effect of vasopressin. Kidney Int 1974;6:379–387.
29. Leaf A, Mamby AR. The normal antidiuretic mechanism in man and dog; its regulation by extracellular fluid tonicity. J Clin Invest 1952;31:54–59.
30. Robertson GL. Thirst and vasopressin function in normal and disordered states of water balance. J Lab Clin Med 1983;101:351–371.
31. Leaf A, Mamby AR. An antidiuretic mechanism not regulated by extracellular fluid tonicity. J Clin Invest 1952;31:60–71.
32. Dunn FL, Brennan TJ, Nelson AE, Robertson GL. The role of blood osmolality and volume in regulating vasopressin secretion in the rat. J Clin Invest 1973;52:3212–3219.
33. Roberston GL, Aycinena P, Zerbe RL. Neurogenic disorders of osmoregulation. Am J Med 1982;72:339–353.
34. Ausiello DA, Skorecki KL, Verkman AS, Bonventre JV. Vasopressin signaling in kidney cells. Kidney Int 1987;31:521–529.
35. Ishikawa S. Cellular actions of arginine vasopressin in the kidney. Endocr J 1993;40:373–386.
36. Johnston CI. Vasopressin in circulatory control and hypertension. J Hypertens 1985;3:557–569.
37. Nemenoff RA. Vasopressin signalling pathways in vascular smooth muscle. Front Biosci 1998;15:d194–207.
38. Moncada S, Palmer RM, Higgs EA. Nitric oxide: physiology, pathophysiology, and pharmacology. Pharmacol Rev 1991;43:109–142.
39. Yanagisawa M, Masaki T. Endothelin, a novel endothelium-derived peptide. Pharmacological activities, regulation and possible roles in cardiovascular control. Biochem Pharmacol 1989;38:1877–1883.
40. Goetzl EJ, An S, Smith WL. Specificity of expression and side effects of eicosanoid mediators in normal physiology and human disease. FASEB J 1995;9:1051–1058.
41. Zeldin DC. Epoxygenase pathways of arachidonic acid metabolism. J Biol Chem 2001;276:36-059-062.
42. Manning DM, Kuchirka C, Kaminski J. Miscuffing: inappropriate blood pressure cuff application. Circulation 1983;68:763–766.
43. Park MK, Menard SM. Accuracy of blood pressure measurement by the Dinamapp monitor in infants and children. Pediatrics 1987;79:907–914.
44. Dannevig I, Dale HC, Liestol K, Lindemann R. Blood pressure in the neonate: three non-invasive oscillometric pressure nomitors com-

pared with invasively measrue blood pressure. Acta Paediatr 2005;94: 191–196.

45. Park MK, Menard SW, Schoolfield J. Oscillometric blood pressure standards for children. Pediatr Cardiol 2005;26:601–607.

46. Sy WP. Ulnar nerv palsy possible related to use of automatically cycled blood pressure cuff. Anesth Analg 1981;60:687–688.

47. Showman A, Betts EK. Hazard of automatic noninvasive blood pressure monitoring. Anesthesiology 1981;55:717–718.

48. Eisenberg S. Blood volume in patients wtih acute glomerulonephritis as determined by radioactive chromium tagged red cells. Am J Med 1959;27:241–245.

49. Powell HR, Rotenberg E, Williams AL, McCredie DA. Plasma renin activity in acute poststreptococcal gomerulonephritis and the haemolytic-uraemic syndrome. Arch Dis Child 1974;49:802–807.

50. Bras H, Oshs HG, Armbruster H, Heintz R. Plasma renin activity (PRA) and aldosterone (PA) in patients with chronic glomerulonephritis (GN) and hypertension. Clin Nephrol 1976;5:57–60.

51. Ishii M, Ikeda T, Takagi M, et al. Elevated plasma catecholamines in hypertensives with primary glomerular diseases. Hypertension 1983; 5:545–551.

52. Grunfeld B, Gimenez M, Leapchuc S, Mendilaharzu J, Gianantonia C. Systemic hypertension and plasma renin activity in childen with the hemolytic-uremic syndrome. Int J Pediatr Nephrol 1982;3:211–214.

53. Yamamoto T, Nagayama K, Satomura K, Honda T, Okada S. Increased serum IL-10 and endothelin levels in hemolytic uremic syndrome caused by *Escherichia coli* O157. Nephron 2000;84:326–332.

54. Amsterdam EA, Albers WH, Christlieb AR, Morgan CL, Nadas AS, Hickler RB. Plasma renin activity in children with coarctation of the aorta. Am J Cardiol 1969;23:396–399.

55. Parker FB Jr, Farrell B, Streeten DH, Blackman JS, Sondheimer HM, Anderson GH Jr. Hypertensive mechanisms in coarctation of the aorta. Further studies of the renin–angiotensin system. J Thorac Cardiovasc Surg 1980;80:568–573.

56. Alpert BS, Bain HH, Balfe JW, Kidd BS, Olley PM. Role of the renin–angiotensin–aldosterone system in hypertensive children with coarctation of the aorta. Am J Cardiol 1979;43:828–834.

57. Stewart JM, Gewitz MH, Woolf PK, Niguidula F, Fish BG, Zeballos GA. Elevated arginine vasopressin and lowered atrial natriuretic factor associated with hypertension in coarctation fo the aorta. J Thorac Cardiovasc Surg 1995;110:900–908.

58. Tenschert W, Baumgart P, Greminger P, Vetter W, Vetter H. Pathogenic aspects of hypertension in Cushing's syndrome. Cardiology 1985;72(Suppl 1):84–90.

59. Schonwetter BS, Libber SM, Jones MD Jr, Park KJ, Plotnick LP. Hypertension in neonatal hyperthyroidism. Am J Dis Child 1983;137: 954–955.

60. Moneta E, Castegnaro E. A case of congenital adrenal hyperplasia with hypertension. Folia Endocrinol 1968;21:603–610.

61. Hague WM, Honour JW. Malignant hypertension in congenital adrenal hyperplasia due to 11 beta-hydroxylase deficiency. Clin Endocrinol 1983;18:505–510.

62. Lauwers P. Promary hyperaldosteronism as a cause of hypertension. Lancet 1967;2:889–890.

63. McVicar M, Carman C, Chandra M, Abbi RJ, Teichberg S, Kahn E. Hypertension secondary to renin-secreting juxtaglomerular cell tumor: case report and review of 38 cases. Pediatr Nephrol 1993;7:404–412.

64. Rosenthal FD, Roy S. Hypertension and hyperthyroidism. BMJ 1972; 4:396–397.

65. Alon US, Monzavi R, Lilien M, Rasoulpour M, Geffner ME, Yadin O. Hypertension in hypophosphatemic rickets—role of secondary hyperparathyroidism. Pediatr Nephrol 2003;18:155–158.

66. Sherrard DJ. Hypercalcemia and hypertension. JAMA 1977;237: 2381.

67. Cushing H. Some experimental and clinical observations concerning state of increased intracranial tension. Am J Med Sci 1902;124: 375.

68. Clifton GL, Robertson CS, Kyper K, Taylor AA, Dhekne RD, Grossma RG. Cardiovascular response to severe head injury. J Neurosu 1983;59:447–454.

69. Goodman JH, Homan RW, Crawford IL. Kindled seizures activa both branches of the autonomic nervous system. Epilepsy Res 1999;3 169–176.

70. Falterman CJ, Kreisberg R. Pheochromocytoma: clinical diagnos and management. South Med J 1982;75:321–328.

71. Seefelder C, Sparks JW, Chirnomas D, Diller L, Shamberger RC Perioperative managemen of a child with severe hypertension from catecholamine secreting neuroblastoma. Paediatr Anaesth 2005;1! 606–610.

72. Shinohara M, Shitara T, Hatakeyama SI, et al. An infant with systemi hypertension, renal artery stenosis, and neuroblastoma. J Pediatr Sur 2004;39:103–106.

73. Virdis R, Balestrazzi P, Zampoli M, Donadio A, Street M, Lorenzet E. Hypertension in children with neurofibromatosis. J Hum Hyper tension 1994;8:395–397.

74. Marosvari I, Kontor E, Kallay K. Renin-secreting Wilms' tumou Lancet 1972;1:1180.

75. Ganguly A, Gribble J, Tune B, Kempson RL, Luetscher JA. Renin secreting Wilms' tumor with severe hypertension. Report of a cas and brief review of renin-secreting tumors. Ann Intern Med 1973 79:835–837.

76. Sheth KJ, Tang TT, Blaedel ME, Good TA. Polydipsia, polyuria, an hypertension associated with renin-secreting Wilms' tumor. J Pediat 1978;92:921–924.

77. Spahr J, Demers LM, Shochat SJ. Renin producing Wilms' tumor. Pediatr Surg 1981;16:32–34.

78. Jones BV, Egelhoff JC, Patterson RJ. Hypertensive encephalopathy i children. Am J Neuroradiol 1997;18:101–106.

79. Tinker JH, Michenfelder JD. Sodium nitroprusside: pharmacology toxicology, and therapeutics. Anesthesiology 1976;45:340–354.

80. Marsh ML, Shapiro HM, Smith RW, Marshall LF. Changes in neuro logic status and intracranial pressure assoiated with sodium nitro prusside administration. Anesthesiology 1979;51:336–338.

81. Morris PJ, Todd M, Philbin D. Changes in canine intracranial pressure in response to infusions of sodium nitroprusside and trinitroglycerin Br J Anaesth 1982;54:991–995.

82. Hartmann A, Buttinger C, Rommel T, Czernicki Z, Trtinjiak F. Alteration of intracranial pressure, cerebral blood flow, autoregulation and carbon dioxide-reactivity by hypotensive agents in baboons with intracranial hypertension. Neurochirurgia 1989;32:37–43.

83. Temple ME, Nahata MC. Treatment of pediatric hypertension. Pharmacotherapy 2000;20:140–150.

84. Grunwald Z, Meyers KEC. Hypertension in infants and children anesthetic implications. Anesthesiol Clin North Am 1999;17:645.

85. Sorkin EM, Clissold SP. Nicardipine. A review of its pharmacodynamic and pharmacokinetic properties, and therapeutic efficacy, in the treatment of angina pectoris, hypertension, and related cardiovascular disorders. Drugs 1987;33:296–345.

86. Treluyer JM. Hubert P, Jouvet P, Couderc S, Cloup M. Intravenous nicardipine in hypertensive children. Eur J Pediatr 1993;152:712–714.

87. Gouyon JB, Gemeste B, Semama DS, Francoise M, Germaine JF. Intravenous nicardipine in hypertensive preterm infants. Arch Dis Child Fetal Neonatal Ed 1997;76:F126–F127.

88. Tenney F, Sakarcan A. Nicardipine is a safe and effective agent in pediatric hypertensive emergencies. Am J Kidney Dis 2000;35:E20.

89. Milou C, Debuche-Benouachkou V, Semama DS, Germaine JF, Gouyon JB. Intravenous nicardipine as a first-line antihypertensive drug in neonates. Intensive Care Med 2000;26:956–958.

90. Tobias JD. Nicardipine to control mean arterial pressure after cardiothoracic surgery in infants and children. Am J Ther 2001;8:3–6.

91. Flynn JT, Mottes TA, Brophy PD, Kershaw DB, Smoyer WE, Bunchman TE. Intravenous nicardipine for treatment of severe hypertension in children. J Pediatr 2001;139:38–43.

92. Nakagawa TA, Sartori SC, Morris A, Schneider DS. Intravenous nicardipine for treatment of postcoarctectomy hypertension in children. Pediatr Cardiol 2004;25:26–30.

93. Halpern NA, Goldberg M, Neely C, Sladen RN, Goldberg JS, Floyd J, Gabrielson G, Greenstein RJ. Postoperative hypertension: a multicenter, prospective, randomized comparison between intravenous nicardipine and sodium nitroprusside. Crit Care Med 1992;20:1637–1643.

94. Neutel JM, Smith DH, Wallin D, et al. A comparison of intravenous nicardipine and sodium nitroprusside in the immediate treatment of severe hypertension. Am J Hypertens 1994;7:623–628.

95. Carter BL. Labetolol. Drug Intell Clin Pharm 1983;17:704–712.

96. Bunchman TE, Lynch RE, Wood EG. Intravenously administered labetalol for treatment of hypertension in children. J Pediatr 1992;120:140–144.

97. Vincent RN, Click LA, Williams HM, Plauth WH, Williams WH. Esmolol as an adjunct in the treatment of systemic hypertension after operative repair of coarctation of the aorta. Am J Cardiol 1990;65:941–943.

98. Smerling A, Gersony WM. Esmolol for severe hypertension following repair of aortic coarctation. Crit Care Med 1990;18:1288–1290.

99. Wiest DB, Garner SS, Uber WE, Sade RM. Esmolol for the management of pediatric hypertension after cardiac operations. J Thorac Cardiovasc Surg 1998;115:890–897.

100. Cuneo BF, Zales VR, Blahunka PC, Benson DW Jr. Pharmacodynamics and pharmacokinetics of esmolol, a short-acting beta-blocking agent, in children. Pediatr Cardiol 1994;15:296–301.

101. Wiest DB, Trippel DL, Gillette PC, Garner SS. Pharmacokinetics of esmolol in children. Clin Pharmacol Ther 1991;49:618–623.

102. Champoux L, Gauthier M. Continuous phentolamine perfusion in the treatment of severe arterial hypertension associated with neuroblastoma. Can Anaesth Soc J 1984;31:206–209.

103. Kubo SH, Cody RJ. Clinical pharmacokinetics of the angiotensin converting enzyme inhibitors. A review. Clin Pharmacokinet 1985;10:377–391.

104. Adelman RD, Coppo R, Dillon MJ. The emergency management of severe hypertension. Pediatr Nephrol 2000;14:422–427.

105. Tohmo H, Karanko M, Korpilahti K, Scheinin M, Viinamaki O, Neuvonen P. Enalaprilat in acute intractable heart failure after myocardial infarction: a prospective, consecutive sample, before–after trial. Crit Care Med 1994;22:965–973.

106. Boldt J Muller M, Heesen M, Harter K, Hempelmann G. Cardiorespiratory effects of continuous i.v. adminiatration of the ACE inhibitor enalaprilat in the critically ill. Br J Clin Pharmacol 1995;40:415–422.

107. Podbregar M, Voga G, Horvat M, Zuran I, Krivec B, Skale R, Pareznik R. Bolus versus continuous low dose of enalaprilat in congestive heart failure with acute refractory decompensation. Cardiology 1999;91:41–49.

108. Singh NC, Kissoon N, al Mofada S, Bennet M, Bohn DJ. Comparison of continuous versus intermittent furosemide administration in postoperative pediatric cardiac patients. Crit Care Med 1992;20:17–21.

109. Luciani GB, Nichani S, Chang AC, Wells WJ, Newth CJ, Starnes VA. Continuous versus inermittent furosemide infusion in critically ill infants after open heart operations. Ann Thorac Surg 1997;64:1133–1139.

110. Sullivan JE, Witte MK, Yamachita TS, Myers CM, Blumer JL. Dose-ranging evaluations of bumetanide pharmacodynamics in critically ill infants. Clin Pharmacol Ther 1996;60:424–434.

111. Howard PA, Dunn MI. Severe musculoskeletal symptoms during continuous infusion of bumetanide. Chest 1997;111:359–364.

24
Heart Transplantation

Shamel Abd-Allah and Paul A. Checchia

Introduction

The first successful heart transplantation was performed by Christian Barnard in 1967 (Table 24.1) [1]. Since then, there have been over 60,000 heart transplantations performed worldwide. The first pediatric cardiac transplantation was attempted by Kantrowitz et al. in 1968 [2]. However, it took another decade until the first series of successful pediatric heart transplantations were reported [3]. Currently, approximately 350 pediatric heart transplantations are performed annually [4]. Still, infant and pediatric cardiac transplantation accounts for only approximately 6% of total cardiac transplantations [5,6]. Improvement in outcomes for infants and children undergoing heart transplantation have now allowed this to be a treatment option for end-stage heart failure or inoperable congenital cardiac defects [7].

Despite the growth in use of pediatric heart transplantation, the volume is still limited compared with the number of procedures performed in adults. Therefore, any discussion of pediatric heart transplantation is complicated by a small experimental base. However, there has been continued enhancement of the care of the pediatric transplant candidate, advances in preservation and surgical techniques, improvement in perioperative critical care practice, and progress in long-term management strategies over the past decades. Additional efforts are being made to increase organ availability and quality through improvement in donor management [8], non-heart-beating protocols, and preservation techniques.

With the growing use of transplantation in the pediatric population, management challenges exist within the intensive care unit. These challenges can be divided into three time periods: the pretransplantation period, the immediate postoperative period, and the long-term management period. This chapter addresses the challenges for the pediatric critical care practitioner within each of these phases. The clinical problems leading to transplantation are discussed, with a focus on the critical management of the listed recipient. A discussion of surgical technique, organ preservation, and donor management concentrates on how these factors impact the postoperative course following transplantation. Immunosuppression and rejection are reviewed as they pertain to critical illness. Finally, the critical care of the transplanted patient as it relates to other disease processes is examined.

The Pretransplantation Period

Indications for Heart Transplantation

Dilated cardiomyopathy (DCM), palliated congenital heart disease with irreversible myocardial dysfunction, life-threatening arrhythmias resistant to conventional medical therapy, and lethal neonatal heart disease are current indications for heart transplantation. The indications for transplantation vary substantially depending on recipient's age. Based on the International Society of Heart and Lung Transplantation Registry data [6], the most common age for pediatric heart transplantation is between 0 and 1 year (Figure 24.1). This group is composed of patients with congenital heart disease as the predominant indication for transplantation. In older pediatric populations, DCM becomes the major indication for transplantation (Table 24.2). In the early years of transplant experience, the ratio of congenital heart disease to DCM overwhelmingly favored congenital heart disease as the indication in this age group. In recent years, this gap has narrowed (Figure 24.2). It is certainly possible that as the number of patients with complex congenital heart disease grows older, they may become candidates for transplantation.

Congenital conditions for which transplantation has been successfully accomplished include hypoplastic left heart syndrome [9], corrected transposition of the great arteries [10], coronary artery fistula [11], cardiac tumor [12], and endocardial fibroelastosis [13]. However, improvements in the outcomes of many surgical palliative and corrective approaches, especially as related to hypoplastic left heart syndrome, have lead to controversy about the best approach to these congenital conditions [14,15]. Many centers that utilized transplantation for these lesions now employ surgical palliation with great success.

D.S. Wheeler et al. (eds.), *Cardiovascular Pediatric Critical Illness and Injury*,
DOI 10.1007/978-1-84800-923-3_24, © Springer-Verlag London Limited 2009

TABLE 24.1. Historical milestones in heart transplantation.

1960	Successful orthotopic cardiac transplantation in the dog by Lower and Shumway
1967	Successful orthotopic cardiac transplantation in a human by Barnard
1972	Development of percutaneous transvenous right ventricular endomyocardial biopsy by Billingham
1974	Development of a standardized grading system for endomyocardial biopsy by Billingham
1979	Cyclosporine A first introduced for use in immunosuppression
1985	Successful orthotopic cardiac transplantation in a human infant by Bailey

TABLE 24.2. Indications for heart transplantation by age.

Age	Myopathy	Congenit…
<1 year	33%	67%
1–10 years	52%	37%
11–17 years	62%	28%

Source: Data are from The Registry of the International Society for Heart and Lung Tran… plantation [6].

Dilated cardiomyopathies represent the other major indication for transplantation. Although progress has been made in understanding the multiple infectious, metabolic, and myocardial protein mutation etiologies that result in a diagnosis of pediatric DCM [16,17], the prognosis of DCM remains guarded [18]. Because of the unpredictable natural history observed in children with DCM, there are no widely accepted clinical or laboratory criteria exist that could help distinguish children who should be listed for transplantation. Many of these patients can demonstrate eventual improvement and resolution of left ventricular dilation and dysfunction [19].

Contraindications to Heart Transplantation

The contraindications to cardiac transplantation are listed in Table 24.3. Although these are general contraindications, a specific factor is elevated pulmonary vascular resistance (PVR) [20]. This is the most difficult preoperative problem to overcome because the donor heart has been exposed to an ischemic injury and the right ventricle may not be able to adequately respond to the increased work required with abnormal pulmonary vasculature. For this reason, a patient with elevated PVR may be best managed by heart–lung transplantation.

Extracardiac anomalies or failure of other organs are also relative contraindications to transplantation. Although renal failure requiring dialysis impacts outcome [21,22], it is not an absolute contraindication to transplantation. Patients with genetic syndromes in which there is diminished longevity are also not candidates for transplantation.

Management of the Transplant Recipient

Once referred for heart transplantation, the potential transplant recipient must undergo a comprehensive, multidisciplinary evaluation, including cardiac, pulmonary, renal, neurologic, socioeconomic, and psychosocial assessment. The pretransplant evaluation must necessarily include extensive laboratory testing (Table 24.4). Once listed for transplantation, children are designated as either status I or status II. Children designated status I take precedence whenever an organ becomes available, and, in order to qualify a status I, children must be hospitalized in the pediatric intensive care unit (PICU) on either mechanical cardiac support or inotropic support. Children designated status II are less critically ill and comprise the remaining children who do not fulfill criteria for status I. One notable exception is that infants less than 6 months of age are automatically designated status I regardless of their severity of illness.

The decisions involved in obtaining suitable candidates for transplantation are difficult. This is especially true for patients admitted to an intensive care unit before transplantation who must have their condition optimized in order to tolerate surgery. This may involve intervention with mechanical respiratory or circulatory support in order to provide a bridge to transplantation.

Circulatory Support

Patients with cardiac failure awaiting transplantation are at high risk for progression to a decompensated shock state. This, obviously, impacts their ability to undergo the transplant procedure. A further complicating factor is that a significant portion of children who present with cardiogenic shock from acute cardiomyopathy eventually recover without the need for transplantation.

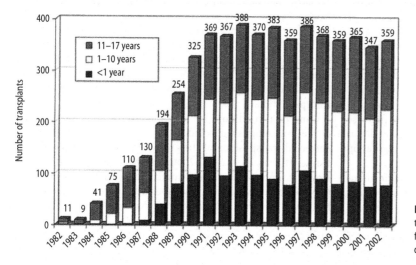

FIGURE 24.1. Age distribution of pediatric heart recipients by year of transplant for transplants done from January 1996 to June 2003. (Data from Boucek et al. [6]. © 2004 with permission from International Society of Heart and Lung Transplanation.)

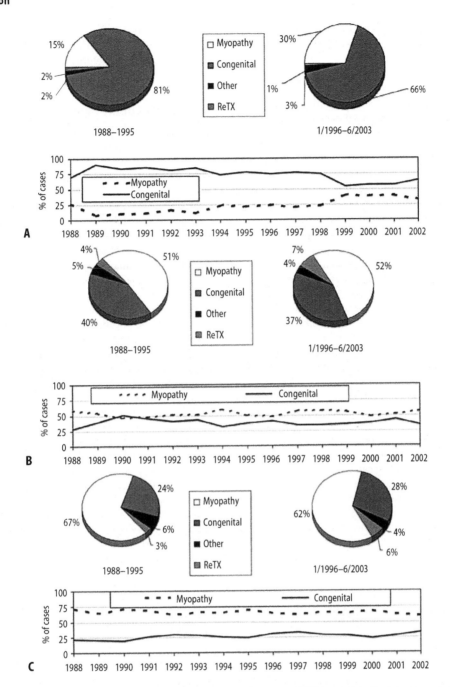

FIGURE 24.2. **(A)** Diagnoses for pediatric heart transplant recipients (aged <1 year) ReTX, retransplantation. **(B)** Diagnoses for pediatric heart transplant recipients (aged 1–10 years). **(C)** Diagnoses for pediatric heart transplant recipients (aged 11–17 years) (Data from Boucek et al. [6]. © 2004 with permission from International Society of Heart and Lung Transplantation.)

TABLE 24.3. Contraindications to cardiac transplantation.

Recent or recurrent malignancy
Serious active infection or recurrent infection (e.g., human immunodeficiency virus, hepatitis B)
Chromosomal, metabolic, or genetic abnormality with poor long-term prognosis
Significant organ system failure
Psychosocial instability

TABLE 24.4. Pretransplant battery of laboratory tests.

ABO type
Electrolytes, blood urea nitrogen/creatinine, liver enzymes
Complete blood count/differential
Viral serologies: human immunodeficiency virus; cytomegalovirus; Epstein-Barr virus; hepatitis A, B, C; herpes simplex virus
HLA typing
Panel reactive antibody
Chest x-ray
Echocardiogram
Electrocardiogram

[17,23]. Again, the goals of intensive care management of these patients are to aid in candidate selection and optimization of the recipient.

Refinements in critical care and inotropic support have improved the survival rate of patients who are critically ill in the PICU and have also helped end-stage patients survive until transplantation. In fact, Tsirka at al. [24] reported the experience with 91 pediatric patients who were diagnosed with DCM during the decade of the 1990s. In their population, PICU admission occurred at the time of presentation for 35% of patients. Interestingly, admission to the PICU at the time of diagnosis was significantly associated with recovery of systolic function. Although this recovery occurs, the advances in heart failure and shock management have contributed to a tendency for more children to be transplanted from a state requiring inotropic or mechanical circulatory support [4]. The successful use of extracorporeal membrane oxygenation (ECMO) in children as a bridge to transplantation has been reported by several centers [25–28]. ECMO support is not without complications. First, infection and bleeding issues develop [29,30]. Second, ECMO bridging to transplantation may require the increased use of marginal donor hearts [4]. Additionally, the need for mechanical circulatory support appears to increase the risk of primary graft failure [31]. Finally, this is not a long-term support. This is of particular concern because the wait for transplantation is likely to be months rather than weeks [32].

In the future it is likely that more permanent mechanical bridges to transplantation will be available [26,33–40]. Within the past few years the use of mechanical support devices to augment cardiac output has dramatically changed the outlook for adult patients who remain unstable despite maximal pharmacologic support. Implantable ventricular assist devices (VAD) can be used with low morbidity and, in adults, can be managed in an outpatient setting [41]. Unfortunately, the sizes of the devices limit their use in children, but they are an attractive option for larger adolescents. External VADs have been used in pediatric patients as small as 20 kg, but ambulation is very difficult.

Respiratory Support

The need for ventilator support in the recipient before transplantation has been identified as a risk factor for primary graft failure in adults [42] and for 1-year mortality for pediatric recipients in the UNOS/ISHLT registry [6]. Its association with the development of isolated right ventricular graft failure in this study suggests that a need for preoperative ventilator support in a transplant candidate may be a sign of increasing PVR. These findings are consistent with other pediatric studies [43–45] suggesting that pediatric patients with PVR >6 Woods units/m^2 who demonstrate evidence of reversibility with medical therapy can undergo successful heart-only transplantation. However, these patients may require more intensive and prolonged postoperative support, including a need for short-term mechanical support, than patients with low pulmonary resistance.

Nutritional Support

In addition to strategies to maximize cardiac output and ventilation, careful attention to nutrition and physical activity is important for patients awaiting transplantation. Children with end-stage heart failure are frequently nauseated and anorexic and have minimal physical activity. This combination can lead to skeletal muscle breakdown and atrophy, which can exacerbate symptoms of heart failure [46–48]. Hyperalimentation may be required maintain adequate nutritional support and a formal physic therapy program is helpful in minimizing muscle weakness a atrophy.

Management of the Potential Organ Donor

As in adult heart transplantation, donor organ availability lim the number of children receiving heart transplantation. Waiti time mortality and morbidity are still significant, ranging fro 10% after 30 days to 20% after 90 days [32]. Although there ha been small increases in the number of available pediatric dono over the past several years, this number remains relative unchanged [49]. Efforts to increase donation rates have focused public education, changes in legislation, and improvements family consenting procedures. Additionally, it has been recognize that the medical management of potential organ donors may infl ence the organs procured [50–53]. Intensivists are intimate involved with each of these efforts.

Standardization of management of organ donors has been pr posed as method of improving recovery rates [50]. Typically, thes management strategies tend to focus on specific organ systems opposed to preserving global function. Furthermore, althoug adult donor management strategies have been investigated an attempts have been made to establish protocols, variations rema [54]. For the pediatric population, little information is availab regarding current donor management practices and their effect o the number of organs recovered. However, the overall recovery ra in the pediatric population is low. Furthermore, this recovery ra does not appear to be influenced by the presence of specialize pediatric care provided at the institutional level [8].

Selection of potential donors is an important factor in the succes of transplantation. The degree of ventricular dysfunction can b evaluated by both echocardiographic indices and cardiac troponi levels [55]. Previous work has found a relationship in infant between degree of donor myocardial injury as determined b cardiac troponin I levels and cause of death in the donor [56 Higher levels of cardiac troponin I in the donor before harvest ar associated with subsequent mortality from primary graft failure i the recipient [57].

Non-Heart-Beating Donors

Efforts to increase potential organs available for transplantatio have included non-heart-beating donation (NHBD). This is define as the surgical recovery of organs after the pronouncement of deat based on cessation of cardiopulmonary function [58]. It is esti mated that NHBD can increase the number of organs available fo transplant by 25% [59]. The process, however, is controversial an carries with it significant ethical considerations. Although NHBI may be viewed as a new donation procedure, it actually provide the foundation for modern clinical transplantation. The procedur has been used most frequently in kidney transplantation, but it als has been utilized in heart transplantation as well [60]. The reevalu ation of NHBD protocols and the pursuit of their implementatio in the pediatric population will be a significant issue facing pedi atric intensivists in the coming years.

Graft Preservation

In addition to donor and recipient factors, graft preservation wi impact the postoperative course of a child undergoing heart trans plantation. In adult heart transplantation, there is evidence that ischemic times greater than 4 hr affect late survival [61]. However, the influence of graft ischemic time is controversial in the adult cardiac transplantation population. Multicenter studies have shown that prolonged ischemic time has a negative effect on early survival [62,63]. Single center studies [64–67] reported that short- and long-term outcomes were not adversely affected by graft ischemic times longer than 4 hr. Two retrospective studies from the pediatric transplantation group at Loma Linda University have analyzed myocardial function using echocardiographic measurements [68] as well as assessing myocardial damage by cardiac myosin light chain efflux [69]. Patients who received donor hearts with long ischemic periods demonstrated diminished cardiac function in the first postoperative week, with functional recovery after the second week. Serum levels of cardiac myosin light chain were higher during the first post-transplant week in patients who received donor hearts with prolonged ischemia; significant differences were not evident beyond the first post-transplant week in patients with either long or short graft ischemia. In both studies, long graft ischemic time was as defined as more than 4 hours, and short ischemic time was defined as less than 4 hours. Additional reports have suggested that ischemic times of greater than 8 hr do not significantly impact short or long-term graft survival [70].

The Surgical Procedure

The nuances of cardiac transplantation pertaining to the surgical technique and procedure are well beyond the intended scope of the current discussion. However, as a general point of reference, the surgical technique is briefly described in the accompanying Figures 24.3 and 24.4. In addition, the interested reader is directed to any of several available pediatric cardiac surgery textbooks for additional information.

The Post-Transplantation Period

Circulatory System

Inotropic Support

Optimal inotropic support after transplantation is critical to support possible primary ventricular dysfunction in the immediate postoperative period. There are elevations in both right- and left-sided filling pressures, which fall over time. The reduction in right-sided pressures may be attributable to a decrease in pulmonary artery pressure, improvement of right ventricular contractility, and a decrease in tricuspid regurgitation [71,72]. Decreasing left-sided filling pressures likely correlate with recovery of the left ventricle

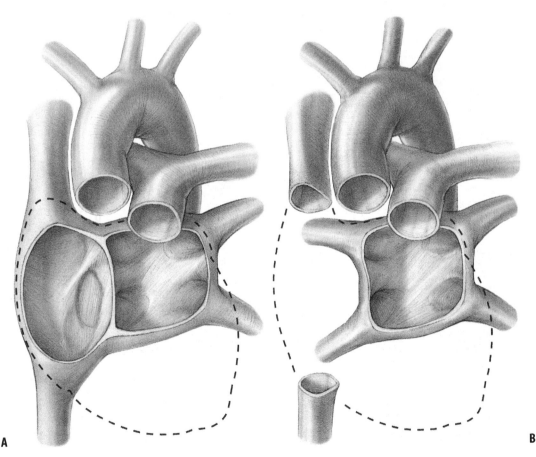

A   **B**

FIGURE 24.3. The recipient heart, **(A)** with hypoplastic left heart syndrome and **(B)** normal heart, has been excised in preparation for transplantation. (Courtesy of James D. St. Louis, MD, Medical College of Georgia.)

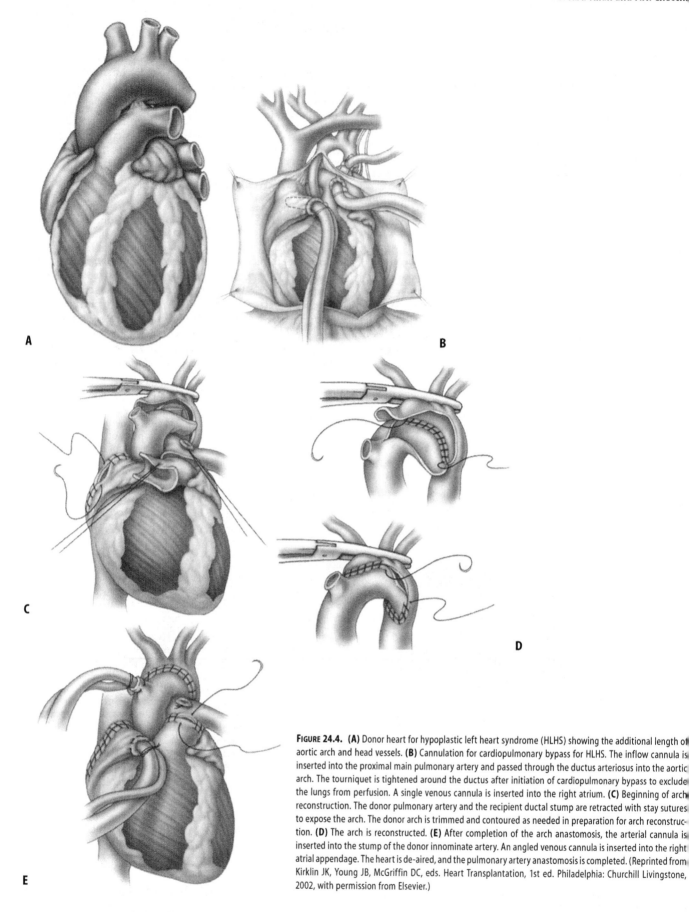

Figure 24.4. **(A)** Donor heart for hypoplastic left heart syndrome (HLHS) showing the additional length of aortic arch and head vessels. **(B)** Cannulation for cardiopulmonary bypass for HLHS. The inflow cannula is inserted into the proximal main pulmonary artery and passed through the ductus arteriosus into the aortic arch. The tourniquet is tightened around the ductus after initiation of cardiopulmonary bypass to exclude the lungs from perfusion. A single venous cannula is inserted into the right atrium. **(C)** Beginning of arch reconstruction. The donor pulmonary artery and the recipient ductal stump are retracted with stay sutures to expose the arch. The donor arch is trimmed and contoured as needed in preparation for arch reconstruction. **(D)** The arch is reconstructed. **(E)** After completion of the arch anastomosis, the arterial cannula is inserted into the stump of the donor innominate artery. An angled venous cannula is inserted into the right atrial appendage. The heart is de-aired, and the pulmonary artery anastomosis is completed. (Reprinted from Kirklin JK, Young JB, McGriffin DC, eds. Heart Transplantation, 1st ed. Philadelphia: Churchill Livingstone, 2002, with permission from Elsevier.)

from its ischemic state during transport and bypass. Additionally, systemic hypertension is frequently seen as a side effect of immunosuppressive therapy and may require afterload reduction.

The choice of inotropic agent for low cardiac output must account for the denervated state of the transplanted heart. Agents that act primarily through the autonomic nervous system may be ineffective in maintaining cardiac output. Similarly, drugs that act both directly on the heart and indirectly via the autonomic nervous system will exert only their direct effects. The loss of the presynaptic neuronal catecholamine update system after denervation leads to a loss of norepinephrine stores beyond the early postoperative period [73]. This affects the action of dopamine, which can no longer be converted to norepinephrine. Dopamine, therefore, will likely manifest only its dopaminergic and β-receptor effects. Additionally, the transplanted heart appears to be supersensitive to exogenous norepinephrine and epinephrine because of a loss of presynaptic reuptake of these drugs [74]. Finally, patients often benefit from a chronotropic stimulus in the perioperative period that can be obtained from the use of isoproterenol.

Nitric Oxide

Pulmonary hypertension before heart transplantation is a major risk factor because of an increased risk of right ventricular failure and death. It is considered desirable for PVR not to exceed 2.5 Wood units or transpulmonary pressure gradient 12 mmHg, although there are no precise thresholds [75]. The management of right-sided heart failure includes the use of inotropes, vasodilators (nitroglycerin, nitroprusside, prostaglandins, and nitric oxide [NO]), and VADs [76]. Specifically, the use of inhaled NO has been examined in this patient population but only in limited series and case reports [77–80]. Auler et al. [81] suggested using inhaled NO immediately after heart transplantation to prevent right ventricular failure. In addition to selective pulmonary vasodilation, inhaled NO can improve hypoxemia by improving the ventilation–perfusion relationship as a result of its delivery as an inhalational agent. This improvement in oxygenation is produced with lower doses of inhaled NO than that required to induce vasodilation.

Mechanical Circulatory Support Following Transplantation

Cardiac transplant recipients may occasionally require mechanical circulatory support following transplantation as a "bridge to recovery" [82]. Similar criteria should be used in deciding to place these children on such support as any other patient, including reversibility of disease, acceptable predicted neurologic function, and failure of other less-invasive therapies. In addition, no significant contraindications should exist, as, for example, multiorgan system failure. It can be difficult to make these decisions and may vary depending on the institution; however, with team discussion, including the patient's family and the gathering of as much objective information as possible regarding the patient's condition, a reasonably informed decision can often be determined. The weight restrictions present for certain VADs and cannula placement will also affect the final conclusion. The child's condition pretransplant may also affect the ultimate result following surgery.

Indications to initiate post-transplant mechanical circulatory support will likely involve significant pulmonary and/or cardiac dysfunction. Timing will vary, with the need arising immediately following cardiac transplantation or years after. Pulmonary failure can be caused by acute respiratory distress syndrome, pneumonia, or intraoperative inability to expand the lungs following pretrans-

plant ECMO. Cardiac indications would include primary graft failure and inability to discontinue cardiopulmonary bypass, acute rejection, unexpected elevated PVR, significant life-threatening dysrhythmias, and cardiac arrest. Sepsis with multiple-organ system dysfunction may also warrant the need for mechanical circulatory support. Failure to recover cardiac function may necessitate retransplantation.

Typically, ECMO is the most common mode of mechanical circulatory support employed; however, as VADs improve technologically, their use may increase. Patients placed on ECMO acutely post-transplant are often cannulated through the chest; late after transplantation, cannulation is mainly through the neck or groin. Significant hemorrhage is the chief disadvantage with chest cannulation, and there is also an increased risk of mediastinitis. Left ventricular distension should be treated promptly with either left atrial drain placement or balloon atrial septostomy. When needed, early institution of mechanical circulatory support is imperative, as prolonged periods of hypoxemia and low cardiac output will contribute to further end-organ damage, decreasing likelihood of recovery [83].

Fenton et al. [82] reported on 20 children who required mechanical circulatory support following cardiac transplantation. Fifteen patients required ECMO less than 6 weeks after transplantation, and five were placed on ECMO up to 7 years post-transplant. Indications included sepsis, elevated PVR, primary graft failure, acute cellular rejection, and pulmonary failure. Overall long-term survival was 50%, but it appeared related to indication for ECMO. In this series, 100% of children survived who required support for rejection, and 83% survived of those with primary graft failure. Similarly, Kirshbom et al. [84] report improved survival (66%) in children requiring late ECMO mainly for rejection compared with a 33% survival rate for those needing early ECMO primarily for immediate graft dysfunction or right heart failure. Two of four patients requiring early ECMO were listed for retransplantation, and both received organs. Merckle et al. [27] include in their series of children treated with the Berlin Heart VAD one patient with early graft failure after transplantation. All patients in this group had at least one episode of cardiopulmonary resuscitation before device implantation. Unfortunately, this specific patient did not survive.

Primary Graft Failure

Primary graft failure can occur at any time. It can be difficult to determine the exact cause in some occasions, as acute rejection will present similarly. In certain patients, the diagnosis is determined on autopsy or on examination of the explanted heart after retransplantation. Elevated pulmonary pressures or hyperacute rejection are often the main factors causing early graft breakdown in children who are unable to wean off cardiopulmonary bypass following cardiac transplantation or who remain on significant support. Other reasons include primary myocardial failure from preoperative myocardial insult in the donor, perioperative preservation, and reperfusion injury [85]. Hoffman et al. [86] report coronary artery injury during harvest or implantation causing acute graft failure in a child who required ECMO support following transplantation. Prolonged donor ischemia time up to 5 hr [87] does not appear to affect graft function and long-term survival, nor does high donor-recipient size mismatches in infants. Previous work has found a relationship in infants between degree of donor myocardial injury as determined by cardiac troponin I levels and primary graft failure in the recipient [56]. With late primary graft failure, coronary artery vasculopathy should be strongly considered.

Cardiac retransplantation remains the best treatment option to recipients with failing grafts. Mechanical circulatory support may be necessary to realize this goal, depending on the degree of graft collapse, and can be achieved with some success [27,82,84,86]. In a series studied by Dearani et al. [88], 32 children were listed for retransplantation, with indications being allograft vasculopathy, primary graft failure, and acute rejection. Ten patients died while on the waiting list, and 22 children underwent cardiac retransplantation. Two patients with primary graft failure underwent retransplantation within 24 hr of the first transplantation procedure while on ECMO. Median time interval to retransplantation for the others was 7.2 years (range 32 days to 9.4 years). There was no significant difference in actuarial survival at 3 years between those children undergoing primary cardiac transplant and those receiving retransplantation. The investigators conclude that elective retransplantation can be performed with acceptable mortality. It is likely this option will become increasingly prevalent with the longer survival of the pediatric heart transplant population.

Dysrhythmias

Dysrhythmias vary following cardiac transplantation in children. In two recent series of patients studied, the incidence of clinically significant dysrhythmias ranged from 19% to 38% [89,90]. Atrioatrial conduction, although rare, can occur as a result of the recipient atrial tissue being anastomosed to the donor organ [91]. It is also known that the donor organ is not initially innervated and typically demonstrates decreased heart rate variability. This may improve over several months; however, the exact mechanism for improvement is unknown, although autonomic "reinnervation" of the donor heart has been proposed [91]. Sinus bradycardia, presumably from sinoatrial node injury, can be seen immediately post-transplant and, if clinically significant, may warrant acute treatment to maintain adequate cardiac output. Other dysrhythmias that can be seen include atrial tachydysrhythmias, ventricular tachycardia, complete atrioventricular block, and Wenckebach periodicity. The atrial disturbances can be further divided into atrial flutter, atrial ectopic tachycardia, atrial fibrillation, and atrioventricular node reentry. Atrial flutter, atrial fibrillation, late episodes of sinus bradycardia, and Wenckebach periodicity appear to be associated with rejection and/or graft vasculopathy. Graft ischemia time does not appear to correlate with the incidence of dysrhythmias [89–92].

Permanent pacemaker placement may be necessary in patients with clinically significant bradydysrhythmias. The incidence of permanent pacemakers in pediatric heart transplant recipients has been reported to be 3%–6% [89,92,93]. Symptoms seen in some patients included syncope and dizziness. In a series described by Cannon et al. (92), those children who required pacemaker placement greater than 3 months following transplantation all eventually required retransplantation secondary to severe graft vasculopathy. The primary rhythms necessitating pacemaker placement in this group were symptomatic sinus pauses with normal average heart rate over a 24-hr period. These patients did not have an increased incidence of rejection. Collins et al. [89] include in their investigation 12 children requiring pacemaker placement for sinus node dysfunction and complete heart block. The majority of these patients died or were retransplanted.

Pulmonary Hypertension

Elevated pulmonary vascular pressure is a major cause of early graft failure in pediatric cardiac transplant recipients. The donor heart is often not adapted to an elevated PVR, and, if suddenly exposed to an extreme right ventricular strain, it may lead to acute right heart failure. Moreover, the postoperative period is complicated by the injury caused by cardioplegia, myocardial ischemia, and postcardiopulmonary bypass inflammatory cascade activation, leading to additional ventricular dysfunction. Determination of preoperative pulmonary arterial resistance is imprecise in infants with complex structural heart defects, and appropriate Wood units before transplantation does not rule out the occurrence of elevated pressures postoperatively [94]. Pulmonary artery systolic pressure >35 mm Hg is associated with increased 1-year mortality, whereas pressures below this are associated with decreased mortality in recipients [6]. A hyperreactive pulmonary vasculature, especially related to simultaneous respiratory infection, will further contribute to pulmonary hypertension crises that can occur at any time. Some suggest that it is the reactivity of the pulmonary vascular bed during cardiac catheterization pretransplantation, not the absolute measures of PVR, that correlate best with outcome [44,95]. Certain centers have proposed the use of oversized donor hearts for recipients with preexisting pulmonary hypertension to ensure adequate right ventricular function after transplantation [44,96]. Others discuss successful transplantation of domino hearts from chronic pulmonary hypertension recipients of heart–lung transplantation [97]. Advantages of the domino heart graft include right ventricular hypertrophy as a result of constant exposure to altered pulmonary vasculature, making the graft better able to function against elevated recipient pulmonary pressures.

Management of pulmonary hypertension in pediatric cardiac transplantation should begin preoperatively. Optimization of oxygen saturations and ventilation should be achieved. If the child is mechanically ventilated, inhaled NO may be necessary. In the operating suite, inhaled NO can be initiated either prophylactically or to successfully wean off cardiopulmonary bypass. This strategy must be continued on return to the PICU. Lung volumes should be adequate, and aggressive treatment of atelectasis is mandatory. Sedation and chemical paralysis can be considered for refractory situations. High-frequency oscillatory ventilation may be necessary to reach acceptable oxygen saturations. Inotropic tactics include minimizing vasoconstrictors and administration of afterload reducers such as milrinone and dobutamine in an attempt to vasodilate the pulmonary vascular bed. In those patients with severe graft dysfunction despite maximum medical measures, mechanical circulatory support can be successful in supporting the myocardium until a decrease in PVR occurs [96,98].

When weaning inhaled NO from the improving patient, a slow decrease in the last 5 ppm over 24 hr may aid in preventing rebound pulmonary hypertension. The use of oral sildenafil has been described to prevent further pulmonary hypertension crisis and to assist in withdrawal of inhaled NO following cardiac surgery in children [99,100]. Additionally, inhaled iloprost and intravenous iloprost have been employed in the treatment of pulmonary hypertension secondary to congenital heart disease with less systemic hypotension seen with the inhaled form [101,102]. Again, for those patients with persistent, diffuse lung congestion and elevated pulmonary pressures post-transplant, pulmonary venous obstruction should be considered, especially in children with underlying diagnoses of situs inversus and total anomalous pulmonary venous return.

Renal System

Acute Renal Insufficiency

Children undergoing heart transplantation may go into surgery with acute renal insufficiency or may develop acute renal insufficiency following transplantation. Cardiac output both before and after transplantation is a major determinant of this parameter. Patients requiring significant inotropic support or ECMO pretransplantation will often have a degree of acute renal insufficiency related to decreased kidney perfusion and the lack of pulsatile flow. Children awaiting heart transplantation placed on a VAD can have full recovery of kidney function before transplantation [103]. Acute hemodialysis or continuous renal replacement therapy (CRRT) may therefore be necessary before transplantation depending on the degree of volume overload, uremia, metabolic acidosis, and hyperkalemia.

Continuous venovenous hemofiltration (CVVH) can be performed while a child is on ECMO if the same conditions persist or occur. In a series of children requiring ECMO as a bridge to cardiac transplantation reported by Gajarski et al. [21], 43% experienced renal failure and required CVVH while listed. These patients did worse than those who did not develop renal failure even after transplantation, with survival to hospital discharge decreasing significantly from 75% to 33%. It is unclear to what extent renal failure directly contributed to the patient deaths versus serving as a marker for multiple-organ dysfunction, because patients requiring CVVH who died also had multiple-organ dysfunction. The ischemia-reperfusion type injury after exposure to cardiopulmonary bypass will add to renal insult [104]. Return of renal function will vary from days to weeks, but it can be rapid with good graft function and close attention to dose adjustment and serum level monitoring of potentially nephrotoxic agents.

The incidence of acute renal insufficiency requiring dialysis or CVVH in the immediate post-transplantation period in children is not clear in the literature. An investigation by Vricella et al. showed 22% of neonates needing peritoneal dialysis postoperatively for acute renal failure [105]. Peritoneal dialysis was begun at a mean of 51 hr after transplantation and continued for a mean of 101 ± 90.5 hr. However, in two separate studies evaluating causes of pediatric acute renal failure leading to renal replacement therapy, approximately 5% were because of heart transplantation [106,107]. There also appears to be an increased use of CRRT in North America and Europe for critically ill children with decreasing use of peritoneal dialysis [108]. Both CRRT and peritoneal dialysis are typically the preferred dialysis modality for hypotensive, mechanically ventilated patients requiring inotropic support except when treatment is necessary for life threatening PO hyperkalemia in which case acute intermittent hemodialysis would be favored. Peritoneal dialysis has a proven history in postoperative pediatric cardiothoracic patients; however, CRRT does appear to offer some advantages over other modes of dialysis in the unstable patient. The gradual, gentle removal of fluid on a continuous basis better mimics normal kidney function and allows greater freedom to provide larger volumes of nutritional support, an always important goal for the postoperative patient [109]. Continuous renal replacement therapy may also assist in the removal of proinflammatory cytokines released during sepsis [110]. In a cohort of 21 critically ill children receiving CVVH,

Goldstein et al. noted that the degree of fluid overload at CVVH initiation was significantly lower in survivors (16.4%) than in nonsurvivors (34%) even when controlled for severity of illness by PRISM score [111]. Similarly, Ronco et al. demonstrated in adult intensive care patients improved survival with escalating CVVH doses in patients who had a lower starting serum urea nitrogen than nonsurvivors [112]. These studies suggest that earlier initiation of CVVH may be beneficial.

Acute Immunosuppression Nephrotoxicity

As mentioned, a large portion of children undergoing heart transplantation will have some amount of renal insufficiency perioperatively. Two nephrotoxic immunosuppressive agents commonly used in the immediate postoperative setting are cyclosporine and tacrolimus, both calcineurin inhibitors. It is imperative that both the intensive care and transplantation teams monitor administration of these two agents closely. These medications cause aberrations in renal microcirculation and can lead to tubulointerstitial fibrosis long term [113,114]. Medications that increase calcineurin inhibitor levels include metoclopramide, verapamil, diltiazem, fluconazole, erythromycin, and corticosteroids. Medications that decrease calcineurin inhibitor levels include rifampin, barbiturates, phenytoin, and carbamazepine.

For survivors within 7 years of pediatric heart transplantation, 10% demonstrated renal dysfunction and 1.2% underwent renal transplantation [6]. These numbers appear to be slowly rising. With hypertension being the most frequent cause of morbidity in this patient population and further renal damage ensuing, uncompromising antihypertensive therapy is also essential. The addition of angiotensin-converting enzyme inhibitors or diltiazem has been shown to have some renal protective effects [104]. Dehydration should be avoided. This applies to both the immediate intensive care setting and long term, as renal insults will be additive. English et al. concluded that the nephrotoxicities of cyclosporine and tacrolimus were comparable over the medium to long term in 123 pediatric heart transplant recipients [114]. They also noted that calculated creatinine clearance consistently overestimated glomerular filtration rate when compared with actual filtration measurement using a triple sample technique with Tc-99m diethylenetriamine pentaacetic acid. Furthermore, the decline in renal function after heart transplantation with early cyclosporine exposure persists even when cyclosporine doses are subsequently reduced [115].

Neurologic System

Acute Neurologic Insult

Children undergoing open heart surgery are at neurologic risk both inherently and extrinsically. Infants with congenital heart disease often have congenital abnormalities involving the central nervous system [116]. Before heart transplantation, children with anatomic cardiac abnormalities and cardiomyopathies are also often chronically hypoxemic and/or in a low cardiac output state. Potential complications of cardiopulmonary bypass include hypoxic-ischemic changes, microembolic phenomena, and reperfusion injury with further neurologic implications for the child who undergoes heart transplantation [117]. No other solid organ transplant patients have this added central nervous system risk as a result of hypothermic circulatory arrest and low-flow cardiopulmonary bypass [118].

In a review of 706 children undergoing open heart surgery at Boston Children's Hospital in 1998, postoperative seizures were most frequent in the acute period after heart transplantation, constituting a seizure rate of 26% in these patients (4 of 15) [119]. All transplant patients had clinical characteristics compatible with seizures caused by cyclosporine neurotoxicity; none had ischemic lesions. Three patients had additional exacerbating factors including high blood pressure and minimal subdural hemorrhage. The cyclosporine levels were elevated in two patients and were within the therapeutic range in another two. The overall seizure incidence in this series was 1.3%. All post-transplant seizures were well controlled with antiepileptic medication. Other acute neurologic complications included mild choreoathetosis seen in two patients, with one having undergone heart transplantation. Transient postoperative seizures following open heart surgery may be associated with worse neurodevelopmental outcomes in later years [120]. Additional neurologic abnormalities that can be seen in the immediate postoperative setting in pediatric heart transplant recipients include strokes, coma, and changes in mental status [121,122]. Such neurologic complications should be treated immediately with appropriate antiseizure medications when indicated for correction of any existing metabolic derangements including clotting parameters, cerebral imaging, and early consultation of the neurology team to prevent further brain injury.

Hypertension is also common in the intensive care setting after heart transplantation unrelated to immunosuppression. If graft function is good, a new efficient pump is now performing in the setting of a chronically underperfused vascular bed that includes the brain. High cerebral blood flow will also be exacerbated by donor–recipient size mismatch, with excessive stroke volumes if the donor was a larger child than the recipient. Increased cardiac output without hypertension perfusing a cerebral vascular bed with abnormal autoregulation following cardiopulmonary bypass could further result in neurologic injury. With this in mind, Martin et al. note a significant decrease in neurologic complications posttransplant with the institution of careful blood pressure control and cautious afterload reduction with high cardiac output states and the elimination of pretransplant cyclosporine [122].

The institution of multimodal neurologic monitoring with nearinfrared cerebral oximetry, transcranial Doppler ultrasound, and electroencephalographic recording during pediatric heart surgery may also decrease the incidence of postoperative neurologic complications and improve developmental outcome [123]. In the intensive care unit after admission from the operating room, tighter control on patient temperature and avoidance of hyperthermia may offer an additional neuroprotective strategy [124].

Cyclosporine Neurotoxicity

Cyclosporine neurotoxicity has been described mainly following other pediatric solid organ transplantation, but similar neuropathology can occur in heart transplant recipients [119,122,125–127]. Abnormalities seen can be mild to severe and include seizures, coma, headaches, depression, focal neurologic deficits, encephalopathy, tremors, peripheral neuropathies, visual and auditory hallucinations, visual field defects, and blindness [128–130]. Common findings on magnetic resonance imaging and computed tomography are cortical leukoencephalopathic changes, especially posteriorly, which are usually reversible. Patients with low cholesterol levels and hypomagnesemia appear to be at increased risk. Cyclosporine levels may be in the therapeutic range with manifestations

of neurologic toxicity. Concomitant medications, particularly highdose glucocorticoid therapy, may also increase the risk of central neurotoxicity. Although the mechanism is unclear, inhibition of cyclosporine transport to the apical pole of brain cells may be the etiology for this neurotoxicity [131]. In the majority of cases, the toxic symptoms resolved following either decrease in cyclosporine dosage or discontinuation. However, in a series of liver transplantation patients, cyclosporine-related postoperative neurologic complications were associated with a higher mortality rate for children than adults [126]. This was true despite the incidence being less in children. Tacrolimus, another calcineurin inhibitor often substituted for cyclosporine, also appears to have similar neurotoxic effects in children undergoing solid organ transplantation [132].

Pulmonary System

In the immediate postoperative period, the majority of children undergoing heart transplantation do not require prolonged mechanical ventilator support. Most patients can be extubated within 24 hr after transplantation with aggressive chest physiotherapy, nutrition, and bronchodilator treatment when indicated, decreasing the likelihood of respiratory failure. Clinical status at time of transplantation is an important factor determining the duration of mechanical ventilation post-transplantation. If the patient was breathing well unassisted before surgery and graft function is good, extubation can be performed successfully in the immediate postoperative period, usually shortly after arrival to the intensive care unit. If the patient required mechanical ventilation and/or ECMO for weakness, low cardiac output, or lung pathology before transplantation, a more prolonged period of mechanical ventilation may be necessary until adequate strength and respiratory parameters are achieved.

On analysis of their current results with pediatric heart transplantation, Kanter et al. noted 24% of the patients being on mechanical ventilation pretransplantation, yet 90% of hospital survivors were weaned from the ventilator within 1 week of surgery [133]. Post-transplantation median time of ventilation was 1 day (mean 3.0 ± 5.7 days). Groetzner et al. recently reported 22% of their patients being intubated pretransplantation, and mean days of mechanical ventilation postoperatively were 4.3 days ± 4.5 for children transplanted for DCM versus 8.3 days ± 8.5 for children transplanted for congenital heart disease [134]. They also commented on the importance of inhaled NO post-transplantation for children with elevated PVR and right ventricular failure. Interestingly, Lamour et al. also demonstrated a mean time to extubation of 4.6 days ± 3.2 postcardiac transplantation for a small group of children with congenital heart disease and a physiologic single lung [135]. These investigations display the resilience of children undergoing cardiac transplantation and the rapid return of respiratory function with strong graft performance. For those patients with persistent, diffuse lung congestion and inability to wean from mechanical ventilation, pulmonary venous obstruction should be considered, especially in children with underlying diagnoses of situs inversus and total anomalous pulmonary venous return. Mediastinal thrombus can also cause venous obstruction in the immediate postoperative period.

Nutritional Support

As for any critically ill, postoperative child, nutrition is essential for the pediatric heart transplant patient. Not only are calories ecessary for adequate healing and return of organ tissue function, ut, unlike adults, children are also growing and these needs must e taken into account. Neonates especially have limited amounts f endogenous nutrient elements. As mentioned, the majority of ediatric heart transplant patients will catch up with somatic rowth [136], indicating that they are capable of utilizing substrate. ostoperative outcome, including long-term neurologic outcome, nd days of mechanical ventilation may depend on patient nutritional status. Preoperatively, many of these children are already malnourished with poor organ tissue perfusion, inability to tolerate enteral intake because of gastrointestinal dysfunction, and nutritional intake being somewhat limited by renal insufficiency. Malnutrition and stress can also lead to decreased host resistance and increased risk of infection [137]. This is in addition to the sudden exogenously applied immunosuppressive agents following transplantation. However, there is evidence that the majority of patients admitted to PICU settings may not receive adequate caloric intake for the majority of their admission. Nutritional delivery was inadequate regardless of route of administration (enteral vs. parenteral). Additionally, once initiated, nutritional delivery is interrupted in the majority of patients during their intensive care course [138].

Nutrition, therefore, should be begun as soon as possible, preferably within 24 hr or so postoperatively. Initial intravenous fluids should include dextrose, especially in neonates, as hypoglycemia can occur rapidly because of poor glycogen stores. Should hyperglycemia occur with the administration of corticosteroids as immunosuppression, insulin can be considered to enhance substrate utilization rather than limit glucose delivery. Electrolytes must be followed closely, including phosphorus, potassium, calcium, and magnesium, to ensure optimal organ tissue function, especially cardiac.

If the child is extubated rapidly or is able while still on mechanical ventilation, enteral nutrition is recommended either orally or via nasogastric tube. For those infants with feeding issues, early consultation with speech therapy and lactation specialists should be obtained to increase success of nipple feeding. Reflux problems and gastric distention can be treated with gastrointestinal motility agents, as well as H_2-receptor blockade, which have the additional consequence of preventing gastrointestinal bleeding. Nutritional consultation should be part of early postoperative care to calculate caloric needs and adequacy of caloric administration. Appropriate protein delivery must be a priority as stress will significantly increase protein breakdown. Postoperative nitrogen loss will be greater in the neonatal age group than in older infants subject to comparable degrees of surgical stress [139]. Lipid, trace element, and vitamin intake must analogously be monitored to enhance organ function. If enteral feeding is not possible, parenteral nutrition should be given. However, even a small amount of enteral feeding may be effective in reducing gastrointestinal mucosal atrophy, thus decreasing bacterial translocation, maintaining enterohepatic enzyme systems, and reducing the incidence of cholestatic jaundice [140,141].

Sakopoulos et al. describe a series of children who developed mainly asymptomatic cholelithiasis following cardiac transplantation [142]. The incidence was 3.2% and predominately (80%) occurred in patients transplanted when younger than 3 months of age. In half the children, the gallstones were detected and treated within 6 months post-transplantation with either open or laparoscopic cholecystectomy. As early gastrointestinal complications following cardiac transplantation in children also include acute

pancreatitis and intestinal pneumatosis [143], these diagnoses should be considered when abdominal distention and/or feeding intolerance occur. With pediatric cardiac transplant patients being at risk for elevated serum cholesterol and triglycerides as well [144], these levels ought to be checked periodically and dietary counseling given early to possibly decrease the incidence of coronary artery vasculopathy.

Immunosuppression

Immunosuppression therapy for pediatric heart transplant patients continues to evolve. Newer agents are constantly being evaluated, and it can be difficult for the pediatric intensivist to be aware of all the complexities encountered with immunosuppression therapy. An involved transplant pharmacist is imperative to a successful program, and those children requiring critical care should be monitored daily as immunosuppression agent blood levels can change rapidly with myriad drug–drug interactions occurring. The balance between prevention of rejection and the iatrogenic side effects of immunosuppressive agents remains challenging. Modern regimens have also had only limited impact on prevention of chronic rejection and graft coronary artery disease, the principal causes of graft loss and death beyond the first 5 years after transplantation in children [145].

Basic Immunosuppression Protocols

A typical immunosuppression strategy involves multiple medications (Table 24.5). Cyclosporine is given pretransplantation when a donor is identified, as well as methylprednisolone and azathioprine. Corticosteroids may be administered during and after cardiopulmonary bypass and are continued for a brief period immediately following transplantation unless the maintenance immunosuppression schedule includes corticosteroids. OKT3 and antithymocyte globulin can be used for induction. Cyclosporine is switched to oral dosing as soon as possible, and in some institutions tacrolimus is substituted for cyclosporine. Intravenous immunoglobulin can also be given postoperatively for further immunomodulation [146]. Mycophenolate mofetil is an additional medication that may be utilized as maintenance immunosuppression.

Based on the 2004 Pediatric Report from the International Society for Heart and Lung Transplantation [6], the percentage of children receiving induction immunosuppression for heart transplantation is increasing (Figure 24.5). The percentage of patients receiving interleukin-2 receptor antagonists has remained relatively stable, but there has been an increase in the number of patients receiving polyclonal antibody preparations against circulating T lymphocytes. The use of OKT3, an anti-CD3 monoclonal antibody, for induction chemotherapy has continued to decrease. This is despite no significant difference being seen overall in the average number of rejection episodes for pediatric heart recipients treated for rejection in the first year between induction agents or no induction therapy (Figures 24.6 and 24.7).

Regarding maintenance immunosuppression, there has been an increase in the use of tacrolimus as the primary T-cell activation inhibitor with roughly equal percentages of patients being on cyclosporine or tacrolimus. Mycophenolate mofetil is now used as the second drug in about 50% of patients at 1 year and 40% at 5 years. Accordingly, azathioprine as the second immunosuppressive agent presently accounts for only about 30% of patients at 1 and

TABLE 24.5. Immunosuppressive drugs.

Medication	Action	Common side effects	Common drug interactions
Azathioprine	Antiproliferative	Bone marrow suppression, elevated liver transaminases, pancreatitis	Allopurinol, co-trimoxazole, angiotensin converting enzyme inhibitors
Mycophenolate mofetil	Antiproliferative	Gastrointestinal bleeding, nausea, vomiting, diarrhea, bone marrow suppression	Ganciclovir, acyclovir, trimethoprim/ sulfamethoxazole, antacids, cholestyramine
Methotrexate	Antiproliferative	Bone marrow suppression, ulcerative stomatitis, encephalopathy, nephrotoxicity, elevated liver transaminases, photosensitivity	Ganciclovir, acyclovir, trimethoprim/ sulfamethoxazole, nonsteroidal antiinflammato agents, penicillin, theophylline
Rapamycin (sirolimus)	Antiproliferative	Hyperlipidemia, nephrotoxicity, bone marrow suppression, aphthous ulcers	Cyclosporine, erythromycin, diltiazem, metoclopramide, fluconazole, phenobarbital, phenytoin
Prednisone	Interleukin-1 inhibitor	Gastrointestinal bleeding, adrenal insufficiency, osteopenia, hyperglycemia, hypertension, growth suppression	Fluconazole, phenobarbital, phenytoin, rifampin, oral contraceptives
Cyclosporine	Calcineurin inhibitor	Nephrotoxicity, neurotoxicity, hyperlipidemia, hirsutism, gingival hyperplasia, elevated liver transaminases	Erythromycin, diltiazem, metoclopramide, fluconazole, phenobarbital, phenytoin
Tacrolimus	Calcineurin inhibitor	Nephrotoxicity, glucose intolerance, neurotoxicity, alopecia, nausea, vomiting, diarrhea	Erythromycin, diltiazem,metoclopramide, fluconazole, phenobarbital, phenytoin
Antithymocyte globulin	Anti-T lymphocyte polyclonal antibody	Chills, fever, arthralgia, leukopenia, thrombocytopenia	
OKT3	Anti-CD3 monoclonal antibody	Cytokine release syndrome, pulmonary edema, nephrotoxicity, aseptic meningitis	
Daclizumab	Interleukin-2 receptor antagonist	Fever, headache, peripheral edema	

5 years. Prednisone use as a third drug in the immunosuppressive regimen is seen in about 60% of patients at 1 year, but by 5 years this is down to about 40% of patients. Some centers have reported successful use of a corticosteroid-free long-term maintenance regimen [147]. Certain genetic polymorphisms appear to predict corticosteroid weaning [148]. Rapamycin is still used infrequently in pediatric heart transplantation. Overall, patients on tacrolimus-based regimens appeared to have a lower percentage treated for rejection [6]. However, a recent preliminary comparison of tacrolimus- versus cyclosporine-based immunosuppression in a small cohort of pediatric heart transplant recipients did not demonstrate a lower incidence of acute cellular rejection in the tacrolimus group [149]. Ganciclovir is typically given intravenously for 2 weeks for

those recipients who are cytomegalovirus positive or who receiv from a cytomegalovirus-positive donor.

Hypertension is the most common morbidity seen in pediatri heart transplant patients, affecting approximately 67% by 7 year after transplantation [6]. Use of prednisone is closely associate with early development of hypertension within the first 3 years c transplant. Both calcineurin inhibitors, cyclosporine and tacrol mus, have known renal toxicity effects but do not contribute to th development of hypertension. Diabetes mellitus and hyperlipid emia also continue to be significant causes of morbidity associate with immunosuppression [6,150]. Coronary artery vasculopath may be linked to the hyperlipidemia, stimulating the increased us of "statins" (3-hydroxy-3-methylglutaryl-coenzyme A reductas

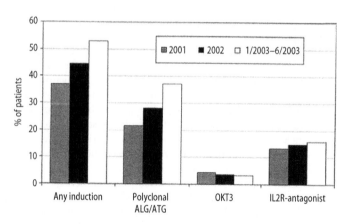

FIGURE 24.5. Pediatric heart recipients. Induction immunosuppression (follow up from January 2001 to June 2003). ALG, antilymphocyte globulin; ATG, antithymocyte globulin; IL2R, interleukin-2 receptor. (Data from Boucek et al. [6]. © 2004 with permission from International Society of Heart and Lung Transplantation.)

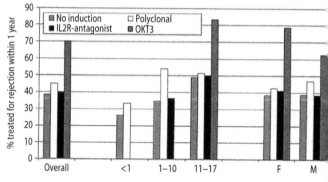

FIGURE 24.6. Percentage of pediatric heart transplant recipients treated for rejection i the first year, stratified by type of induction (transplants from January 1, 2000, to June 30 2002). IL2R, interleukin-2 receptor; 1–10, no induction versus polyclonal ($p = 0.015$); 11–1 no induction versus OKT3 ($p = 0.006$); polyclonal versus OKT3 ($p = 0.02$); IL2R versus OKT ($p = 0.03$); Female: No induction versus OKT3 ($p = 0.003$); polyclonal versus OKT ($p = 0.014$); IL2R versus OKT3 ($p = 0.03$). (Data from Boucek et al. [6]. © 2004 with permis sion from International Society of Heart and Lung Transplantation.)

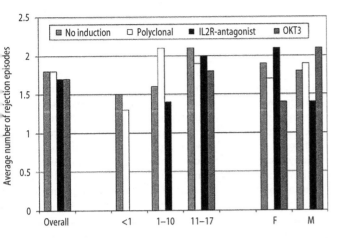

FIGURE 24.7. Number of rejection episodes for pediatric heart transplant recipients treated for rejection in the first year, stratified by type of induction (transplants from January 1, 2000, to June 30, 2002). No within-age group or within-gender comparisons were statistically significant. IL-2R, interleukin-2 receptor. (Data from Boucek et al. [6]. © 2004 with permission from International Society of Heart and Lung Transplantation.)

inhibitors) in children following heart transplantation. Statins also have immunosuppressive properties unrelated to their lipid-lowering effect that have been proposed to reduce post-transplant coronary artery disease in adults [151]. Little, however, is known about the safety profile of these agents in children [144,145].

Elevated Panel Reactive Antibody and ABO Incompatibility

The child with an elevated panel reactive antibody (PRA) poses a more challenging immunosuppression task. The PRA test combines the potential recipient's serum with samples of antigen-containing cells taken from 60 different individuals within the community, representative of the potential donor pool. The percentage PRA is the percentage of these 60 combinations that react positively. A level greater than or equal to 10% is considered elevated. These patients are considered to be at greater risk for acute cellular and humeral rejection, transplant vasculopathy, and mortality. Common risk factors for elevated PRA in the pediatric population include previous blood transfusions, previous exposure to allograft material, and previous transplantations [152]. As the use of mechanical circulatory support increases, additional children undergo palliative surgery before transplantation, and the pediatric cardiac retransplantation incidence rises, it is likely that more children will exhibit elevated PRA in the future. Rather than wait even longer for a compatible donor with possible increased associated morbidity and mortality, some centers have adopted a more aggressive immunosuppression regimen and proceeded with transplantation. Various protocols involve preoperative and postoperative intravenous immunoglobulin, cyclophosphamide or mycophenolate, and exchange transfusion or plasmapheresis [152]. Such intensive strategies may help lower the risks for these patients.

Similarly, cardiac transplantation with ABO incompatibility between the recipient and donor can be done in young infants with some alteration in the typical immunosuppression regimen. Because of mortality among infants waiting for transplantation and the continued short supply of donor organs, this becomes an attractive alternative. Infants have immature immune systems with low levels of complement and antibody, fewer natural killer cells, antigenically naïve thymocytes, and decreased cytokine production. Therefore, they appear to have better tolerance of foreign antigens, exhibiting less rejection rates, better late survival, and decreased graft vasculopathy [153]. The groups in both Toronto and New Castle upon Tyne report good results with cardiac transplantation of 13 infants with ABO incompatibility. The major difference in immunosuppression was plasma exchange being performed during cardiopulmonary bypass [154,155].

Long-Term Management

Acute Rejection/Graft Failure

Up to 3 years post-transplantation, acute rejection and graft failure are the most common causes of death in pediatric heart transplant recipients [6]. The risk of rejection is greatest in the first 3 to 6 months after transplantation. Most recipients in childhood experience at least one episode of moderate or severe acute cellular rejection [104]. Therefore, it is imperative that acute rejection and graft failure be high on the differential when these patients are ill. Risk factors for rejection include older age at transplant and African-American race. Hemodynamically significant rejection episodes predict a particularly devastating outcome, with approximately 40% mortality following the first episode [156]. In children developing recurrent rejection requiring inotropic support, mortality increases to >50% within 1 year. The highest risk of recurrent rejection occurs within 1 month of a previous rejection episode [157].

Most episodes of mild and moderate acute rejection present on surveillance biopsy in asymptomatic children. Serious rejection episodes, however, usually are accompanied by increased tiredness, decreased appetite, nausea, a sudden drop in blood pressure, abdominal pain, a rapid increase in weight gain, or a low-grade temperature for more than 2 days. Infants may present with prolonged periods of fussiness or poor feeding over several days [104]. Tachycardia or irregular rhythm is also a sensitive marker for acute rejection [89]. A gallop may be heard on cardiac examination. Chest x-ray findings may include increased cardiomegaly, pulmonary edema, and pleural effusions. Echocardiogram can reveal new pericardial effusion, poor ventricular function, thickening of the left ventricle posterior wall and septum, new mitral insufficiency, and decreasing left ventricular fiber-shortening fraction [158]. Electrocardiogram is relatively insensitive, but when findings such as conduction defects, dysrhythmias, or ectopy are present they should be taken seriously [159].

Endomyocardial biopsy specimens are graded according to the criteria of the International Society for Heart and Lung Transplantation (Table 24.6) [160], with most centers only treating biopsies

TABLE 24.6. International Society for Heart and Lung Transplantation categories of acute cellular rejection.

Classification	Description
Grade 0	No evidence of cellular rejection
Grade 1A	Focal perivascular or interstitial infiltrate *without myocyte injury*
Grade 1B	Multifocal or diffuse sparse infiltrate *without myocyte injury*
Grade 2	Single focus of *dense* infiltrates *with myocyte injury*
Grade 3A	Multifocal, *dense* infiltrates *with myocyte injury*
Grade 3B	Diffuse, *dense* infiltrates *with myocyte injury*
Grade 4	Diffuse and extensive polymorphous infiltrate *with myocyte injury*; may have hemorrhage, edema, and microvascular injury

Source: Adapted from Billingham et al. [160].

with a 3A (i.e., lymphocyte infiltration with myocyte degeneration) or greater histology. Periodic endomyocardial biopsy and echocardiogram are the main modalities used for screening and diagnosing acute graft rejection in children. Serum vascular endothelial growth factor, B-type natriuretic peptide, and genetic polymorphisms linked with TNF-α and IL-10 production have also been investigated in children to identify an association with acute rejection [161–163]. On polymerase chain reaction analyses of over 500 endomyocardial biopsy samples, Shirali et al. noted that the identification of viral genome, particularly adenovirus, in the myocardium of pediatric transplant recipients is predictive of adverse clinical events, including graft loss due to acute rejection [164].

Children with serious rejection often die precipitously with little warning. The final cause of death is typically severely depressed graft function and/or a sudden irrecoverable dysrhythmia. Diagnosis and treatment of the rejection episode in a timely manner is therefore crucial. These are not patients who should be waiting in the clinic or in the emergency department for admission. It is the practice at Loma Linda University Children's Hospital to initially admit all pediatric heart transplant patients in acute rejection directly to the cardiac intensive care unit for at least 24 hr. If there is evidence of hemodynamic compromise, central venous access is obtained and inotropes begun. Early tracheal intubation and mechanical ventilation are initiated when necessary. Tracheal intubation is performed cautiously in these patients as cardiac arrest can occur during the procedure. Concomitant benzodiazepine and narcotic administration may precipitate severe hypotension. Ketamine can be employed as an adjunct sedative to increase systemic mean arterial pressure [165]. An arterial catheter may be placed to monitor blood pressure continuously. In the presence of significant dysrhythmias, prompt electrophysiology consultation should be obtained. Immediate start of acute rejection immunotherapy is also vital with closely coordinated management between the transplant and critical care services. Most protocols involve bolus corticosteroid therapy and antithymocyte agents. Tacrolimus and mycophenolate mofetil can be used, as well as intravenous immunoglobulin and plasmapheresis [166,167]. Total lymphoid irradiation has been employed for refractory rejection [168]. As mentioned, mechanical circulatory support with ECMO can be utilized as "bridge to recovery" with good success for those children with severe graft failure secondary to acute rejection requiring mechanical circulatory support [82,84].

In a retrospective, cohort study by Ringewald et al., late rejection after pediatric heart transplantation occurred primarily during adolescence, was associated with late mortality, and was frequently associated with nonadherence [169]. Nonadherence was suspected by nontherapeutic concentration of cyclosporine, the voluntary admission of irregular medication administration, or both. The authors conclude that adherence with transplant care is especially difficult during the vulnerable period of adolescence and emphasize the importance of increased interventions before and long after transplantation, such as more frequent home nursing visits, increased outpatient visits, and teen peer support groups to improve behavior in this high-risk population. The adolescent fraction will naturally continue to grow as children transplanted during infancy age because of improved survival rates.

Post-Transplant Coronary Artery Disease

After 3 years and at 5 years post-transplantation, coronary artery vasculopathy is the leading cause of death in children undergoing heart transplantation. The incidence is increasing and was most recently seen in about 14% of 7-year survivors with a worsening predicted trend [6]. The pathology differs from ischemic heart disease in the normal adult population [170]. Typical graft vasculopathy consists of myointimal proliferation that is concentric and involves the entire length of the vessel, including intramyocardial branches with eventual luminal occlusion. Because discrete stenoses are rare, coronary angioplasty is usually ineffective. Subsequent development of myocyte hypertrophy and disarray resulting in fibrosis and scarring with progressive myocardial dysfunction greatly increase the incidence of sudden death in these children [88]. As with rejection, most patients are asymptomatic until significant obstruction is present. The signs and symptoms seen with pending sudden death are similar to those manifesting with post-transplantation coronary artery disease [104]. These characteristics make this entity difficult to treat. Early rejection, as well as late rejection frequency and severity, are predictors of development of graft vasculopathy [6,171]. Certain dysrhythmias and late pacemaker requirement can also indicate the presence of coronary artery compromise [90,92]. Coronary artery involvement has been identified as early as 2 months after transplantation [172].

Coronary angiography, the primary screening tool for post-transplantation coronary artery disease, is a relatively insensitive marker of mild disease secondary to the diffuse nature of the disease; however, it seems to be a strong predictor of severe disease if positive [173]. Intravascular ultrasound may also be employed for disease detection. This modality appears to be more sensitive in children for detecting graft vasculopathy but is somewhat limited because of catheter size [174,175]. Additionally, dobutamine stress echocardiography has been utilized successfully with less age and size restrictions to detect coronary artery disease in pediatric heart transplant patients without the associated invasive morbidity [176,177]. Unlike coronary angiography and intravascular ultrasound, myocardial ischemia can also be identified.

Retransplantation is the only definitive therapeutic option of long-term benefit for children with significant post-transplantation coronary artery disease [88,178]. Survival rates are similar to those of primary transplantation. Early relisting should be considered for children identified with significant disease, as the risk of death is high. For those children admitted to the intensive care unit while awaiting retransplantation, vigilant monitoring is important. Inotropes may be required to improve contractility, as well as antidysrhythmic agents. Optimizing the balance between these prodysrhythmogenic and cardiac depressant medications can be challenging. Nitroglycerin can be considered to augment coronary artery perfusion. Pacemaker placement may be necessary. Mechanical circulatory support as bridge to retransplantation is an option. Unfortunately, when these children suffer cardiac arrest, it is often impossible to resuscitate them.

Several pharmacologic approaches have been used for prevention of graft vasculopathy following transplantation. These agents include calcium antagonists, angiotensin-converting enzyme inhibitors, vitamin E, statins, aspirin, and antiproliferative agents such as mycophenolate mofetil and rapamycin [104].

Sudden Death

Sudden death occurs in a minority of pediatric heart transplant recipients but is obviously a devastating event. In the literature, timing of sudden death ranges from the day of transplant to years post-transplant [85,171,179]. The causes of sudden death in these hildren include dysrhythmias, severe graft dysfunction, and myocardial infarction. Acute rejection can produce these conditions in the early post-transplantation period; however, later episodes are usually related to graft vasculopathy secondary to chronic rejection. Because all transplanted hearts are denervated, chest pain is an unlikely presentation of coronary ischemia [104]. Therefore, there will be no forewarning of increasing coronary compromise until luminal obstruction is complete. Heralds of sudden death include ectopy, presyncope, syncope, intermittent edema, and exercise intolerance. The presence of such signs and symptoms may indicate that graft vascular supply is becoming significantly compromised and/or chronic rejection is worsening. Again, the exact anatomic cause of the sudden death may not be recognized until autopsy. In a small portion of patients an etiology is never identified [179]. In 10 children who died suddenly as described by Mulla et al., graft vasculopathy was diagnosed at autopsy in all patients with percentage narrowing of epicardial coronary arteries being ≥50% [171]. Coronary angiograms were all normal 3 to 9 months before their deaths. Moderate rejection was also present in six of these patients and may have contributed to their demise. Additionally in this series, three patients died suddenly 10 days to 3 months after the angiographic diagnosis of graft vasculopathy was made. One patient demonstrated autopsy evidence of a recent myocardial infarction.

A large, multicenter survey complied by Pahl et al. reported only 9 of 58 children with post-transplantation coronary artery disease surviving, including 5 who underwent retransplantation [180]. Many deaths were sudden and unexpected; however, the exact incidence of sudden death was unable to be determined. Increased surveillance angiograms and biopsies in long-term survivors may be warranted, particularly in patients with a history of frequent rejection. Warning signs and symptoms of potential sudden death must be taken seriously by the pediatric intensivist, with extensive workup and appropriate consultation in an attempt to prevent this grim outcome.

Post-Transplantation Lymphoproliferative Disease

Post-transplantation lymphoproliferative disorders (PTLDs) are a spectrum of conditions between infection and malignant neoplasia. The majority of cases in pediatric heart recipients are associated with Epstein-Barr virus (EBV) infection in the first 3 years after transplantation, although EBV infection can lead to PTLD at any time after transplantation. Epstein-Barr virus–negative cases usually arise beyond five years [181]. Most cases of PTLD occur in children who are seronegative for EBV at the time of transplantation and who subsequently develop primary EBV infection [182]. Primary EBV infection after transplantation can come from several potential sources, including donor organs, perioperative blood products, or community acquisition. Epstein-Barr virus–associated disease, including PTLD, develops in more than 20% of patients who experience primary infection after transplantation. Additional risk factors associated with an increased risk of developing PTLD include cytomegalovirus disease and the use of antilymphocyte antibodies for prevention or treatment of rejection. The greater the level of T-lymphocyte suppression, the greater the risk of developing PTLD [181]. The incidence of PTLD in pediatric heart transplant recipients ranges from 4% to 10% [182,183]. Histologic disease was noted within a mean time of 29 months (range 3–72 months) from heart transplantation in a series of children with PTLD described by Zangwill et al. [182].

The diagnosis of EBV disease in pediatric organ transplant recipients is based on clinical history, physical examination, and laboratory confirmation. Earlier diagnosis appears to correlate with more successful outcome; therefore, there should be a high index of suspicion at all times. Critically ill children with disseminated disease that involves multiple extranodal sites often die within days or weeks of presentation. Symptoms of PTLD include fever, malaise, weight loss, sore throat, abdominal pain, nausea, vomiting, gastrointestinal bleeding, swollen glands, headache or focal neurologic symptoms, and symptoms of graft dysfunction. Physical signs include pallor, lymphadenopathy, subcutaneous nodules, tonsillar enlargement, hepatosplenomegaly, and focal neurologic findings. Pulmonary disease is especially common in cardiac transplant recipients. Laboratory analysis often reveals leukopenia, anemia, atypical lymphocytosis, thrombocytopenia, and elevated uric acid and lactate dehydrogenase. There may be evidence of liver and kidney dysfunction. Stool can be positive for occult blood. Immunoglobulin, particularly IgE, levels may be elevated. Various imaging studies are also helpful in the evaluation of suspected PTLD.

The most informative study is computed tomographic evaluation of the chest, abdomen, and pelvis. Small pulmonary nodules or enlarged mediastinal lymph nodes may be apparent. In the abdomen, disease may be found at normal lymph node sites, within the gastrointestinal tract, or extranodal, including the liver, spleen, and kidney. Head computed tomographic scanning should be performed when there is clinical evidence of central nervous system involvement. Upper or lower gastrointestinal endoscopy is warranted for children with gastrointestinal symptoms. Other studies utilized for the diagnosis of PTLD consist of core needle or excision biopsy, bone scan, bone marrow biopsy, and lumbar puncture [181]. Magnetic resonance imaging may also be valuable in better delineating specific lesions. Epstein-Barr viral load measurement in the peripheral blood with polymerase chain reaction has also been employed for screening and measuring of response to therapy for PTLD patients [184]. Histologic evaluation is required to confirm the diagnosis of PTLD [181].

The initial mainstay of treatment for children with PTLD is reduction in immunosuppression. This allows the host to recover natural immune surveillance and subsequently gain control over the EBV-infected B cells. The use of acyclovir or ganciclovir is also routine initial treatment in most centers. Additionally, chemotherapy is a first-line remedy for overt malignancy such as Burkett's lymphoma. Secondary therapies include intravenous immunoglobulin and anti-B-cell monoclonal antibodies (rituximab). Chemotherapy is again administered for refractory and relapsed PTLD. Surgery and/or radiation therapy can be utilized for isolated lesions in some patients [181]. For the pediatric intensivist, in addition to the critical care management of children with PTLD, it is essential to involve all necessary consultants early in the hospitalization to optimize outcomes. This would include the transplant team, gastrointestinal subspecialists, appropriate surgical staff, and the hematology/oncology group when necessary. Most pediatric solid organ transplant recipients respond well to early initiation of PTLD treatment. By seven years after cardiac transplantation, >90% of pediatric recipients were free of morbidity from a new malignancy, according to the latest pediatric registry report [6].

Infections

Although most infections in pediatric heart transplant recipients are successfully treated, infection is an important cause of post-

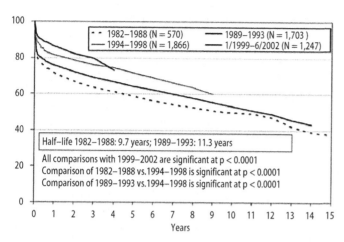

FIGURE 24.8. Pediatric heart transplantation Kaplan-Meier survival data by era (January 1982 to June 2002). (Data from Boucek et al. [6]. © 2004 with permission from International Society of Heart and Lung Transplantation.)

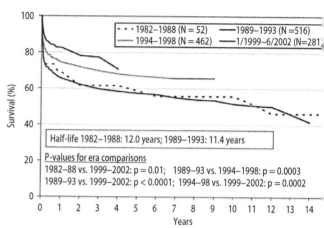

FIGURE 24.9. Pediatric heart transplantation Kaplan-Meier survival data (January 1982 June 2002). (Data from Boucek et al. [6]. © 2004 with permission from International Society of Heart and Lung Transplantation.)

transplantation morbidity and death, especially in infants. In a multiinstitutional analysis performed by Schowengerdt et al. involving 332 patients, the risk for development of the first infection of any type was highest during the first month after transplantation [185]. There was an average of 0.84 infections per child during the study period, with approximately 40% of patients having one or more infections. Bacterial infections were the most common type of infection identified (60%), followed by viral (31%), fungal (7%), and protozoan (2%). Bacterial infections accounted for over 70% of the infections in infants younger than 6 months of age. The most common bacterial pathogens isolated included *Staphylococcal* species, *Pseudomonas* species, and *Enterobacter cloacae*. The most common sites of bacterial infection were the lung and blood. Of the bacterial lung infections identified, approximately 40% were in patients on mechanical ventilation at the time of transplantation, with a mortality rate of 30%. Fifteen percent of bacterial blood infections were associated with infection-related death. Surgical wound infection occurred in only eight cases.

Cytomegalovirus was the most common single infectious agent identified, accounting for about 60% of all viral infections, and was most frequently isolated in the blood. As expected, donor and recipient serologic status had an impact on risk of cytomegalovirus infection, with the greatest risk occurring in the case of a cytomegalovirus-positive donor organ transplanted into a cytomegalovirus-negative recipient. Fungal and protozoan (*Pneumocystis* species) infections most commonly affected the lung. Death related to infection constituted one third of all deaths occurring during the study period. Although fungal infections were rare, death occurred in over half of cases in which fungal infection was identified. Conversely, cytomegalovirus-associated demise was low, occurring in only 6% of cases in which cytomegalovirus was diagnosed. Significant risk factors for death from infection demonstrated in this study included younger recipient age, use of a ventilator at time of transplantation, and history of previous sternotomy. Longer donor ischemic time, particularly those longer than 300 minutes, also correlated with increased risk of earlier infection. For the critical care practitioner, vigilance regarding removal of unnecessary indwelling catheters and other invasive monitoring devices, early extubation, aggressive pulmonary toilet, and prompt initiation of antibiotic or antiviral therapy when indicated may assist in improving infection incidence and

outcome for pediatric heart transplant recipients in the intensive care unit.

Developmental Outcome

With increased survival rates of children undergoing heart transplantation (Figures 24.8 through 24.12), focus has recently moved to developmental outcomes of these children. Physical growth while awaiting transplantation is poor, but beyond 5 years most children (88%) have undergone adequate catch-up growth and achieve weights and heights in the normal range [136]. Risk factors for short stature include rejection history, degree of illness, and especially parental height. In a series of children aged 2–38 months transplanted in infancy, Freier et al. noted on formal testing normal cognitive development in the majority of patients with only 11.8% being significantly delayed, but motor function was overall mildly delayed, with 27.4% being significantly delayed [186]. However, in the 36–38 month age group, mean motor function was within normal limits, showing a trend toward improvement. Among the hypotheses for these findings was the use of immunosuppressive agents. Increased acute and serous otitis media as a result of

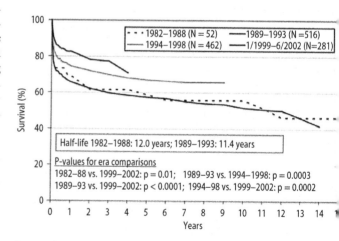

FIGURE 24.10. Pediatric heart transplantation Kaplan-Meier survival by era (January 1982 to June 2002) for patients aged less than 1 year old. (Data from Boucek et al. [6]. © 2004 with permission from International Society of Heart and Lung Transplantation.)

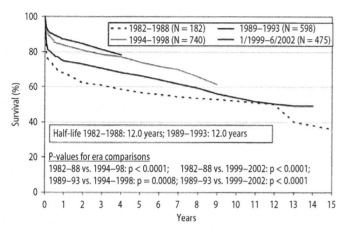

FIGURE 24.11. Pediatric heart transplantation Kaplan-Meier survival by era (January 1982 to June 2002) for patients aged 1 to 10 years. (Data from Boucek et al. [6]. © 2004 with permission from International Society of Heart and Lung Transplantation.)

immunosuppression, direct cyclosporine ototoxicity, and cyclosporine-induced hypertrichosis in the ear canal may affect language development in these children. In addition, the cyclosporine-induced gingival hyperplasia may further affect auditory processes and speech development by blocking the eustachian tube and negatively impacting eating, speech, and general appearance. In a similar study, Baum et al. found IQ and achievement levels within the normal range in infant heart transplant recipients, but there was a significant amount of variability with more children than would be expected scoring in the lower ranges [187].

Children with heart transplantation also appeared to be at risk for visual-spatial skill deficits. Young children were additionally susceptible to social isolation, and symptoms of depression were seen in older children. In another investigation, Baum et al. demonstrated low-average long-term neuropsychological functioning in infant heart transplant recipients [188]. Intraoperative and postoperative variables (bypass time, hospital course, and lowest post-transplant pH), long-term medical complications (serious infections and post-transplantation surgical procedures), and socioeconomic factors (paternal education, birth order) were associated with cognitive functioning. Visual-motor functioning was also related to cardiopulmonary bypass and total support time. In a small population of

children treated for hypoplastic left heart syndrome with heart transplantation, Ikle et al. described similar cognitive deficits and adaptive/behavioral abnormalities [189]. They concluded that early recognition of the deficits identified with appropriate referral for services could potentially enhance the outcomes for these children.

Transplant Patients and Other Diseases

The success of heart transplantation in children has lead to patients being readmitted to the PICU for issues not immediately related to their transplanted organ. For example, children are now readmitted for respiratory insufficiency from viral infection such as respiratory syncytial virus, routine surgical procedures, and trauma. It is known that respiratory failure requiring intubation and mechanical ventilation represents a particularly poor prognostic indicator, approaching futility, in other forms of transplantation [190]. There is, however, little information dealing with mechanical ventilator support of heart transplant recipients in the nonperioperative period.

In a study examining the Loma Linda University transplant population, survival after tracheal intubation and mechanical ventilation is significantly affected in cardiac transplant recipients [191]. However, at 29%, survival is greater than that found in bone marrow transplant recipients (0%–20%) [192,193] and far exceeds definitions of medical futility [194]. Attempts have been made to develop criteria that would allow identification of those recipients who would most benefit from interventions such as tracheal intubation [192,195]. In the present study, age at transplantation, age at tracheal intubation, or elapsed time from transplantation to first tracheal intubation did not affect survival. In fact, the elapsed time from transplantation to first tracheal intubation is longer (1.7 years) when compared with published reports of the same measurement in other transplant populations, suggesting a favorable complication-free survival following cardiac transplantation compared with other organs [196–198]. Additionally, the requirement of multiple episodes of tracheal intubation and mechanical ventilation did not impact mortality. However, interpretation of these data is limited by their small size.

Conclusion

Heart transplantation is a treatment option for end-stage heart failure or inoperable congenital cardiac defects in children. The pediatric critical care practitioner is intimately involved in every aspect of transplantation management. With the growing use of transplantation in the pediatric population, management challenges exist within the intensive care unit. However, by ensuring close cooperation of the transplantation, cardiology, cardiothoracic surgery, and critical care teams, outcomes for these patients can be optimized. The development of more selective and less toxic immunosuppressive agents and strategies may be of further benefit.

References

1. Barnard CN. The operation. A human cardiac transplant: an interim report of a successful operation performed at Groote Schuur Hospital, Cape Town. S Afr Med J 1967;41(48):1271–1274.
2. Kantrowitz A, Haller JD, Joos H, et al. Transplantation of the heart in an infant and an adult. Am J Cardiol 1968;22(6):782–790.

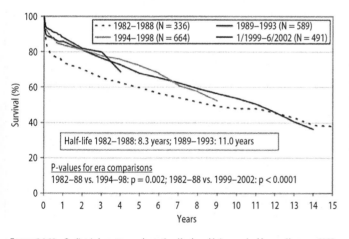

FIGURE 24.12. Pediatric heart transplantation Kaplan–Meier survival by era (January 1982 to June 2002) for patients aged 11 to 17 years. (Data from Boucek et al. [6]. © 2004 with permission from International Society of Heart and Lung Transplantation.)

3. Oyer PE, Stinson EB, Reitz BA, et al. Cardiac transplantation: 1980. Transplant Proc 1981;13(1 Pt 1):199–206.

4. Burch M, Aurora P. Current status of paediatric heart, lung, and heart–lung transplantation. Arch Dis Child 2004;89(4):386–389.

5. Trulock EP, Edwards LB, Taylor DO, et al. The Registry of the International Society for Heart and Lung Transplantation: twenty-first official adult heart transplant report—2004. J Heart Lung Transplant 2004;23(7):804–815.

6. Boucek MM, Edwards LB, Keck BM, et al. Registry for the International Society for Heart and Lung Transplantation: Seventh Official Pediatric Report—2004. J Heart Lung Transplant 2004;23(6):933–947.

7. Fricker FJ, Addonizio L, Bernstein D, et al. Heart transplantation in children: indications. Report of the Ad Hoc Subcommittee of the Pediatric Committee of the American Society of Transplantation (AST). Pediatr Transplant 1999;3(4):333–342.

8. Donkin M, Kolovos NS, Checchia PA. The effect of specialized pediatric management on organ recovery from potential pediatric transplant donors. Crit Care Med 2004;32(12 Suppl):82.

9. Bailey LL, Nehlsen-Cannarella SL, Doroshow RW, et al. Cardiac allotransplantation in newborns as therapy for hypoplastic left heart syndrome. N Engl J Med 1986;315(15):949–951.

10. Reitz BA, Jamieson SW, Gaudiani VA, et al. Method for cardiac transplantation in corrected transposition of the great arteries. J Cardiovasc Surg 1982;23(4):293–296.

11. Fricker FJ, Griffith BP, Hardesty RL, et al. Experience with heart transplantation in children. Pediatrics 1987;79(1):138–146.

12. Jamieson SW, Gaudiani VA, Reitz BA, et al. Operative treatment of an unresectable tumor of the left ventricle. J Thorac Cardiovasc Surg 1981;81(5):797–799.

13. Cooley DA, Frazier OH, Van Buren CT, et al. Cardiac transplantation in an 8-month-old female infant with subendocardial fibroelastosis. JAMA 1986;256(10):1326–1329.

14. Checchia PA, Larsen R, Sehra R, et al. Effect of a selection and postoperative care protocol on survival of infants with hypoplastic left heart syndrome. Ann Thorac Surg 2004;77(2):477–483.

15. Quintessenza JA, Morell VO, Jacobs JP. Achieving a balance in the current approach to the surgical treatment of hypoplastic left heart syndrome. Cardiol Young 2004;(14 Suppl 1):127–130.

16. Lipshultz SE, Sleeper LA, Towbin JA, et al. The incidence of pediatric cardiomyopathy in two regions of the United States [see comment]. N Engl J Med 2003;348(17):1647–1655.

17. Nugent AW, Daubeney PE, Chondros P, et al. The epidemiology of childhood cardiomyopathy in Australia [see comment]. N Engl J Med 2003;348(17):1639–1646.

18. Arola A, Tuominen J, Ruuskanen O, et al. Idiopathic dilated cardiomyopathy in children: prognostic indicators and outcome. Pediatrics 1998;101(3 Pt 1):369–376.

19. Lewis AB. Late recovery of ventricular function in children with idiopathic dilated cardiomyopathy. Am Heart J 1999;138(2 Pt 1):334–338.

20. Erickson KW, Costanzo-Nordin MR, O'Sullivan EJ, et al. Influence of preoperative transpulmonary gradient on late mortality after orthotopic heart transplant. J Heart Transplant 1990;9(5):526–537.

21. Gajarski RJ, Mosca RS, Ohye RG, et al. Use of extracorporeal life support as a bridge to pediatric cardiac transplantation. J Heart Lung Transplant 2003;22(1):28–34.

22. Vossler MR, Ni H, Toy W, et al. Pre-operative renal function predicts development of chronic renal insufficiency after orthotopic heart transplantation. J Heart Lung Transplant 2002;21(8):874–881.

23. Burch M, Siddiqi SA, Celermajer DS, et al. Dilated cardiomyopathy in children: determinants of outcome. Br Heart J 1994;72(3):246–250.

24. Tsirka AE, Trinkaus K, Chen SC, et al. Improved outcomes of pediatric dilated cardiomyopathy with utilization of heart transplantation. J Am Coll Cardiol 2004;44(2):391–397.

25. Fiser WP, Yetman AT, Gunselman RJ, et al. Pediatric arteriovenous extracorporeal membrane oxygenation (ECMO) as a bridge to cardiac transplantation. J Heart Lung Transplant 2003;22(7):770–777.

26. Levi D, Marelli D, Plunkett M, et al. Use of assist devices and ECMO to bridge pediatric patients with cardiomyopathy to transplantation. J Heart Lung Transplant 2002;21(7):760–770.

27. Merkle F, Boettcher W, Stiller B, et al. Pulsatile mechanical cardiac assistance in pediatric patients with the Berlin heart ventricular assist device. J Extra-Corpor Technol 2003;35(2):115–120.

28. Pennington DG, Smedira NG, Samuels LE, et al. Mechanical circulatory support for acute heart failure. Ann Thorac Surg 2001;71(3 Suppl):S56–S85.

29. Ishino K, Weng Y, Alexi-Meskishvili V, et al. Extracorporeal membrane oxygenation as a bridge to cardiac transplantation in children. Artif Organs 1996;20(6):728–732.

30. Muntean W. Coagulation and anticoagulation in extracorporeal membrane oxygenation. Artif Organs 1999;23(11):979–983.

31. Huang J, Trinkaus K, Huddleston CB, et al. Risk factors for primary graft failure after pediatric cardiac transplantation: importance of recipient and donor characteristics. J Heart Lung Transplant 2004;23(6):716–722.

32. Rosenthal DN, Dubin AM, Chin C, et al. Outcome while awaiting heart transplantation in children: a comparison of congenital heart disease and cardiomyopathy. J Heart Lung Transplant 2000;19(8):751–755.

33. Hetzer R, Loebe M, Potapov EV, et al. Circulatory support with pneumatic paracorporeal ventricular assist device in infants and children [see comment]. Ann Thorac Surg 1998;66(5):1498–1506.

34. Ishino K, Loebe M, Uhlemann F, et al. Circulatory support with paracorporeal pneumatic ventricular assist device (VAD) in infants and children. Eur J Cardio-Thorac Surg 1997;11(5):965–972.

35. Konertz W, Hotz H, Schneider M, et al. Clinical experience with the MEDOS HIA–VAD system in infants and children: a preliminary report. Ann Thorac Surg 1997;63(4):1138–1144.

36. Laliberte E, Cecere R, Tchervenkov C, et al. The combined use of extracorporeal life support and the Berlin Heart pulsatile pediatric ventricular assist device as a bridge to transplant in a toddler. J Extra-Corpor Technol 2004;36(2):158–161.

37. Samuels L. Biventricular mechanical replacement. Surg Clin North Am 2004;84(1):309–321.

38. Stiller B, Hetzer R, Weng Y, et al. Heart transplantation in children after mechanical circulatory support with pulsatile pneumatic assist device. J Heart Lung Transplant 2003;22(11):1201–1208.

39. Taenaka Y, Takano H, Noda H, et al. Experimental evaluation and clinical application of a pediatric ventricular assist device. ASAIO Trans 1989;35(3):606–608.

40. Throckmorton AL, Allaire PE, Gutgesell HP, et al. Pediatric circulatory support systems. ASAIO J 2002;48(3):216–221.

41. Goldstein DJ, Oz MC, Rose EA. Implantable left ventricular assist devices. N Engl J Med 1998;339(21):1522–1533.

42. Young JB, Hauptman PJ, Naftel DC, et al. Determinants of early graft failure following cardiac transplantation, a 10-year, multi-institutional, multivariable analysis. J Heart Lung Transplant 2001;20(2):212.

43. Addonizio LJ, Gersony WM, Robbins RC, et al. Elevated pulmonary vascular resistance and cardiac transplantation. Circulation 1987;76(5 Pt 2):V52–V55.

44. Gajarski RJ, Towbin JA, Bricker JT, et al. Intermediate follow-up of pediatric heart transplant recipients with elevated pulmonary vascular resistance index. J Am Coll Cardiol 1994;23(7):1682–1687.

45. Zales VR, Pahl E, Backer CL, et al. Pharmacologic reduction of pretransplantation pulmonary vascular resistance predicts outcome after pediatric heart transplantation. J Heart Lung Transplant 1993;12(6 Pt 1):965–973.

46. Anker SD, Clark AL, Teixeira MM, et al. Loss of bone mineral in patients with cachexia due to chronic heart failure. Am J Cardiol 1999;83(4):612–615.

47. Anker SD, Coats AJ. Cardiac cachexia: a syndrome with impaired survival and immune and neuroendocrine activation. Chest 1999;115(3):836–847.

48. Ponikowski P, Piepoli M, Chua TP, et al. The impact of cachexia on cardiorespiratory reflex control in chronic heart failure [see comment]. Eur Heart J 1999;20(22):1667–1675.

49. Renlund DG, Taylor DO, Kfoury AG, et al. New UNOS rules: historical background and implications for transplantation management. United Network for Organ Sharing. J Heart Lung Transplant 1999; 18(11):1065–1070.

50. Dosemeci L, Yilmaz M, Cengiz M, et al. Brain death and donor management in the intensive care unit: experiences over the last 3 years. Transplant Proc 2004;36(1):20–21.

51. Phongsamran PV. Critical care pharmacy in donor management. Prog Transplant 2004;14(2):105–113.

52. Sacristan-Lista F, Mosquera-Reboredo J, Vazquez-Martul E, et al. Influence of the management of asystolic donors on kidney transplantation outcome. Transplant Proc 2004;36(3):745–746.

53. Smith M. Physiologic changes during brain stem death–lessons for management of the organ donor. J Heart Lung Transplant 2004;23(9 Suppl):S217–S222.

54. Cantin B, Kwok BW, Chan MC, et al. The impact of brain death on survival after heart transplantation: time is of the essence. Transplantation 2003;76(9):1275–1279.

55. Checchia PA, Sehra R, Moynihan J, et al. Myocardial injury in children following resuscitation after cardiac arrest. Resuscitation 2003;57(2): 131–137.

56. Grant JW, Canter CE, Spray TL, et al. Elevated donor cardiac troponin I. A marker of acute graft failure in infant heart recipients [erratum appears in Circulation 1995;91(12):3027]. Circulation 1994;90(6): 2618–2621.

57. Potapov EV, Ivanitskaia EA, Loebe M, et al. Value of cardiac troponin I and T for selection of heart donors and as predictors of early graft failure. Transplantation 2001;71(10):1394–1400.

58. Edwards JM, Hasz RD Jr, Robertson VM. Non-heart-beating organ donation: process and review. AACN Clinical Issues 1999;10(2): 293–300.

59. Whetstine L, Bowman K, Hawryluck L. Pro/con ethics debate: is non-heart-beating organ donation ethically acceptable? Critical Care (Lond) 2002;6(3):192–195.

60. DeVita MA, Snyder JV, Grenvik A. History of organ donation by patients with cardiac death. Kennedy Inst Ethics J 1993;3(2):113–129.

61. Del Rizzo DF, Menkis AH, Pflugfelder PW, et al. The role of donor age and ischemic time on survival following orthotopic heart transplantation. J Heart Lung Transplant 1999;18(4):310–319.

62. Bourge RC, Naftel DC, Costanzo-Nordin MR, et al. Pretransplantation risk factors for death after heart transplantation: a multiinstitutional study. The Transplant Cardiologists Research Database Group. J Heart Lung Transplant 1993;12(4):549–562.

63. Kobashigawa JA, Kirklin JK, Naftel DC, et al. Pretransplantation risk factors for acute rejection after heart transplantation: a multiinstitutional study. The Transplant Cardiologists Research Database Group. J Heart Lung Transplant 1993;12(3):355–366.

64. de Begona JA, Gundry SR, Razzouk AJ, et al. Transplantation of hearts after arrest and resuscitation. Early and long-term results. J Thorac Cardiovasc Surg 1993;106(6):1196.

65. Mullen JC, Bentley MJ, Modry DL, et al. Extended donor ischemic times and recipient outcome after orthotopic cardiac transplantation. Can J Cardiol 2001;17(4):421–426.

66. Ott GY, Herschberger RE, Ratkovec RR, et al. Cardiac allografts from high-risk donors: excellent clinical results. Ann Thorac Surg 1994;57(1):76–82.

67. Pflugfelder PW, Singh NR, McKenzie FN, et al. Extending cardiac allograft ischemic time and donor age: effect on survival and long-term cardiac function. J Heart Lung Transplant 1991;10(3):394–400.

68. Kawauchi M, Gundry SR, de Begona JA, et al. Prolonged preservation of human pediatric hearts for transplantation: correlation of ischemic time and subsequent function. J Heart Lung Transplant 1993;12(1 Pt 1):55–58.

69. Kawauchi M, Gundry SR, Beierle F, et al. Myosin light chain efflux after heart transplantation in infants and children and its correlation with ischemic preservation time. J Thorac Cardiovasc Surg 1993; 106(3):458–462.

70. Scheule AM, Zimmerman GJ, Johnston JK, et al. Duration of graft cold ischemia does not affect outcomes in pediatric heart transplant recipients. Circulation 2002;106(12 Suppl 1):I163–I167.

71. Bhatia SJ, Kirshenbaum JM, Shemin RJ, et al. Time course of resolution of pulmonary hypertension and right ventricular remodeling after orthotopic cardiac transplantation. Circulation 1987;76(4): 819–826.

72. Young JB, Leon CA, Short HD 3rd, et al. Evolution of hemodynamics after orthotopic heart and heart–lung transplantation: early restrictive patterns persisting in occult fashion. J Heart Lung Transplant 1987;6(1):34–43.

73. Vatner DE, Lavallee M, Amano J, et al. Mechanisms of supersensitivity to sympathomimetic amines in the chronically denervated heart of the conscious dog. Circ Res 1985;57(1):55–64.

74. Gilbert EM, Eiswirth CC, Mealey PC, et al. Beta-adrenergic supersensitivity of the transplanted human heart is presynaptic in origin. Circulation 1989;79(2):344–349.

75. Hosenpud JD, Bennett LE, Keck BM, et al. The Registry of the International Society for Heart and Lung Transplantation: seventeenth official report—2000. J Heart Lung Transplant 2000;19(10):909–931.

76. Stobierska-Dzierzek B, Awad H, Michler RE. The evolving management of acute right-sided heart failure in cardiac transplant recipients. J Am Coll Cardiol 2001;38(4):923–931.

77. Carrier M, Blaise G, Belisle S, et al. Nitric oxide inhalation in the treatment of primary graft failure following heart transplantation. J Heart Lung Transplant 1999;18(7):664–667.

78. Girard C, Durand PG, Vedrinne C, et al. Case 4-1993. Inhaled nitric oxide for right ventricular failure after heart transplantation [see comment]. J Cardiothorac Vasc Anesth 1993;7(4):481–485.

79. Mosquera I, Crespo-Leiro MG, Tabuyo T, et al. Pulmonary hypertension and right ventricular failure after heart transplantation: usefulness of nitric oxide. Transplant Proc 2002;34(1):166–167.

80. Williams TJ, Salamonsen RF, Snell G, et al. Preliminary experience with inhaled nitric oxide for acute pulmonary hypertension after heart transplantation. J Heart Lung Transplant 1995;14(3):419–423.

81. Auler Junior JO, Carmona MJ, Bocchi EA, et al. Low doses of inhaled nitric oxide in heart transplant recipients. J Heart Lung Transplant 1996;15(5):443–450.

82. Fenton KN, Webber SA, Danford DA, et al. Long-term survival after pediatric cardiac transplantation and postoperative ECMO support. Ann Thorac Surg 2003;76(3):843–847.

83. Duncan BW. Extracorporeal life support for infants and children with cardiac disease. Overview and examples. In: Zwischenberger JB, Steinhorn RH, Bartlett RH, eds. ECMO: Extracorporeal Cardiopulmonary Support in Critical Care, 2nd ed.

84. Kirshbom PM, Bridges ND, Myung RJ, et al. Use of extracorporeal membrane oxygenation in pediatric thoracic organ transplantation. J Thorac Cardiovasc Surg 2002;123(1):130–136.

85. Canter C, Naftel D, Caldwell R, et al. Survival and risk factors for death after cardiac transplantation in infants. A multi-institutional study. The Pediatric Heart Transplant Study. Circulation 1997;96(1): 227–231.

86. Hoffman TM, Spray TL, Gaynor JW, et al. Survival after acute graft failure in pediatric thoracic organ transplant recipients. Pediatr Transplant 2000;4(2):112–117.

87. Morgan JA, John R, Park Y, et al. Successful outcome with extended allograft ischemic time in pediatric heart transplantation. J Heart Lung Transplant 2005;24(1):58.

88. Dearani JA, Razzouk AJ, Gundry SR, et al. Pediatric cardiac retransplantation: intermediate-term results. Ann Thorac Surg 2001;71(1): 66–70.

89. Collins KK, Thiagarajan RR, Chin C, et al. Atrial tachyarrhythmias and permanent pacing after pediatric heart transplantation. J Heart Lung Transplant 2003;22(10):1126–1133.

90. Kertesz NJ, Towbin JA, Clunie S, et al. Long-term follow-up of arrhythmias in pediatric orthotopic heart transplant recipients: incidence and correlation with rejection. J Heart Lung Transplant 2003;22(8): 889–893.

91. Sanatani S, Chiu C, Nykanen D, et al. Evolution of heart rate control after transplantation: conduction versus autonomic innervation. Pediatr Cardiol 2004;25(2):113–118.

92. Cannon BC, Denfield SW, Friedman RA, et al. Late pacemaker requirement after pediatric orthotopic heart transplantation may predict the presence of transplant coronary artery disease. J Heart Lung Transplant 2004;23(1):67–71.

93. Chinnock RE, Torres VI, Jutzy RV, et al. Cardiac pacemakers in pediatric heart transplant recipients: incidence, indications, and associated factors. Pediatric Heart Transplant Group-Loma Linda. Pacing Clin Electrophysiol 1996;19(1):26–30.

94. Bauer J, Dapper F, Demirakca S, et al. Perioperative management of pulmonary hypertension after heart transplantation in childhood. J Heart Lung Transplant 1997;16(12):1238–1247.

95. Kimberling MT, Balzer DT, Hirsch R, et al. Cardiac transplantation for pediatric restrictive cardiomyopathy: presentation, evaluation, and short-term outcome. J Heart Lung Transplant 2002;21(4): 455–459.

96. Tamisier D, Vouhe P, Le Bidois J, et al. Donor-recipient size matching in pediatric heart transplantation: a word of caution about small grafts. J Heart Lung Transplant 1996;15(2):190–195.

97. Luckraz H, Charman SC, Parameshwar J, et al. Are non-brain stem-dead cardiac donors acceptable donors? J Heart Lung Transplant 2004;23(3):330.

98. Bauer J, Thul J, Valeske K, et al. Pediatric management in pediatric heart transplantation. Thorac Cardiovasc Surg 2005;53(Suppl 2): S155–S158.

99. Atz AM, Lefler AK, Fairbrother DL, et al. Sildenafil augments the effect of inhaled nitric oxide for postoperative pulmonary hypertensive crises. J Thorac Cardiovasc Surg 2002;124(3):628–629.

100. Laquay N, Levy ML, Vaccaroni L, et al. Interet du sildenafil (Viagra) per os en cas d'hypertension arterielle pulmonaire apres chirurgie cardiaque pediatrique. Ann Fr Anesth Reanimation 2003;22(2): 140–143.

101. Hallioglu O, Dilber E, Celiker A. Comparison of acute hemodynamic effects of aerosolized and intravenous iloprost in secondary pulmonary hypertension in children with congenital heart disease. Am J Cardiol 2003;92(8):1007–1009.

102. Rimensberger PC, Spahr-Schopfer I, Berner M, et al. Inhaled nitric oxide versus aerosolized iloprost in secondary pulmonary hypertension in children with congenital heart disease: vasodilator capacity and cellular mechanisms. Circulation 2001;103(4):544–548.

103. El-Banayosy NR, Arusoglu L, Kleikamp G, et al. Recovery of organ dysfunction during bridging to heart transplantation in children and adolescents. Int J Artif Organs 2003;26(5):395–400.

104. Blume ED. Current status of heart transplantation in children: update 2003. Pediatr Clin North Am 2003;50(6):1375–1391.

105. Vricella LA, de Begona JA, Gundry SR, et al. Aggressive peritoneal dialysis for treatment of acute kidney failure after neonatal heart transplantation. J Heart Lung Transplant 1992;11(2 Pt 1):320–329.

106. Bunchman TE, McBryde KD, Mottes TE, et al. Pediatric acute renal failure: outcome by modality and disease. Pediatr Nephrol 2001;16(12): 1067–1071.

107. Stickle S, Brewer ED, Goldstein SL. Pediatric acute renal failure update: epidemiology and outcome from a three and one-half year experience [abstr]. J Am Soc Nephrol 2002;13:649.

108. Warady BA, Bunchman T. Dialysis therapy for children with acute renal failure: survey results. Pediatr Nephrol 2000;15(1–2):11–13.

109. Flynn JT. Choice of dialysis modality for management of pediatric acute renal failure. Pediatr Nephrol 2002;17(1):61–69.

110. Hoffmann JN, Hartl WH, Deppisch R, et al. Hemofiltration in hum sepsis: evidence for elimination of immunomodulatory substanc Kidney Int 1995;48(5):1563–1570.

111. Goldstein SL, Currier H, Graf C, et al. Outcome in children receivi continuous venovenous hemofiltration. Pediatrics 2001;107(6):130 1312.

112. Ronco C, Bellomo R, Homel P, et al. Effects of different doses in co tinuous veno-venous haemofiltration on outcomes of acute ren failure: a prospective randomised trial [see comment]. Lancet 200 356(9223):26–30.

113. Alonso EM. Long-term renal function in pediatric liver and hea recipients. Pediatr Transplant 2004;8(4):381–385.

114. English RF, Pophal SA, Bacanu SA, et al. Long-term comparison tacrolimus- and cyclosporine-induced nephrotoxicity in pediatr heart-transplant recipients. Am J Transplant 2002;2(8):769–773.

115. Hornung TS, de Goede CG, O'Brien C, et al. Renal function aft pediatric cardiac transplantation: the effect of early cyclospori dosage. Pediatrics 2001;107(6):1346–1350.

116. van Houten JP, Rothman A, Bejar R. High incidence of cranial ultr sound abnormalities in full-term infants with congenital hea disease. Am J Perinatol 1996;13(1):47–53.

117. Ferry PC. Neurologic sequelae of open-heart surgery in children. A "irritating question." Am J Dis Child 1990;144(3):369–373.

118. Baum M, Freier MC, Chinnock RE. Neurodevelopmental outcome solid organ transplantation in children. Pediatr Clin North A 2003;50(6):1493–1503.

119. Menache CC, du Plessis AJ, Wessel DL, et al. Current incidence of acu neurologic complications after open-heart operations in childre Ann Thorac Surg 2002;73(6):1752–1758.

120. Rappaport LA, Wypij D, Bellinger DC, et al. Relation of seizures aft cardiac surgery in early infancy to neurodevelopmental outcom Boston Circulatory Arrest Study Group. Circulation 1998;97(8):773 779.

121. Lynch BJ, Glauser TA, Canter C, et al. Neurologic complications pediatric heart transplantation. Arch Pediatr Adolesc Med 199 148(9):973–979.

122. Martin AB, Bricker JT, Fishman M, et al. Neurologic complications heart transplantation in children. J Heart Lung Transplant 1992;11(5 933–942.

123. Andropoulos DB, Stayer SA, Diaz LK, et al. Neurological monitorin for congenital heart surgery. Anesth Analg 2004;99(5):1365–1375.

124. Cottrell SM, Morris KP, Davies P, et al. Early postoperative body tem perature and developmental outcome after open heart surgery i infants. Ann Thorac Surg 2004;77(1):66–71.

125. Faraci M, Lanino E, Dini G, et al. Severe neurologic complication after hematopoietic stem cell transplantation in children [erratu appears in Neurology 2003;60(6):1055]. Neurology 2002;59(12):1895 1904.

126. Menegaux F, Keeffe EB, Andrews BT, et al. Neurological complication of liver transplantation in adult versus pediatric patients. Transplan tation 1994;58(4):447–450.

127. Wong M, Mallory GB Jr, Goldstein J, et al. Neurologic complication of pediatric lung transplantation. Neurology 1999;53(7):1542–1549.

128. Al-Rasheed AK, Blaser SI, Minassian BA, et al. Cyclosporine A neuro toxicity in a patient with idiopathic renal magnesium wasting [se comment]. Pediatr Neurol 2000;23(4):353–356.

129. Schowengerdt KO Jr, Gajarski RJ, Denfield S. Progressive visual dete rioration leading to blindness after pediatric heart transplantation Texas Heart Inst J 1993;20(4):299–303.

130. Tweddle DA, Windebank KP, Hewson QC, et al. Cyclosporin neuro toxicity after chemotherapy [see comment]. BMJ 1999;318(7191):1113

131. Taque S, Peudenier S, Gie S, et al. Central neurotoxicity of cyclospo rine in two children with nephrotic syndrome. Pediatr Nephro 2004;19(3):276–280.

132. Staatz CE, Taylor PJ, Lynch SV, et al. A pharmacodynamic investiga tion of tacrolimus in pediatric liver transplantation. Liver Transplan 2004;10(4):506–512.

133. Kanter KR, Tam VK, Vincent RN, et al. Current results with pediatric heart transplantation. Ann Thorac Surg 1999;68(2):527–531.

134. Groetzner J, Reichart B, Roemer U, et al. Cardiac transplantation in pediatric patients: fifteen-year experience of a single center. Ann Thorac Surg 2005;79(1):53.

135. Lamour JM, Hsu DT, Quaegebeur JM, et al. Heart transplantation to a physiologic single lung in patients with congenital heart disease. J Heart Lung Transplant 2004;23(8):948–953.

136. Chinnock R, Baum M. Somatic growth in infant heart transplant recipients [see comment]. Pediatr Transplant 1998;2(1):30–34.

137. Wesley JR. Nutrient metabolism in relation to the systemic stress response. In: Fuhrman BP, Zimmerman JJ, eds. Pediatric Critical Care, 2nd. ed. St. Louis: Mosby; 1998:799–819.

138. Ngo K, Fry-Bowers E, Sehra R, et al. Inadequate caloric delivery in pediatric patients in intensive care unit settings. Crit Care Med 2001;29(12):A125.

139. Grewal RS, Mampilly J, Misra TR. Postoperative protein metabolism and electrolyte changes in pediatric surgery. Int Surg 1969;51(2):142–148.

140. Merritt RJ. Cholestasis associated with total parenteral nutrition. J Pediatr Gastroenterol Nutr 1986;5(1):9–22.

141. Wildhaber BE, Yang H, Spencer AU, et al. Lack of enteral nutrition—effects on the intestinal immune system. J Surg Res 2005;123(1):8.

142. Sakopoulos AG, Gundry S, Razzouk AJ, et al. Cholelithiasis in infant and pediatric heart transplant patients. Pediatr Transplant 2002;6(3):231–234.

143. Rakhit A, Nurko S, Gauvreau K, et al. Gastrointestinal complications after pediatric cardiac transplantation. J Heart Lung Transplant 2002;21(7):751.

144. Seipelt IM, Crawford SE, Rodgers S, et al. Hypercholesterolemia is common after pediatric heart transplantation: initial experience with pravastatin. J Heart Lung Transplant 2004;23(3):317–322.

145. Russo LM, Webber SA. Pediatric heart transplantation: immunosuppression and its complications. Curr Opin Cardiol 2004;19(2):104–109.

146. Kirklin J, Chinnock RE, Pearce FB. Pediatric heart transplantation. In: Kirklin J, Young JB, McGiffin DC, eds. Heart Transplantation, 1st ed. Philadelphia: Churchill Livingston; 2002:717–770.

147. Leonard H, Hornung T, Parry G, et al. Pediatric cardiac transplant: results using a steroid-free maintenance regimen. Pediatr Transplant 2003;7(1):59–63.

148. Zheng H, Webber S, Zeevi A, et al. The MDR1 polymorphisms at exons 21 and 26 predict steroid weaning in pediatric heart transplant patients. Hum Immunol 2002;63(9):765–770.

149. Pollock-BarZiv SM, Dipchand AI, McCrindle BW, et al. Randomized clinical trial of tacrolimus- vs cyclosporine-based immunosuppression in pediatric heart transplantation: preliminary results at 15-month follow-up. J Heart Lung Tranplant 2005;24(2):190.

150. Hathout EH, Chinnock RE, Johnston JK, et al. Pediatric post-transplant diabetes: data from a large cohort of pediatric heart-transplant recipients. Am J Transplant 2003;3(8):994–998.

151. Kobashigawa JA. Statins as immunosuppressive agents. Liver Transplant 2001;7(4):559–561.

152. Jacobs JP, Quintessenza JA, Boucek RJ, et al. Pediatric cardiac transplantation in children with high panel reactive antibody. Ann Thorac Surg 2004;78(5):1703–1709.

153. Boucek MM. Breaching the barrier of ABO incompatibility in heart transplantation for infants [comment]. N Engl J Med 2001;344(11):843–844.

154. Rao JN, Hasan A, Hamilton JR, et al. ABO-incompatible heart transplantation in infants: the Freeman Hospital experience. Transplantation 2004;77(9):1389–1394.

155. West LJ, Pollock-Barziv SM, Dipchand AI, et al. ABO-incompatible heart transplantation in infants [see comment]. N Engl J Med 2001;344(11):793–800.

156. Pahl E, Naftel DC, Canter CE, et al. Death after rejection with severe hemodynamic compromise in pediatric heart transplant recipients: a multi-institutional study. J Heart Lung Transplant 2001;20(3):279–287.

157. Chin C, Naftel DC, Singh TP, et al. Risk factors for recurrent rejection in pediatric heart transplant: a multicenter experience. J Heart Lung Transplant 2004;23(2):178–185.

158. Chinnock R, Sherwin T, Robie S, et al. Emergency department presentation and management of pediatric heart transplant recipients. Pediatr Emerg Care 1995;11(6):355–360.

159. Johnston J, Mathis C. Determination of rejection using noninvasive parameters after cardiac transplantation in very early infancy: the Loma Linda experience. Progr Cardiovasc Nurs 1988;3(1):13–18.

160. Billingham ME, Cary NR, Hammond ME, et al. A working formulation for the standardization of nomenclature in the diagnosis of heart and lung rejection: Heart Rejection Study Group. The International Society for Heart and Lung Transplantation. J Heart Transplant 1990;9(6):587–593.

161. Abramson LP, Pahl E, Huang L, et al. Serum vascular endothelial growth factor as a surveillance marker for cellular rejection in pediatric cardiac transplantation [erratum appears in Transplantation 2002;73(2):321]. Transplantation 2002;73(1):153–156.

162. Awad MR, Webber S, Boyle G, et al. The effect of cytokine gene polymorphisms on pediatric heart allograft outcome. J Heart Lung Transplant 2001;20(6):625–630.

163. Lan YT, Chang RK, Alejos JC, et al. B-type natriuretic peptide in children after cardiac transplantation. J Heart Lung Transplant 2004;23(5):558–563.

164. Shirali GS, Ni J, Chinnock RE, et al. Association of viral genome with graft loss in children after cardiac transplantation [see comment]. N Eng J Med 2001;344(20):1498–1503.

165. Oklu E, Bulutcu FS, Yalcin Y, et al. Which anesthetic agent alters the hemodynamic status during pediatric catheterization? Comparison of propofol versus ketamine [see comment]. J Cardiothorac Vasc Anesth 2003;17(6):686–690.

166. Jordan SC, Quartel AW, Czer LS, et al. Posttransplant therapy using high-dose human immunoglobulin (intravenous gammaglobulin) to control acute humoral rejection in renal and cardiac allograft recipients and potential mechanism of action. Transplantation 1998;66(6):800–805.

167. Pahl E, Crawford SE, Cohn RA, et al. Reversal of severe late left ventricular failure after pediatric heart transplantation and possible role of plasmapheresis. Am J Cardiol 2000;85(6):735–739.

168. Asano M, Gundry SR, Razzouk AJ, et al. Total lymphoid irradiation for refractory rejection in pediatric heart transplantation. Ann Thorac Surg 2002;74(6):1979–1985.

169. Ringewald JM, Gidding SS, Crawford SE, et al. Nonadherence is associated with late rejection in pediatric heart transplant recipients. J Pediatr 2001;139(1):75–78.

170. Billingham ME. Histopathology of graft coronary disease. J Heart Lung Transplant 1990;119:538–544.

171. Mulla NF, Johnston JK, Vander Dussen L, et al. Late rejection is a predictor of transplant coronary artery disease in children. J Am Coll Cardiol 2001;37(1):243–250.

172. Berry GJ, Rizeq MN, Weiss LM, et al. Graft coronary disease in pediatric heart and combined heart–lung transplant recipients: a study of fifteen cases. J Heart Lung Transplantation 1993;12(6 Pt 2):S309–S319.

173. Dent CL, Canter CE, Hirsch R, et al. Transplant coronary artery disease in pediatric heart transplant recipients. J Heart Lung Transplant 2000;19(3):240–248.

174. Costello JM, Wax DF, Binns HJ, et al. A comparison of intravascular ultrasound with coronary angiography for evaluation of transplant coronary disease in pediatric heart transplant recipients. J Heart Lung Transplant 2003;22(1):44–49.

175. Kuhn MA, Jutzy KR, Deming DD, et al. The medium-term findings in coronary arteries by intravascular ultrasound in infants and children after heart transplantation. J Am Coll Cardiol 2000;36(1):250–254.

176. Di Filippo S, Semiond B, Roriz R, et al. Non-invasive detection of coronary artery disease by dobutamine-stress echocardiography in children after heart transplantation. J Heart Lung Transplant 2003; 22(8):876–882.

177. Larsen RL, Applegate PM, Dyar DA, et al. Dobutamine stress echocardiography for assessing coronary artery disease after transplantation in children. J Am Coll Cardiol 1998;32(2):515–520.

178. Razzouk AJ, Chinnock RE, Dearani JA, et al. Cardiac retransplantation for graft vasculopathy in children: should we continue to do it? Arch Surg 1998;133(8):881–885.

179. Webber SA, Naftel DC, Parker J, et al. Late rejection episodes more than 1 year after pediatric heart transplantation: risk factors and outcomes. J Heart Lung Transplant 2003;22(8):869–875.

180. Pahl E, Zales VR, Fricker FJ, et al. Posttransplant coronary artery disease in children. A multicenter national survey. Circulation 1994;90(5 Pt 2):II56–II60.

181. Green M, Webber S. Posttransplantation lymphoproliferative disorders. Pediatr Clin North Am 2003;50(6):1471–1491.

182. Zangwill SD, Hsu DT, Kichuk MR, et al. Incidence and outcome of primary Epstein-Barr virus infection and lymphoproliferative disease in pediatric heart transplant recipients. J Heart Lung Transplant 1998;17(12):1161–1166.

183. Harwood JS, Gould FK, McMaster A, et al. Significance of Epstein-Barr virus status and post-transplant lymphoproliferative disease in pediatric thoracic transplantation [see comment]. Pediatr Transplant 1999;3(2):100–103.

184. Orentas RJ, Schauer DW Jr, Ellis FW, et al. Monitoring and modulation of Epstein-Barr virus loads in pediatric transplant patients. Pediatr Transplant 2003;7(4):305–334.

185. Schowengerdt KO, Naftel DC, Seib PM, et al. Infection after pediatric heart transplantation: results of a multiinstitutional study. The Pediatric Heart Transplant Study Group. J Heart Lung Transplant 1997;16(12):1207–1216.

186. Freier MC, Babikian T, Pivonka J, et al. A longitudinal perspective on neurodevelopmental outcome after infant cardiac transplantation. J Heart Lung Transplant 2004;23(7):857–864.

187. Baum M, Freier MC, Freeman K, et al. Developmental outcomes and cognitive functioning in infant and child heart transplant recipients. Progr Pediatr Cardiol 2000;11:159–163.

188. Baum M, Freier MC, Freeman K, et al. Neuropsychological outcome of infant heart transplant recipients. J Pediatr 2004;145(3):365–372.

189. Ikle L, Hale K, Fashaw L, et al. Developmental outcome of patients with hypoplastic left heart syndrome treated with heart transplantation [comment]. J Pediatr 2003;142(1):20–25.

190. Faber-Langendoen K, Caplan AL, McGlave PB. Survival of adult bone marrow transplant patients receiving mechanical ventilation: a case for restricted use. Bone Marrow Transplant 1993;12(5):501–507.

191. Checchia PA, Sehra R, Daher N, et al. An examination of the incidence of intubation and mechanical ventilation beyond the peri-operative period in pediatric heart transplant recipients. J Heart Lung Transplant 2004;23(3):379–382.

192. Gale GB. Pediatric stem cell transplantation and critical care (an outcome evaluation). Front Biosci 2001;6:G33–G37.

193. Keenan HT, Bratton SL, Martin LD, et al. Outcome of children who require mechanical ventilatory support after bone marrow transplantation. Crit Care Med 2000;28(3):830–835.

194. Schneiderman L, Jecker N, Jonsen A. Medical futility: Its meaning and clinical implications. Ann Intern Med 1990;112:949–954.

195. Huaringa AJ, Leyva FJ, Giralt SA, et al. Outcome of bone marrow transplantation patients requiring mechanical ventilation. Crit Care Med 2000;28(4):1014–1017.

196. Afessa B, Gay PC, Plevak DJ, et al. Pulmonary complications of orthotopic liver transplantation. Mayo Clin Proc 1993;68(5):427–434.

197. Afessa B, Tefferi A, Hoagland HC, et al. Outcome of recipients of bone marrow transplants who require intensive-care unit support. Mayo Clin Proc 1992;67(2):117–122.

198. Dawkins KD, Jamieson SW, Hunt SA, et al. Long-term results, hemodynamics, and complications after combined heart and lung transplantation. Circulation 1985;71(5):919–926.

ndex

Lightning Source UK Ltd.
Milton Keynes UK
UKOW07f0007161116

287710UK00001B/4/P